TWELFTH EDITION

EMERGENCY
MEDICAL RESPONDER
FIRST ON SCENE

Christopher J. Le Baudour
Kaitlyn Laurélle

MEDICAL REVIEWER
Keith Wesley, MD

LEGACY AUTHOR
J. David Bergeron

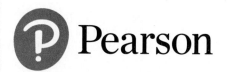

Library of Congress Cataloging-in-Publication Data

Names: Le Baudour, Chris, author.
Title: Emergency medical responder : first on scene / Christopher J. Le Baudour;
   Medical Reviewer, Keith Wesley; Legacy author, J. David Bergeron.
Description: 12th edition. | Hoboken, NJ : Pearson, [2024] | Includes
   bibliographical references and index. | Summary: "The foundation of this text
   is the National Emergency Medical Services Education Standards for Emergency
   Medical Responders and includes the 2023 Focused Updates from the American
   Heart Association Guidelines for Cardiopulmonary Resuscitation and First Aid.
   Unique among Emergency Medical Responder textbooks, this edition again
   includes references to some of the most current medical literature. This edition
   places a stronger focus on the language of inclusiveness, recognizing that
   Emergency Medical Responders and our patients come from a variety of cultures,
   socioeconomic backgrounds, and life experiences. The new 12th edition retains
   many of the features found to be successful in previous editions and includes
   some new topics and concepts that have recently become part of most Emergency
   Medical Responder programs"-- Provided by publisher.
Identifiers: LCCN 2023035752 (print) | LCCN 2023035753 (ebook) |
   ISBN 9780138100407 (paperback) | ISBN 0138100403 (paperback) |
   ISBN 9780138101244 (ebook)
Subjects: MESH: Emergency Medical Services | Emergencies | Emergency
   Responders | Emergency Treatment
Classification: LCC RC86.7 (print) | LCC RC86.7 (ebook) | NLM WX 215 |
   DDC 616.02/5--dc23/eng/20230829
LC record available at https://lccn.loc.gov/2023035752
LC ebook record available at https://lccn.loc.gov/2023035753

Content Management: Kevin Wilson
Content Production: Maria Reyes
Product Management: Katrin Beacom and John Goucher
Product Marketing: Brooke Imbornone
Rights and Permissions: Ben Ferriini, Matthew Perry,
   and Joan Diaz
Content Development: Tanya Martin

Please contact https://support.pearson.com/getsupport/s/ with
any queries on this content

Cover image by Derek O. Hanley

About the cover:
The cover image is from the book *Photos From the Front Lines:
A Year on the Streets of Alameda County* (dohp.net/books)
written and photographed by Derek O. Hanley and features
Katy Farinacci-Magee, an EMT from the Royal Ambulance in
the field during the height of the global COVID-19 pandemic.

Notice on Care Procedures

It is the intent of the authors and publisher that this textbook be used as part of a formal Emergency Medical Responder education program taught by qualified instructors and supervised by a licensed physician. The procedures described in this textbook are based on consultation with first responder and medical authorities. The authors and publisher have taken care to make certain that these procedures reflect currently accepted clinical practice; however, they cannot be considered absolute recommendations.

The material in this textbook contains the most current information available at the time of publication. However, federal, state, and local guidelines concerning clinical practices, including, without limitation, those governing infection control and universal precautions, change rapidly. The reader should note, therefore, that new regulations may require changes in some procedures.

It is the responsibility of the reader to familiarize himself or herself with the policies and procedures set by federal, state, and local agencies as well as the institution or agency where the reader is employed. The authors and the publisher of this textbook and the supplements written to accompany it disclaim any liability, loss, or risk resulting directly or indirectly from the suggested procedures and theories, from any undetected errors, or from the reader's responsibility to stay informed of any new changes or recommendations made by any federal, state, or local agency as well as by his or her employing institution or agency.

11 2024

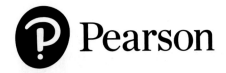

ISBN-10: 0-13-810040-3
ISBN-13: 978-0-13-810040-7

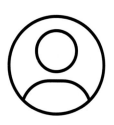

Pearson's Commitment to Diversity, Equity, and Inclusion

Pearson is dedicated to creating bias-free content that reflects the diversity, depth, and breadth of all learners' lived experiences.

We embrace the many dimensions of diversity, including but not limited to race, ethnicity, gender, sex, sexual orientation, socioeconomic status, ability, age, and religious or political beliefs.

Education is a powerful force for equity and change in our world. It has the potential to deliver opportunities that improve lives and enable economic mobility. As we work with authors to create content for every product and service, we acknowledge our responsibility to demonstrate inclusivity and incorporate diverse scholarship so that everyone can achieve their potential through learning. As the world's leading learning company, we have a duty to help drive change and live up to our purpose to help more people create a better life for themselves and to create a better world.

Our ambition is to purposefully contribute to a world where:

- Everyone has an equitable and lifelong opportunity to succeed through learning.
- Our educational content accurately reflects the histories and lived experiences of the learners we serve.

- Our educational products and services are inclusive and represent the rich diversity of learners.
- Our educational content prompts deeper discussions with students and motivates them to expand their own learning (and worldview).

Accessibility

We are also committed to providing products that are fully accessible to all learners. As per Pearson's guidelines for accessible educational Web media, we test and retest the capabilities of our products against the highest standards for every release, following the WCAG guidelines in developing new products for copyright year 2022 and beyond.

 You can learn more about Pearson's commitment to accessibility at
https://www.pearson.com/us/accessibility.html

Contact Us

While we work hard to present unbiased, fully accessible content, we want to hear from you about any concerns or needs with this Pearson product so that we can investigate and address them.

 Please contact us with concerns about any potential bias at
https://www.pearson.com/report-bias.html

 For accessibility-related issues, such as using assistive technology with Pearson products, alternative text requests, or accessibility documentation, email the Pearson Disability Support team at **disability.support@pearson.com**

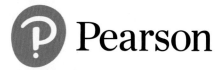

DEDICATION

To the memory and legacy of our photographer Michal Heron, who passed away during the revision of this textbook. Michal's quest for realism and attention to detail single-handedly raised the bar for photography in EMS publications. We are fortunate to have called Michal both a colleague and a dear friend. May you rest in peace.

CONTENTS

12 Obtaining a Medical History and Vital Signs 224

13 Principles of Patient Assessment 248

14 Caring for Cardiac Emergencies 283

15 Caring for Respiratory Emergencies 297

KEY SKILLS

SKILLS VIDEOS
available in **MyLab BRADY**

Airway

Complete Ventilation Sequence for a Nonbreathing Patient with a Pulse

Head-Tilt Chin-Lift

Jaw-Thrust

Jaw-Thrust with Mask: Mouth-to-Mask with Suspected Spinal Injury

Mouth-to-Shield Ventilation for a Nonbreathing Patient with a Pulse

Nasal Suction: Electric

Nasopharyngeal Airway: Measuring and Insertion for Adults

One Rescuer Bag-Valve-Mask Ventilation

Oral Suction: Electric

Oropharyngeal Airway: Measuring and Insertion for Infants and Children

Oropharyngeal Airway: Measuring and Insertion in Adults

Oxygen Administration: Nasal Cannula

Oxygen Administration: Nonrebreather Mask

Oxygen Tank Set Up

Recovery Position or Lateral Recumbent Position

Two Rescuer Bag-Valve-Mask Ventilation

Ventilation: Mouth-to-Mask

Assessment

Blood Pressure: Placement of Cuff and Obtaining Reading

Counting Respirations

Locating Radial, Carotid, Brachial, and Pedal Pulses

Obtaining a Medical History

Primary Assessment

Pupils: With and without Light Source

Reassessment

Secondary Assessment: Medical

Secondary Assessment: Trauma

Stethoscope Use

Medical

Applying 12-Lead Electrodes

Automated External Defibrillator

Blood Glucose Monitor

Complete Cardiac Arrest Management Sequence

Epinephrine Auto Injector

Inhaler Use with and without Holding Chamber

Intramuscular Injection

Naloxone Administration

Nitroglycerin Administration

Oral Glucose Administration

Stroke Assessment: Cincinnati Prehospital Stroke Scale (CPSS)

Stroke Assessment: Los Angeles Prehospital Stroke Screen (LAPSS)

Trauma

Arm Sling

Assessment for Spinal Injury: Ambulatory Patient

Bleeding Control with Hemostatic Agent

Bleeding Control: Direct Pressure

Bleeding Control: Tourniquet

Cervical Collar: Sizing and Application

Log Roll: Three Person with Spine Motion Restriction

Shock Management

Spine Motion Restriction: Ambulatory Patient

Splinting a Long Bone

Splinting Joints

Other

Clamping and Cutting an Umbilical Cord

Neonatal Resuscitation

Removal of Gloves

Routine Care of the Newborn

As the authors of this textbook, we want to personally congratulate you on your decision to become an Emergency Medical Responder. Your decision to serve others, especially in times of great need, is one of the most rewarding opportunities anyone can experience.

This textbook has been an important component of thousands of training programs over the past 40 years and has contributed to the success of hundreds of thousands of students just like you. The new 12th edition retains many of the features found to be successful in previous editions and includes some new topics and concepts that have recently become part of most Emergency Medical Responder programs. The foundation of this text is the National Emergency Medical Services Education Standards for Emergency Medical Responders and includes the 2023 Focused Updates from the American Heart Association Guidelines for Cardiopulmonary Resuscitation and First Aid. Unique among Emergency Medical Responder textbooks, this edition again includes references to some of the most current medical literature.

Your decision to become an Emergency Medical Responder is significant. We believe strongly that being able to assess and care for patients requires much more than just technical skills. It requires you to be a good leader, and good leaders demonstrate characteristics such as integrity, compassion, accountability, respect, and empathy. Our team has enhanced components in the 12th edition that we believe will help you become the best Emergency Medical Responder you can be; one such component is the "First on Scene" scenarios woven throughout each chapter. In these scenarios, we throw you right in the middle of a real-life emergency and offer you a perspective that you will not get with any other training resource. You will see firsthand how individuals just like you make decisions when faced with an emergency situation. You will feel the fear and anxiety that is such a normal part of being a new Emergency Medical Responder. Not everyone you meet will make the best decisions, so we want you to consider each scenario carefully and discuss it with your classmates and instructor. At the end of each chapter is the "First on Scene Run Review." Here you will have a chance to answer specific critical-thinking questions relating to the First on Scene scenario and consider how you might have done things differently.

This edition places a stronger focus on the language of inclusiveness, recognizing that Emergency Medical Responders and our patients come from a variety of cultures, socioeconomic backgrounds, and life experiences. To emphasize this, unless the gender of a person is relevant to the content, we use "they/them" pronouns throughout this text.

Becoming an Emergency Medical Responder is just the first step in what is likely to be a lifetime of service. Just a warning to you: The feeling you get when you are able to help those in need is contagious. We encounter students all across the country who have discovered that their passion is helping others. I hope that we can be part of helping you discover your passion. We welcome you to EMS and a life of service!

Improving patient care, one student at a time.

Chris Le Baudour
Kaitlyn Laurélle
Keith Wesley

The publication of the 12th edition of *Emergency Medical Responder* marks the 41st anniversary of the publication of the first edition back in 1982. This new edition is driven by the National Emergency Medical Services Education Standards. These standards represent the work of leading EMS educators across the nation as well as internationally. The majority of the changes are the result of evidence-based research conducted by many individuals and organizations.

The contents of the 12th edition are summarized below, followed by notes on what's new to each chapter. Note that, within each chapter, the cognitive objectives are updated and reorganized to more effectively match the flow of chapter content, and the Quick Quizzes were revised to better assess the cognitive objectives. The chapters also include a number of new photos.

Chapters 1–5

The first few chapters set the foundation for all that follow by introducing the basic concepts, information, and framework for someone entering the profession. The EMS system and the role of the Emergency Medical Responder within the system are introduced. Legal and ethical principles of emergency care are covered, as well as basic anatomy, physiology, and medical terminology. Each chapter includes new elements related to justice, equity, diversity, and inclusion (JEDI), and crew resource management (CRM).

WHAT'S NEW?

- *Chapter 1, Introduction to EMS Systems*, includes updates to the EMS timeline and introduces the EMS Agenda for the Future 2050 and the six guiding principles for EMS system design. The alliance model for EMS design and the concept of people-centered care are introduced.

- *Chapter 2, Legal and Ethical Principles of Emergency Care*, includes an expanded discussion related to patients who are deemed not competent and the addition of information related to COVID-19.

- *Chapter 3, Wellness and Safety of the Emergency Medical Responder*, now includes a discussion of crew resource management, information related to COVID and MPOX vaccines, CDC tips for resiliency, and expanded information related to coping with stress and resources for improved mental health.

- *Chapter 4, Introduction to Medical Terminology, Human Anatomy, and Lifespan Development*, includes updates to terminology related to lifespan development.

- *Chapter 5, Introduction to Pathophysiology*, includes updated statistics related to diabetes; the chapter also contains expanded coverage of blood vessel structure, cardiac output, and tidal volume.

Chapters 6–8

These three chapters introduce many of the fundamental skills necessary to be an effective Emergency Medical Responder, covering the proper techniques for lifting, moving, and positioning ill and injured patients. They also address important principles related to proper verbal and written communication and documentation. Each chapter includes new elements related to justice, equity, diversity, and inclusion (JEDI), and crew resource management (CRM).

WHAT'S NEW?

- *Chapter 6, Principles of Lifting, Moving, and Positioning of Patients*, provides updated data that reinforces the importance of proper lifting technique to avoid injury.

- *Chapter 7, Principles of Effective Communication*, provides updated information on establishing patient rapport, and communication with patients with hearing loss, cognitive disabilities, or who require a service animal. This chapter also addresses communication across linguistic and cultural differences, including the use of translation services. Health care literacy and family-centered care are defined and discussed.

- *Chapter 8, Principles of Effective Documentation*, reinforces the importance of providing excellent patient care first and documenting once you've completed a proper patient handoff. It also includes information on the privacy of patient health information as it relates to HIPAA, correcting errors on both an electronic and paper PCR, an expanded description of subjective patient information, and the use of smart phone apps for patient documentation.

Chapters 9–11

No patient will survive without an open and clear airway, which is why Chapters 9 and 10 may be considered the most important. Basic airway management techniques are covered in detail, as is proper ventilation and oxygen administration. Chapter 11 contains the most recent updates related to cardiopulmonary resuscitation (CPR) and the use of the automated external defibrillator (AED). Each chapter includes new elements related to justice, equity, diversity, and inclusion (JEDI), crew resource management (CRM), and patient handoff.

WHAT'S NEW?

- *Chapter 9, Principles of Airway Management and Ventilation*, now includes crew resource management sections. Also added are the latest American Heart Association guidelines for airway management.

- *Chapter 10, Principles of Oxygen Therapy*, includes updated features, including scene safety, crew resource management, and the patient handoff. It also further explains the proper technique for connecting a regulator to an oxygen cylinder.

- *Chapter 11, Principles of Resuscitation*, retains the newest information on CPR as well as the use of the automated external defibrillator according to the American Heart Association's guidelines and recommendations. Updates to the chapter include updates to the adult and pediatric chains of survival and current recommendations for ventilation rates for patients of all ages. It also differentiates the most common causes of cardiac arrest in adults vs. pediatric patients.

Chapters 12–13

These two chapters are all about patient assessment, the foundation for the care Emergency Medical Responders will provide. Each chapter includes new elements related to justice, equity, diversity, and inclusion (JEDI), crew resource management (CRM), and patient handoff.

WHAT'S NEW?

- *Chapter 12, Obtaining a Medical History and Vital Signs*, includes updated blood pressure guidelines from the American Hospital Association. It also provides best practices for communicating with patients, including across language barriers.

- *Chapter 13, Principles of Patient Assessment*, offers expanded information on multisystem trauma, significant versus nonsignificant mechanisms of injury, and rapid trauma assessment.

Chapters 14–17

These chapters cover many of the most common medical emergencies encountered in the field and the most up-to-date recommendations for patient care. Each chapter includes new elements related to justice, equity, diversity, and inclusion (JEDI), crew resource management (CRM), and patient handoff.

WHAT'S NEW?

- *Chapter 14, Caring for Cardiac Emergencies*, expands the discussion of congestive heart failure, and discusses atypical signs of a cardiac event.

- *Chapter 15, Caring for Respiratory Emergencies*, reinforces the signs and symptoms of respiratory compromise and the importance of utilizing bystanders to assist with patient assessment when the patient is having difficulty speaking. It also includes updates on contraindications for metered-dose inhalers.

- *Chapter 16, Caring for Common Medical Emergencies*, introduces the "last known normal" and the FAST assessment tool for patients experiencing stroke. It also includes important strategies for assessing patients with an altered mental status and discusses its potential causes.

- *Chapter 17, Caring for Environmental Emergencies*, now includes updated information on rewarming a local cold injury, heat cramps, and the amount of air to provide during rescue breaths. It also includes updated images for cold injuries to the feet.

Chapters 18–22

These chapters address many of the more common emergencies related to trauma and bleeding. Each chapter includes new elements related to justice, equity, diversity, and inclusion (JEDI), crew resource management (CRM), and patient handoff.

WHAT'S NEW?

- *Chapter 18, Caring for Soft Tissue Injuries and Bleeding*, includes updated information on the following topics: tourniquet and roller bandage applications, hemostatic dressing use, signs and symptoms of internal bleeding, impaled object removal, open chest wound care, and burn treatment based on affected body surface area. It also includes tips on involving the patient in their own care.

- *Chapter 19, Recognition and Care of Shock*, now includes additional examples of distributive shock, updated information on signs and symptoms of shock, and more detailed definitions of septic shock, hypoperfusion, and shock.

- *Chapter 20, Caring for Muscle and Bone Injuries*, reinforces the various methods for immobilization of an elbow injury and for determining treatment priorities.

- *Chapter 21, Caring for Head and Spinal Injuries*, now defines and explains traumatic brain injury (TBI) and concussion and their causes. It also includes a detailed description of spinal motion restriction (SMR).

- *Chapter 22, Caring for Chest and Abdominal Emergencies*, now offers an expanded section on management of open chest injuries along with updates on treatment of patients with a flail chest, the care of open chest wounds, spontaneous pneumothorax, and the management of evisceration.

Chapter 23

This chapter covers normal pregnancy and childbirth. It also discusses many of the common emergencies related to pregnancy and childbirth. Each chapter includes new elements related to justice, equity, diversity, and inclusion (JEDI), crew resource management (CRM), and patient handoff.

WHAT'S NEW?

- *Chapter 23, Care During Pregnancy and Childbirth*, retains all the most up-to-date information regarding Emergency Medical Responder care of the mother and child before, during, and after delivery.

Chapters 24 and 25

Chapters 24 and 25 cover the unique differences in the special populations of pediatric and geriatric patients. They also introduce specific assessment strategies for each group. Each chapter includes new elements related to justice, equity, diversity, and inclusion (JEDI), crew resource management (CRM), and patient handoff.

WHAT'S NEW?

- *Chapter 24, Caring for Infants and Children*, retains past updates to the definitions of newborn and infant decompensated shock. It also includes updated strategies for caring for parents/caregivers who are in distress at the scene of an incident involving an infant or child.

- *Chapter 25, Special Considerations for the Geriatric Patient*, provides an overview of special considerations when caring for the geriatric patient. It also provides statistics on the aging population, along with discussions of suicide in older adults, the causes of pressure sores, definitions of mechanical falls, and an expanded discussion on multiple medications and side effects of some common medications.

Chapters 26 and 27

These two chapters cover many of the topics related to EMS operations, such as the phases of an emergency response, responding to a hazardous materials incident, and responding to multiple-casualty incidents. The principles of the incident management system (IMS) and triage are also addressed. Both chapters retain information important to the roles of Emergency Medical Responders during hazardous materials and multiple-casualty responses. Each chapter includes new elements related to justice, equity, diversity, and inclusion (JEDI), crew resource management (CRM), and patient handoff.

WHAT'S NEW?

- *Chapter 26, Introduction to EMS Operations and Hazardous Response*, includes updates to education standards and on managing patients who are contaminated; it also includes new information on safety awareness related to working around electric and hybrid vehicles.

- *Chapter 27, Introduction to Multiple-Casualty Incidents, the Incident Command System, and Triage*, includes information about online FEMA training, the SALT triage system, and the use of colored ribbons to replace triage tags.

Appendices

There are four appendices in this edition: "Patient Monitoring Devices"; "Principles of Pharmacology"; "Air Medical Transport Operations"; and an "Introduction to Terrorism Response and Weapons of Mass Destruction." Each includes an overview of its topic relevant to the role of the Emergency Medical Responder.

ACKNOWLEDGMENTS

It takes the efforts of many to render care efficiently and appropriately during an emergency. Assembling a project such as this requires similar efforts. Without the coordinated work of many people spread throughout the United States, this project would not have been possible. I'd like to acknowledge the key players who helped create the end product that you see before you.

I'd like to begin with Audrey Le Baudour, my personal assistant, copy editor, travel coordinator, and, most importantly, my wife. She is the one who keeps me organized, focused, and on schedule.

I'd like to extend a special thank you to photographer, Michal Heron, who has single-handedly raised the bar for the way EMS is depicted in textbooks across the country. Michal, you brought something no other artist did when shooting for these books. Your work is clearly head and shoulders above the rest, and you really challenged authors to do it better.

A very special thank you is in order for my team at Pearson, Kevin Wilson and Maria Reyes, along with freelance development editor Tanya Martin. I simply could not ask for a more professional and passionate team to be working with.

A special thanks to the entire sales team at Pearson Education, who provide the support and infrastructure to make these projects happen and get them to those who need them. The skill and teamwork it takes to choreograph a project such as this is truly amazing.

Medical Director

Keith Wesley, MD, FACEP

Our special thanks to Dr. Keith Wesley. His reviews were carefully prepared, and we appreciate the thoughtful advice and keen insight offered.

Dr. Keith Wesley is board certified in emergency medicine with subspecialty board certification in emergency medical services. Dr. Wesley is the EMS medical director for HealthEast Medical Transportation in St. Paul, Minnesota. He has served as the state EMS medical director for both Minnesota and Wisconsin and chair of the National Council of State EMS Medical Directors. Dr. Wesley is the author of many articles and EMS textbooks and a frequent speaker at EMS conferences across the nation.

Contributors to Previous Editions

We would like to extend our sincere appreciation and thanks to the following individuals who contributed to the completion of the 10th edition, as well as previous editions. Thank you for your ideas, feedback, and contributions.

Lorenzo J. Alviso,
CHT, NREMT; Instructional Assistant, Santa Rosa Junior College EMT Program, Santa Rosa, CA

Lt. John L. Beckman,
AA, BS, FF/EMT-P; Fire Science Instructor, Technology Center of Dupage, Addison, IL

Ted Williams,
NREMT-P; Faculty, Santa Rosa Junior College, Santa Rosa, CA

Todd Janssen,
NREMT; Falck Northern California, Petaluma, CA

Photo Acknowledgments

All photographs not credited in the photo caption were photographed on assignment by Michal Heron for Pearson Education, Inc.

Organizations

We wish to thank the following organizations for their assistance in creating the photo program for this edition:

Windsor Fire Department, Windsor, California, Chief Doug Williams

Falck Northern California, Gary Tennyson—CEO, and Sean Sullivan—COO

Santa Rosa Junior College–Public Safety Training Center, April Chapman—Dean

Sonoma County Regional Parks, Mark Norman—Park Ranger/EMT, Sabrina Spear—Lifeguard/EMT, John Menth—Lifeguard/EMT

Sonoma County Search and Rescue Team, Steve Freitas—Sheriff

Photo Coordinators/Subject Matter Experts

Thanks to Paramedic Ted Williams for his valuable assistance directing the medical accuracy of the shoots and coordinating models, props, and locations for our photo shoots.

Models

Thanks to the following people who portrayed patients and EMS providers in our photographs:

Rachel Abravaya	Jacob Garrison	John Menth
Joseph Armbruster	Brandon Hefele	Molly Muldoon
Veronique Asti	Mark Hubenette	Mark Norman
Amanda Baker	Melissa Keck	Ryan Opiekun
Michael Baker	Mina Kiani	Fredrick Presler
Kevin Beans	Nathan Koman	James Renegar
Breanne Benward	Misty Landeros	Tyler Reynolds
Irene Calzada-Bickham	Katy Le Baudour	Sabrina Spear
Andrea Bordignon	Matt Marshall	Morgan Stameroff
Rebecca Calleja	John "JR" Maricich	Lana Trapp
Breanna Cheatham	John Martin	Cody Whitmore
Don Chigazola	Mike McDonald	Steve Whitmore
Jesus Diaz	Addison Meints	Bradley Williams
Mark Diaz	Casey Meints	Ted Williams
Jason Freyer	Kayla Meints	

Photo Assistants/Digital Postproduction

Maria Lyle

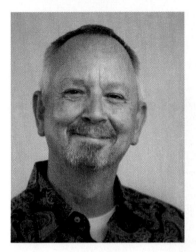

Chris Le Baudour

Chris Le Baudour has been working in the EMS field since 1978. In 1984, Chris began his teaching career in the Department of Public Safety—EMS Division at Santa Rosa Junior College in Santa Rosa, California.

Chris holds a Bachelor's Degree in Communications and a Master's Degree in Education with an emphasis in online teaching and learning as well as numerous EMS and instructional certifications. Chris has spent the past 40 years mastering the art of experiential learning in EMS and is well known for his innovative classroom techniques and his passion for both teaching and learning in both traditional and online classrooms.

Chris is involved in EMS education at the national level, having served six years as a board member of the National Association of EMS Educators, and actively advises many organizations throughout the country. Chris is a frequent presenter at both state and national conferences and a prolific EMS writer. Along with numerous articles, he is the author of *Emergency Care for First Responders*, and coauthor of *EMT Complete: A Basic Worktext*, and the Active Learning Manual for the EMT. Chris currently serves as the EMS Administrator for the County of Marin in Northern California. Chris and his wife, Audrey, have two adult children and reside in Northern California.

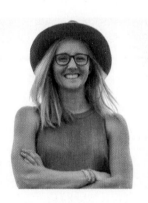

Kaitlyn Laurélle

Kaitlyn began her career in EMS in 2015 as a way to enhance her preparedness for her outdoor and remote adventures. She has worked as both a clinical and wilderness EMT and as an emergency first responder instructor for the wilderness context.

Kaitlyn holds a Master's Degree from the University of California, Davis, as well as numerous professional certificates. From the corporate boardroom, to the classroom, to the mountain summit, she is passionate about managing high-impact projects focused on innovative, long-term solutions to improving the quality of life for resource-limited communities around the globe.

She is an avid outdoor adventurer, spending much of her free time rock climbing, mountaineering, mountain biking, or kayaking in and around the Sierra Nevada mountains. Kaitlyn has been both the rescuer and the patient in the first responder context (her frostbite injuries are featured in Chapter 17). Kaitlyn brings her passion for educating adult learners with empathetic and tolerant teaching methodologies into her work as a writer, most notably through her influence as a JEDI strategist on this 12th edition.

Derek O. Hanley is a longtime paramedic, prior military combat medic, author, published photographer, multi-instrumentalist, noted video producer, and CEO and creative director of DOHP (dohp.net).

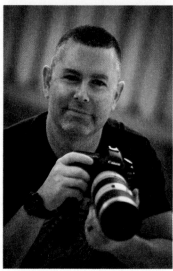

(Anthony Dimaano; adimaanophotography.com)

Emergency Medical Response Certification Program

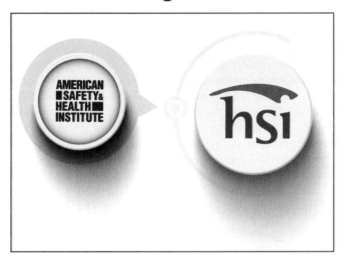

Health & Safety Institute (HSI) is a nationally recognized training provider in emergency care, workplace safety, first responder continuing education, and a variety of compliance and safety solutions. HSI's mission is *Making the Workplace and Community Safer™*. HSI authorizes qualified individuals to offer Emergency Medical Response training and certification programs for corporate America, government agencies, and emergency responders. *Emergency Medical Responder: First on Scene*, is the required textbook of the HSI Emergency Medical Response training program. To learn more, visit hsi.com.

In the early 1970s, officials at the U.S. Department of Transportation National Highway Traffic Safety Administration (NHTSA) recognized a gap between basic first aid training and the training of Emergency Medical Technicians (EMTs). Their solution was to create "Crash Injury Management: Emergency Medical Services for Traffic Law Enforcement Officers," an emergency medical care course for "patrolling law enforcement officers." As it evolved, the course expanded to include other "First Responders"—public and private safety and service personnel who, in the course of performing other duties, are likely to respond to emergencies (firefighters, highway department personnel, etc.). The Crash Injury Management course provided the basic knowledge and skills necessary to perform lifesaving interventions while waiting for EMTs to arrive. The original program was never intended for training EMS personnel. Because the Crash Injury Management course was designed to fill the gap between basic first aid training and EMT, it was considered "advanced first aid

training." In 1978, the Crash Injury Management course was renamed *Emergency Medical Services First Responder Training Course* and was specifically targeted at "public service law enforcement, fire, and EMS rescue agencies that did not necessarily have the ability to transport patients or carry sophisticated medical equipment." Then, in 1995, the course went through a major revision and its name was changed to *First Responder: National Standard Curriculum*. At that time, the First Responder was described as "an integral part of the Emergency Medical Services System." Later, in 2006, a FEMA EMS Working Group recommended a new job title for first responders working within the EMS system—the **Emergency Medical Responder (EMR)**. This title is meant to specify a state-licensed and credentialed individual responding within an EMS-providing entity, organization, or agency. Specifically, the use of the word "medical" in the EMR title is intended to help distinguish those persons who have successfully completed a state-approved EMR program from other first responders such as law enforcement officers, public health workers, and search and rescue personnel (to name a few).

HSI Emergency Medical Response for Non-EMS Personnel

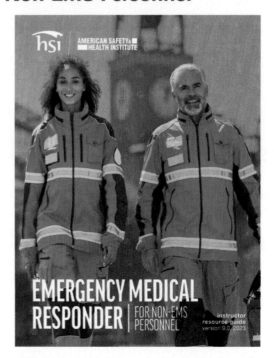

The gap between basic first aid training and the training of EMS professionals that was recognized more than 30 years ago remains. There is still a need for advanced first aid and emergency care training for non-EMS providers who, in the course of performing other duties, are likely (or expected) to respond to emergencies. These individuals, including law enforcement officers, firefighters, and other public and private safety and service personnel, are part of a network of resources—people, communications, and equipment—prepared to provide emergency care to victims of sudden illness or injury. These individuals are not, and in most cases do not wish to be, state-licensed and credentialed EMS professionals. The original first responder program was intended to provide these first-on-the-scene responders with the basic knowledge and skills necessary for lifesaving interventions while waiting for the EMS professionals to arrive. That original intent (filling the knowledge and skill gap between basic first aid training and EMS) is the intent of HSI's Emergency Medical Response for Non-EMS Personnel program. Additionally, because this program uses the same textbooks and related instructional tools as those used to train EMRs, it serves to encourage a continuum in care for the ill or injured person as they are transitioned from care provided by the first responder to care provided by the EMS professional.

Certification in HSI Emergency Medical Response

Evaluation of knowledge and skill competence is required for certification in HSI Emergency Medical Response. The learner must successfully complete the HSI Emergency Medical Response for Non-EMS Personnel Exam and demonstrate the ability to work as a lead first responder in a scenario-based team setting, adequately directing the initial assessment and care of a responsive and unresponsive medical and trauma patient.

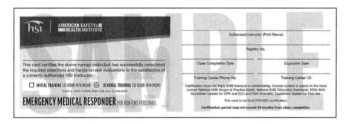

State Licensure and Credentialing

State EMS agencies have the legal authority and responsibility to license, regulate, and determine the scope of practice of EMS providers within the state EMS system. HSI's Emergency Medical Response program is designed to allow properly qualified and authorized HSI instructors to train and certify individuals as first responders consistent with the National EMS Education Standards and Instructional Guidelines. It is not the intent of HSI's Emergency Medical Response program to cross the EMS scope of practice threshold. An individual who has been trained and certified in HSI Emergency Medical Response is NOT licensed and credentialed to practice emergency medical care as an EMS provider within an organized state EMS system. EMS

provider licensing and credentialing are legal activities performed by the state, not HSI. Individuals who require or desire licensure and credentialing within the state EMS system must complete specific requirements established by the regulating authority.

International Use of HSI Emergency Medical Response for Non-EMS Personnel

Given the current state of globalization and the increasing international reach of authorized HSI instructors, the HSI Emergency Medical Response program has expanded outside of the United States. As appropriate actions by first responders alleviate suffering, prevent disability, and save lives, HSI encourages this international expansion, particularly in areas with emerging but undeveloped EMS systems. However, as in the United States, the scope of practice for medically trained persons is often subject to federal, state, provincial, or regional laws and regulations. It is not the intent of HSI's Emergency Medical Response program to cross the EMS (or medical) scope of practice threshold in any country.

Health & Safety Institute (HSI)

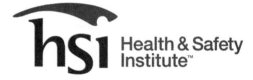

HSI is a family of well-known and respected brands in the Environmental, Health, and Safety (EH&S) space. Our brands span the broad range of needs in EH&S—from emergency care training to facilitating workplace safety training, tracking, and reporting, to the management of chemical inventories. HSI's emergency care training and emergency medical service (EMS) continuing education programs are currently accepted, approved, or recognized as meeting the requirements of more than 5,200 state and federal regulatory agencies, occupational licensing boards, national associations, commissions, and councils in more than 550 occupations and professions. Since 1978, HSI authorized instructors have certified nearly 33 million emergency care providers in the United States and more than 100 countries throughout the world. HSI is an accredited organization of the Commission on Accreditation of Pre-Hospital Continuing Education (CAPCE), the national accreditation body for Emergency Medical Service Continuing Education programs, and a member of the American National Standards Institute (ANSI) and ASTM International, two of the largest voluntary standards development and conformity assessment organizations in the world.

Health & Safety Institute
1450 Westec Drive, Eugene, OR 97402
800-447-3177
response@hsi.com

WALK THROUGH

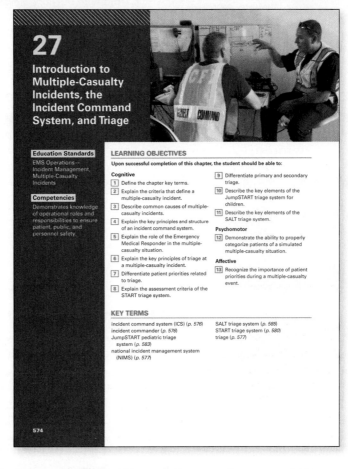

Education Standards and Competencies ▶

Provides standards and competencies that are addressed in each chapter.

◀ Learning Objectives

A list of the cognitive, psychomotor, and affective goals for you to master following completion of a chapter.

◀ First on Scene and First on Scene Run Review

You will experience a new medical emergency at the start of each chapter as you follow the actions of an Emergency Medical Responder who is first on the scene, then follow the EMR and their patients throughout the chapter as the case develops. Finally, you'll have a chance to debrief at the end of the chapter as you respond to Run Review questions, thinking about the steps the EMR took and what might have gone differently.

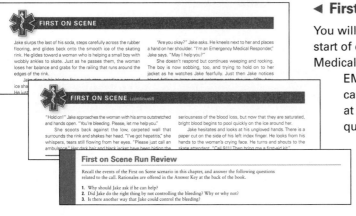

Remember ▶

Appearing throughout the chapters, these boxes highlight important or critical concepts that are important take-aways from your reading.

REMEMBER

As a new member of the EMS team who will be caring for patients, it is best to make it a habit to wear gloves for all patient contacts. While it is true that not all patients pose a risk of exposure to a pathogen, you do not yet have enough experience to know the difference. Play it safe and always don gloves prior to making

Scene Safety ▶

These stop-and-think boxes reinforce the idea that the safety—of the patient, the Emergency Medical Responder, bystanders, or others—is of paramount importance when responding to the scene.

SCENE SAFETY

One of the most important concepts you can learn and live by is that Emergency Medical Responders are usually not trained to deal with a hazardous materials spill. If you suspect that a hazardous material is involved at a scene to which you are responding, stay clear and call in a specialized hazmat team to secure the scene before you ent...

JEDI ▶

Tips on caring for patients representing diverse populations.

▼ Crew Resource Management

Guidance on making the best use of team resources at the emergency scene.

CREW RESOURCE MANAGEMENT

Efficiency is especially important when working as a team to resuscitate a patient in cardiac arrest. Each team member should know their role and perform it in concert with other members of the team. This approach is often called "pit crew CPR" because it requires the same kind of synchronized activity that is characteristic of race car pit crews.

▼ Key Skills

These are the key skills the Emergency Medical Responder performs when assisting a patient at the scene of an emergency.

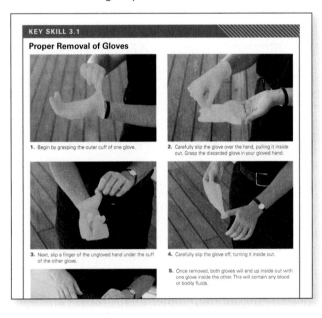

KEY SKILL 3.1

Proper Removal of Gloves

1. Begin by grasping the outer cuff of one glove.
2. Carefully slip the glove over the hand, pulling it inside out. Grasp the discarded glove in your gloved hand.
3. Next, slip a finger of the ungloved hand under the cuff of the other glove.
4. Carefully slip the glove off, turning it inside out.
5. Once removed, both gloves will end up inside out with one glove inside the other. This will contain any blood or bodily fluids.

▼ First on Scene Run Review

As described previously, these questions give you a chance to think through the events and actions that occurred in the chapter case study and evaluate what happened, what went well, what needed work, and how you might have responded differently if you were the Emergency Medical Responder in that situation.

First on Scene Run Review

Recall the events of the First on Scene scenario in this chapter, and answer the following questions related to the call. Rationales are offered in the Answer Key at the back of the book.

1. Why should Jake ask if he can help?
2. Did Jake do the right thing by not controlling the bleeding? Why or why not?
3. Is there another way that Jake could control the bleeding?

▼ First on Scene Patient Handoff

Examples of information conveyed when transferring patients to a higher level of care.

First on Scene Patient Handoff

We have a 36-year-old female named Emily who experienced a mechanical fall backward onto the ice, striking her head. The fall was witnessed, and Emily did not have any loss of consciousness immediately following the fall. She has an open wound to the back of her head with obvious bleeding. Emily states that she is positive for hepatitis and was reluctant to have anyone assist her at first. I instructed Emily to hold pressure on the back of her head while I waited for gloves. Emily then became unresponsive, and we carefully laid her supine on the ice with a blanket beneath her for insulation. Her son is here with her and would like to go with her if she is transported...

▼ Summary

A bulleted list of the key points from the chapter.

Summary

- Prior to beginning work as an Emergency Medical Responder, it is important for you to establish a baseline health status to ensure that you are healthy and prepared. Part of this health assessment includes receiving appropriate immunizations.
- Standard precautions are those precautions all health care professionals must follow to minimize exposure to infectious pathogens. This includes maintaining a philosophy that all patients are potentially infectious and donning all necessary personal protective equipment (PPE).
- Proper body substance isolation (BSI) precautions should be taken prior to making contact with all patients. BSI precautions include wearing PPE such as gloves, eye protection, and protective gowns when necessary.
- Pathogens can enter the body one of four ways: injection, absorption, inhalation, or ingestion.
- Know your company/agency procedure should you sustain an exposure to a patient's blood or bodily fluids. At a minimum, you must immediately wash the area with warm soap and water and contact your supervisor.
- Exposure to pathogens is just one potential hazard when caring for patients. Emergency scenes are full of other hazards, such as moving traffic, downed power lines, spilled fuel or chemicals, and violent patients. You must always keep personal safety as your top priority and use appropriately trained resources to help mitigate these hazards.
- Stress is an emotionally disruptive or upsetting condition that occurs in response to adverse external influences. Stressors are those factors that cause stress. As an Emergency Medical Responder, you must be aware of the common causes of stress and the typical ways that stress may exhibit itself.
- If not properly managed, stress can become very disruptive. It can cause negative changes in behavior and attitude as well as physical changes that negatively affect health.
- You must learn to develop good coping mechanisms for many of the common stressors of the job. Eating a healthy, balanced diet; getting regular exercise; and maintaining work-life balance are all important.
- Critical incident stress management (CISM) can be helpful for many when trying to manage the effects of stress following a critical incident.

Take Action

Slippery When Wet

Learning to put on and remove protective gloves is an important skill for all Emergency Medical Responders. One way you can practice this skill is to don a pair of disposable gloves and spread a generous portion of shaving cream over both gloved hands. The shaving cream is used to simulate blood or other bodily fluids. Now carefully try to remove the gloves, one at a time, without splattering the shaving cream. The gloves will be difficult to remove when they are wet but, with enough practice, you will become skilled at safely removing them.

Stressed Out

Most EMS systems around the country have specialized teams of people who are trained to assist EMS personnel who have responded to a critical incident. These teams will provide support and assistance for those who were directly involved in the incident and help them understand the reactions they may be experiencing. Ask your instructor or another EMS professional in your area how to access these resources.

First on Scene Patient Handoff

We have a 36-year-old female named Emily who experienced a mechanical fall backward onto the ice, striking her head. The fall was witnessed, and Emily did not have any loss of consciousness...

▼ Quick Quiz

These multiple choice questions check your understanding of the chapter's content.

Quick Quiz

To check your understanding of the chapter, answer the following questions. Then, compare your answers to those in the Answer Key at the back of the book.

1. All of the following are routes through which pathogens may enter the body EXCEPT:
   a. ingestion.
   b. mentation.
   c. inhalation.
   d. injection.

2. Which of the following is NOT a commonly recommended immunization for health care providers?
   a. Rabies
   b. Pertussis
   c. Hepatitis
   d. Tetanus

3. Which of the following types of PPE would be most important to use when caring for a patient with tuberculosis?
   a. Gloves
   b. Eyeglasses
   c. HEPA mask
   d. Gown

4. You have arrived at the scene of a vehicle collision, and there are downed power lines across the road. Which of the following resources is most appropriate to manage this hazard?
   a. Law enforcement
   b. Fire department
   c. Hazmat team
   d. Utility company

8. All of the following are terms used for the stages of death and dying EXCEPT:
   a. denial.
   b. anger.
   c. bargaining.
   d. refusal.

9. When caring for family members after the death of a loved one, you should:
   a. avoid talking directly to the patient's family.
   b. not tolerate angry reactions.
   c. try your best to understand their feelings.
   d. tell them everything will be okay.

10. All of the following are common signs and symptoms of stress EXCEPT:
   a. irritability.
   b. difficulty sleeping.
   c. increased appetite.
   d. difficulty concentrating.

11. A broad-based approach involving several strategies designed to help emergency personnel cope with stress is called:
   a. Critical Incident Stress Management.
   b. Emergency Stress Reduction Protocol.

◀ Take Action

Hands-on activities that give you an opportunity to practice some of the skills and concepts you learned in a chapter.

What Is MyLab BRADY with Pearson eText?

MyLab BRADY is a comprehensive online program that gives you—the student—the opportunity to test your understanding of information and concepts to see how well you know the material. The added benefit of the embedded Pearson eText for *Emergency Medical Responder: First on Scene, 12th edition*, gives you access to your textbook anytime, anywhere, on the device of your choice—even offline!

With *MyLab BRADY for Emergency Medical Responder*, you can track your own progress through your entire emergency medical responder course.

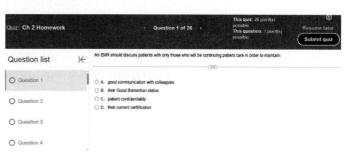

How Do Students Benefit?

Here's how *MyLab BRADY for Emergency Medical Responder* helps you:

- Keep up and get unstuck by providing immediate feedback on homework.
- Apply your knowledge with case studies of situations you may encounter in the field.
- Review videos of key skills so you can be ready anywhere, anytime.
- Use the mobile eText to help you learn on your terms, wherever you are.

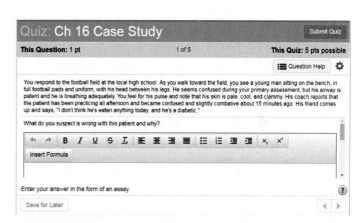

Key Features of *MyLab BRADY for Emergency Medical Responder, 12th Edition*

- **Chapter Audio Review** from expert author, Chris Le Baudour, points you in the direction of the chapter's key concepts.
- **Homework** covers all chapter objectives and consists of multiple-choice questions with study aids to assist when you are uncertain.
- **Case Studies** with questions help with application of knowledge and retention for situations you may encounter in the field.
- **Skills Videos** of more than 50 critical skills allow you to watch and review at a moment's notice.
- **Multimedia Library** gathers all media items in one searchable location so you don't have to struggle finding what you need.

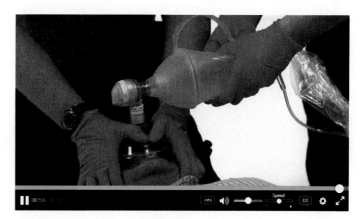

How Do Instructors Benefit?

- Keep students with different learning styles engaged through a variety of interactive components.
- Track student progress and understanding of course content through Homework and Case Studies.
- Save time through auto-grading.
- Enliven classroom presentations by working through a case study or displaying an animation or skill video.
- Deliver tests/exams online with auto-grading so you can eliminate the time to tabulate results.
- MyLab BRADY can be fully integrated into the majority of commercially available Learning Management Systems, so the experience can be completely seamless. Ask for details.

Pearson eText

The **Pearson eText** provides a fully-integrated electronic experience so users can read, study, and take notes anytime, anywhere on the device of their choice—even offline.

How Do Students Benefit?

Standard Pearson eText features include the ability to highlight, take notes, bookmark pages, and search. In addition, the eText for *Emergency Medical Responder, 12th edition* includes interactivity and multimedia that enhances the learning experience:

- Full audio book
- Flashcards
- End-of-chapter self-study review questions
- Application review questions included as part of the "First on Scene" scenarios

How Do Instructors Benefit?

Instructors can push notes and highlights directly to students so they can provide embellishment or focus on key concepts within the text.

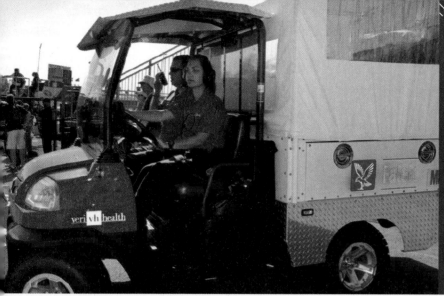

1

Introduction to EMS Systems

Education Standards

Preparatory—EMS Systems, Research, Public Health

Competencies

Uses knowledge of the EMS system and the safety/well-being of the Emergency Medical Responder at the scene of an emergency while awaiting a higher level of care.

Develops an awareness of local public health resources and their role in public health.

LEARNING OBJECTIVES

Upon successful completion of this chapter, the student should be able to:

Cognitive

1. Define the chapter key terms.

2. Explain the role of the National Highway Traffic Safety Administration (NHTSA) and its relationship to EMS.

3. Differentiate the various attributes of an EMS system and describe the function of each.

4. Identify the six guiding principles of the EMS Agenda 2050.

5. Explain the roles that the National EMS Education Standards and the National Scope of Practice Model play in shaping the EMS system across the United States.

6. Differentiate the four nationally recognized levels of EMS provider.

7. Differentiate the roles and responsibilities of the Emergency Medical Responder from those of other EMS providers.

8. Differentiate the various EMS models in practice across the United States.

9. Explain the roles that state and local EMS offices, medical oversight, and local credentialing play in an EMS system.

10. Explain how state and local statutes and regulations affect how an Emergency Medical Responder might function.

11. Explain the various methods used to access the EMS system.

12. Explain the various types of medical direction and how the Emergency Medical Responder might interact with each.

13. Describe the characteristics of professionalism as they relate to the Emergency Medical Responder.

14. Explain the role of the Emergency Medical Responder with regard to continuous quality improvement (CQI).

15. Explain the role of public health systems and their relationship to EMS, disease surveillance, and injury prevention.

16. Explain the role that Disaster Medical Assistance Teams (DMATs) play and how they integrate with EMS systems.

17. Explain the role that research plays in the EMS system and the ways that an Emergency Medical Responder might seek out and support research.

Psychomotor

18. Participate in simple research activities facilitated by the instructor.

Affective

19. Demonstrate appreciation of the importance of accepting and upholding the responsibilities of an Emergency Medical Responder.

20 Support the rationale for always maintaining a high degree of professionalism when performing the duties of an Emergency Medical Responder.

21 Demonstrate commitment to providing the best possible care for all patients regardless of culture, gender, age, or socioeconomic status.

22 Model a desire for continuous quality improvement (CQI) both personally and professionally.

23 Demonstrate appreciation of the importance of quality research and its connection to high-quality patient care.

KEY TERMS

Advanced Emergency Medical Technician (AEMT) (*p. 9*)
chief complaint (*p. 14*)
continuous quality improvement (CQI) (*p. 16*)
Disaster Medical Assistance Team (DMAT) (*p. 17*)
emergency care (*p. 3*)
Emergency Medical Dispatcher (EMD) (*p. 9*)
Emergency Medical Responder (EMR) (*p. 8*)
emergency medical services (EMS) system (*p. 4*)
Emergency Medical Technician (EMT) (*p. 9*)

evidence-based practice (*p. 6*)
medical director (*p. 6*)
medical oversight (*p. 6*)
National EMS Education Standards (*p. 8*)
off-line medical direction (*p. 10*)
on-line medical direction (*p. 10*)
Paramedic (*p. 9*)
protocols (*p. 10*)
public health system (*p. 17*)
public safety answering point (PSAP) (*p. 9*)
research (*p. 17*)
scope of practice (*p. 9*)
Scope of Practice Model (*p. 8*)
specialty hospital (*p. 10*)
standing orders (*p. 10*)

You have made a great choice in deciding to become a member of the EMS team and train as an Emergency Medical Responder. An estimated 240 million calls are made to 911 in the United States each year,[1] and many of those calls are responded to by individuals trained at the Emergency Medical Responder level.

Thousands of people become ill or are injured every day, and many are far from a hospital at the time of their emergency. EMS systems have been developed for this very reason. Their purpose is to get trained medical personnel to the patient as quickly as possible and provide emergency care at the scene. Emergency Medical Responders are an essential part of a community and the EMS team.

Realizing that people will depend on you to provide assistance during an emergency can be overwhelming. To gain confidence in your knowledge and skills, it is very important that you learn and understand what is expected of you in this new role. When you do, you can act more quickly to provide efficient and effective emergency care.

This chapter will introduce the EMS system, its components, and how they work together to deliver care to the ill and injured. We will also discuss the roles and responsibilities you will be expected to embrace as an Emergency Medical Responder.

FIRST ON SCENE

It's a bright, sunny spring day and you have just left what you feel was one of your best interviews yet. If all goes well, you will soon be working as a senior camp counselor for the largest summer camp in the state. Things are looking up, and there is a noticeable bounce in your step as you descend the stairs to the visitor parking lot. As you reach the sidewalk, you hear someone shouting for help from across the lot. You hesitate for a moment and look around. Again, you hear a female voice yelling for help, but you cannot see anyone. You decide to investigate and run toward the voice.

Two rows over, you see a middle-aged woman leaning over a young boy on the ground. He appears to be shaking and a white, foamy substance is coming from his mouth. The woman sees you and, in a panicked voice, asks you to call an ambulance.

You reach for your cell phone and call 911 for help. You then run into the building to tell the receptionist what is going on. She alerts the building's Medical Emergency Response Team. Nervously, you return to the scene in the parking lot.

The EMS System

LO2 Explain the role of the National Highway Traffic Safety Administration (NHTSA) and its relationship to EMS.

LO3 Differentiate the various attributes of an EMS system and describe the function of each.

LO4 Identify the six guiding principles of the EMS Agenda 2050.

LO5 Explain the role that the National EMS Education Standards and the National Scope of Practice Model play in shaping the EMS system across the United States.

LO6 Differentiate the four nationally recognized levels of EMS provider.

LO7 Differentiate the roles and responsibilities of the Emergency Medical Responder from other EMS providers.

It is likely that people have been providing **emergency care** for one another since humans first walked the Earth. Many of those early treatments would seem primitive by today's standards, but the awareness that some kind of care is often needed at the scene of the emergency has not changed. A formal system for responding to emergencies has existed only since the late 18th century (Figure 1.1).

During the American Civil War, the Union Army began training soldiers to provide first aid to the wounded on the battlefield. These *corpsmen*, as they were known, were trained to provide care for the most immediate life threats, such as bleeding. After their initial care, the injured were transported by horse-drawn carriage to awaiting physicians. Thus, the first formal ambulance system in the United States had begun.

The first civilian ambulance services began in the late 1800s with the sole purpose of transporting injured and ill patients to the hospital for care. It was not until 1928 that the concept of civilian on-scene care was first implemented, with the organization of the Roanoke Life Saving and First Aid Crew in Roanoke, Virginia.

In 1966, the National Academy of Sciences released a report called "Accidental Death and Disability: The Neglected Disease of Modern Society." That report revealed for the first time the inadequacies of prehospital care. It also provided suggestions for the development of formal EMS systems.

emergency care ▶ assessment and basic care for an ill or injured patient in an emergency situation.

1790s	Napoleon's chief physician, Dominique Jean Larrey, develops a system designed to triage and transport injured soldiers from the battlefield to established aid stations.
1805–1815	Dominique Jean Larrey formed the Ambulance Volante (flying ambulance). It consisted of a covered horse-drawn cart designed to bring medical care closer to the injured on the battlefields of Europe.
1861–1865	Clara Barton coordinates the care of sick and injured soldiers during the American Civil War.
1869	New York City Health Department Ambulance Service begins operation out of what was then known as the Free Hospital of New York, now Bellevue Hospital.
1915	First recorded air medical transport occurred during the retreat of the Serbian army from Albania.
1928	The concept of "on-scene care" was first initiated when Julian Stanley Wise started the Roanoke Life Saving and First Aid Crew in Roanoke, Virginia.
1950–1973	The first use of helicopters to evacuate injured soldiers and deliver them to waiting field hospitals occurred in the Korean and Vietnam wars.
1966	The report entitled "Accidental Death and Disability: The Neglected Disease of Modern Society," commonly referred to as the "White Paper," is published. The study concludes that many of the deaths occurring every day were unnecessary and could be prevented through better prehospital treatments. The report resulted in Congress passing the National Highway Safety Act.
1968	On February 16, 1968, Senator Rankin Fite completed the first 911 call made in the United States in Haleyville, Alabama. The serving telephone company was then Alabama Telephone Company. This Haleyville 911 system is still in operation today. On February 22, 1968, Nome, Alaska implemented 911 service.
1973	Congress passes the Emergency Medical Services Act, which provides funding for a series of projects related to trauma care.
1988	The National Highway Traffic and Safety Administration (NHTSA) defines elements necessary for all EMS systems.
1990	The Trauma Care Systems Planning and Development Act of 1990 encourages development of improved trauma systems.
1995	An update to the EMT Basic and First Responder National Standard curricula is released.
1996	The EMS Agenda for the Future outlines the most important directions for the future of EMS development.
1998	An update to the EMT Paramedic National Standard Curriculum is released.
1999	An update to the EMT Intermediate National Standard Curriculum is released.
2000	NHTSA publishes "EMS Education Agenda for the Future: A Systems Approach."
2005	NHTSA publishes the National EMS Core Content.
2007	NHTSA publishes the National EMS Scope of Practice Model, redefining the four levels of EMS certification and licensure.
2009	NHTSA publishes the new EMS Education Standards.
2019	NHTSA publishes EMS Agenda 2050.
2019	NHTSA publishes new EMS Scope of Practice Model.
2021	NHTSA updates National Education Standards.

Figure 1.1 Timeline of significant events in the history of Emergency Medical Services.

emergency medical services system ▶ chain of human resources and services linked together to provide continuous emergency care at the scene and during transport to a medical facility. Abbrev: EMS.

Fortunately, it has become possible to extend lifesaving care through a chain of resources known as the **emergency medical services (EMS) system** (Key Skill 1.1). Once the EMS system is activated, care begins at the emergency scene and continues during transport to a medical facility. At the hospital, a formal transfer of care to the emergency department staff ensures a smooth continuation of care. (The emergency department may still be referred to as the emergency room or ER in some areas.)

Understand the EMS System

An effective EMS system depends on both trained and untrained resources.

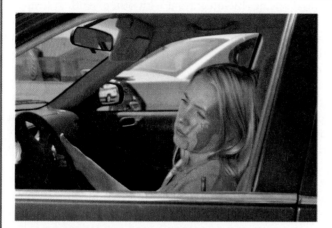

1. An individual becomes injured in a vehicle collision.

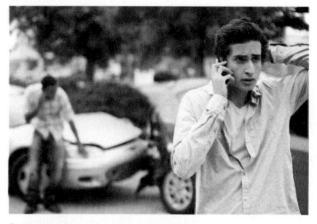

2. A witness to the incident calls 911.
(MBI/Shutterstock)

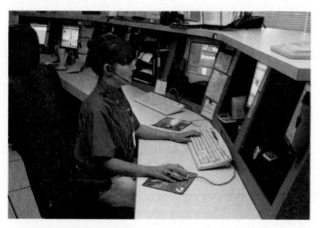

3. The Emergency Medical Dispatcher sends the appropriate resources.

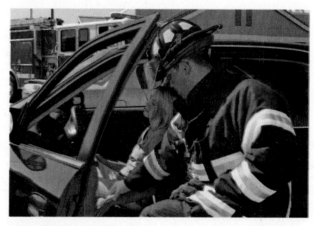

4. Emergency Medical Responders arrive to assist the patient.

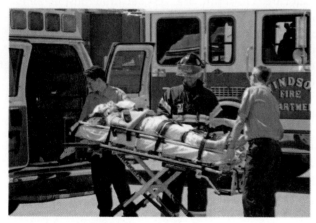

5. EMTs and Paramedics continue care and transport the patient to the hospital.

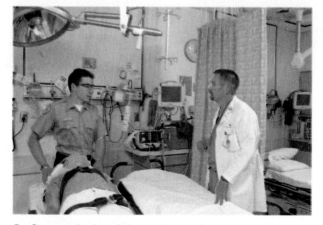

6. Once at the hospital, care is transferred to emergency department personnel.

In 1996, the National Highway Traffic Safety Administration (NHTSA) identified 14 key attributes of an integrated EMS system that assists states in developing and assessing these components.[2] They are:

- *Integration of health services.* Historically, EMS has always focused on only the care provided in the prehospital setting. By integrating with other health system components, EMS can improve health care for the entire community. The future of EMS includes EMTs and Paramedics working closely with public health departments and health care networks to identify non-emergent health needs in the community and to assist in providing for those needs.

- *EMS research.* EMS has evolved relatively fast over the past 50 years despite the slow progress of EMS-related research. Only in recent years has the importance of EMS-related research gained the attention of the federal government. The National Institutes of Health are more committed than ever to funding EMS research. EMS systems are placing a greater emphasis on **evidence-based practice** when developing policies and protocols.

- *Legislation and regulation.* To provide a quality, effective system of emergency medical care, each state must have legislation and regulations that identify and support a lead EMS agency. This agency has the authority to plan and implement an effective EMS system. It can also create appropriate rules and regulations for each recognized component of the EMS system.

- *System finance.* Emergency medical services systems must be financially stable to provide services for the community and continue to improve those services. EMS systems must develop new and creative relationships with health care insurance companies and other health care providers to become more financially efficient and sustainable.

- *Human resources.* The ability to provide high-quality EMS care depends heavily on the availability of qualified, competent, and compassionate personnel. To attract and retain these personnel, EMS must strive to develop a strong career ladder like other health care professions.

- *Medical direction.* Each state must ensure that physicians are involved in all aspects of the EMS system. The role of the state EMS **medical director** must be clearly defined. It should have legislative authority and responsibility for EMS system standards, protocols, and evaluation of patient care. **Medical oversight** for all EMS providers must be used to evaluate medical care as it relates to patient outcomes, training programs, and medical direction.

- *Education systems.* Quality training and education of the EMS workforce is the foundation of excellent patient care. The future of EMS education must maximize the use of technology. Technology will allow those in rural areas more convenient access to quality EMS education resources.

- *Public education.* EMS can play an important role in educating members of the community on topics such as system function, access, bystander care, and prevention.

- *Prevention.* In addition to education about injury prevention, EMS systems can collect data to identify trends related to illness and injury rates in a community. Education programs and other systems can then be developed to target those prevention needs.

- *Public access.* The 911 number has been in service since 1968 and today serves approximately 96 percent of the population of the United States.[3] Barriers to accessing prompt EMS care still exist for many communities in the United States. EMS systems must continue to expand the reach of the 911 system in the communities they serve.

- *Communication systems.* As you are well aware, effective and efficient communication is an essential component of any high-performing system or process. As more and more agencies and institutions become integrated in an overall health care delivery model, the need for efficient communications becomes more important. All components of the health care system must be able to communicate and share information to ensure the best patient care possible.

evidence-based practice ▶ integrating clinical expertise with the best available clinical evidence from systematic research.

medical director ▶ physician who assumes the ultimate responsibility for medical oversight of the patient care aspects of the EMS system.

medical oversight ▶ supervision related to patient care provided for an EMS system or one of its components by a licensed physician.

- *Clinical care.* The care provided by EMS professionals has evolved significantly over the past 40 years and must continue to do so. The care the EMS professionals provide must continue to be driven by evidence and maximize the use of technology and advances in science.
- *Information systems.* The federal government has mandated that EMS systems collect data on many aspects of their performance within the communities they serve. The ability to collect, link, and analyze this data will allow EMS systems to respond more appropriately to the needs of the community.
- *Evaluation.* Each state EMS system is responsible for evaluating the effectiveness of its services. A uniform, statewide data-collection system must exist to capture the minimum data necessary to measure compliance with standards. It also must ensure that all EMS providers consistently and routinely provide data to the lead agency. The lead agency performs routine analysis of that data. Your participation in the evaluation process will help drive the improvement of the EMS system and the care that patients receive.

In January 2019, NHTSA published its updated vision for the future in a document titled EMS Agenda 2050: A People-Centered Vision for the Future of Emergency Medical Services. This document is the culmination of a collaborative and inclusive two-year effort to create a bold plan for the next several decades. Building on the foundation established by the 1996 EMS Agenda for the Future, EMS Agenda 2050 lays out a vision for EMS systems that serve the needs of patients, families, clinicians, and communities. To achieve that goal, EMS Agenda 2050 describes six guiding principles (Figure 1.2) that need to be at the heart of efforts to implement the vision. EMS systems must be: inherently safe and effective, integrated and seamless, reliable and prepared, socially equitable, sustainable and efficient, and adaptable and innovative.

The events that occurred on September 11, 2001, as well as the many subsequent terrorist attacks and natural disasters that have occurred in recent years, have increased public awareness of our EMS systems. These events have also brought to the public's attention rescue personnel called *first responders* who are trained medical care providers.

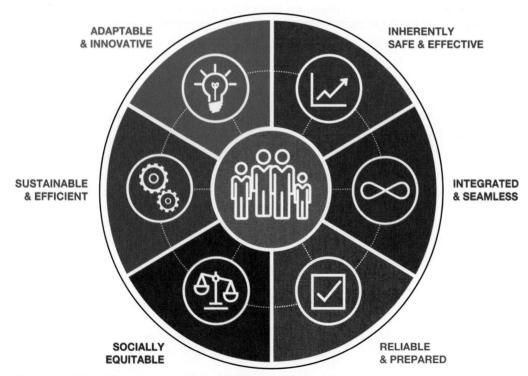

Figure 1.2 Six guiding principles of the EMS Agenda 2050.
(www.ems.gov/projects/ems-agenda-2050.html)

Emergency Medical Responder (EMR). This level of EMS training is designed specifically for the individual who is often first to arrive at the scene. Many police officers, firefighters, industrial workers, and other public service providers are trained as Emergency Medical Responders. This training emphasizes scene safety and how to provide immediate care for life-threatening injuries and illnesses as well as how to assist ambulance personnel when they arrive.

Emergency Medical Technician (EMT). In most areas of the United States, an EMT is considered the minimum level of education and certification for ambulance personnel. The training emphasizes assessment, care, and transportation of the ill or injured patient. The EMT may also assist with the administration of certain common medications. (This was previously called the *EMT-Basic* level of training.)

Advanced Emergency Medical Technician (AEMT). An Advanced EMT is a basic-level EMT who has completed additional education and training in specific areas, allowing a minimal level of advanced life support. Some of the additional skills an Advanced EMT may be able to perform are starting intravenous (IV) lines, inserting certain advanced airways, and administering certain medications. (This was previously called the *EMT-Intermediate* level of training.)

Paramedic. Paramedics are trained to perform what is commonly referred to as advanced life support care, such as inserting advanced airways and starting IV lines. They also administer a large list of medications, interpret electrocardiograms, monitor cardiac rhythms, and perform cardiac defibrillation. (This was previously called the *EMT-Paramedic* level of training.)

Figure 1.3 Levels of EMS Education and Training.

Scope of Practice Model ▶ national model that defines the scope of care for the four nationally recognized levels of EMS provider.

National EMS Education Standards ▶ education and training standards developed by the National Highway Traffic Safety Administration (NHTSA) for the four nationally recognized levels of EMS training.

Emergency Medical Responder ▶ member of the EMS system who has been trained to render first-aid care for a patient and to assist higher-level providers at the emergency scene. Abbrev: EMR.

The National Highway Traffic Safety Administration (NHTSA) is the lead-coordinating agency for EMS on a national level and defines all levels of EMS providers. These definitions are included in two documents called the **Scope of Practice Model**[4] and the **National EMS Education Standards**[5]. In support of the definitions established in these two documents, this textbook addresses the level of training known as **Emergency Medical Responder (EMR)**.

Figure 1.3 summarizes the four levels of EMS training and compares the responsibilities of professionals in each of these roles. These descriptions are based on NHTSA's National Scope of Practice Model but may vary slightly from state to state and region to region. Your instructor will explain variations in your area. The framework for this text and all EMS education and training is guided by the National EMS Education Standards. These standards are the culmination of many years of work and will serve as the basis for EMS education at all levels for many years to come.

EMS Models

LO8 | Differentiate the various EMS models in practice across the United States.

Emergency medical services are delivered in a variety of models throughout the United States. These include:

- *Fire-based EMS model.* In this system, much of the EMS service and infrastructure are operated by a local fire department or group of organized fire departments within a city or region.
- *Third-service or public utility model.* In this model, services are typically operated by non-fire-based government entities within cities or counties. The EMS provider agency reports directly to governmental authorities.
- *Hospital-based EMS system.* Typically, this is operated by a large hospital or group of hospitals serving a particular region.
- *Private EMS model.* EMS services are provided by a privately owned company. The private entity often contracts with a municipality to provide services for a specific area.
- *Alliance model.* This is a relatively recent EMS delivery model that typically involves a partnership between a fire service and a private ambulance service.

Many of these models overlap and can operate together within a given EMS system. Regardless of the model, all EMS systems are designed to deliver the best care possible in the most efficient manner possible.

CREW RESOURCE MANAGEMENT

Regardless of the type or model of EMS system, the principles of crew resource management will play a big part in ensuring a safe and efficient response to every patient. We like to say that EMS is a team sport, and every player is important to the outcome of the game.

Scope of Practice

LO9 Explain the roles that state and local EMS offices, medical oversight, and local credentialing play in an EMS system.

LO10 Explain how state and local statutes and regulations affect how an Emergency Medical Responder might function.

The term **scope of practice** identifies the duties and skills an EMS provider is legally allowed to perform. Quite often, the scope of practice is defined by state and/or regional statutes and regulations. Those statutes and regulations will also define any related licensing, credentialing, and certification that may be required. While a scope of practice typically is defined at the state level, local counties and/or EMS agencies may further define the scope of practice based on local needs. Most EMS providers are licensed or certified by a state or local EMS agency to practice in the EMS system.

Activating the EMS System

LO11 Explain the various methods used to access the EMS system.

Once someone at the scene recognizes an emergency, it is necessary to activate the EMS system. Most citizens activate it by way of a 911 phone call to an emergency dispatcher. The dispatcher then sends available responders—Emergency Medical Responders (EMRs), **Emergency Medical Technicians (EMTs)**, **Advanced Emergency Medical Technicians (AEMTs)**, and **Paramedics**—to the scene. Some areas of the country may not have a 911 system. In those areas, the caller may need to dial a 7- or 10-digit number for ambulance, fire, police, or rescue personnel.

Most 911 calls are automatically directed to a designated **public safety answering point (PSAP)**. Most primary PSAPs are operated by city or county agencies. Many 911 dispatch centers are staffed with **Emergency Medical Dispatchers (EMDs)**, who receive specialized training. In addition to taking the call and dispatching appropriate resources, EMDs provide prearrival care instructions to callers, thereby helping to initiate lifesaving care before EMS personnel arrive.

Once the EMS system is activated, personnel and vehicles are dispatched. EMS personnel will provide care at the scene and during transport. They also deliver the patient to the most appropriate medical facility.

The most desirable 911 activation service is referred to as an *enhanced 911* (E911) system. An enhanced 911 system enables the call to be selectively routed to the most appropriate dispatch center (PSAP) for the caller's location. In addition, the E911 system enables the communications center to automatically receive caller information, such as phone number and address, making it easier to confirm location and reconnect should the call be dropped.

As of June 2017, it is estimated that nearly 51 percent of all U.S. households currently rely on cellular service as their primary telephone service.[6] The widespread use of cellular phones has had a huge impact on how people access the 911 system. Recent developments in technology and wireless communications have required that 911 systems be enhanced to accommodate cellular access. The Federal Communications Commission (FCC) has developed a two-phase plan for how E911 systems must accommodate cell phone users:

- Phase I requires that wireless carriers deliver the phone number of the cellular caller and the location of the cell site/sector receiving the 911 call to the appropriate PSAP.
- Phase II requires that wireless providers deliver the latitude and longitude of the caller.

scope of practice ► care that an Emergency Medical Responder, an Emergency Medical Technician, or Paramedic is allowed to provide according to local, state, or regional regulations or statutes. Also called *scope of care*.

Emergency Medical Technician ► member of the EMS system whose training emphasizes assessment, care, and transportation of the ill or injured patient. Depending on the level of training, emergency care may include starting IV (intravenous) lines, inserting certain advanced airways, and administering some medications. Abbrev: EMT.

Advanced Emergency Medical Technician ► member of the EMS system whose training includes basic-level EMT training plus responsibility for a minimal level of advanced life support. Additional skills include starting IV (intravenous) lines, inserting certain advanced airways, and administering certain medications. Abbrev: AEMT.

Paramedic ► member of the EMS system whose training includes advanced life support care, such as inserting advanced airways and starting IV lines. Paramedics also administer medications, interpret electrocardiograms, monitor cardiac rhythms, and perform cardiac defibrillation.

public safety answering point ► designated 911 emergency dispatch center. Abbrev: PSAP.

Emergency Medical Dispatcher ► specially trained member of the EMS system dispatch team capable of providing prearrival instructions to callers, thereby helping to initiate lifesaving care before EMS personnel arrive. Abbrev: EMD.

In-Hospital Care System

Most patients assisted by EMS personnel are taken to a hospital emergency department. Hospital staff stabilize all immediate life threats and provide the appropriate care before the patient is discharged. If necessary, the patient may be transferred to the most appropriate in-hospital resources, such as the medical/surgical or intensive care units, or the patient may be transferred to a more specialized hospital for more advanced care.

Some hospitals handle all routine and emergency cases and have a medical specialty that sets them apart from other hospitals. One type of **specialty hospital** is a trauma center. A trauma center is where specific trauma services and surgery teams are available 24 hours a day. Some hospitals specialize in the care of certain conditions, such as burns (Burn Center), cardiac problems (Cardiac [STEMI] Receiving Hospital), or strokes (Stroke Receiving Hospital). Other hospitals may specialize in a particular type of patient, such as pediatric and neonatal patients.

specialty hospital ▶ hospital that is capable of providing specialized services, such as trauma care, pediatric care, cardiac care, stroke care, or burn care.

FIRST ON SCENE

By the time you return to the scene, you can tell that the young boy has stopped shaking. Within seconds, two women arrive and introduce themselves as Christine and Jessica, members of the company's Medical Emergency Response Team. They have equipment with them and seem to know what they are doing. Christine kneels beside the patient and appears to be listening for something. Jessica takes the woman aside and asks questions about the boy.

Medical Direction

LO12 Explain the various types of medical direction and how the Emergency Medical Responder might interact with each.

Each EMS system has a medical director. The medical director is a licensed physician who assumes the ultimate responsibility for direction and oversight of all patient care delivered by EMS personnel. The medical director also oversees training and assists in the development of treatment **protocols**. Protocols are clearly defined guidelines that describe how to manage the most common types of conditions, such as chest pain, cardiac arrest, difficulty breathing, and severe allergic reactions. Some protocols contain **standing orders**. Standing orders give the EMS provider permission to administer specific interventions, such as oxygen and medications. Protocols and standing orders are a type of medical direction known as **off-line medical direction**.

protocols ▶ written guidelines that direct the care EMS personnel provide for patients.

standing orders ▶ component of a protocol that allows EMS personnel to provide specific interventions to a patient.

off-line medical direction ▶ EMS system's written standing orders and protocols, which authorize personnel to perform particular skills in certain situations without actually speaking to the medical director or their designated agent.

on-line medical direction ▶ orders to perform a skill or administer care from the on-duty physician given to the rescuer in person by radio or by phone.

While quite rare for the Emergency Medical Responder, procedures not covered by protocols or standing orders require EMS personnel to contact medical direction by radio or telephone prior to performing a particular skill or intervention. Orders from medical direction given in this manner—by radio or phone—are known as **on-line medical direction**. The primary role of medical direction is to ensure that the quality of care is standardized and consistent throughout the local EMS system.

As an Emergency Medical Responder at the scene of an emergency, you may have limited access to the medical director. It will be necessary for you to adhere to the training you've completed and, in some cases, to follow the orders of on-scene EMS providers with a higher level of training or certification.

Like all EMS personnel, you must only provide the care that is within your scope of practice, defined as the care an Emergency Medical Responder is allowed and expected to provide according to local, state, or regional regulations or statutes. The scope of practice is outlined in protocols and guidelines approved by your medical director. The scope of practice may vary from state to state and region to region. Your instructor will inform you of any local protocols and policies that may define your scope of practice. Always follow your local protocols.

The Emergency Medical Responder

The lack of people with enough training to provide care before more highly skilled EMS providers arrive at a scene is the weakest link in the chain of any EMS system. Training Emergency Medical Responders will help overcome this challenge.

Emergency Medical Responders are trained to reach patients, find out what is wrong, and provide emergency care at the scene. They are also trained to move patients when necessary and without causing further injury (Key Skill 1.2). They are usually the first medically trained personnel to reach the patient. Many police officers and firefighters are trained to this level. In addition, many private and public organizations have trained employees as Emergency Medical Responders. The more individuals trained as Emergency Medical Responders, the stronger the EMS system becomes.

FIRST ON SCENE

Within minutes, the sirens of responding emergency vehicles can be heard. At this point, five members of the Medical Emergency Response Team are caring for the young boy. The team of responders places the boy on his side, clears out his mouth with a suction device, and gives him oxygen. That must be what he needed because after they clear his mouth, he wakes up and begins to cough.

Roles and Responsibilities

Emergency Medical Responders carry out a wide range of roles and responsibilities. These vary depending on your level of training, agency, and local/regional protocols.

CREW RESOURCE MANAGEMENT

One principle of CRM is that rank has no place when it comes to safety. Regardless of your rank or experience on the team, you must be willing and able to point out safety issues that could affect the patient or the team. You must be able to do so without fear of being reprimanded by others on the team.

Personal Safety Your primary concern as an Emergency Medical Responder at an emergency scene is your own personal safety. The desire to help those in need of care may tempt you to ignore hazards at the scene. You must make certain that you can safely reach the patient and that you will remain safe while providing care.

Part of this concern for personal safety must include the proper protection from infectious diseases. All Emergency Medical Responders who assess or provide care for patients *must* take steps to avoid direct contact with blood, saliva, and other bodily fluids. Personal protective equipment (PPE) that minimizes contact with infectious material includes the following:

- Disposable gloves
- Barrier devices, such as face masks with one-way valves
- Protective eyewear such as goggles or face shields
- Specialized face masks (HEPA, N95, N100) with filters that minimize contact with airborne microorganisms
- Gowns or aprons that minimize contact of splashed blood and other bodily fluids

SCENE SAFETY

Each year, many people are injured and even killed when they rush into an unsafe scene to help an injured victim. Take the time to stop and observe the scene before rushing in. Do your best to identify any obvious hazards that could endanger you or others arriving at the scene.

Understand the Roles of Emergency Medical Responders

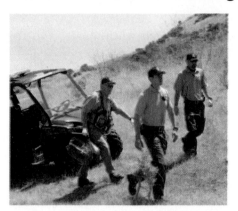

1. Emergency Medical Responders working as part of a search-and-rescue team.

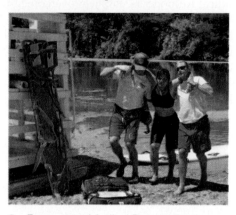

2. Emergency Medical Responders serving as lifeguards at a recreational area.

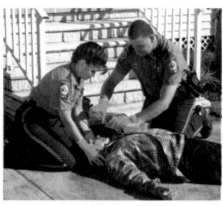

3. Many members of law enforcement receive Emergency Medical Responder training.

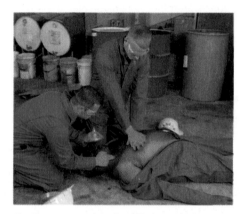

4. Emergency Medical Responders serve on industrial Medical Emergency Response Teams.

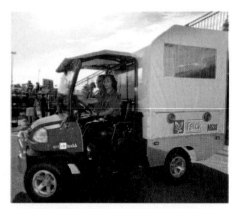

5. Emergency Medical Responders often work in support of large events, such as NASCAR races.

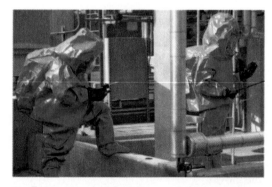

6. Emergency Medical Responders serve on specialized response teams, such as hazmat and rescue teams.

For most patient care situations, you will need only protective gloves and eye protection. However, all the items listed on page 11 should be on hand so you can protect yourself and provide care safely. We will talk more about infectious diseases and personal protection in Chapter 3.

Keep in mind that Emergency Medical Responders who are in law enforcement, the fire service, or private industry may be required to carry out their specific job tasks before they provide patient care (such as controlling traffic, stabilizing vehicles, or shutting down machinery). If this applies to you, always follow department or company standard operating procedures.

Patient-Related Duties   Prior to receiving care, the ill or injured individual may be referred to as a *victim* of an event such as a stroke or vehicle accident. Once you start to carry out your duties as an Emergency Medical Responder, the victim becomes your *patient*. Your presence at the scene means that the EMS system has begun its first phase of care (Key Skill 1.3). The patient may need the skills of a physician and care team at the hospital to survive, but their chances of reaching the hospital alive are greatly improved

---

KEY SKILL 1.3

Patient-Related Duties

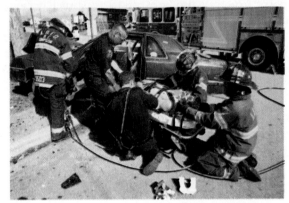

1. One of the duties of an Emergency Medical Responder is to safely gain access to the patient.

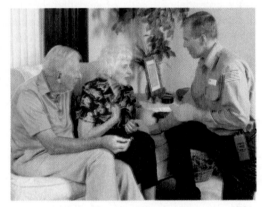

2. Emergency Medical Responders must act quickly to find out what is wrong with the patient.

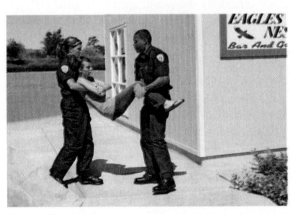

3. Emergency Medical Responders must learn to safely lift and move patients when necessary.

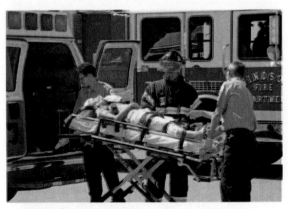

4. The Emergency Medical Responder will often assist EMTs and other transport personnel at the scene of an emergency.

when proper care is provided at the scene. Emergency Medical Responders have six main patient-related duties to carry out at the scene:

- *Size up the scene.* Scene safety is your first concern, even before patient care. Before rendering care, evaluate how to protect yourself, those helping you, bystanders, and the patient. You must also try to determine what caused the patient's illness or injury, the number of patients, and what kind of assistance you will need. You must remain alert for changing conditions at the scene to protect yourself and the patients and to minimize additional injuries.

- *Determine the patient's* **chief complaint.** Gather information from the patient, from the scene, and from bystanders. Using the supplies you have, provide emergency care to the level of your training. Remember, emergency care deals with both illness and injury. It can be as simple as providing emotional support to someone who is frightened because of a crash or mishap. Or it can be more complex, requiring you to deal with life-threatening emergencies, such as providing basic life-support measures for an individual experiencing a heart attack. In later chapters, you will learn how to provide a combination of emotional support and physical care to help the patient until more highly trained personnel arrive.

- *Lift, move, or reposition the patient when necessary.* You need to judge when safety or care requires you to move or reposition the patient. When you must move a patient, use techniques that minimize the chance of injuring yourself or the patient.

- *Transfer the patient and patient information.* Provide for an orderly transfer of the patient and all patient-related information to more highly trained personnel. This is often called the "patient handoff." You may also be asked to assist such personnel and work under their direction.

- *Protect the patient's privacy and maintain confidentiality.* You have a responsibility both morally and legally to protect the privacy of your patient. You may not share any information relating to the patient or the situation unless it is with other EMS professionals who are taking over care of the patient.

- *Be the patient's advocate.* You must be willing to be an advocate for the patient and do what is best for them as long as it is safe to do so.

chief complaint ▶ primary problem that causes a patient to seek or need medical care.

> **REMEMBER**
>
> In addition to proper hand washing/sanitizing and the use of PPE to prevent being exposed to infectious agents, an often overlooked precaution is to be vaccinated against the more common agents you may encounter. Blood has the potential of exposing you to hepatitis B and C, while an individual with a fever or cough may expose you to COVID-19, pneumonia, influenza (flu), or meningitis. The influenza vaccine is released yearly based on assumptions of what type of flu will be most prevalent, and many EMS systems require field personnel to get an annual vaccine. Being vaccinated provides you with one more layer of protection against disease.

Traits

LO13 Describe the characteristics of professionalism as they relate to the Emergency Medical Responder.

To be an Emergency Medical Responder, you must be willing to take on certain duties and responsibilities. It takes hard work and study to be an Emergency Medical Responder. Since you must keep your emergency care skills sharp and current (Figure 1.4), you may also be required to obtain continuing education and to recertify or relicense periodically.

It is quite common today for a state or local EMS authority to require criminal background checks for anyone seeking certification or licensing to practice. Those processes are designed to protect the patient and ensure the quality of patient care delivered within an EMS system.

You must also be willing to deal with difficult situations and people. Individuals who are ill or injured are not at their best. You must be able to overlook rude behavior and unreasonable demands, realizing that patients may act this way because of fear, uncertainty, or pain. Dealing with patient reactions is often the hardest part of the job. You have a responsibility to remain professional and compassionate even when it is difficult to do so.

All patients have the same right to the very best of care. Your respect for others and acceptance of their rights are essential parts of the total patient care that you provide as an

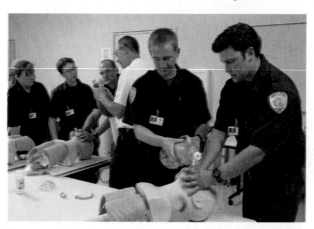

Figure 1.4 Frequent training promotes a high standard of care for your patients.

Emergency Medical Responder. You must not modify the care you provide or discriminate based on your view of another individual's religious beliefs, cultural expression, age, gender, sexual orientation, social behavior, socioeconomic background, or geographic origin. Every patient is unique and deserves to have their needs met by a consistent standard of care.

To be an Emergency Medical Responder, you must be honest and realistic. When assisting patients, you cannot tell them they are okay if they are truly sick or hurt. You cannot tell them that everything is all right when they know that something is wrong. Telling someone not to worry is not realistic. When an emergency occurs, there is truly something to worry about. Your conversations with patients can help them relax, if you are honest. By telling patients that you are trained in emergency care and that you will help them, you ease their fears and gain their confidence. Letting patients know that additional aid is on the way also will help them relax.

As an Emergency Medical Responder, you may have limits on what you can say to a patient or their loved ones. Telling a patient that a loved one is dead may not be appropriate if you are still providing care for the patient. In such circumstances, it is necessary for you to be tactful. You also don't want to provide false hope by telling a family member that a loved one is fine when they are not. Remember, people under the stress of illness or injury often do not tolerate additional stress well.

Being an Emergency Medical Responder also requires that you control your feelings at the emergency scene. You must learn how to care for patients while controlling your emotional reactions to their illness or injuries. Patients do not need sympathy and tears. They need your professional care, compassion, and empathy.

As an Emergency Medical Responder, you are required to be a highly disciplined professional. You must not make inappropriate comments about patients or the horror of the incident. You must maintain your focus on the patient and avoid unnecessary distractions.

Providing appropriate care requires you to admit that the stress of responding to emergency scenes will affect you. You may have to speak with a respected peer, counselor, other EMS professionals, or a specialist within the EMS system to resolve the stress and emotional challenges caused by responding to emergencies.

No one can demand that you change your lifestyle to be an Emergency Medical Responder. However, first impressions are very important and your appearance alone can earn a patient's confidence. So, keep your uniform neat and clean at all times. How you approach the patient and the respect you show are very important. Refer to the patient in a manner that is appropriate for their age. All adults should be referred to as "Sir" or "Ma'am" until you clarify their name and ask them what they would like to be called. Children respond well to their first names and working with them from a kneeling position rather than standing over them. How you address a patient can greatly affect their willingness to share information and their ability to feel comfortable in your care.

Skills

In addition to learning the knowledge that is the foundation of emergency care, you will be required to perform certain skills as part of your training. Those skills vary from course to course. The list below is an example of the skills learned by the typical Emergency Medical Responder. Read the list and check off each skill as you learn it in your course.

As an Emergency Medical Responder, you will learn how to:

- Assess for and manage potential hazards at the scene
- Gain access to patients in vehicles, buildings, and outdoor settings
- Evaluate the possible cause of an illness or injury
- Properly use all items of personal safety
- Evaluate and manage a patient's airway and breathing status
- Conduct an appropriate patient assessment
- Obtain and record accurate vital signs

- Properly document assessment findings
- Relate signs and symptoms to illnesses and injuries
- Perform cardiopulmonary resuscitation (CPR) for adults, children, and infants
- Operate an automated external defibrillator (AED)
- Control all types of bleeding
- Assess and manage a patient who is showing signs of shock
- Perform basic dressing and bandaging techniques
- Assess and care for injuries to bones and joints
- Assess and care for possible head and face injuries
- Assess and care for possible injuries to the neck and spine
- Assess and care for possible heart attacks, strokes, seizures, and diabetic emergencies
- Identify and care for poisonings
- Assess and care for burns
- Assess and care for heat- and cold-related emergencies
- Assist a woman in delivering her baby
- Provide initial care for the newborn
- Identify and care for patients who are experiencing drug- or alcohol-related emergencies
- Perform standard and emergent patient moves when required
- Perform triage at a multiple-patient emergency scene
- Work under the direction of an Incident Commander in an incident command system (ICS) or incident management system (IMS) operation
- Work under the direction of more highly trained personnel to help them provide patient care, doing what you have been trained to do at your level of care

In some systems, Emergency Medical Responders may be required to perform some or all of the following:

- Administer oxygen
- Apply specialized splints
- Apply cervical collars
- Assist with the application of specialized extrication devices
- Assist in securing a patient to a long spine board (backboard) or another device used to immobilize a patient's spine

Equipment, Tools, and Supplies

Most Emergency Medical Responders carry very few pieces of equipment, tools, and supplies. Some may carry specialized kits for trauma emergencies, medical emergencies, and childbirth. If you are assigned to a special event, such as a concert, sporting event, or carnival, you may want to include items that will meet the needs of that event in addition to the standard dressings and bandages. For instance, if you were providing medical support for a football game, it would be appropriate to have cervical collars and a backboard handy, given the likelihood of head, neck, and spine injuries.

Continuous Quality Improvement

LO14 Explain the role of the Emergency Medical Responder with regard to continuous quality improvement (CQI).

One of the goals of the evaluation component of an EMS system is **continuous quality improvement (CQI)**. CQI is exactly what the name implies—a continuous improvement in the quality of the product or service being delivered. In the case of EMS, that product is patient care. As a trained Emergency Medical Responder working within an EMS system, you will be accountable for and expected to participate in the CQI process.

A properly designed CQI program is based on the philosophy that every component within a system can be improved. It is a process that expects and allows everyone in the

continuous quality improvement ▶ continuous improvement in the quality of the product or service being delivered. Abbrev: CQI.

system to participate and contribute to its improvement. It should focus more on the systems and processes and less on the people within the system.

As an Emergency Medical Responder, you will be an important component of the CQI system and will be expected to submit accurate and complete patient care reports that will be audited by trained individuals. Those audits are meant to reveal many characteristics of the care being provided including, but not limited to, types of illnesses and injuries, ages of patients, geographic location of calls, and many other factors.

You may be asked to participate in training or serve on a quality committee as part of the CQI process. Whatever your role or level of participation, everyone in the system plays an important part in the CQI process.

The Role of the Public Health System

LO15 Explain the role of public health systems and their relationship to EMS, disease surveillance, and injury prevention.

Each county, region, and state has people and resources that serve as part of the **public health system**. Those resources are dedicated to promoting optimal health and quality of life for the communities they serve. Public health systems monitor the health of the population they serve, provide health care to certain population groups, and educate members of the community about disease and injury prevention. They also work to advance population-based health programs and policies.

public health system ▶ local resources dedicated to promoting optimal health and quality of life for the people and communities they serve.

Disaster Assistance

LO16 Explain the role that Disaster Medical Assistance Teams (DMATs) play and how they integrate with EMS systems.

Each state has identified specific individuals already working in its EMS systems to participate as members of specialized teams that provide medical care following a natural or human-caused disaster. This type of team is called a **Disaster Medical Assistance Team (DMAT)**. The individuals who make up DMATs are highly experienced, trained EMS personnel. They can be deployed on a moment's notice should a disaster strike anywhere in the United States. For example, DMATs from across the nation descended on Northern California during the wildfires that devastated much of California in 2017, 2018, 2019, and 2021. DMATs arrive in an area during and after a disaster and are quickly integrated into the local EMS resources.

Disaster Medical Assistance Team ▶ specialized team that provides medical care following a disaster. Abbrev: DMAT.

research ▶ systematic investigation to establish facts.

The Role of Research in EMS

LO17 Explain the role that research plays in the EMS system and the ways that an Emergency Medical Responder might seek out and support research.

Research is the systematic investigation to establish facts (Figure 1.5). Each year, new research is being conducted and old research is being challenged. Several organizations around the globe have spent years gathering and verifying research that is defining how EMS providers practice emergency care. Every few years, the American Heart Association and the International Liaison Committee on Resuscitation (ILCOR) release new guidelines that define how EMS providers should perform resuscitation and emergency care.[7] The military is constantly conducting research that is influencing how EMS providers care for those who are ill or injured in the civilian world.

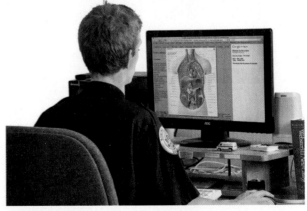

Figure 1.5 Staying current with the latest research is an important aspect of being a good Emergency Medical Responder.

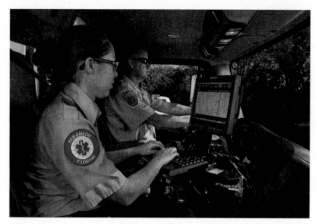

Figure 1.6 A typical device with GPS capability installed in an emergency vehicle.

This book includes many of the changes in emergency care that are being recommended as a result of this new research. Be sure to play an active role in searching for, reading, and evaluating research that affects your job as an Emergency Medical Responder.

Advances in Technology

In recent years, several advances in technology have made the job of the EMS team more effective and efficient. One of the most important advances is the introduction of the global positioning system (GPS) to the civilian marketplace (Figure 1.6). GPS is a standard tool in all types of public safety vehicles, such as police cars, fire engines, and ambulances. The use of GPS technology allows emergency personnel to more easily navigate to the location of the emergency, thus reducing response time. It also gives dispatch personnel the ability to track the location of emergency vehicles and to use resources more efficiently.

FIRST ON SCENE WRAP-UP

It looks like the cavalry is arriving; there are so many vehicles with lights and sirens. First, two fire trucks pull up. Then, an ambulance shows up and behind that is an SUV-type vehicle, painted just like the ambulance. Before you know it, nearly a dozen people are hovering over the young boy.

You stick around to observe the excitement and even forget for a minute why you are actually there. You hear Christine give a report to the ambulance team about the boy. She says she thinks he might have had a seizure.

Wow, what an exciting day! You can't stop thinking about the boy and how he must have felt when he awoke to see so many people hovering over him. The woman with the boy turns out to be his mother. She takes the time to thank you for making the call to 911 so quickly.

Summary

The emergency medical services (EMS) system is a chain of resources established to provide care to the patient at the scene of an emergency and during transport to the hospital emergency department. Review these key concepts related to working within an EMS system:

- There are four levels of nationally recognized EMS education and training: Emergency Medical Responder (EMR), Emergency Medical Technician (EMT), Advanced Emergency Medical Technician (AEMT), and Paramedic.
- EMS personnel are dispatched to the scene of an emergency when a dispatcher receives an emergency call. Dispatchers may be specially trained as Emergency Medical Dispatchers (EMDs) who offer prearrival care instructions to bystanders at the scene.
- Every EMS system is required to designate a medical director—a physician who assumes the ultimate responsibility for medical oversight of the patient care aspects of the EMS system.
- The Emergency Medical Responder's primary responsibility is personal safety. No one should enter or approach an emergency scene until it is safe to do so.

- An Emergency Medical Responder's main duties are scene safety, gaining access to the patient, assessing the patient, providing emergency care, moving patients (when necessary), and transferring care to more highly trained personnel.
- You must be mindful of maintaining the patient's privacy and being sensitive to any cultural differences that may affect the care you provide.
- Patient confidentiality is an important concept; you may not discuss details of the call or any patient information with those not directly involved in care of the patient.
- Being a patient advocate means putting the patient's needs before your own.
- Emergency Medical Responders have a duty to maintain skills, keep up to date with the latest trends and research, and maintain a professional demeanor at all times.
- As an Emergency Medical Responder, you play an important part in the quality of the EMS system and may participate in specific duties related to the CQI process.
- More than ever before, research is defining the way that EMS personnel deliver care to patients. As an Emergency Medical Responder, you have a duty to stay informed about the latest research findings.

Take Action

Know Your System

No two EMS systems are exactly the same. To provide the best care possible, you must know what resources are available within your system. Find someone who is currently working with EMS and ask them the following questions:

- Where are 911 calls answered?
- Does the system use an enhanced 911 system?
- Which of the four levels of EMS providers are recognized by your local EMS system?
- What levels of providers are utilized in your EMS system?
- What types of EMS models exist in your area or region: fire-based, third-service, hospital-based, other types?
- Are there any specialty hospitals in your local or regional system?
- Are there helicopter resources operating in your local system?

If possible, try to arrange a tour of a 911 dispatch center. A good place to begin is by asking your instructor. Most dispatch centers allow people to sit in and observe during certain times. This experience will give you a good appreciation for how the dispatch side of things works.

First on Scene Patient Handoff

Jesus is a 12-year-old boy who appears to have had a generalized seizure based on the report we received from his mother who is with him. According to his mother, his convulsions lasted approximately 90 seconds. Jesus was unresponsive and post-ictal when we arrived on scene about 10 minutes ago. His mother states he has no prior history of seizure activity. Following the seizure activity, we positioned him in the recovery position, suctioned his airway, and placed him on oxygen by non-rebreather mask at 10 pm. He began to become more responsive just before EMS arrived.

First on Scene Run Review

Recall the events of the First on Scene scenario in this chapter and answer the following questions related to the call. Rationales are provided in the Answer Key at the back of the book.

1. Prior to calling 911, what important information should you have obtained from the woman who was with the boy? Why was this information needed?
2. What equipment should the company's Medical Emergency Response Team have with them when responding to a call?
3. When caring for this patient, how would each of the six patient-related duties apply?
4. How would protocols and standing orders apply to this call?

Quick Quiz

To check your understanding of the chapter, answer the following questions. Then compare your answers to those in the Answer Key at the back of the book.

1. Which of the following is NOT an attribute of an integrated EMS system?
   a. EMS Research
   b. Medical direction
   c. Health insurance companies
   d. Education systems

2. The licensed physician who assumes the ultimate responsibility for oversight of all patient care provided by EMS personnel is the:
   a. medical director.
   b. fire chief.
   c. ambulance supervisor.
   d. nursing supervisor.

3. Which of the following best describes the role of the Emergency Medical Responder in an EMS system?
   a. Decontaminates hazardous materials
   b. Cares for immediate life threats and assists EMTs
   c. Serves as an Incident Commander and directs other personnel
   d. Assists Paramedics with advanced skills

4. Emergency Medical Dispatchers receive training that allows them to:
   a. control the scene via the radio.
   b. triage patients via the radio.
   c. declare a mass-casualty incident.
   d. provide pre-arrival care instructions.

5. Which of the following receives the highest level of training in an EMS system?
   a. Emergency Medical Responder
   b. Emergency Medical Technician
   c. Advanced Emergency Medical Technician
   d. Paramedic

6. Clearly defined, written guidelines that describe how to manage the most common types of conditions are called:
   a. dispatches.
   b. protocols.
   c. on-line direction.
   d. prescriptions.

7. Specialized teams of experienced EMS personnel who respond on short notice during disasters are called:
   a. Rapid Response Work Groups.
   b. Disaster Medical Assistance Teams.
   c. Disaster Care Response Teams.
   d. Rapid Response Task Force.

8. Protocols and standing orders are forms of:
   a. off-line medical direction.
   b. on-line medical direction.
   c. pre-arrival instructions.
   d. stand-by guidelines.

9. The care that an Emergency Medical Responder is allowed and supposed to provide according to local, state, or regional regulations or statutes is known as:
   a. scope of practice.
   b. standard of care.
   c. national standard curricula.
   d. Emergency Medical Responder care.

10. Protocols and patient care decisions should be based on:
    a. current EMS research.
    b. which options are cheapest.
    c. the opinion of EMRs.
    d. traditions and historical practice.

Endnotes

1. "9-1-1 Statistics," National Emergency Number Association website, n.d. Accessed December 10, 2017, at https://www.nena.org/?page=911Statistics

2. "Emergency Medical Services: Agenda for the Future," National Highway Traffic Safety Administration website, August 1996. Accessed July 2, 2014, at http://www.ems.gov/pdf/2010/EMSAgendaWeb_7-06-10.pdf

3. "9-1-1 Statistics," National Emergency Number Association Website, n.d. Accessed December 10, 2017, at https://www.nena.org/?page=911Statistics

4. https://www.ems.gov/pdf/National_EMS_Scope_of_Practice_Model_2019.pdf

5. https://www.ems.gov/pdf/EMS_Education_Standards_2021_v22.pdf

6. https://www.npr.org/sections/alltechconsidered/2015/12/03/458225197/the-daredevils-without-landlines-and-why-health-experts-are-tracking-them

7. Nolan, J. P., Maconochie, I., Soar, J., Olasveengen, T. M., Greif, R., Wyckoff, M. H., Singletary, E. M., Aickin, R., Berg, K. M., Mancini, M. E., Bhanji, F., Wyllie, J., Zideman, D., Neumar, R. W., Perkins, G. D., Castrén, M., Morley, P. T., Montgomery, W. H., Nadkarni, V. M., Billi, J. E., Merchant, R. M., de Caen A., Escalante-Kanashiro, R., Kloeck, D., Wang, T.L., Hazinski, M.F. (2020). Executive summary: 2020 international consensus on cardiopulmonary resuscitation and emergency cardiovascular care science with treatment recommendations. *Circulation*, 142(16, Suppl. 1): S2–S27.

2

Legal and Ethical Principles of Emergency Care

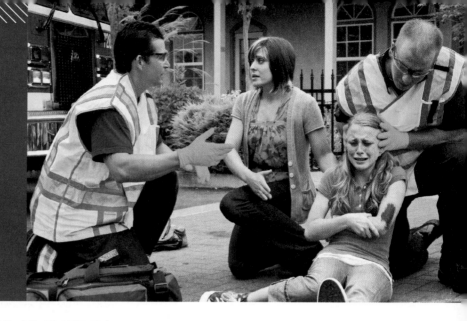

Education Standards

Preparatory—Medical/ Legal and Ethics

Competencies

Uses knowledge of the EMS system and medical, legal, and ethical issues at the scene of an emergency while awaiting a higher level of care.

LEARNING OBJECTIVES

Upon successful completion of this chapter, the student should be able to:

Cognitive

1. Define the chapter key terms.
2. Differentiate between *scope of practice* and *standard of care*.
3. Explain the term *ethics* and how it relates to the Emergency Medical Responder.
4. Differentiate the various types of consent used by the Emergency Medical Responder.
5. Explain the role of the Emergency Medical Responder for patients who refuse care.
6. Differentiate civil (tort) versus criminal litigation.
7. Describe the common elements of an advance directive.
8. Explain the role of the Emergency Medical Responder in regard to an advance directive.
9. Explain the concepts of *duty* and *breach of duty* as they relate to the Emergency Medical Responder.
10. Explain *Good Samaritan laws* and how these laws relate to the Emergency Medical Responder.
11. Explain the role of the Emergency Medical Responder in regard to patient confidentiality.
12. Explain the term *mandated reporter* and how it relates to the Emergency Medical Responder.
13. Explain the role of the Emergency Medical Responder in regard to evidence preservation when working in or around an actual or potential crime scene.

Psychomotor

There are no psychomotor objectives for this chapter.

Affective

14. Consistently model ethical behavior in all aspects of Emergency Medical Responder training and job performance.
15. Demonstrate compassion and empathy toward all classmates, coworkers, and actual and simulated patients.
16. Participate willingly as a team member in all class/training activities.
17. Value the importance of maintaining patient confidentiality.
18. Demonstrate a desire to always do what is right for the patient.

KEY TERMS

abandonment (*p. 32*)
advance directive (*p. 29*)
battery (*p. 28*)
capacity (*p. 26*)
competence (*p. 26*)
confidentiality (*p. 32*)
consent (*p. 26*)
criminal law (*p. 28*)
duty (*p. 24*)
duty to act (*p. 31*)
emancipated minor (*p. 27*)
ethics (*p. 25*)

expressed consent (*p. 26*)
Good Samaritan laws (*p. 24*)
Health Insurance Portability and
   Accountability Act (HIPAA) (*p. 32*)
implied consent (*p. 27*)
informed consent (*p. 26*)
mandated reporter (*p. 33*)
negligence (*p. 30*)
standard of care (*p. 24*)
unresponsive (*p. 27*)
values (*p. 25*)

One of the most common reasons a person would be hesitant to stop and render aid at the scene of an emergency is the fear of being held liable for doing something wrong. The reality is that lawsuits are relatively rare in EMS, and proper training greatly reduces the likelihood of doing something wrong.

As an Emergency Medical Responder, you must make many decisions when responding to an emergency and while caring for patients. For example, should you, as an off-duty Emergency Medical Responder, stop to assist victims of an automobile crash? Should you release information about your patient to an attorney over the telephone? May a child with a suspected broken arm be treated, even if a parent is not present? What should you do if a patient who needs emergency medical care refuses it? Understanding the legal and ethical issues related to your decisions and actions will help you make the best choices possible for the patient.

FIRST ON SCENE

They're moving fast on the open road when Sameer yells, "Hold on!" and she feels his body tense under the leather jacket. The motorcycle leans far to the right and then quickly back to the left, causing the tires to squeal and wobble as the bike comes to a stop. Manpreet looks over Sameer's shoulder and feels her stomach grow cold. Two deep gouges scar the asphalt all the way to the far side of the road where a small sports car is overturned and partially wrapped around a tree. The object they were avoiding on the road behind her suddenly begins to register as a person lying in a heap.

In a matter of seconds, the entire Emergency Medical Responder class that Manpreet took two months ago flashes through her head. She quickly pulls her wind-whipped hair back into a ponytail. "That person in the road needs help right now!"

Legal Duties

Most of us have heard stories about people being sued because of something they did or did not do when they stopped to help someone at the scene of an emergency. In reality, successful lawsuits of this type are extremely rare. Most states have established **Good Samaritan laws** that minimize exposure to liability and encourage passersby, whether medically trained or not, to provide emergency care to those in need.[1] Most of these laws require the individual providing care to be doing so without compensation and to remain within a specified standard of care (as explained in the following section).

Depending on the specific role you play as an Emergency Medical Responder, you may have a legal and/or ethical duty to assist those in need. **Duty** is a legal term that means that one is legally obligated to act in some way, usually to provide assistance. An Emergency Medical Responder who works normal shifts or is on call as a volunteer and is expected to respond to dispatches has a legal duty to respond and provide care to those who are ill or injured. In addition to the duty to respond, you also have a duty (obligation) to provide care as you have been trained and to the expected standard of care in your local area, region, or state.

Standard of Care

LO2 Differentiate between *scope of practice* and *standard of care*.

The term **standard of care** is somewhat subjective and deals with questions such as, "Did you do the right thing, at the right time, and for the right reasons?" It is defined by several factors, such as your level of training, common practice, current research, and sometimes juries in court cases. Standard of care can and does vary from county to county, state to state, and region to region (Figure 2.1). Another way to think of standard of care is to ask, "What would a similarly trained individual do, given the same or similar circumstances?"

A standard of care allows you to be judged based on what is expected of someone with your training and experience working under similar conditions. Your Emergency Medical Responder course follows guidelines developed by the U.S. Department of Transportation and other authorities that have studied what is needed to provide the most appropriate standard of care required at your level in your region. You will be trained to provide this standard of care.

As discussed in the previous chapter, each agency that provides care within an EMS system receives direction and guidance from a physician known as the Medical Director.

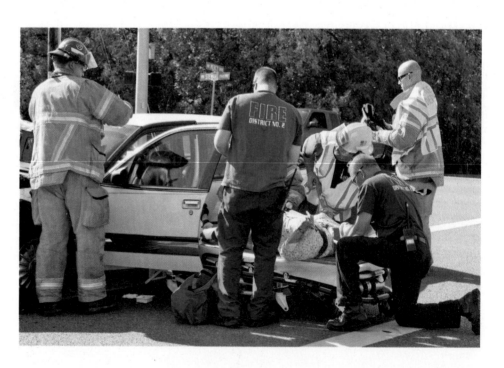

Figure 2.1 Various emergency personnel may be assisting during an emergency, including police, firefighters, and EMTs. Each must practice the standard of care expected of professionals at their level of training.
(TFoxFoto/Shutterstock)

The standard of care your agency provides is largely defined by your Medical Director. While it is relatively uncommon for the EMR to interact directly with medical direction from the field, you will be expected to follow approved protocols developed by your Medical Director for your EMS system.

Most EMS systems require employees rendering care at the scene to complete forms detailing the care provided. These forms are often called field treatment forms or patient care reports (PCR). It is your duty to complete these forms thoroughly and in a timely manner. Your documentation must be able to show that you provided an appropriate standard of care.

Scope of Practice

LO2 Differentiate between *scope of practice* and *standard of care*.

You may recall from Chapter 1 that the term *scope of practice* refers to what is legally permitted to be done by some or all individuals trained or licensed at a particular level, such as an Emergency Medical Responder, Emergency Medical Technician, or Paramedic. The scope of practice, however, does *not* define what must be done for a given patient or in a particular situation. That is more often defined by the standard of care.

The scope of practice for a layperson might be based on nothing more than common sense or an 8-hour first-aid class taken many years ago. However, the scope of practice for Emergency Medical Responders and other EMS personnel is based in part on the U.S. Department of Transportation's education standards for EMS and, in most cases, is more clearly defined by local and state statutes and regulations.

In short, scope of practice is what one is allowed to do by training and/or statute, and standard of care is what one is supposed to do for any given situation based on more local standards and expectations.

Ethical Responsibilities

LO3 Explain the term *ethics* and how it relates to the Emergency Medical Responder.

Ethics can be defined as the moral principles that guide our behavior. However, it is not just any behavior, but behavior that is right, good, and proper. As an Emergency Medical Responder, you have an ethical obligation to behave in a way that puts your patient's needs before your own, so long as it is safe to do so. You have a responsibility to see that your patient receives the most appropriate medical care possible, even when they do not think they need any care.

ethics ▶ moral principles that define behavior as right, good, and proper.

As an Emergency Medical Responder, you will be caring for people of all social, economic, and cultural backgrounds. You must maintain an open mind and develop an understanding of those differences. You have an ethical responsibility to treat all people equally and provide the highest standard of care for your patients.

Another ethical responsibility as a member of the EMS team is to maintain your skills and continue to grow your knowledge related to your duties as an EMR. This includes keeping abreast of current research by reading professional publications and attending conferences when practical. It means practicing your skills to maintain confidence and the required level of competency. You must also attend continuing education and refresher programs to keep yourself ready to perform at all times. Remember, every patient deserves the best care possible.

JEDI

You have an ethical responsibility to treat all people equally and provide the highest standard of care for your patients.

It is also important for you to be honest in reporting the care you provided to a patient, even if a mistake was made. While all EMS providers should provide the appropriate care at all times, mistakes do happen. Errors should be reported immediately so corrective steps, if needed, may be taken as soon as possible.

Your behavior (guided by ethics) is always being influenced by your personal values. **Values** are core beliefs that you hold to be true. Doing the right thing is not always easy and can cause you internal struggles. Many groups and professions have a common set of shared values. Those values serve as a moral compass and help guide an individual's and an organization's decision-making processes. Because EMS personnel must frequently

values ▶ personal beliefs that determine how an individual actually behaves.

make difficult decisions, several EMS groups, agencies, and institutions have adopted the following set of core values for the EMS profession[2]:

- Integrity
- Compassion
- Accountability
- Respect
- Empathy

Consent

LO4 | Differentiate the various types of consent used by the Emergency Medical Responder.

consent ▶ legal term that means to give formal permission for something to happen.

Consent is a legal term that means to give formal permission for something to happen. In the case of the Emergency Medical Responder, you must receive permission from every patient before you can legally provide care. The individual providing consent must have the legal capacity to do so as well as be competent to make rational decisions about their health care.[3] Consent may come in several different forms, depending on the situation.

Capacity

capacity ▶ refers to patients' legal rights and ability to make decisions concerning their medical care.

The term **capacity** refers to patients' legal rights and ability to give consent for their care. In the United States, most individuals under the age of 18 do not have the legal capacity to provide consent for care. In these instances, a parent or legal guardian provides consent for treatment based on a legal concept called "implied consent" (will be discussed further in a later section).

An individual's capacity to legally grant consent for treatment may be affected by factors such as incarceration or mental illness. For instance, an incarcerated prisoner or an individual with a severe mental illness may not have the legal capacity to grant or deny consent because their rights have been taken away or assumed by the state.

Competence

competence ▶ patient's mental ability to comprehend the situation and make rational decisions regarding their medical care.

Competence is defined as the patient's ability to understand what is going on around them, your questions, and the implications of the decisions they are making. For an Emergency Medical Responder to obtain consent or accept a refusal of care, the EMR must establish, to the extent possible, that the patient is competent to make such decisions.

A patient may not be competent to make medical decisions in certain cases, such as intoxication, drug ingestion, serious injury, or mental illness. To determine competency, the Emergency Medical Responder may begin by asking questions that a competent individual should be able to answer, such as where the patient is at the time, what day or month it is, and what has happened to them. If you suspect for any reason that the person you are caring for is not competent, you should seek the opinion of more experienced providers such as members of law enforcement, EMTs, or paramedics.

Expressed and Informed Consent

An adult patient of legal age, when alert and competent, can give you consent to provide care. In an emergency situation, a patient's consent is usually oral (spoken, not written) and commonly referred to as **expressed consent**.

expressed consent ▶ competent adult's decision to accept emergency care.

informed consent ▶ consent granted by a patient after they have been appropriately informed of the care being suggested and associated consequences.

Another type of consent common to medicine is known as **informed consent**. To qualify as informed consent, the patient must be given enough information to make an informed decision regarding the care that is being offered (Figure 2.2). Informed consent is most often used in hospitals prior to procedures such as surgery.

For a patient to make an informed decision, you need to advise them of the following:

- Your level of training
- Why you think care may be necessary
- What care you plan to provide
- Any consequences related to providing that care or the refusal of care

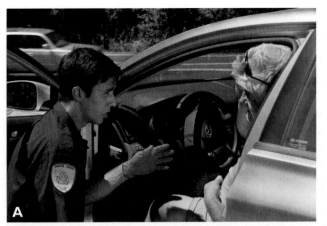
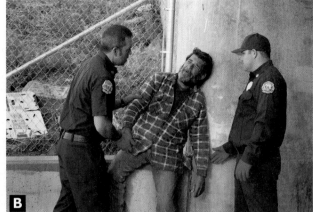

Figure 2.2 (A) Once the scene is safe, you must obtain consent to care for the patient. (B) Always show respect when obtaining consent.

You must receive consent before caring for any patient. A simple way to gain this consent may be by stating something like, "Hi, my name is Kaitlyn. I'm an Emergency Medical Responder. May I help you?" A patient who is responsive may answer verbally, nod, or simply allow you to continue your care. Expressed consent does not need to be verbal. By not pulling away or stopping you and by allowing you to initiate care, the patient is providing expressed consent.

There are occasions when a child refuses care. By law, only a parent or guardian of the child may give consent or refuse care. Of course, gaining the child's confidence and easing any fears should be part of your care.

Implied Consent

In emergency situations in which a patient is **unresponsive**, confused, or so severely ill or injured that expressed consent cannot be given, you may legally provide care based on the concept of **implied consent**. It can be implied that the patient would want to receive care and treatment if they were aware of the situation and able to respond appropriately.

Since children are not legally allowed to grant consent or to refuse medical care, a form of implied consent is used in most states when parents or guardians are not on the scene and cannot be reached quickly. The law assumes that the parents would want care to be provided for their child (Figure 2.3).

The same holds true in cases involving individuals with a developmental disability and/or mental illness. It is assumed that the patient's parents or legal guardians would give consent for treatment if they knew of the emergency situation.

unresponsive ▸ having no reaction to verbal or painful stimuli; also referred to as *unconscious*.

implied consent ▸ legal form of consent that assumes that a patient who lacks the capacity or competency to provide consent would consent to receiving emergency care if they were able. This form of consent may apply in situations where the patient is a minor, is unresponsive, or lacks capacity.

emancipated minor ▸ minor whose parents or guardian(s) have surrendered the right to their care, custody, and earnings and no longer are obligated to support the minor.

Emancipated Minor

Not all individuals under the age of 18 are considered minors in the traditional sense. Some have become legally emancipated and have been released from the control of their parents or legal guardian. **Emancipated minors** are legally allowed to make their own decisions regarding medical care. Minors may become legally emancipated if they are married, pregnant, a parent, a member of the armed forces, or financially independent and living away from their parents or guardian. It is not common for an Emergency Medical Responder to encounter an emancipated minor. Should this situation occur, simply provide care as you would for an adult patient in the same situation. You may not have any real way of verifying if the patient is indeed an emancipated minor, so you may have to take their word for it. If in doubt, allow someone of higher authority to decide.

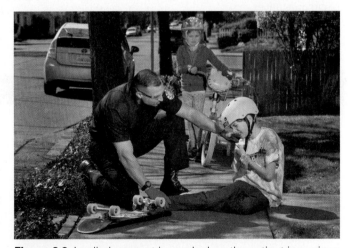

Figure 2.3 Implied consent is used when the patient is a minor.

Refusal of Care

LO5 Explain the role of the Emergency Medical Responder for patients who refuse care.

LO6 Differentiate civil (tort) versus criminal litigation.

Alert and competent adults have the right to refuse care. Their refusal may be based on a variety of reasons, including their economic situation or religious views. They may even base it on a lack of trust. In fact, they may have reasons that you find difficult to understand. You may not force care on competent adults, nor may you restrain them against their wishes. Restraining or threatening to restrain a patient against his or her wishes could result in a violation of **criminal law** and a charge of assault and/or **battery**. Your only course of action is to try to gain a patient's confidence and trust through conversation. If this fails and you feel the patient is at risk, you may have to call in law enforcement.

A patient does not have to speak to refuse your care. If the patient shakes his or her head to signal "no" or if they hold up their hand to signal you to stop, the patient has refused your help. If the patient pulls away from you, that should also be viewed as refusal of care.

It is important to understand the laws that govern patient refusal in your area. In many jurisdictions, an Emergency Medical Responder may not leave a patient who is refusing care until someone with higher training has arrived and taken over care.

How to Handle Refusal of Care   When your care is refused:

- Stay calm and professional and do your best to explain the situation to the patient.
- Inform them of the potential dangers of refusal.
- Do your best to identify and address their reasons for refusal.
- Engage the help of someone the patient trusts to try to convince them to accept care.
- Carefully document the refusal of care.

Documenting a Refusal of Care   Situations that involve a refusal of care can be some of the riskiest from a legal standpoint. There may be an accusation of negligence if the patient becomes worse or dies following your contact, despite a refusal of care. Carefully document your offer of help, your explanation of your level of training, why you think care is needed, the consequences of not accepting care, and the patient's refusal to accept your care. Also document the names of anyone who witnessed your efforts to assist the patient. If your EMS system provides you with release forms, ask the patient to read and sign the form. Make certain that you ask the patient if they understand what they have read before signing the form. Whenever possible, have someone such as the patient's spouse or a member of another agency sign as a witness to the refusal of care.

A parent or legal guardian can refuse to let you care for a child. If the reason is fear or lack of confidence, simple conversation may change the individual's mind. In cases involving children, if the adult takes the child from the scene before EMTs arrive, you must report the incident to the EMTs or to the police. All states have laws protecting the welfare of children. Know the laws in your state and jurisdiction regarding reporting such events. In all cases, know and follow local protocols.

criminal law ▶ body of law dealing with crimes and punishment.

battery ▶ unlawful physical contact.

REMEMBER

When providing care to the ill and injured, you are more likely to be sued for what you DON'T DO rather than for what you DO. For this reason, refusal of care is a source of legal risk for an Emergency Medical Responder. Your medical director and service director should provide guidelines and protocols to follow in these circumstances.

FIRST ON SCENE *(continued)*

Manpreet approaches the person lying in the road and finds him to be unresponsive. With each raspy breath, blood pours from his mouth and collects on the pavement in a shining pool. Unsure of what to do, Manpreet walks over to the overturned car where she finds a woman pinned between the passenger door and the tree. "Hello?" she says. "Are you okay?"

The woman moans softly, but her eyes remain closed.

Sameer is now off the motorcycle and is staring at the man in the road. "My cell phone has no signal," he shouts to Manpreet. "Give your phone a try!" Manpreet replies, "No signal here either!"

Advance Directives

| LO7 | Describe the common elements of an advance directive. |

| LO8 | Explain the role of the Emergency Medical Responder in regard to an advance directive. |

There have been many high-profile medical cases based on the right to die and end-of-life decisions. These decisions are often left up to the surviving family members, who do not always agree on the most appropriate action. Many of these cases take years to resolve. One solution to the dilemma of end-of-life decisions is a legal document called an **advance directive**, which allows a person to define in advance what their wishes are should they become incapacitated due to illness or injury.

advance directive ▶ legal document that allows a patient to define in advance what their wishes are should they become incapacitated due to a medical illness or severe injury.

Advance directives are relatively simple documents that allow an individual to define their wishes and to appoint another individual to make health care decisions on their behalf. They can be created for any individual age 18 and older to provide instructions for future treatment. Keep in mind that advance directives do *not* provide guidance for EMS personnel.

Advance directives commonly address issues such as:

- Designation of an agent or representative (spouse, family member, or friend) to make health care decisions on the patient's behalf
- Choice to prolong or not prolong life
- How pain will be managed as a person's health declines
- Wishes regarding donation of organs after death

Many states have laws governing living wills, a type of advance directive. Living wills are the patient's signed statements of their wishes about the use of long-term life support, ventilators, intravenous feedings, and comfort measures such as pain medications.

Another form of advanced directive is known as Physician's Orders for Life-Sustaining Treatment (POLST). A POLST form is used for a seriously ill patient near the end of their life (regardless of age). It does not replace a general advance directive but can accompany one. The POLST provides specific instructions regarding the immediate care of a patient of any age and should guide the actions of EMS personnel.

At some point, you will encounter a patient who has a do-not-resuscitate (DNR) order, a type of advance directive. It is typically in the form of a written document, usually signed by the patient and their health care provider (Figure 2.4). It often states that, due to specific medical reasons such as a terminal illness, the patient does not wish to prolong life through resuscitative efforts. The DNR is generally a written document that expresses wishes of the patient, but in some cases, the patient will be wearing a piece of medical identification jewelry containing a DNR order.

The presence of a DNR order does not mean "do not provide care." As an Emergency Medical Responder, you have a duty to provide appropriate comfort and care within the bounds of the DNR. It is also within the patient's rights and those of the person holding Power of Attorney (if such a person has been named) to withdraw the DNR order at any time.

REMEMBER

Be sure to understand the laws in your state regarding advance directives and DNR orders so you can provide the patient with the most appropriate and compassionate care. If in doubt as to whether the documents presented to you are valid or pertain to the patient's condition, it is better to err on the side of treating them until those with a higher level of certification arrive.

Negligence

| LO9 | Explain the concepts of *duty* and *breach of duty* as they relate to the Emergency Medical Responder. |

| LO10 | Explain *Good Samaritan laws* and how these laws relate to the Emergency Medical Responder. |

The basis for many civil (tort) lawsuits involving prehospital emergency care is the concept of negligence. Tort law involves a wrongful act, whether intentional or unintentional, that causes an injury. **Negligence** is a term often used to indicate either that a care provider did

PREHOSPITAL DO NOT RESUSCITATE ORDERS

ATTENDING PHYSICIAN

In completing this prehospital DNR form, please check part A if no intervention by prehospital personnel is indicated. Please check Part A and options from Part B if specific interventions by prehospital personnel are indicated. To give a valid prehospital DNR order, this form must be completed by the patient's attending physician and must be provided to prehospital personnel.

A) _____**Do Not Resuscitate (DNR):**
No Cardiopulmonary Resuscitation or Advanced Cardiac Life Support be performed by prehospital personnel

B) _____**Modified Support:**
Prehospital personnel administer the following checked options:
_____Oxygen administration
_____Full airway support: intubation, airways, bag/valve/mask
_____Venipuncture: IV crystalloids and/or blood draw
_____External cardiac pacing
_____Cardiopulmonary resuscitation
_____Cardiac defibrillator
_____Pneumatic anti-shock garment
_____Ventilator
_____ACLS meds
_____Other interventions/medications (physician specify)
_____

Prehospital personnel are informed that (print patient name)_____
should receive no resuscitation (DNR) or should receive Modified Support as indicated. This directive is medically appropriate and is further documented by a physician's order and a progress note on the patient's permanent medical record. Informed consent from the capacitated patient or the incapacitated patient's legitimate surrogate is documented on the patient's permanent medical record. The DNR order is in full force and effect as of the date indicated below.

_____   _____
Attending Physician's Signature

                                          _____

_____   _____
Print Attending Physician's Name   Print Patient's Name and Location
                                          (Home Address or Health Care Facility)

_____
Attending Physician's Telephone

_____   _____
Date   Expiration Date (6 Mos from Signature)

Figure 2.4 A DNR order is an example of one type of advance directive.

negligence ▶ failure to provide the expected standard of care.

not do what was expected or did something carelessly. For a lawsuit alleging negligence to be successful, the following four elements must be established:

- *Duty to act.* The Emergency Medical Responder had a legal duty to provide care.
- *Breach of duty.* Care for the patient was not provided to an acceptable standard of care.
- *Damages.* The patient was injured (damaged) in some way as a result of improper care or lack of care.
- *Causation.* A direct link can be established between the damages to the patient and the breach of duty on the part of the Emergency Medical Responder.

In many cases, Emergency Medical Responders have a legal **duty to act**. Those functioning as part of a fire service, rescue squad, police force, or formal response team may be legally obliged to respond and render care. This means they are required, at least while on duty, to provide care according to their agency's standard operating procedures. In some localities, this duty to act also may apply to Emergency Medical Responders when they are off duty.

duty to act ▶ requirement that Emergency Medical Responders, at least while on duty, must provide care according to a set standard.

The concept of duty to act can be less clear when Emergency Medical Responders work in a business office or industrial environment. When in doubt, it is best to provide care and call for help.

Since the laws governing the duty to act vary from state to state, your instructor can inform you about the specifics in your state or region. In most cases, Emergency Medical Responders are considered to have a duty to act once they begin caring for a patient. If care is offered and accepted by the patient, a legal duty to act has been established, and the Emergency Medical Responder must remain at the scene until someone of equal or higher training takes over.

After a duty to act has been established, the second condition for negligence would be applicable if the care provided was substandard. The same would apply if the care rendered was beyond the scope of the Emergency Medical Responder.

Finally, if there was a duty to act and the standard of care was not met, a suit for negligence may be successful if the patient was injured (damaged) in some way due directly to the inappropriate actions of the Emergency Medical Responder. This is a complex legal concept, made more difficult by the fact that the damage may be physical, emotional, or psychological.

Physical damage is the easiest to understand. For example, if an Emergency Medical Responder moved a patient's injured leg before applying a splint and the standard of care states that the Emergency Medical Responder should have suspected a fracture and placed a splint on the limb, then the responder may be negligent if this action worsened the existing injury.

The same case becomes much more involved when the patient claims that the Emergency Medical Responder's inappropriate action caused emotional or psychological problems. The court could decide that the patient has been damaged and establish the third requirement for negligence.

Inappropriate care does not always involve some type of physical skill. As a general rule, you should always advise a patient to seek treatment by EMTs and to go to the hospital. If you tell an ill or injured patient that they do not need to be seen by more highly trained personnel, you could be negligent if you had a duty to act and the patient accepted your care, but:

- The standard of care stated that you should have alerted or had someone activate the EMS system to request an EMS response, and you failed to do so.
- An avoidable delay in providing care led to additional injury.

As previously noted, a requirement for proof of negligence is the failure of the Emergency Medical Responder to provide care to a recognized and acceptable standard of care. There is no guarantee that you will not be sued, but a successful suit is unlikely if you provide care to an acceptable standard.

If your state has Good Samaritan laws, you may be protected from civil liability if you act in good faith to provide care to the level of your training and to the best of your ability. You will be trained to deliver the standard of care expected of Emergency Medical Responders in your area. Your instructor will explain the laws specific to your locality.

Abandonment

Once you begin to help someone who is sick or injured, you have established a legal duty and must continue to provide care until you transfer patient care to someone of equal or higher training (such as an EMT, paramedic, or physician). If you leave the scene before more highly trained personnel arrive, you may be guilty of abandoning the patient and

REMEMBER

One of the most common places abandonment is likely to occur is at an emergency scene, before EMTs or paramedics arrive. This can occur if the Emergency Medical Responder leaves the patient and the scene before providing an appropriate handoff to EMTs. It is not considered abandonment if you are leaving to call 911 or retrieve an AED and then return to the scene.

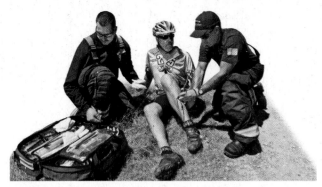

Figure 2.5 Once care is initiated, the Emergency Medical Responder assumes responsibility for the patient until relieved by more highly trained personnel.

may be subject to legal action under specific civil (tort) laws of **abandonment** (Figure 2.5). If the scene becomes unsafe and you must leave the patient to ensure your own safety, it is unlikely that you will be accused of abandonment.

Because you are not trained in medical diagnosis or how to predict the stability of a patient, you should avoid leaving a patient even if someone with training equal to your own arrives at the scene. The patient may develop more serious problems that would be better handled by two Emergency Medical Responders.

Some legal authorities consider abandonment to include the failure to turn over patient information during the transfer of the patient to more highly trained personnel. You must inform those providers of the facts you gathered, the assessment made, and the care rendered.

Confidentiality

LO11 Explain the role of the Emergency Medical Responder in regard to patient confidentiality.

abandonment ▶ to leave a sick or injured patient before equal or more highly trained personnel can assume responsibility for care.

confidentiality ▶ refers to the treatment of information that an individual has disclosed in a relationship of trust and with the expectation that it will not be divulged to others.

Health Insurance Portability and Accountability Act ▶ law that dictates the extent to which protected health information can be shared. Abbrev: HIPAA.

Confidentiality is an important concept for those who care for patients. As an Emergency Medical Responder, you should not speak to your friends, family, or other members of the public (including the press and media) about the details of care you have provided to a patient. You should not name the individuals who received your care. If you speak of the emergency, you should not relate specifics about what a patient may have said, any unusual aspects of behavior, or any descriptions of personal appearance. To do so may violate the confidentiality of the patient. Your state may not have specific laws regarding these issues, but most individuals in emergency care are committed to protecting the patient's right to privacy.

Information about an emergency and patient care should be released only if the patient has authorized you to do so in writing or if you receive an appropriate request from a court or law enforcement agency. In all other cases, refer requests for patient information to your supervisor or other appropriate individual within your agency or institution.

Authorization is not required for you to pass on patient information to other health care providers who are part of the continued care of the patient (Figure 2.6). This sharing of information with those involved in the care of the patient is a necessary and important part of good patient care (Figure 2.7).

The **Health Insurance Portability and Accountability Act (HIPAA)** is a federal law that went into effect in 1996 that dictates the extent to which protected health information may be shared. HIPAA gives patients more control over their health care information and dictates how confidential patient information is stored and shared with others. It also establishes strong accountability for the protection, use, and sharing of patient information, and provides significant fines for violating these regulations.

Figure 2.6 To maintain patient confidentiality, discuss your patient only with those who will be continuing patient care.

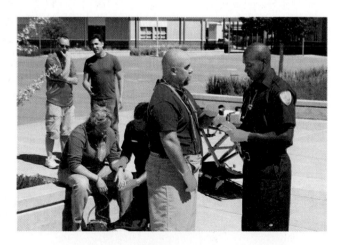

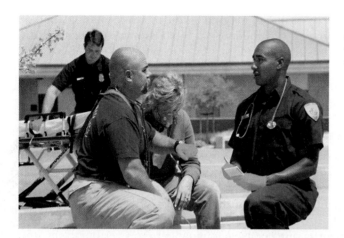

Figure 2.7 You must provide an accurate report to the EMS team who will be taking over care of the patient.

A good rule of thumb regarding the sharing of patient information is, when in doubt, don't. Your instructor will explain in detail what types of information may be shared and in what situations.

Reportable Events

LO12 Explain the term *mandated reporter* and how it relates to the Emergency Medical Responder.

All 50 states have laws that define **mandated reporters** and what types of events they must report.[4] What differs from state to state is who is considered a mandated reporter. For example, all Emergency Medical Responders must report certain events or conditions that they know or suspect have occurred. These events may include things such as exposures to certain infectious diseases, injuries that result from a crime, child and elder physical abuse, domestic violence, and sexual abuse. Check with your instructor, service director, or state and federal agencies to learn which incidents are reportable in your area and to whom or to which agency you should report them.

mandated reporter ▸ any individual required by law to report (or cause a report to be made) whenever financial, physical, sexual, or other types of abuse or neglect have been observed or are suspected.

FIRST ON SCENE (continued)

Manpreet realizes that she can't safely reach the woman pinned in the car and decides to try to help the man in the road. She shakes off her backpack, rummages through it, and pulls out two large beach towels. "Help me roll him onto his side," she says to Sameer. "Slow and careful!"

They are able to get the man onto his side and clear much of the blood from his mouth and nose. "Hey, here comes a car," Sameer says as he holds the man's head still. "Let's ask them to stay here with these people while we go get help."

"I've already started helping them," Manpreet says and grabs one of her beach towels to flag down the oncoming car. "I can't leave now."

The approaching car slows to a stop, and the windows are suddenly filled with curious faces. Manpreet runs to the driver's side. "Listen, these people are seriously hurt. I need you to find a landline or get to a place with a cell signal and call 911!"

Special Situations

You may encounter certain situations in which a patient's wishes or special needs or law enforcement policies will dictate your actions.

Organ Donors

You may respond to a call where a critically injured patient is near death and has been identified as an organ donor. An organ donor is a patient who has completed a legal document that allows for donation of the patient's organs and tissues in the event of their death.

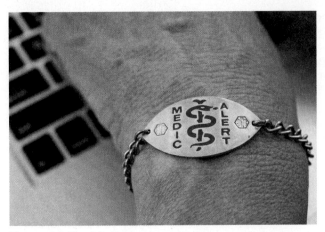

Figure 2.8 The MedicAlert bracelet is one example of a medical identification device.

A family member may give you this information, or you may find an organ donor card in a patient's personal effects. Sometimes organ donor status is indicated on the patient's driver's license. Emergency care of a patient who is an organ donor must not differ in any way from the care of a patient who is not a donor.

Medical Identification Devices

Another special situation involves the patient who wears a medical identification device (Figure 2.8). This device—a card, necklace, or wrist or ankle bracelet—is meant to alert EMS personnel that the patient has a particular medical condition, such as a heart problem, allergies, diabetes, or epilepsy. If the patient is unresponsive or unable to answer questions, this device may provide important medical information.

In some areas of the country, the Vial of Life program is currently in use. This program includes a special vial where important medical information is stored and a window sticker that alerts EMS personnel to the presence of the vial. The vial is kept in the patient's refrigerator, where it can easily be found by rescuers.

Crime Scenes

LO13 Explain the role of the Emergency Medical Responder in regard to evidence preservation when working in or around an actual or potential crime scene.

A crime scene is defined as the location where a crime has been committed or any place where evidence relating to a crime may be found. Many crime scenes involve injuries to people and therefore require the assistance of EMS personnel. If you suspect a crime has been committed, do not enter the scene until it is safe to do so or you are instructed to by law enforcement personnel.

When an Emergency Medical Responder is providing care at a crime scene, certain actions should be taken to preserve evidence. Make as little impact on the scene as possible, moving items only as necessary for patient care. Take special care to note the position of the patient and preserve any clothing you may remove or damage. Try not to cut through holes in clothing from gunshot wounds or stabbings. Remember to report any items you move or touch.

FIRST ON SCENE WRAP-UP

About 15 minutes later, just when Manpreet is beginning to think that the people in the car might have just kept on driving, she hears sirens approaching. *What a comforting sound!* she thinks. Within moments, the scene is filled with firefighters and EMTs in bulky yellow coats and pants, carrying multicolored bags and shouting orders to each other.

The man on the road is quickly loaded into an ambulance, which rushes away with sirens blaring. Manpreet turns and walks over to see what they are doing to help the woman

trapped in the car. The firefighters have peeled most of the car away using large, noisy power tools. Once the woman is finally freed, Manpreet sees that her left leg is nearly severed at about mid-thigh.

With a sigh, Manpreet makes her way past the blood and bent pieces of the small car and finds Sameer standing by the motorcycle. She hugs him and they both watch silently as the second ambulance pulls away and disappears around the bend.

Summary

As an Emergency Medical Responder, you must become well informed regarding the legal and ethical responsibilities that come with your new role. Here is a summary of some of these key principles:

- You may have a legal duty to provide care and must do so within your scope of practice.
- You must understand the difference between your scope of practice and the expected standard of care for your area, region, or state.
- You must maintain a high degree of integrity as well as ethical and moral standards when caring for patients.
- You have a responsibility to keep your knowledge and skills up to date.

- You must obtain consent from every patient you encounter and apply the principles of expressed and implied consent appropriately.
- It is especially important to properly manage and document all patients who refuse care and enlist the assistance of EMS personnel and/or law enforcement when necessary.
- You could be accused of negligence if you do not provide an acceptable level of care or if you abandon your patient.
- You must respect the privacy and confidentiality of all patients and refrain from sharing information about patients unless legally allowed or required to do so.

Take Action

My Wishes

Most states have a standard advance directive form that can be found online. Download this form and study it to become familiar with what it looks like and its contents. Take it one step further and complete the form with your own information. Going through the steps of deciding your own end-of-life choices is a good exercise for all EMS professionals. Share your wishes with family members, and ask them to share theirs as well.

Company/Agency Values

Ethics and values were briefly discussed in this chapter. Consider doing some research to determine if the company or agency you work or volunteer for has a common set of shared values. If so, what are they, and do you feel you can embrace them? Perhaps they have a code of ethics. Read this code of ethics and ask yourself how such a document may have been developed. Compare these values with your own. Do they complement or perhaps conflict with one another? For a fun activity that allows you to identify your own personal core values, go to www.icarevalues.org.

First on Scene Patient Handoff

We have two victims of what appears to have been a vehicle roll over. The first victim is an adult male who appears to have been ejected from his vehicle. The second victim is an adult female who is semi responsive and still trapped in the vehicle. Victim number one was found lying supine in the road, unresponsive, and bleeding from the nose and mouth. We carefully rolled him onto his side to clear his airway and have been monitoring his pulse and breathing. We were unable to reach the woman in the car but we have continued to reassure her that help was on the way, and she has been responsive to verbal stimulus the entire time.

First on Scene Run Review

Recall the events of the First on Scene scenario in this chapter, and answer the following questions related to the call. Rationales are offered in the Answer Key at the back of the book.

1. Why do you think Sameer wanted to leave the scene so quickly?
2. Of the patients described, who is your first priority and why?
3. Should you leave the scene after you start treatment? Why or why not?
4. What information will you want to give the ambulance crew when they arrive on scene?

Quick Quiz

To check your understanding of the chapter, answer the following questions. Then compare your answers to those in the Answer Key at the back of the book.

1. The actions that a similarly trained individual would do, given the same or similar circumstances, are referred to as the:
   a. standard of care.
   b. scope of practice.
   c. duty.
   d. negligence.

2. A document that allows a patient to define in advance what their wishes are should they become incapacitated is called a(n):
   a. power of attorney.
   b. advance directive.
   c. individual protocol.
   d. doctor's directive.

3. Which type of consent is necessary to obtain from responsive, competent adult patients?
   a. Implied
   b. Applied
   c. Absentee
   d. Expressed

4. Which of the following is NOT true about expressed consent?
   a. The patient may withdraw it at any time.
   b. It may be given via nonverbal communication.
   c. It can be given by parents of minors on their behalf.
   d. It requires a signed form to be valid.

5. You are caring for a patient who has overdosed and is unresponsive. You are legally allowed to provide care based on which type of consent?
   a. Implied
   b. Expressed
   c. Assumed
   d. Informed

6. Which of the following patients may legally refuse care at the scene of an emergency?
   a. 11-year-old boy who was hit by a car while riding his bicycle
   b. 26-year-old unresponsive patient who has overdosed
   c. 46-year-old intoxicated driver of a vehicle involved in a collision
   d. 68-year-old alert woman having chest pain

7. Which of the following is NOT an element required for a claim of negligence?
   a. Duty
   b. Abandonment
   c. Damages
   d. Causation

8. Most states require Emergency Medical Responders and other EMS personnel to report incidents involving known or suspected:
   a. seizure activity.
   b. accidental overdose.
   c. abuse or neglect.
   d. pregnancy.

9. When caring for a patient at a crime scene, you should:
   a. allow the patient to shower prior to transport if they wish.
   b. avoid moving objects at the scene when possible.
   c. question the patient about the crime and report information to law enforcement.
   d. refuse to enter without an armed police escort.

10. An Emergency Medical Responder fails to protect patient privacy when he or she:
    a. provides detailed information about the patient to the nurse in the emergency department.
    b. returns to the station and shares the patient's name with colleagues.
    c. shares details of the patient's condition with the EMTs who are taking over care.
    d. provides details about the emergency after being subpoenaed to court.

Endnotes

1. Eboni Morris, "Liability under 'Good Samaritan' Laws," AAOS Now Web site, Vol. 8, No. 1 (January 2014). Accessed July 3, 2014, at https://www.aaos.org/aaosnow/2014/jan/managing/managing3/
2. United States Department of Veterans Affairs Web site. Accessed August 30, 2022, at https://www.va.gov/icare/core-values.asp
3. King, K.C., Martin Lee, L.M., and Goldstein, S. EMS Capacity and Competence. 2021 Sep 28. In: StatPearls [Internet]. Treasure Island (FL): StatPearls Publishing; 2022 Jan–. PMID: 29261953.
4. Child Welfare Information Gateway, "Mandatory Reporters of Child Abuse and Neglect," U.S. Department of Health and Human Services Children's Bureau Web site, 2014. Accessed July 3, 2014, at https://www.childwelfare.gov/topics/systemwide/laws-policies/statutes/manda/

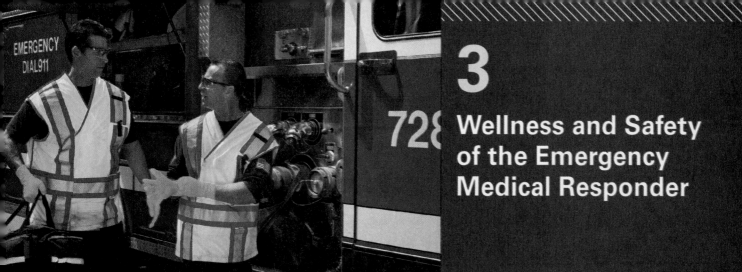

3

Wellness and Safety of the Emergency Medical Responder

LEARNING OBJECTIVES

Upon successful completion of this chapter, the student should be able to:

Cognitive

1 Define the chapter key terms.

2 Explain the importance of a baseline health assessment for new EMS providers.

3 Describe the various immunizations recommended for health care providers.

4 Explain the term *standard precautions* as it relates to the Emergency Medical Responder.

5 Explain what body substance isolation (BSI) precautions are and when they should be used.

6 Identify the four routes by which pathogens enter the body.

7 List examples of personal protective equipment (PPE) and the purpose of each.

8 Differentiate between cleaning and disinfection, and state when each should be performed.

9 Explain the procedure the Emergency Medical Responder should follow after a possible pathogen exposure.

10 Describe common hazards at the scene of an emergency.

11 Explain the steps the Emergency Medical Responder should take to mitigate common scene hazards.

12 Explain the terms *stress* and *stressor* as they relate to the Emergency Medical Responder.

13 Describe several sources of stress commonly encountered by the Emergency Medical Responder.

14 Describe common physical, emotional, and psychological responses to stress.

15 Describe common responses to death and dying and strategies to assist oneself and others in coping with death.

16 Describe strategies for minimizing the effects of stress on the Emergency Medical Responder.

17 Describe the key components of critical incident stress management (CISM).

Psychomotor

18 Describe and demonstrate proper handwashing technique.

19 Describe and demonstrate the proper application and removal of personal protective equipment (PPE).

Affective

20 Maintain a high regard for safety in all aspects of Emergency Medical Responder training.

21 Value the importance of body substance isolation (BSI) precautions.

Education Standards

Preparatory—Workforce Safety and Wellness

Medicine—Infectious Diseases

Competencies

Uses knowledge of the EMS system, safety and well-being of the Emergency Medical Responder, and medical, legal, and ethical issues at the scene of an emergency while awaiting a higher level of care.

Caring for others in their time of need is a tremendous responsibility and one that brings great rewards. It requires a considerable amount of mental, physical, and emotional conditioning that is sometimes difficult to balance due to the demands of the job. As you will soon learn, your personal well-being is an essential component for a long and healthy career in EMS. In this chapter, you will be introduced to the steps necessary to keep yourself in top shape, some of the common stressors that can weaken your defenses, and strategies for keeping yourself healthy and safe during your career in EMS.

FIRST ON SCENE

Jake slurps the last of his soda, steps carefully across the rubber flooring, and glides back onto the smooth ice of the skating rink. He glides toward a woman who is helping a small boy with wobbly ankles to skate. Just as he passes them, the woman loses her balance and grabs for the railing that runs around the edges of the rink.

Jake digs in his blades for a quick stop, sending a spray of ice shavings into the air, and grabs for the woman's flailing arms. He just misses her fingers and watches as she crashes onto her back, her head bouncing off the ice with a hollow thud. She sits up, laces her hands together on the back of her head, and begins to rock back and forth. Her cries of pain echo across the rink.

"Are you okay?" Jake asks. He kneels next to her and places a hand on her shoulder. "I'm an Emergency Medical Responder," Jake says. "May I help you?"

She doesn't respond but continues weeping and rocking. The boy is now sobbing, too, and trying to hold on to her jacket as he watches Jake fearfully. Just then Jake notices blood falling in large round splatters onto the ice. "Oh, hey, you're bleeding."

The woman suddenly looks wide-eyed at Jake, then at the boy. She frantically scoots backward away from both of them. "Don't touch me!" she cries. "Stay away!"

Personal Well-Being

LO2 Explain the importance of a baseline health assessment for new EMS providers.

It is not uncommon for an employer to require a medical exam before an individual starts a new job. In most cases, the purpose is to establish a **baseline health status**. It also will help you and your new employer to be certain that you are physically ready to handle the job.

As an Emergency Medical Responder, you will be exposed to risks to which the average individual is not typically exposed. For example, you will be caring for patients who are ill and/or injured, which can expose you to a wide variety of diseases. You will also be exposed to some unsafe scenes where people have been injured. If you hope to stay healthy enough to help others, you must be able to recognize these and other stressors unique to the EMS profession and learn how to manage them appropriately.

baseline health status ▶ preemployment medical examination to determine overall health status prior to beginning a job.

Immunizations

LO3 Describe the various immunizations recommended for health care providers.

One way Emergency Medical Responders can minimize the risk of acquiring an infectious disease is by becoming immunized. Vaccines commonly administered to health care providers include:

- COVID-19
- Hepatitis A and B
- Influenza
- Measles
- Meningitis
- Mumps
- Tetanus

While most people receive recommended vaccines as part of childhood wellness checks, additional vaccines are available to adults and those with a high risk of **exposure** to pathogens. In 1992, the **Occupational Safety and Health Administration (OSHA)** mandated that all employees who have a reasonable risk of becoming exposed to blood or other potentially infectious materials (OPIM) must be offered hepatitis B vaccinations. Employers are required to offer the vaccine at no charge.

Scientists are constantly developing new vaccines that could greatly decrease the likelihood of acquiring an infectious disease. Some vaccines are given only once in a lifetime. Others may need to be given more often. It is a good idea to consult with your personal health care provider before receiving vaccinations.

The worldwide COVID pandemic has raised the awareness of the importance of vaccines for all citizens and not just for EMS personnel. Given the fact that as an EMR you will be responding to both vaccinated and unvaccinated patients in need, it is especially important to ensure your own defenses are as strong as possible. Some EMS systems require that all providers receive vaccines while others allow personal choice. It is important that you know the requirements of your local system and those of your potential employer.

Prior to employment, you will likely be asked to have a thorough medical exam, which may include a simple test to ensure that you are not a carrier of tuberculosis (TB). A physical agility test may be required as well. Regardless of what your employer might require, it is your responsibility to ensure that you are as prepared as you can be before beginning your job as an Emergency Medical Responder.

exposure ▶ condition of being subjected to a fluid or substance capable of transmitting an infectious agent.

Occupational Safety and Health Administration ▶ U.S. government agency charged with ensuring a safe work environment. Abbrev: OSHA.

pathogen ▶ disease-causing organism such as a virus or bacterium.

standard precautions ▶ steps to take to protect against exposure to bodily fluids.

Centers for Disease Control and Prevention ▶ U.S. government agency charged with identifying, preventing, and controlling diseases and other health problems. Abbrev: CDC.

Standard Precautions

LO4 Explain the term *standard precautions* as it relates to the Emergency Medical Responder.

The likelihood for exposure to **pathogens**, such as bacteria or viruses that cause infectious diseases, is very high when caring for ill and injured persons. The term **standard precautions** refers to the guidelines recommended by the **Centers for Disease Control and Prevention (CDC)**.

universal precautions ▶
component of standard
precautions that involves the
philosophy that all patients
are considered infectious until
proven otherwise.

They are steps designed to reduce the risk of transmission of disease in the health care setting. The term **universal precautions** refers to the approach that *all* patients are considered infectious until proven otherwise. In other words, the use of precautions should be universal when you are unsure about a patient's infectious status.

Body Substance Isolation (BSI) Precautions

| LO5 | Explain what body substance isolation (BSI) precautions are and when they should be used. |

One component of standard precautions is the use of **body substance isolation (BSI) precautions**, which are specific steps that help minimize exposure to a patient's blood and bodily fluids. BSI involves using **personal protective equipment (PPE)** to minimize the chances of being exposed to bodily fluids. Examples of BSI precautions include wearing protective gloves, masks, gowns, and eyewear. In recent years, the term PPE has become a part of our daily vocabulary, and the use of PPE such as face masks is now a common sight.

Consider the following situations that represent possible exposures:

- A police officer puts handcuffs on a suspect who has a small open wound on her hand.
- A firefighter finds his leather gloves soaked with blood after extricating a patient from a wrecked car.
- A lifeguard touches dried blood while cleaning equipment after an emergency.
- A sheriff's deputy is searching the front seat of a suspect's car and is stuck by a needle that the suspect dropped the night before.
- An EMT is caring for a patient in the back of an ambulance who begins to vomit.
- A security guard arrives first on the scene to care for a patient who has suddenly become ill and is exposed to the patient's heavy coughing spell.

> **REMEMBER**
>
> Even dried bodily fluids are potentially infectious. Take the appropriate measures to prevent contact with any material that could possibly contain infectious pathogens.

body substance isolation precautions ▶ practice of using specific personal protective equipment to minimize contact with a patient's blood and bodily fluids. Abbrev: BSI.

personal protective equipment ▶ equipment such as gloves, masks, eyewear, gowns, turnout gear, and helmets that protect rescuers from infection and/or from exposure to hazardous materials and the dangers of rescue operations. Abbrev: PPE.

In each situation, the Emergency Medical Responder may be at risk of exposure to an infectious disease. What BSI precautions should be taken in each case described above? At the start of each shift, Emergency Medical Responders should check their hands for breaks in the skin and cover any areas that are not intact. If unprotected hands come in contact with blood (wet or dry) or any other bodily fluids, they should be washed with soap and warm water or a commercially produced antiseptic hand cleanser (Figure 3.1).

Make sure you wear disposable gloves before touching any patient and before handling equipment that may have been exposed to blood and bodily fluids (Figure 3.2). Your hands are very vulnerable to exposure and should be protected any time there is a chance of contact with a patient's blood or other bodily fluid.

Wear gloves, mask, and eye protection with any patient who is coughing, sneezing, spitting, or otherwise spraying bodily fluids. Finally, to dispose of blood-soaked equipment (including gloves), follow OSHA or **National Fire Protection Association (NFPA)** guidelines.

Emergency Medical Responders frequently face unpredictable, uncontrollable, and life-threatening circumstances. Anything can happen in an emergency. You might help a heart-attack victim. You might carry a child from a burning building. You might break up a brawl or help deliver a baby. Each situation has the potential to expose you to infectious diseases. Use good judgment. Always take proper protective precautions. By being consistent and thorough, you reduce risk and become a role model for your colleagues and peers.

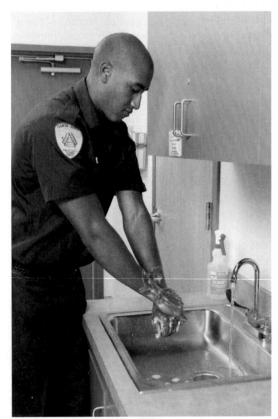

Figure 3.1 The CDC states that handwashing is one of the most effective means of minimizing the spread of infection.

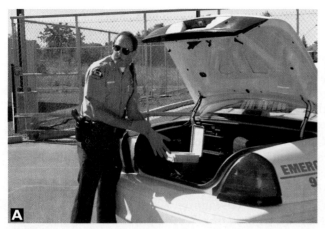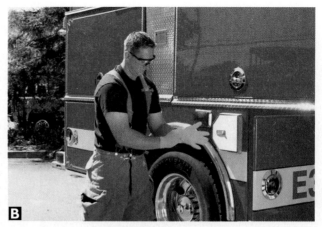

Figure 3.2 (A) Law enforcement officers must take precautions against exposure to blood. (B) Many of the incidents that a firefighter will face require appropriate protection from bodily fluids.

Routes of Exposure

| LO6 | Identify the four routes by which pathogens enter the body.

The very nature of work in EMS means that exposure to pathogens is likely. Under the right conditions, pathogens can enter the body, multiply, and produce harmful effects. They enter the body in one of four ways:

- *Ingestion*—by swallowing
- *Injection*—through a needle stick, puncture, sting, or bite
- *Absorption*—through the skin
- *Inhalation*—breathed in through the upper respiratory system and entering the lungs

You must be aware of each of the routes of exposure and learn the appropriate precautions to take when faced with a variety of known diseases.

Managing Risk

| LO7 | List examples of personal protective equipment (PPE) and the purpose of each.

| LO8 | Differentiate between cleaning and disinfection, and state when each should be performed.

Regardless of the risk of **infection**, all EMS personnel must follow the rules for their own safety and the safety of others. The way disease is spread and develops is a subject so complicated that its study is a specialty unto itself. Do not take chances with whether or not to wear protective gloves and a face mask. You are obtaining this training in order to help care for patients who are sick or injured. You can begin by not becoming a patient yourself and by not spreading infections.

Infections are caused by pathogens such as viruses and bacteria. The term *pathogen* refers to something that generates suffering (*patho-*, suffering; *-gen*, create or form). Viruses cause illnesses such as colds, flu, HIV, hepatitis, and COVID. Bacteria cause food poisoning, rheumatic fever, gonorrhea, and tuberculosis, to name a few. There are both viral and bacterial forms of pneumonia and meningitis. Pathogens are spread by exposure to bodily fluids such as blood and vomitus, as well as exposure to airborne droplets such as those spread when a person coughs, sneezes, spits, or even just breathes close to someone's face.

The COVID outbreak that began in late 2019 reinforced the importance of using proper PPE when caring for all patients. As a result, EMS systems around the world began reevaluating their current practices, and many began requiring increased training related to the evaluation of ill patients and the use of PPE (Figure 3.3).

Infectious diseases are a real danger to EMS personnel. However, if you follow basic safety procedures and use the PPE provided by your agency, the risks can be

National Fire Protection Association ▶ nonprofit organization that develops codes and standards for the prevention of fire, electrical, and related hazards. Abbrev: NFPA.

infection ▶ condition in which the body is invaded by a disease-causing agent.

REMEMBER

Your first step following an exposure to a patient's bodily fluids is to wash with warm water and soap. If water and soap are not immediately available, use an alcohol-based disinfectant until you can get to soap and water.

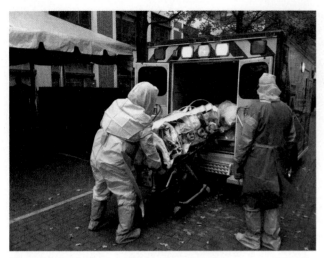

Figure 3.3 Medical staff in protective gear escort a COVID-positive patient from an ambulance in the early days of the COVID pandemic.
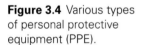
(Pearson Education)

greatly minimized for both you and the patient. Types of PPE include (Figure 3.4):

- *Synthetic gloves.* It is best practice to don protective gloves before any patient contact. It is also best practice to change gloves when moving from one patient to the next. Be careful not to touch common surfaces, equipment, door handles, steering wheels, or portable radios with contaminated gloves. Microorganisms on your hands will multiply quickly in the warm, moist environment within the glove. Therefore, it is important to wash hands with soap and warm water after removing protective gloves.
- *Face shields or masks.* Wear a protective face mask to minimize the potential for blood or fluid splatter entering your nose or mouth. A simple surgical-style mask will usually work well. To minimize exposure to fine particles of airborne droplets, wear a high-efficiency particulate air (HEPA), N-95, or N-100 mask. In addition, a surgical-type mask may be placed on the patient if they are alert and cooperate.
- *Eye protection.* The mucous membranes of your eyes can absorb fluids and are an easy route for pathogens to enter the body. Use eyewear that protects your eyes from both the front and sides. Prescription glasses or sunglasses are adequate for most situations but be aware that most do not have good protection from an exposure to the side of the face.
- *Gowns.* Protect your clothing and bare skin in situations involving spurting blood, childbirth, or multiple injuries with heavy bleeding.

Since you cannot tell if patients have infectious diseases just by looking at them, it is important to wear PPE for any contact with a patient. This includes wearing gloves at all times. In addition, wear face shields and eye protection whenever you may be exposed to splattering fluids or airborne droplets. This protection builds a barrier between you and the patient.

Your instructor will show you how to properly put on and use protective equipment in a way that maximizes effectiveness and maintains its cleanliness. You will also learn how and where to properly remove and dispose of all contaminated materials (Key Skill 3.1).

Figure 3.4 Various types of personal protective equipment (PPE).

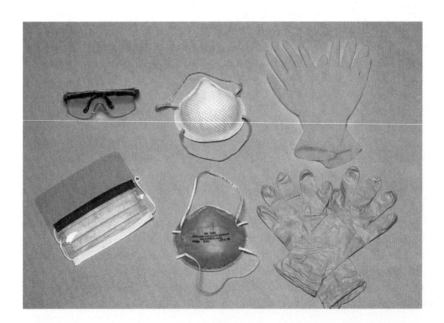

Proper Removal of Gloves

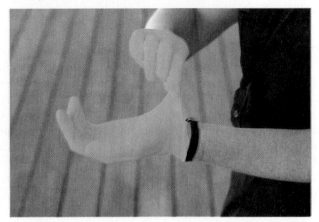

1. Begin by grasping the outer cuff of one glove.

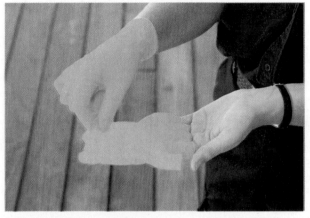

2. Carefully slip the glove over the hand, pulling it inside out. Grasp the discarded glove in your gloved hand.

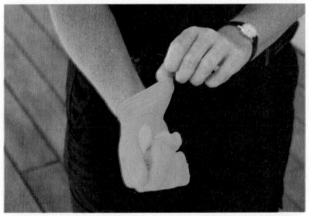

3. Next, slip a finger of the ungloved hand under the cuff of the other glove.

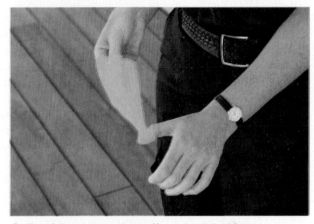

4. Carefully slip the glove off, turning it inside out.

5. Once removed, both gloves will end up inside out with one glove inside the other. This will contain any blood or bodily fluids.

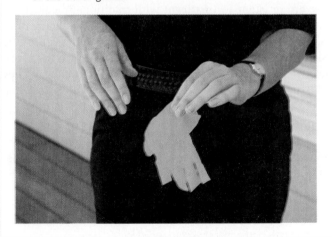

It is important that all reusable equipment be cleaned after each use to minimize the spread of disease. First, equipment must be cleaned thoroughly with soap and water to remove all visible blood, vomit, and other bodily fluids. Then it must be properly disinfected using an appropriate solution. Cleaning with soap and water alone will not disinfect and eliminate pathogens. Disposable equipment must be discarded as soon as practical in a designated hazardous waste receptacle.

You must learn and practice infection-control procedures to reduce your risk of infection. They are based on guidelines from OSHA and the CDC. Practicing them is part of your responsibility as an Emergency Medical Responder.

Bloodborne and Airborne Pathogens

Infectious diseases range from such mild conditions as the common cold to life-threatening diseases such as COVID, hepatitis, and tuberculosis. The four diseases of most concern to Emergency Medical Responders today are COVID-19, human immunodeficiency virus (HIV), hepatitis, and tuberculosis (Table 3.1).

COVID-19 has demonstrated to the world just how quickly a pathogen travels and spreads throughout a population. COVID-19 is a respiratory virus that spreads from person to person via close contact with an infectious person, particularly with droplets from an infected person's cough or sneeze. Proper PPE, minimizing close contact with infected persons, and frequent handwashing will go a long way to protect you from becoming infected.

An estimated 250 health care workers die each year from hepatitis or its complications, more than from any other infectious disease.[1] Other viruses, such as HIV—the virus that causes acquired immunodeficiency syndrome (AIDS)—are far less likely to infect you. HIV does not survive well outside the body and is not as highly concentrated in bodily fluids as are the hepatitis B and C viruses.

The routes of exposure to HIV are limited to direct contact with nonintact (open) skin or mucous membranes and with blood, semen, or other bodily fluids. Thus, it is very unlikely that a rescuer taking proper BSI precautions will acquire the HIV infection on the job.

In contrast to HIV, hepatitis B and C are very tough and aggressive viruses that damage the liver. They are both transmitted through contact with blood or bodily fluids and can survive on clothing, newspaper, or other objects for at least seven days or longer after infected blood has dried. HBV and HCV may cause permanent liver damage and, in some cases, can be fatal. In November 2017, the Federal Advisory Committee on Immunization Practices endorsed a new hepatitis B vaccine for use in adults. This is the first new hepatitis B vaccine in more than 25 years.

Tuberculosis (TB), a disease most often affecting the lungs, can also be fatal. Thought to have been nearly eradicated in 1985, incidents of TB are on the rise once again. Even worse, new strains of the disease are resistant to treatment with traditional medications. Unlike HIV and hepatitis, TB is spread by aerosolized droplets in the air, usually the result of coughing and sneezing. Thus, TB can be contracted even without direct physical contact with a carrier. Use a face mask with a one-way valve or a bag-mask device for rescue breathing. Use a HEPA, N-95, or P-100 mask when TB is suspected (Figure 3.5). These masks greatly reduce the risk of exposure to TB and other airborne diseases.

> **REMEMBER**
>
> As a new member of the EMS team who will be caring for patients, it is best to make it a habit to wear gloves for all patient contacts. While it is true that not all patients pose a risk of exposure to a pathogen, you do not yet have enough experience to know the difference. Play it safe and always don gloves prior to making patient contact.

TABLE 3.1 **Diseases of Concern to Emergency Medical Responders**

Disease	How Transmitted	Vaccine
COVID-19	Close contact with an infectious person; contact with droplets from an infected person's cough or sneeze	Yes
HIV/AIDS	Needle sticks, blood splash on mucous membranes (eye, mouth), or blood contact with open skin	No
Hepatitis B & C viruses	Needle sticks, blood splash on mucous membranes (eye, mouth), or blood contact with open skin; some risk during mouth-to-mouth CPR and exposure to contaminated equipment and dried blood	B—Yes; C—No
Tuberculosis (TB)	Airborne aerosolized droplets	No

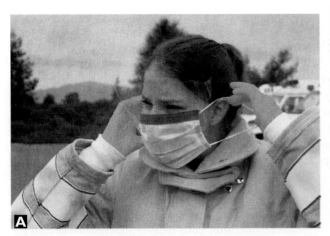
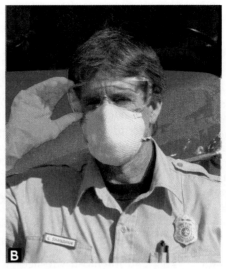

Figure 3.5 (A) A simple surgical-style mask with eye shield or (B) an N-95/N-100 mask will minimize your chances of being exposed to an airborne pathogen.

Not all pathogens are well understood. In fact, there are new pathogens emerging all the time. The following is a list of pathogens that have received significant attention in recent years from the CDC and the media:

- *Zika.* A virus spread by the bite of a certain species of mosquito. In otherwise healthy adults, the Zika virus causes signs and symptoms similar to the common flu. Zika is especially dangerous for pregnant women as it can be transmitted to the fetus from the mother. Zika is known to cause birth defects, including brain damage in unborn fetuses.
- *Ebola.* A virus spread by human-to-human contact that causes an acute, serious illness that is often fatal if untreated. Ebola virus disease (EVD) first appeared in Africa in 1976 and was responsible for the deaths of tens of thousands during an outbreak in 2014–2016.
- *Swine flu (H1N1).* This is a form of influenza. It is common in pigs and has been known to spread to humans. In 2009, the strain known as H1N1 became a pandemic among humans.
- *Severe acute respiratory syndrome (SARS).* First reported in Asia in 2003, the SARS virus quickly spread to more than 8,000 people in two dozen countries in North America, South America, Europe, and Asia. According to the World Health Organization (WHO), a total of 774 died before the SARS global outbreak of 2003 was contained.
- *West Nile virus (WNV).* A potentially serious illness, WNV is a seasonal epidemic in North America. It flares up in the summer and continues into the fall.
- *Avian influenza.* This form of influenza is common in birds; it is also called bird flu. In rare cases, it has been known to spread to humans, resulting in a high mortality rate.
- *Methicillin-resistant Staphylococcus aureus (MRSA).* This bacterium is resistant to certain antibiotics, including oxacillin, penicillin, and amoxicillin. MRSA and

FIRST ON SCENE *(continued)*

"Hold on!" Jake approaches the woman with his arms outstretched and hands open. "You're bleeding. Please, let me help you."

She scoots back against the low, carpeted wall that surrounds the rink and shakes her head. "I've got hepatitis," she whispers, tears still flowing from her eyes. "Please just call an ambulance." Her dark hair and black jacket have been hiding the seriousness of the blood loss, but now that they are saturated, bright blood begins to pool quickly on the ice around her.

Jake hesitates and looks at his ungloved hands. There is a paper cut on the side of his left index finger. He looks from his hands to the woman's crying face. He turns and shouts to the skate attendant, "Call 911! Then bring me a first-aid kit."

other staph infections occur most frequently in hospitals and health care facilities (such as nursing homes and dialysis centers) among people who have weakened immune systems.

Employee Responsibilities

An infection-control program will work only if you learn and follow correct procedures. As an Emergency Medical Responder, you have an obligation to adhere to safe work practices to protect yourself, your family, and the public. Washing hands regularly, using gloves and other personal protective equipment, and making safe work practices a habit are good ways to start.

Following an Exposure

LO9 Explain the procedure the Emergency Medical Responder should follow after a possible pathogen exposure.

First and foremost, you need to understand the difference between an exposure and an infection. All infections come from an exposure to a pathogen. However, not all exposures result in an infection. In fact, the vast majority of exposures do not. To help minimize the chances of becoming infected following an exposure, follow these simple steps:

- For an exposure to the skin, immediately wash the area with warm water and soap.
- If exposure is to the eyes, flush with clean water for 20 minutes.
- Document the details of the exposure on the appropriate form included in your employer's exposure-control plan.
- Report the exposure to your company/agency infection-control plan administrator.
- Schedule a follow-up medical evaluation with an appropriate health care provider.

The follow-up evaluation will include an assessment of the exposure and the development of a plan of action to minimize the likelihood of an infection. In some cases, it may include an immediate test for infection as well as post-exposure medications. Your health care provider will help develop a plan of action based on the facts surrounding your exposure.

Scene Safety

LO10 Describe common hazards at the scene of an emergency.

LO11 Explain the steps the Emergency Medical Responder should take to mitigate common scene hazards.

Scene safety begins long before Emergency Medical Responders actually arrive at the scene. En route, get as much information about the emergency as possible from dispatch. The nature of the call will help to determine what type of personal protective equipment may be needed. It also will tell you what type of precautions to take as you approach the scene.

Dispatchers will not always have complete or accurate details about an incident. Often, people who report an emergency are excited, nervous, confused, in pain, or in a panic. They may even hang up before they finish giving all the details.

Approaching and Managing the Scene

When approaching an emergency scene, always look around for hazards. For many first responders, one of your first decisions will be where to position your vehicle. (Should it be facing the scene to provide lighting? Should it be beyond the scene to provide quick and easy supply access? Should it be on the street to block traffic? Should it be off the street to protect yourself and your partner?) When deciding where to position the vehicle, consider that placement must provide for access to equipment and continued traffic flow where possible or at least rerouting of traffic around the scene.

Before approaching the patient, ensure scene safety for yourself, the patient, and bystanders. Observe for hazardous materials, toxic substances, downed power lines, or unstable vehicles at the scene. Environmental conditions such as icy and slippery roads, steep grades, rocky terrain, or heavy traffic and a crowd of onlookers must all be considered in your approach and care of your patient.

Violent situations may involve weapons—not just guns but knives or bats, boards, chains, and other items. All can be used to harm you, just as they harmed the victim. In addition, you must be aware of the potential for violence to continue at the scene (Figure 3.6). Do not approach the scene until it is safe. When the scene is safe to enter, do not disturb evidence any more than you must while caring for the patient. Look for the presence of weapons. Do not attempt to provide care if you see them. Contact law enforcement immediately.

Crowds can be potentially dangerous. When necessary, notify dispatch that you need assistance from law enforcement for crowd control, protection, and scene security.

Keeping yourself safe is your first responsibility. Once you can ensure your own safety, approach and take care of the patient.

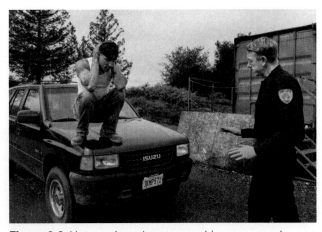

Figure 3.6 Use caution when approaching anyone who appears to be agitated or aggressive.

Crew Resource Management

Crew resource management (CRM) is a concept borrowed from the aviation profession, giving everyone on the team a shared responsibility for safety. CRM has been adapted for many professions in which human error can have serious negative outcomes. CRM is most often seen among specialty teams such as air medical flight teams, neonatal transport teams, and critical care transport teams.

CRM is based on these key concepts:

crew resource management ▶ effective use of all available resources, allowing on-scene personnel to ensure a safe operation, increase efficiency, reduce/prevent errors, and avoid stress. Abbrev: CRM.

- Communication
- Situational awareness
- Problem solving
- Decision making
- Teamwork

A foundation of CRM is that rank cannot get in the way of safety. If anyone on the EMS team sees a safety issue or has a safety concern, they are encouraged to speak up and share their concern regardless of rank. Decisions related to patient care, such as which patient care priority should be addressed first, if a patient should be moved, how a patient should be moved, or which medication should be administered, are all decisions requiring good situational awareness, problem solving, and communication. The goal is to make decisions about managing the scene and the patient that will ensure the safety of all responders and the patient.

Hazardous Materials Incidents

Some chemicals can cause serious illness or death, even if your exposure is brief. Some chemicals may be transported by truck or rail. Some may be stored in warehouses or used in local industries.

In a collision involving chemicals, damaged or leaking containers should be considered a hazard to the community and responding EMS personnel. A safe distance should be maintained and the scene treated as a **hazardous materials incident**.

Placards identify hazardous materials with coded colors and numbers. All placard codes are listed in the U.S. Department of Transportation's *Emergency Response Guidebook*. This book should be placed in every emergency response vehicle. It provides important information about hazardous substances, as well as information on safe distances, emergency care, and suggested procedures in the event of a spill or chemical release.

As an Emergency Medical Responder, your most important duty in a hazardous materials incident is to recognize potential problems and take action to preserve your

REMEMBER

The most common exposures occur in the home. It often happens when various cleaning products, mixed together, produce dangerous fumes. Many home garages are full of hazardous materials that are often not properly labeled or stored.

hazardous materials incident ▶ release of a harmful substance into the environment. Also called a *hazmat incident*.

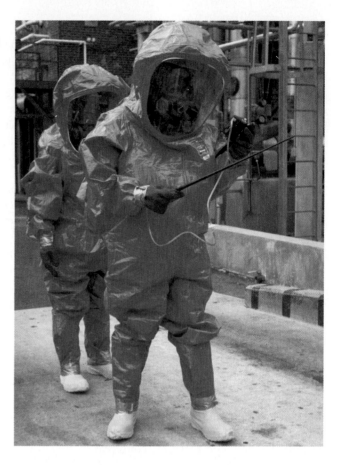

Figure 3.7 Do not enter any scene that may be unsafe unless you are properly trained and equipped.

own safety and that of others. (See more in Chapter 25.) You should also make sure that a specially trained hazardous materials response team is notified (Figure 3.7). Leave the handling of the incident to them. Do not take any action other than to protect yourself, your patients, and bystanders. Many emergency response agencies require hazardous materials training at the awareness level. Your instructor can inform you of the requirements in your area.

Rescue Operations

Rescue scenes may include dangers from electricity, fire, explosion, hazardous materials, traffic, or water and ice. It is important to evaluate each situation and request the appropriately trained teams to assist as necessary. You may need the police, fire services, utility company, or other specialized personnel. Never perform rescues for which you are not properly trained. Secure the scene to the best of your ability. Then, wait for the help you have requested to arrive.

Remember that whenever you are working at a rescue operation, you must use personal protective equipment. PPE at rescue scenes may include firefighter turnout gear, protective eyewear, helmets, puncture-proof gloves, and disposable synthetic gloves.

Crime Scenes and Acts of Violence

Emergency Medical Responders may respond to scenes involving victims of violence or crimes. In some areas, EMS providers are issued bulletproof vests for their protection along with other PPE. No matter what area you work in, your first priority—even before patient care—is to be certain the scene is safe before you enter it.

Threatening people or animals, people with weapons, intoxicated people, and others may present problems you are not prepared to handle. Recognize those situations early and request the necessary help. Do not enter the scene until help arrives to secure it and makes it safe for you to perform your duties.

Emotional Wellness of Emergency Medical Personnel

Responding to emergencies and caring for people who are suddenly ill or injured can carry a heavy emotional toll. It is important to understand how your role as an Emergency Medical Responder may affect you personally. It also is important to develop strategies for coping with stress.

Emergency Medical Responders and Stress

Almost everyone must deal with some type of stress on a daily basis, whether driving in traffic, coping with work and family problems, meeting school or office deadlines, or waiting for an appointment. **Stress** is an emotionally disruptive or upsetting condition that occurs in response to adverse external influences. It is capable of affecting one's physical health. Stress can cause an increased heart rate, a rise in blood pressure, muscular tension, irritability, and depression.

Surveys and research reports over the past two decades have revealed that a large percentage of all adults sustain adverse health effects from stress.[2] Recent research confirms that stress contributes to cardiovascular disease, stroke, diabetes, cancer, and arthritis, as well as to gastrointestinal, skin, neurological, and emotional disorders.

Another Side of Personal Safety

Stress is a concern for all Emergency Medical Responders. The job makes intense physical and psychological demands on your well-being. Police officers, firefighters, and disaster response personnel must respond quickly to emergencies and react appropriately in situations in which lives are at risk. The need to make immediate decisions about patient care is a big responsibility. They know that a mistake caused by their reaction to stress can cause harm to patients as well as to other rescuers.

Three of the best ways to minimize the stress associated with responding to emergencies and caring for patients are:

- Work closely with other, more experienced responders.
- Practice your skills often.
- Talk with trusted friends and/or family members about your stress (without violating patient confidentiality).

Causes of Stress

LO12 Explain the terms *stress* and *stressor* as they relate to the Emergency Medical Responder.

LO13 Describe several sources of stress commonly encountered by the Emergency Medical Responder.

Emergencies are stressful events, some more than others. The following are examples of very stressful situations, or **critical incidents**, encountered in EMS. The stress of any one of these events can continue long after the event is over. They include:

- *Multiple-casualty incidents.* An emergency that involves multiple patients is referred to as a **multiple-casualty incident (MCI)**. MCIs range from a motor-vehicle crash that injures two drivers and a passenger to a large hurricane that causes injury to hundreds of people (Figure 3.8).
- *Pediatric patients.* Emergencies involving infants or children are considered some of the most stressful that EMS providers are required to handle (Figure 3.9).
- *Untimely death.* It can be difficult for a health care provider to deal with the death of a patient, and even more so if the patient is young or someone the provider knows. The death or injury of another provider, even if you do not personally know that individual, can also cause a stress response.

stress ▶ emotionally disruptive or upsetting condition that occurs in response to adverse external influences.

REMEMBER

The *Emergency Response Guidebook* is now available as a smartphone application. It can be downloaded free from the app store appropriate for your device. Having access to an electronic version of the guidebook will help ensure that the resource is available when you need it and that you are referencing the most accurate and up-to-date information.
You also would be wise to carry a pair of binoculars in your vehicle. Use them to identify hazardous materials placards from a safe distance, thus ensuring your own safety.

critical incident ▶ any situation that causes a rescuer to experience unusually strong emotions that interfere with the ability to function either during the incident or after a highly stressful incident.

multiple-casualty incident ▶ single incident that involves multiple patients. Also called a *mass-casualty incident*. Abbrev: MCI.

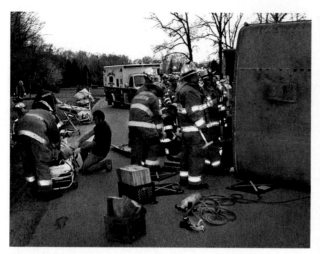

Figure 3.8 Emergency scenes that involve multiple patients are some of the most stressful for responders.
(© Edward T. Dickinson, MD)

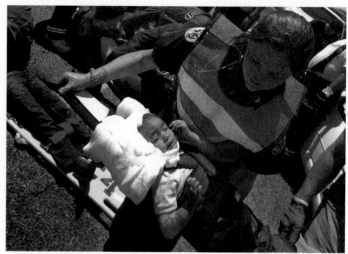

Figure 3.9 Injured and ill children are particularly challenging for many responders.

- *Violence.* Not only is it difficult to witness violence against others, but it is also dangerous. Take steps to protect yourself when responding to a violent situation or when a situation suddenly becomes violent.
- *Abuse and neglect.* As an Emergency Medical Responder, you may be called upon to provide care for an infant, child, adult, or an older adult patient who exhibits signs of abuse or neglect. Remember that abuse and neglect occur in all social and economic levels of society.

Although everyone responds to stress a little differently, having a stress reaction is common to all emergency personnel. It pays to stay aware of the stress factors you are exposed to every day, as well as your immediate and long-term reactions to them. Just as important is the ability to recognize stress in your coworkers. Keep an eye out and offer assistance as appropriate.

Burnout

stressor ▶ any emotional or physical demand that causes stress.

EMS personnel are trained to handle difficult situations, but **stressors**—factors that cause wear and tear on the body's physical or mental resources—can take their toll. Stressors in EMS work can be as obvious as a fatal collision or the unexpected death of a child. Sometimes stress can accumulate over months or even years of responding to ordinary injuries and illnesses.

burnout ▶ extreme emotional state characterized by emotional exhaustion, a diminished sense of personal accomplishment, and cynicism.

Some EMS providers suffer from **burnout**, a reaction to cumulative stress or to multiple critical incidents. Emergency Medical Responders are at increased risk for burnout because of the demands and activities of the job. The signs of burnout include a loss of enthusiasm and energy replaced by feelings of frustration, hopelessness, low self-esteem, isolation, and mistrust. Many factors contribute to burnout. They include multiple or back-to-back emergency events involving serious medical problems, injuries, or death; facing public hostility; struggling with bureaucratic obstacles; long hours; and poor working conditions.

Shift work—12, 24, or even 48 hours at a time—can be a significant source of stress, particularly when combined with other stress factors. This pattern of work is common in EMS. It may be even more stressful for partners in dual-income families, who often miss time shared with their children and each other. The need for continuing education also contributes to already strained schedules. For example, evening meals that could be restful times are too often replaced with high-caffeine beverages and high-fat fast food consumed on the run. A healthier diet and lifestyle can help Emergency Medical Responders combat the stressors that are an unavoidable part of the job.

Both short-term and long-term stressors are occupational hazards for Emergency Medical Responders. Fortunately, research in the past 15 years has found ways to help reduce both kinds of stress. We will discuss strategies for helping you manage the stressors of being an EMR later in this chapter.

Signs and Symptoms of Stress

LO14 Describe common physical, emotional, and psychological responses to stress.

The way you handle stress can affect both your emotional health and the way you respond to emergencies. Emergency Medical Responders have a duty to confront the psychological effects of the work they do. Ignoring stress does not make it go away. Instead, it may crop up in unexpected forms, such as insomnia, fatigue, alcohol abuse, increased incidence of illnesses, heart disease, or other disruptive responses. You may find yourself doing less well at work and having difficulties in your relationships with others. Those who do not find ways to cope with stress can become depressed, sustain physical disorders, experience burnout, and may even have to leave the field permanently.

Recognize the signs and symptoms of stress. They include irritability with family, friends, and coworkers; inability to concentrate; changes in daily activities, such as difficulty sleeping or nightmares, loss of appetite, and loss of interest in sexual activity; and anxiety, indecisiveness, guilt, isolation, and loss of interest in work or poor performance. You might also experience constipation, diarrhea, headaches, nausea, and hypertension.

FIRST ON SCENE (continued)

The woman's sobs slowly taper off and, as her bloody hands drop to the ice, Jake sees that she is losing consciousness. Her eyes are shifting groggily from him to the crowd of onlookers and to the small boy who is now being comforted by a teenage girl. Jake wants so badly to help the woman somehow, to apply pressure to stop her bleeding, to hug her, and to tell her that she'll be okay—anything. But hepatitis. *Wow*, he thinks. He doesn't want to get hepatitis. Just then, one of the employees reaches over the wall and hands Jake the first-aid kit. Jake quickly opens the bag and searches for a pair of gloves.

As the small mumbling crowd watches, the woman's eyes slowly close and she slumps over onto the red ice.

Death and Dying

LO15 Describe common responses to death and dying and strategies to assist oneself and others in coping with death.

As an Emergency Medical Responder, you will at some time have to deal with a patient who has a terminal illness or injury. Some patients with terminal illnesses who are expected to live 6 months or less will be receiving hospice care, or care that helps relieve their symptoms rather than treat their conditions. Such patients and their families will have many different reactions to the death of a loved one. A basic understanding of what they are going through will help you deal with the stress they are experiencing, as well as that of your own.

When individuals learn that they or a loved one is dying, they will often experience several stages of response, each varying in duration and magnitude. Sometimes those stages are not experienced in the same order given below, and sometimes the stages overlap one another. Whatever the length or order of the stages, they all affect both the patient and their loved ones. The stages of grief first described by Dr. Elisabeth Kübler-Ross in 1969 include the following:

- *Denial.* The patient often denies that he or she is dying and thus puts off having to deal with the situation. Often the patient displays strong disbelief. Thoughts and statements such as, "Not me," or "This can't be happening to me," are common.

- *Anger.* The patient is angry about the situation. This anger is often vented upon family members or even EMS personnel. Thoughts and statements such as, "Why me?" are common.
- *Bargaining.* The patient feels that making bargains will postpone the inevitable. Statements such as, "Okay, but first let me . . . " are common in this stage.
- *Depression.* The patient often becomes sad and depressed and frequently mourns things that he or she has not accomplished. The patient then may become unwilling to communicate with others. Statements such as, "Okay, but I haven't . . . " are common in this stage.
- *Acceptance.* The patient, having worked through all the stages, is finally able to accept death, even though he or she may not welcome it. Frequently, the patient will reach this stage before family members do, in which case the patient may find themselves comforting their loved ones. Thoughts and statements such as, "It's going to be okay. I'm not afraid," are common at this stage.

Many times, a patient's family member or loved one will respond by going through these same stages. Do not neglect their need for information and compassion. Several approaches are appropriate when dealing with situations such as these. The following strategies may be helpful when confronted with grieving friends and family members:

- *Recognize patient needs.* Treat your patient with respect and do whatever is possible to preserve his or her dignity and sense of control. Speak directly to the patient and avoid talking about them to family members or friends in their presence. Try to respond to the patient's choices about how to handle the situation. Allow the patient to talk about feelings, even though it may make you uncomfortable. Respect the patient's privacy if they do not want to express personal feelings.
- *Remain tolerant.* There may be angry reactions from the patient or family members. Sometimes they will direct their anger at you, but do not take it personally. The patient and family need a chance to vent, and they will often choose whoever is nearby as a target.
- *Listen empathetically.* Try to understand the feelings of the patient or family member. There is seldom anything you can do to fix the situation, but sometimes just listening is very helpful.
- *Do not give false hope or reassurance.* Avoid saying things such as, "Everything will be all right." The family knows things will not be all right, and they do not want to try to justify what is happening. A simple, "I'm sorry" is sufficient.
- *Offer comfort.* Let both the patient and the family know that you will do everything you can to help and/or that you will help them find assistance from other sources, if needed. Remember, a gentle tone of voice and possibly a reassuring touch, if appropriate, can be very helpful.

Dealing with Stress

Stress may be caused by a single traumatic event, or it may result from the combined effects of several incidents. It is important to remember that a traumatic event can cause different reactions in different people. Stress may also be caused by a combination of factors, including personal problems, such as friends and family members who just do not understand the job. It is frequently necessary for health care providers to work on holidays, weekends, and during important family events. This can be frustrating to friends and family members, which may cause stress for the provider. It can also be difficult when family and friends do not understand the strong emotions involved in responding to a critical incident.

The Emergency Medical Responder can use many strategies to deal with stress, ranging from making simple lifestyle changes to seeking professional counseling.

Lifestyle Changes

LO16 Describe strategies for minimizing the effects of stress on the Emergency Medical Responder.

It is often difficult to make changes in the habits or the lifestyle you have developed, but it is essential to consider the effects that current conditions have on your well-being. Remember that your health is of primary importance. Look carefully at your habits and consider making simple but important adjustments.

There are several strategies you can use to enhance your ability to cope with stress. They include:

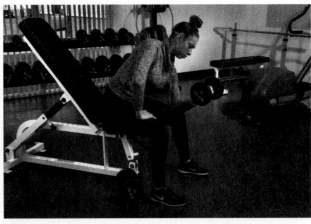

Figure 3.10 Establishing a consistent exercise routine is one step toward developing good coping mechanisms for stress.

- *Develop healthier dietary habits.* Avoid fatty foods and focus on a more balanced diet. Also, reduce your consumption of alcohol, sugar, and caffeine, which can negatively affect sleep patterns and cause irritability.
- *Exercise regularly.* Regular exercise helps reduce stress (Figure 3.10). It can also help you to deal with the physical aspects of your responsibilities, such as carrying equipment and performing other physically demanding emergency procedures.
- *Devote time to relaxing.* Consider trying relaxation techniques, such as deep-breathing exercises, meditation, or simply reading a good book.
- *Change your work environment or shifts.* If possible, reduce the number of hours you are on call or the amount of overtime worked. You may also consider asking for a rotation to a less-stressful assignment for a brief time.
- *Seek professional help.* Consider meeting with a mental health professional or a member of the clergy. It is important to develop a healthy perspective about what you do. Being an Emergency Medical Responder is what you do, not who you are.

Critical Incident Stress Management

LO17 Describe the key components of critical incident stress management (CISM).

Critical incident stress management (CISM) is a broad-based approach involving several strategies designed to help emergency personnel cope with critical incident stress. The **critical incident stress debriefing (CISD)** is one tool in the larger CISM plan. CISD is a process in which teams of trained peer counselors and mental health professionals meet with rescuers and health care providers who have been involved in a critical incident. These meetings are usually held 24 to 72 hours after the incident. The goal is to assist the providers in dealing with the stress related to that incident.

Participation in a CISD is strictly voluntary. No one should ever be forced or coerced to attend. Participants are encouraged to talk about their reactions to the incident. It is *not* a critique. All participants should be made aware that whatever is said during a debriefing will be held in the strictest confidence by the participants and by the debriefing team. CISDs can be helpful in assisting EMS personnel to better understand their reactions and feelings both during and after an incident. Attendees will also come to understand that other members of the team were very likely experiencing similar reactions.

In the opening discussion, everyone is encouraged to share but not forced to do so. Then, the debriefing teams offer suggestions on how to deal with and prevent further stress. It is important to realize that stress reactions following a critical incident are both normal and expected. The CISD process can be very helpful for some in learning how to cope with stress. Your instructor will inform you of situations in which CISD should be requested and how to access the local system.

critical incident stress management ▶ broad-based approach involving several strategies designed to help emergency personnel cope with critical incident stress. Abbrev: CISM.

critical incident stress debriefing ▶ formal process in which teams of professional and peer counselors provide emotional and psychological support to those who have been involved in a critical incident. Abbrev: CISD.

REMEMBER

While CISD is a valuable tool to help individuals cope with stress, it cannot stand alone. Follow-up care may be needed for some providers, and an ongoing assessment of affected providers should be done to determine if additional personal assistance is indicated. Do not be afraid to speak to your personal health care provider about any unusual or concerning symptoms and recognize that even the most experienced health care providers may need emotional and psychological care at some point in their careers.

Resources to Help Cope with Stress

In recent years there has been an increased awareness of the stressors that affect frontline health care workers, including Emergency Medical responders. This awareness has led to the development of a variety of resources directed at helping frontline workers cope with these stressors. The CDC has developed a list of tips for health care workers to help them take better care of themselves. This list can be found at https://emergency.cdc.gov/coping/responders.asp.

CrewCare is a mobile phone app developed by ImageTrend, a leading health care company that supports the EMS profession and engages the frontline worker with daily updates and wellness check ins. They have also published a report based on data collected through their app that reveals just how big a need there is for these resources. This report can be found at https://www.crewcarelife.com/crewcare-results/. CrewCare can be found at both the Apple Store and Google Play.

ResilientFirst is another valuable resource developed by the team at FirstWatch (firstwatch.net). ResilientFirst is a neuroscience-based tool that is a convenient, affordable, and effective way to build resilience for yourself or your team. It is a mobile phone app that engages the frontline worker in daily check-ins and provides resources to help with the development of healthy coping mechanisms.

FIRST ON SCENE WRAP-UP

Ten minutes after the woman fell, a group of firefighters and EMTs are walking gingerly across the ice. They slide a cot piled high with equipment toward her. Jake explains to the first uniformed rescuer what happened and lowers his voice as he mentions the hepatitis.

The crews, already wearing gloves, quickly put an oxygen mask on the woman, control her bleeding, and place a cervical collar around her neck. As they are lifting her onto the gurney, she wakes.

"I think she'll be okay," the EMT at the head of the gurney says to Jake. "It was the right thing to call us."

Jake accompanies them to the edge of the rink and watches the crews take her and the boy out of the arena. He again looks down at his hands and decides never again to be caught without a pair of protective gloves.

Summary

- Prior to beginning work as an Emergency Medical Responder, it is important for you to establish a baseline health status to ensure that you are healthy and prepared. Part of this health assessment includes receiving appropriate immunizations.
- Standard precautions are those precautions all health care professionals must follow to minimize exposure to infectious pathogens. This includes maintaining a philosophy that all patients are potentially infectious and donning all necessary personal protective equipment (PPE).
- Proper body substance isolation (BSI) precautions should be taken prior to making contact with all patients. BSI precautions include wearing PPE such as gloves, eye protection, and protective gowns when necessary.
- Pathogens can enter the body one of four ways: injection, absorption, inhalation, or ingestion.
- Know your company/agency procedure should you sustain an exposure to a patient's blood or bodily fluids. At a minimum, you must immediately wash the area with warm soap and water and contact your supervisor.
- Exposure to pathogens is just one potential hazard when caring for patients. Emergency scenes are full of other hazards, such as moving traffic, downed power lines, spilled fuel or chemicals, and violent patients. You must always keep personal safety as your top priority and use appropriately trained resources to help mitigate these hazards.
- Stress is an emotionally disruptive or upsetting condition that occurs in response to adverse external influences. Stressors are those factors that cause stress. As an Emergency Medical Responder, you must be aware of the common causes of stress and the typical ways that stress may exhibit itself.
- If not properly managed, stress can become very disruptive. It can cause negative changes in behavior and attitude as well as physical changes that negatively affect health.
- You must learn to develop good coping mechanisms for many of the common stressors of the job. Eating a healthy, balanced diet; getting regular exercise; and maintaining work-life balance are all important.
- Critical incident stress management (CISM) can be helpful for many when trying to manage the effects of stress following a critical incident.

Take Action

Slippery When Wet

Learning to put on and remove protective gloves is an important skill for all Emergency Medical Responders. One way you can practice this skill is to don a pair of disposable gloves and spread a generous portion of shaving cream over both gloved hands. The shaving cream is used to simulate blood or other bodily fluids. Now carefully try to remove the gloves, one at a time, without splattering the shaving cream. The gloves will be difficult to remove when they are wet but, with enough practice, you will become skilled at safely removing them.

Stressed Out

Most EMS systems around the country have specialized teams of people who are trained to assist EMS personnel who have responded to a critical incident. These teams will provide support and assistance for those who were directly involved in the incident and help them understand the reactions they may be experiencing. Ask your instructor or another EMS professional in your area how to access these resources.

First on Scene Patient Handoff

We have a 36-year-old female named Emily who experienced a mechanical fall backward onto the ice, striking her head. The fall was witnessed, and Emily did not have any loss of consciousness immediately following the fall. She has an open wound to the back of her head with obvious bleeding. Emily states that she is positive for hepatitis and was reluctant to have anyone assist her at first. I instructed Emily to hold pressure on the back of her head while I waited for gloves. Emily then became unresponsive, and we carefully laid her supine on the ice with a blanket beneath her for insulation. Her son is here with her and would like to go with her if she is transported by ambulance.

First on Scene Run Review

Recall the events of the First on Scene scenario in this chapter, and answer the following questions related to the call. Rationales are offered in the Answer Key at the back of the book.

1. Why should Jake ask if he can help?
2. Did Jake do the right thing by not controlling the bleeding? Why or why not?
3. Is there another way that Jake could control the bleeding?

Quick Quiz

To check your understanding of the chapter, answer the following questions. Then, compare your answers to those in the Answer Key at the back of the book.

1. All of the following are routes through which pathogens may enter the body EXCEPT:
   a. ingestion.
   b. mentation.
   c. inhalation.
   d. injection.

2. Which of the following is NOT a commonly recommended immunization for health care providers?
   a. Rabies
   b. Pertussis
   c. Hepatitis
   d. Tetanus

3. Which of the following types of PPE would be most important to use when caring for a patient with tuberculosis?
   a. Gloves
   b. Eyeglasses
   c. HEPA mask
   d. Gown

4. You have arrived at the scene of a vehicle collision, and there are downed power lines across the road. Which of the following resources is most appropriate to manage this hazard?
   a. Law enforcement
   b. Fire department
   c. Hazmat team
   d. Utility company

5. All of the following are common emotional reactions of an Emergency Medical Responder who has faced serious trauma, illness, or death, EXCEPT:
   a. depression.
   b. burnout.
   c. excessive energy.
   d. insomnia.

6. The best definition of the term *stressor* is:
   a. a situation involving death or dying.
   b. something that consumes the attention of the individual experiencing stress.
   c. anything that puts pressure on the body.
   d. any emotional or physical demand that causes stress.

7. Common causes of stress for Emergency Medical Responders include all of the following EXCEPT:
   a. documenting each call.
   b. multiple casualty incidents.
   c. severely injured pediatric patients.
   d. the scene of a violent crime.

8. All of the following are terms used for the stages of death and dying EXCEPT:
   a. denial.
   b. anger.
   c. bargaining.
   d. refusal.

9. When caring for family members after the death of a loved one, you should:
   a. avoid talking directly to the patient's family.
   b. not tolerate angry reactions.
   c. try your best to understand their feelings.
   d. tell them everything will be okay.

10. All of the following are common signs and symptoms of stress EXCEPT:
    a. irritability.
    b. difficulty sleeping.
    c. increased appetite.
    d. difficulty concentrating.

11. A broad-based approach involving several strategies designed to help emergency personnel cope with stress is called:
    a. Critical Incident Stress Management.
    b. Emergency Stress Reduction Protocol.
    c. Stress Prevention Strategy.
    d. Incident Emotional Response Program.

12. After caring for a trauma patient, you notice that there is dried blood on your blood pressure cuff. You should:
    a. sterilize the BP cuff prior to further use.
    b. clean the cuff with soap and water and then disinfect.
    c. report the exposure to your supervisor.
    d. throw the cuff away and replace it with a new one.

13. Proper body substance isolation (BSI) precautions should be taken:
    a. for TB and HBV patients only.
    b. for any ill or injured patient.
    c. only for patients who have a known infection.
    d. only for patients who are bleeding.

Endnotes

1. Kent A. Sepkowitz and Leon Eisenberg, "Occupational Deaths among Healthcare Workers," *Emerging Infectious Diseases*, Vol. 11, No. 7 [serial on the Internet], (July 2005). doi:10.3201/eid1107.041038

2. Schonfeld I.S. and Chang C.H., *Occupational health psychology: Work, stress, and health*. New York: Springer Publishing Company, 2017.

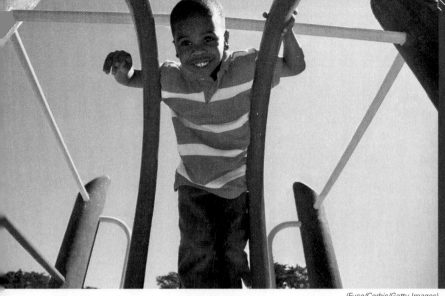

(Fuse/Corbis/Getty Images)

4

Introduction to Medical Terminology, Human Anatomy, and Lifespan Development

LEARNING OBJECTIVES

Upon successful completion of this chapter, the student should be able to:

Cognitive

1. Define the chapter key terms.

2. Apply knowledge of basic medical terminology to interpret common medical terms and conditions.

3. Describe the standard anatomical position and its purpose.

4. Identify the four major body cavities.

5. Describe the major anatomy contained in each of the body cavities.

6. Describe the major anatomical structures and function of the respiratory system.

7. Describe the major anatomical structures and function of the cardiovascular system.

8. Describe the major anatomical structures and function of the musculoskeletal system.

9. Describe the major anatomical structures and function of the nervous system.

10. Describe the major anatomical structures and function of the digestive system.

11. Describe the major anatomical structures and function of the reproductive system.

12. Describe the major anatomical structures and function of the urinary system.

13. Describe the major anatomical structures and function of the skin.

14. Describe the major anatomical structures and function of the endocrine system.

15. Name and describe the phases of lifespan development.

Psychomotor

16. Given an illustration of the human body, properly describe the location of random injuries as presented by the instructor.

Affective

17. Demonstrate an awareness of and respect for cultural differences and diversity with respect to the human body.

18. Value the importance of using standard anatomical and medical terms when describing and documenting illnesses and injuries.

Education Standards

Anatomy and Physiology, Medical Terminology, Pathophysiology, Lifespan Development

Competencies

Uses knowledge of the anatomy and function of the upper airway, heart, vessels, blood, lungs, skin, muscles, and bones as the foundation of emergency care.

Uses medical and anatomical terms.

Uses knowledge of age-related differences to assess and care for patients.

KEY TERMS

abdominal cavity (*p. 64*)

abdominal quadrants (*p. 66*)

anatomical position (*p. 59*)

anatomy (*p. 59*)

anterior (*p. 59*)

cranial cavity (*p. 64*)

distal (*p. 61*)

inferior (*p. 61*)

lateral (*p. 61*)

lateral recumbent (*p. 61*)

medial (*p. 61*)

midline (*p. 61*)

ovulation (*p. 74*)

palpate (*p. 66*)

pelvic cavity (*p. 66*)

perfusion (*p. 67*)

physiology (*p. 62*)

posterior (*p. 59*)

prone (*p. 61*)

proximal (*p. 61*)

superior (*p. 61*)

supine (*p. 61*)

thoracic cavity (*p. 64*)

tidal volume (*p. 69*)

As an Emergency Medical Responder, your ability to provide the most appropriate care for an ill or injured patient depends on your being able to perform a complete and accurate patient assessment. To do so, you must be familiar with human anatomy and physiology and how the body changes throughout an individual's lifespan. You also must know the language used to describe anatomy, along with common medical terminology. This knowledge will make it possible for you to communicate accurately with other health care providers about your patient. It will also help you properly document the care that you provide.

This chapter introduces you to the anatomy of the human body, including its major systems and their basic functions. You'll also learn basic medical terminology and the phases of lifespan development.

 FIRST ON SCENE

"George 14, George 1-4," says the dispatcher, interrupting State Trooper Marnie's cell phone call.

"Go ahead for George 14," Marnie says after quickly ending her call.

"George 14, respond to Highway 4 between Ottoman and West Carlin for a check on the welfare of Adam 9. He was on a traffic stop about four minutes ago, and we can't get a response now."

"Copy." Marnie puts her cruiser into drive and activates the lights and siren. "George 14 responding from Okalusa Drive and Southwest 14th." She realizes her stomach is tight, and she's feeling nauseated as she covers the distance to Eric's location.

He was having radio trouble earlier in the day, so she thinks it's probably nothing. Then again, the department has been making an increasing number of drug-related arrests now that summer is here, and the lake is attracting visitors at a record pace. She forces herself to focus on the road ahead as she travels along Highway 4.

Cresting the hill just past the West Carlin exit, she sees a patrol car on the shoulder of the highway, takedown lights still flashing but nothing else—no other vehicles, no movement, and no police officer. As she pulls up to the empty, idling car, her stomach drops. She has to force her hand to stop trembling as she grabs the radio mic. Eric lies on the side of the road, not moving.

Medical Terminology

LO2 Apply knowledge of basic medical terminology to interpret common medical terms.

Every profession has its own language. It consists of a unique set of terms, jargon, and phrases that must be learned to ensure clear, concise, and efficient communication among all members. Medical terminology is a very specialized language used by medical professionals. You might be surprised to discover how much of it you already know. Thanks to movies and television and the popularity of medical reality programs, many of us hear this language nearly every day.

One of the first steps in your journey to become an Emergency Medical Responder is to learn the language of medicine. This chapter provides a general overview of common terms used in medicine. Once you begin caring for patients and experience how these terms are used during patient care, it will become much easier to remember them.

There are two categories of anatomical terms:

- Descriptive terms describe shape, size, color, and function.
- Eponyms honor the individual who first discovered or described an anatomical structure or developed a procedure or instrument. For example, the fallopian tubes are the structures that connect the uterus to the ovaries. They are named after the 16th-century Italian anatomist Gabriello Fallopio.

There are three basic parts to many descriptive medical terms—the root, the prefix, and the suffix. We can use the medical term *myocarditis* as an example:

Prefix: **myo** = muscle
Root: **card** = heart
Suffix: **itis** = inflammation

By understanding the prefix, root, and suffix, you can determine that *myocarditis* means inflammation of the heart muscle.

Table 4.1 lists some common medical word roots. It is not essential that you memorize them all. However, the more you learn, the more you will understand about your patients' conditions and ailments. Notice that some words have two roots. This is because some have both a Latin and a Greek origin.

Tables 4.2 and 4.3 list common prefixes and suffixes. They are just a small sampling of the prefixes and suffixes that make up the world of medical terminology. You do not have to memorize them all, but learning some will ensure a good head start on building your medical vocabulary.

> **REMEMBER**
>
> Medical terminology can be confusing and sometimes intimidating. It is more important that your description is understood than it is to try to impress the listener. If you are speaking to a patient, their family, or even a fellow provider who may not have your level of knowledge, using medical terminology does not improve your care. If you are not sure of the proper medical term to use, there is no shame in using common terms to describe your findings.

Positional and Directional Terms

LO3 Describe the standard anatomical position and its purpose.

The following are some basic terms that may be used to refer to the human body (Figure 4.1):

- *Anatomical position.* Whenever you describe anything related to human **anatomy**, the location of injuries, or related signs and symptoms, it is always assumed that the patient is in what is called **anatomical position** or standard anatomical position. In this position, the patient is standing upright, facing forward with arms down at the sides, and the palms of the hands turned forward. References to all body structures and locations assume that the body is in this position.
- *Right and left.* When referring to the human body, right and left are always described as seen from the patient's perspective. Even though you may think this is simple, it is easy to get confused and make references to your own left and right.
- *Anterior and posterior.* The term **anterior** refers to the front of the body, and **posterior** refers to the back of the body.

anatomy ▶ the study of body structure.

anatomical position ▶ standard reference position for the body in the study of anatomy; the body is standing upright (erect), facing the observer, arms are down at the sides, and the palms of the hands are facing forward.

anterior ▶ front of the body or body part.

posterior ▶ back of the body or body part.

TABLE 4.1 Common Medical Word Roots

Root	Meaning	Example
stomat	mouth	stomatitis (inflammation of the lining of the mouth)
dent	teeth	dentist
gloss/lingu	tongue	glossitis (inflammation of the tongue), lingual nerve
gingiv	gums	gingivitis (inflammation of the gums)
encephal	brain	encephalitis (inflammation of the brain)
gastr	stomach	gastritis (inflammation of the stomach)
enter	intestine	gastroenteritis (inflammation of the lining of the stomach and intestines)
col	large intestine	colitis (inflammation of the colon)
proct	anus/rectum	proctitis (inflammation of the rectum)
hepat	liver	hepatitis (inflammation of the liver)
nephr/rene	kidney	nephritis, renal artery (inflammation of the kidney)
orchid	testis	orchiditis (inflammation of the testes)
oophor	ovary	oophoritis (inflammation of an ovary)
hyster	uterus	hysterectomy (removal of the uterus)
derm	skin	dermatitis (inflammation of the skin)
mast/mamm	breast	mammography (image of the breast)
oste	bones	osteoporosis (disease that causes weakening of the bones)
cardi	heart	electrocardiogram (ECG) (electrical tracing of the heart)
cyst	bladder	cystitis (inflammation of the bladder)
rhin	nose	rhinitis (inflammation of the nasal membranes)
phleb/ven	veins	phlebitis (inflammation of a vein)
pneum/pulm	lung	pneumonitis (inflammation of a lung)
hem/emia	blood	hematoma (localized swelling caused by blood)

TABLE 4.2 Common Medical Word Prefixes

Prefix	Meaning	Example
arterio-	artery	arteriosclerosis (hardening of the arteries)
brady-	slow	bradycardia (slow heart rate)
cardio-	heart	electrocardiogram (ECG)
hemo-	blood	hematology (the study of the blood)
hyper-	over, above, beyond	hyperglycemia (high blood sugar levels)
hypo-	below, under	hypothermia (low body core temperature)
naso-	nose	nasopharyngeal airway (airway placed in the nose)
neuro-	nerve	neuropathy (disease of the nervous system)
oro-	mouth	oropharyngeal airway (airway placed in the mouth)
tachy-	rapid	tachycardia (rapid heart rate)
thermo-	heat	thermometer (instrument for measuring temperature)
vaso-	blood vessel	vasoconstriction (constriction of the blood vessels)

TABLE 4.3 **Common Medical Word Suffixes**

Suffix	Meaning	Example
-ectomy	to cut out, remove	appendectomy (removal of the appendix)
-emia	blood	anemia (deficiency of red blood cells)
-graphy/graph	recording an image	mammography (X-ray of the soft tissue of the breast)
-gram	the image (X-ray)	mammogram
-itis	inflammation	tonsillitis (inflammation of the tonsils)
-ology/ologist	to study, specialize in	cardiologist (physician who specializes in diseases of the heart and cardiovascular system)
-osis	abnormal condition	cyanosis (bluish coloration of the skin)
-ostomy	to make an opening	colostomy (a surgical opening in the colon)
-otomy	to cut into	tracheotomy (surgical hole placed in the trachea)
-scopy/scopic	to look, observe	colonoscopy (examination of the inner colon)

Note: The suffixes -graphy, -graph, and -gram are very common and generally refer to the recording of a diagnostic image such as an X-ray, ultrasound, CT scan, or MRI scan.

- *Midline.* The **midline** is an imaginary vertical line that divides the body into right and left halves. Anything toward the midline is said to be **medial**. Anything away from the midline is said to be **lateral**. For example, when considering the anatomical position with the palms forward, the thumbs can be described as being on the lateral (away from midline) side of the hand.

midline ▸ imaginary vertical line used to divide the body into right and left halves.

medial ▸ toward the midline of the body.

lateral ▸ to the side, away from the midline of the body.

Other directional terms are also useful. **Superior** means toward the top of the head, as in "the eyes are superior to the nose." **Inferior** means toward the feet, as in "the mouth is inferior to the nose." Superior and inferior are usually reserved for structures in the head, neck, and torso. Note that you cannot say something is superior or inferior unless you are comparing at least two points of reference, for example, the heart is superior to the stomach. Because you are using the anatomical position for all your references to the body, most medical professionals will understand what you mean when you say a wound is just above the right eye. For this reason, terms such as *superior* and *inferior* may be optional.

superior ▸ toward the head.

inferior ▸ toward the feet.

Proximal and *distal* are most commonly used to describe anatomy related to the limbs. You must have a point of reference and two structures that can be compared. The point closest to the torso is said to be **proximal**, while the point farthest away is **distal**. Thus, the elbow is proximal (closer to the torso) to the wrist and the hand is distal (farther from the torso) to the wrist. The knee is proximal to the ankle, and the foot is distal to the ankle. Trying to remember all this in an emergency situation can be confusing. Take the opportunity to use the classroom setting to practice the proper use of these terms.

proximal ▸ closer to the torso.

distal ▸ farther away from the torso.

In addition to directional terms, there are specific positional terms with which you should become familiar (Figure 4.2A–F). Positional terms include the following:

- **Supine** means lying face up.
- **Prone** means lying face down.
- The **lateral recumbent** position, also called the recovery position, means lying on one's side.
- Semi-Fowler's position refers to the patient sitting up at an angle.
- Trendelenburg position refers to the patient lying supine on a firm surface such as a bed or backboard with the foot end higher than the head.
- Shock position refers to the patient lying supine with feet elevated. Legs will be bent at the hips.

supine ▸ patient is lying face up.

prone ▸ patient is lying face down.

lateral recumbent ▸ patient is lying on their side, also called *recovery position*.

Figure 4.1 Common anatomical terms of direction.

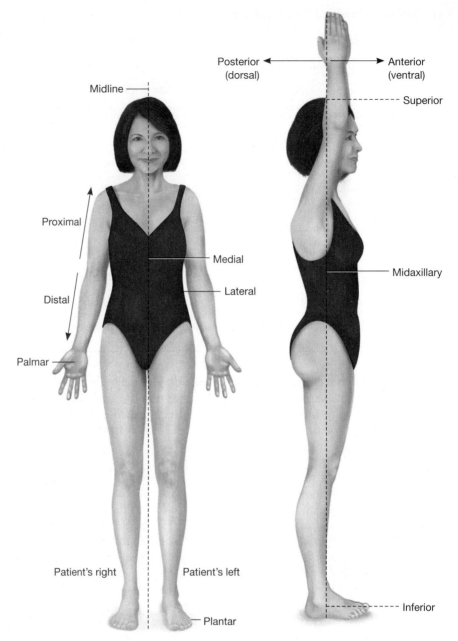

Posterior (dorsal) ← → Anterior (ventral)

Midline

Superior

Proximal

Medial

Lateral

Midaxillary

Distal

Palmar

Patient's right | Patient's left

Plantar

Inferior

Documentation of the patient's position may be of medical significance and also may become part of the legal record of how a patient was first found. As with directional terms, positional terms should be learned and practiced so they become part of your normal vocabulary and documentation.

Most Emergency Medical Responders do not deal with emergencies on a daily basis. Unless you review and use anatomical terms often, you may forget them over time. Be aware that medical and rescue personnel are trained to take your information. They will not be confused if you use terms such as *front, back, above,* and *below.* Never let terminology stand in the way of clear communication with EMS providers, physicians, and other medical professionals.

Overview of the Human Body

Human anatomy refers to the structure of the human body. **Physiology** refers to the function of the body and its many systems. Students beginning training in Emergency Medical Responder courses are often a little worried about having to learn anatomy and

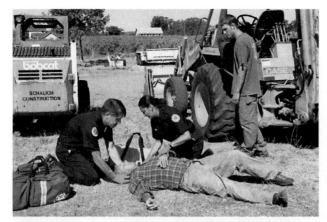

Figure 4.2A A patient lying in the supine position.

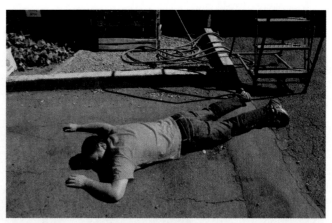

Figure 4.2B A patient lying in the prone position.

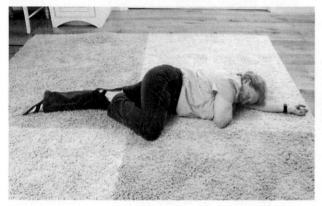

Figure 4.2C A patient placed in the lateral recumbent (recovery) position.

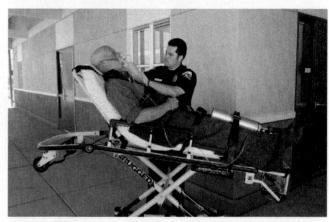

Figure 4.2D A patient placed in the semi-Fowler's position.

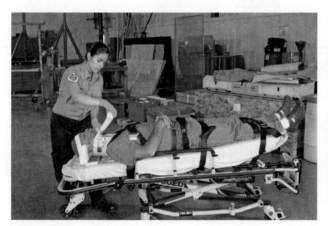

Figure 4.2E A patient placed in the Trendelenburg position.

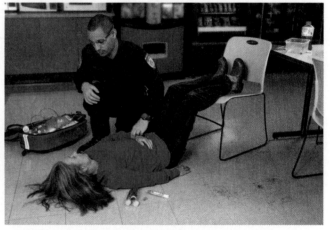

Figure 4.2F A patient placed in the shock position.

physiology. Don't be. As an Emergency Medical Responder, you must know basic body structures but not in as much detail as more highly trained medical personnel.

Regions of the Body

To be an Emergency Medical Responder, you must be able to look at an individual's body and know the major internal structures and the general location of each (Figure 4.3). Your concern is not how a dissected body looks or how the body looks on an anatomical wall chart. You must be concerned with living bodies and knowing generally where things are located as you look from the outside.

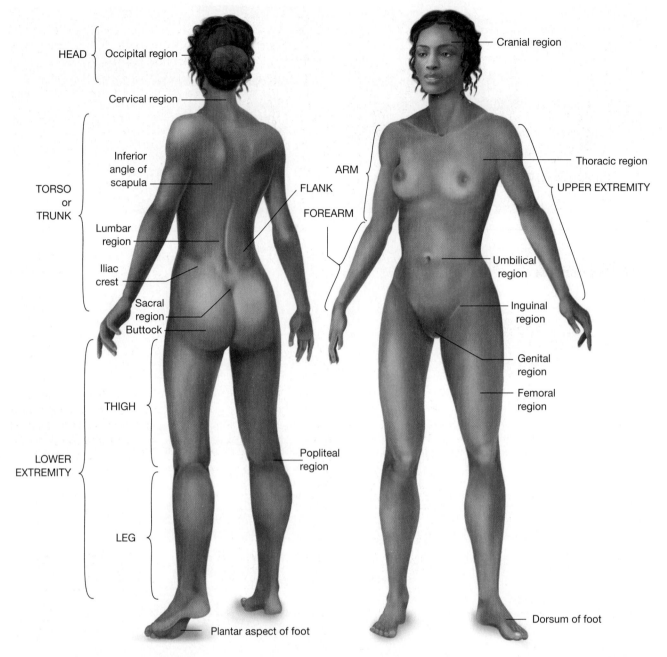

Figure 4.3 Anatomical body regions.

Body Cavities

LO4 Identify the four major body cavities.

LO5 Describe the anatomy contained in each of the body cavities.

There are four major body cavities: cranial, thoracic, abdominal, and pelvic (Figure 4.4). Housed in these cavities are the major organs (Key Skill 4.1), blood vessels, and nerves.

cranial cavity ▸ space inside the skull that houses the brain.

thoracic cavity ▸ anterior body cavity that is above (superior to) the diaphragm, also called the *chest cavity*.

abdominal cavity ▸ anterior body cavity that extends from the diaphragm to the pelvic cavity.

- *Cranial cavity.* The **cranial cavity** houses the brain and its specialized membranes.
- *Thoracic cavity.* The **thoracic cavity**, also known as the chest cavity, is enclosed by the rib cage (Figure 4.5). It holds and protects the lungs, heart, aorta and vena cava, part of the trachea (windpipe), and part of the esophagus. The diaphragm is the muscle that separates the chest cavity from the abdominal cavity.
- *Abdominal cavity.* The **abdominal cavity** lies between the chest and the pelvic cavities. The stomach, liver, gallbladder, pancreas, spleen, small intestine, and most

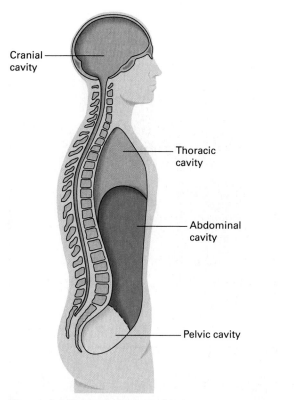

Figure 4.4 The main body cavities.

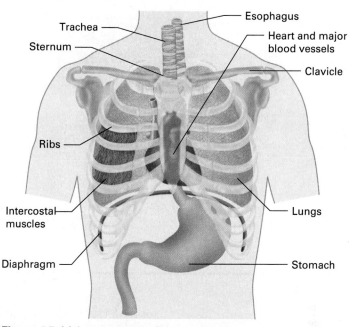

Figure 4.5 Major structures of the chest cavity.

Understanding the Major Body Organs

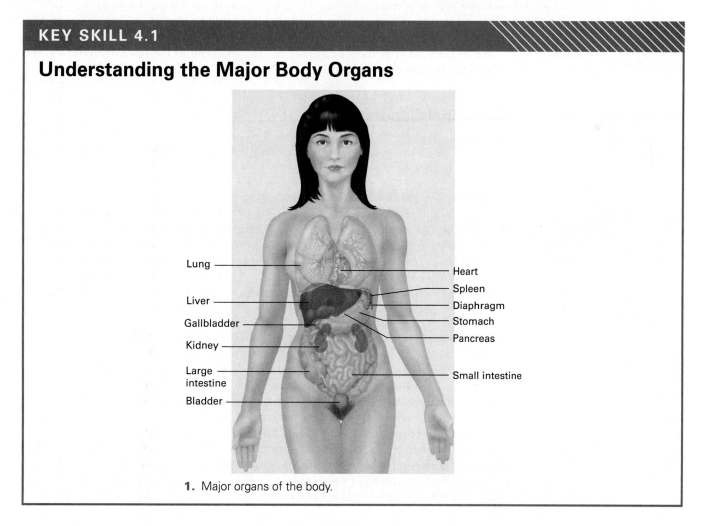

1. Major organs of the body.

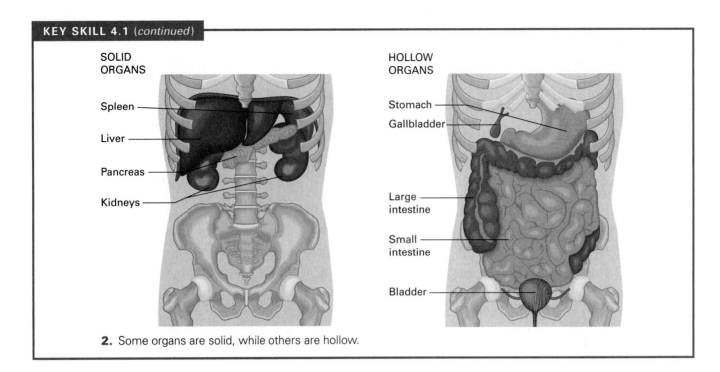

SOLID
ORGANS

Spleen

Liver

Pancreas

Kidneys

HOLLOW
ORGANS

Stomach

Gallbladder

Large
intestine

Small
intestine

Bladder

2. Some organs are solid, while others are hollow.

of the large intestine (colon) can be found in the abdominal cavity. Unlike other body cavities, the abdominal cavity is not surrounded by bones. If you consider the major organs in this cavity and the lack of bony protection, it is easy to see why trauma to the abdomen can result in severe injury.

- *Pelvic cavity.* The **pelvic cavity** is protected by the bones of the pelvis or pelvic girdle. This cavity houses the urinary bladder, portions of the large intestine, and the internal reproductive organs.

pelvic cavity ▶ anterior body cavity surrounded by the bones of the pelvis.

Abdominal Quadrants

The abdomen is a large body region that contains many vital organs. The umbilicus (navel) is the main point of reference when describing the abdomen, which is divided into four **abdominal quadrants** (Figure 4.6):

- *Right upper quadrant (RUQ).* Contains most of the liver, the gallbladder, and part of the small and large intestines.
- *Left upper quadrant (LUQ).* Contains most of the stomach, the spleen, part of the small and large intestines, and part of the liver.
- *Right lower quadrant (RLQ).* Contains the appendix, part of the small and large intestines, and the urinary bladder.
- *Left lower quadrant (LLQ).* Contains part of the small and large intestines and the urinary bladder.

Some organs are located in more than one quadrant, as you can see from the preceding list. Pelvic organs are also included in these quadrants.

When assessing a patient's abdominal area, be sure to **palpate** the soft areas of the abdomen on the patient's posterior (back) side, as well. These areas are located superior to (above) the iliac crest. Use three fingers to press in firmly on these soft areas to attempt to elicit a painful response. This area contains the kidneys and is susceptible to injury because it is not protected by bone. The kidneys are not contained within the abdominal cavity because they are located behind a membrane that lines the cavity. The location of the kidneys makes them subject to injury from blows to the midback. Any pain or ache in the back may involve the kidneys. The abdominal aorta and vena cava are two major vessels that are also located behind this membrane.

> **REMEMBER**
>
> Because the pelvic and abdominal cavities do not have any structure that separates them, we generally speak of the abdominopelvic cavity because some of the abdominal organs, such as the large and small intestines, extend into the pelvis. Likewise, the pregnant uterus extends into the abdominal cavity.

abdominal quadrants ▶ four divisions of the abdomen used to pinpoint the location of pain or injury: right upper quadrant (RUQ), left upper quadrant (LUQ), right lower quadrant (RLQ), and left lower quadrant (LLQ).

palpate ▶ to examine by feeling with one's hands.

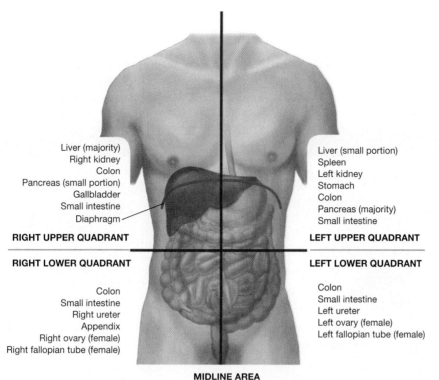

Figure 4.6 The four abdominal quadrants and associated anatomy.

Liver (majority)
Right kidney
Colon
Pancreas (small portion)
Gallbladder
Small intestine
Diaphragm

RIGHT UPPER QUADRANT

Liver (small portion)
Spleen
Left kidney
Stomach
Colon
Pancreas (majority)
Small intestine

LEFT UPPER QUADRANT

RIGHT LOWER QUADRANT

LEFT LOWER QUADRANT

Colon
Small intestine
Right ureter
Appendix
Right ovary (female)
Right fallopian tube (female)

Colon
Small intestine
Left ureter
Left ovary (female)
Left fallopian tube (female)

MIDLINE AREA
Bladder - Uterus (female) - Prostate (male)

Body Systems

Now that you have been introduced to some common anatomical terms, it is time to explore the anatomy and physiology (essential processes, activities, and functions) of each major body system. Throughout this text, specific anatomy and some basic functions are covered as they apply to illness, injury, and Emergency Medical Responder care.

 FIRST ON SCENE *(continued)*

"Eric!" Marnie drops to her knees in the dirt next to her colleague, pulls on a pair of gloves, and tears open his bloody uniform shirt. There is a perfectly round hole in his chest just below the right nipple, and blood is dripping steadily from the wound. She rolls him onto his side to check his back and he moans, grabbing weakly at her arms. There is a large, ragged hole just below his right shoulder blade, and blood is bubbling thickly out onto the ground.

She grabs her portable radio and keys the mic. "Control, George 14, officer down, I repeat, officer down. Adam 9 has

been shot. I need you to let the responding ambulance know that Adam 9 has an entrance wound just inferior to the right nipple and an exit wound just medial to the right shoulder blade. He is responsive to pain and has noisy breathing. I don't see anything else."

Marnie drops the radio and runs back to her patrol car to grab the first aid kit. She places an occlusive dressing over both wounds and applies steady pressure the best she can. "Help is on the way Eric, hang in there," Marnie states, trying to keep the panic from showing through in her voice.

To function properly, all body systems must have adequate **perfusion**, which is the supply of well-oxygenated blood and nutrients to all body systems and the removal of cellular waste. When a body system stops functioning properly due to inadequate perfusion such as from an illness or injury, it becomes less efficient and eventually will fail completely. It can have an immediate and often life-threatening effect on the rest of the body. The term *pathophysiology* refers to the abnormal function of the body or one of its systems due to disease or injury.

perfusion ▶ circulation of blood through tissues.

Respiratory System

LO6 Describe the major anatomical structures and function of the respiratory system.

The primary structures associated with the respiratory system include the nasopharynx (nose), oropharynx (mouth), trachea, lungs, bronchi, bronchioles, alveoli, and associated muscles related to breathing (Key Skill 4.2). The respiratory system is primarily responsible

---

KEY SKILL 4.2

Understanding the Respiratory System

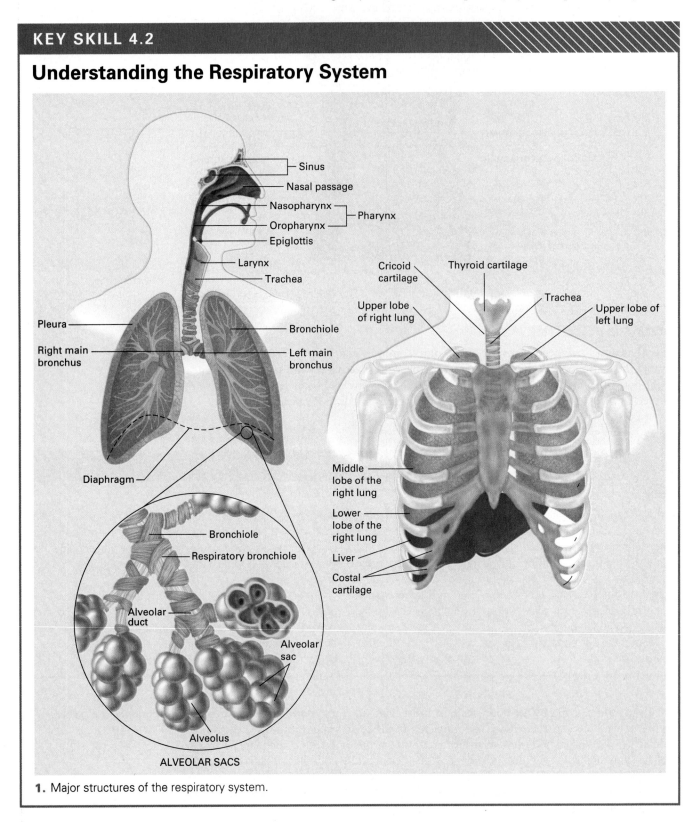

1. Major structures of the respiratory system.

for the exchange of oxygen and carbon dioxide. It also warms, filters, and moisturizes air as it enters the body. In addition, structures such as the epiglottis help minimize the possibility of choking by blocking off the opening of the trachea when we swallow.

The respiratory system is divided into two sections: the upper and lower respiratory tracts. The upper tract consists of the nose, mouth, pharynx, and larynx. All structures of the upper tract are located outside of the chest cavity.

The lower respiratory tract consists of the trachea and the bronchi, bronchioles, alveoli (air sacs), and connective tissues of the lungs. The diaphragm is the primary muscle of respiration and contracts and relaxes to move air in and out of the lungs.

Respirations are normally controlled by the autonomic nervous system through signals originating deep within the brain stem. Specialized receptors located in the aorta and carotid arteries measure the level of carbon dioxide (CO_2) and will cause an increase in respiratory rate when carbon dioxide levels increase.

After air enters the body through the nose and mouth, it passes down the trachea and enters the lungs through the right and left bronchi. From there, the air passes through smaller passages called bronchioles and eventually ends up at the alveoli. It is deep within the lungs at the alveoli that the exchange of oxygen and carbon dioxide takes place. Perfusion can be adversely affected if the patient is not able to take in adequate amounts of oxygen or eliminate carbon dioxide.

Numerous diseases can affect the respiratory system. Many disrupt the delivery of oxygen all the way down to the alveoli. When this happens, blood circulates but the body systems that rely on a fresh supply of oxygen begin to fail.

Trauma can also affect respiratory system function. When the chest wall becomes damaged or a lung collapses, the **tidal volume** (the, amount of air that can be taken in) is decreased. If the injury is not cared for promptly, other body systems become starved for oxygen and will eventually fail.

tidal volume ▶ amount of air being moved in and out of the lungs with each breath.

Cardiovascular System

LO7 Describe the major anatomical structures and function of the cardiovascular system.

The primary components of the cardiovascular system are the heart, blood vessels, and blood (Key Skill 4.3). There are two pathways within the cardiovascular system. The arterial system carries oxygenated blood to the body, and the venous system returns deoxygenated blood to the heart and lungs. The main jobs of the cardiovascular system are to carry blood and other nutrients to the body's cells and assist with the removal of wastes and carbon dioxide from the cells.

The heart is a hollow, muscular organ that pumps approximately 55 million gallons of blood in the average lifetime. Its two upper chambers are the atria, and the two lower chambers are the ventricles.

The right atrium receives deoxygenated blood from the body. The blood is then moved into the right ventricle before it is pumped to the lungs, where it passes off carbon dioxide and receives oxygen. The oxygenated blood then returns to the left atrium before being pumped into the left ventricle. The left ventricle is the largest and strongest chamber of the heart and pumps blood out of the heart and to the rest of the body.

The myocardium (heart muscle) receives its blood supply by way of the coronary arteries. When the coronary arteries become blocked, a heart attack can occur.

All three components of the cardiovascular system (heart, vessels, blood) must be functioning properly to maintain good perfusion. First and foremost, there must be an adequate supply of blood within the system. Damaged tissues and open wounds can cause life-threatening bleeding. Next, the blood vessels must remain intact and functioning normally (constricting and dilating). The function of blood vessels can be affected by both illness and injury. Last, the heart, which serves as the pump for the whole system, must be functioning normally. It must be pumping at a good rate and with enough force to maintain adequate blood pressure. The heart's function can be affected by both illness and injury, thus causing poor perfusion.

Understanding the Cardiovascular System

Cardiovascular System

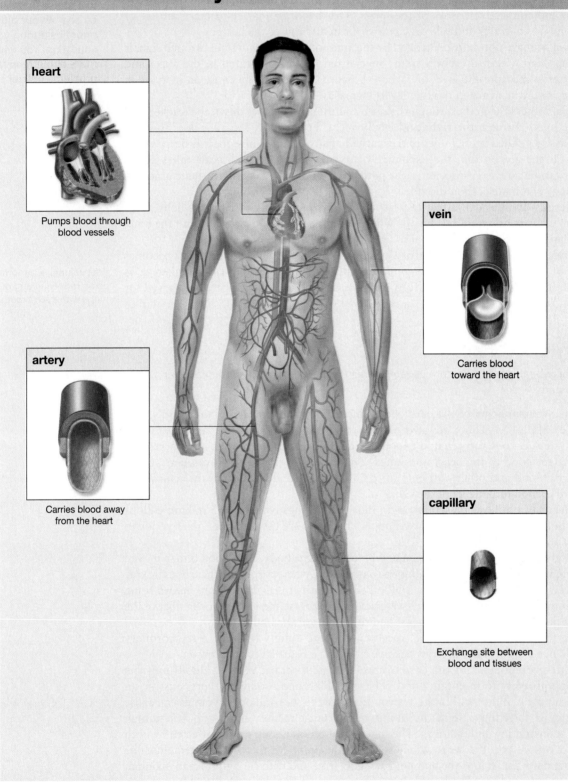

heart

Pumps blood through blood vessels

vein

Carries blood toward the heart

artery

Carries blood away from the heart

capillary

Exchange site between blood and tissues

1. The cardiovascular system.

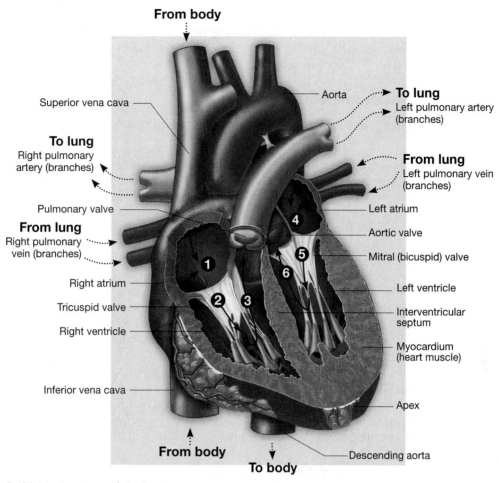

From body

Superior vena cava

Aorta

To lung
Left pulmonary artery
(branches)

To lung
Right pulmonary
artery (branches)

From lung
Left pulmonary vein
(branches)

Pulmonary valve

From lung
Right pulmonary
vein (branches)

Left atrium

Aortic valve

Mitral (bicuspid) valve

Right atrium

Left ventricle

Tricuspid valve

Interventricular
septum

Right ventricle

Myocardium
(heart muscle)

Inferior vena cava

Apex

From body

Descending aorta

To body

2. Major structures of the heart.

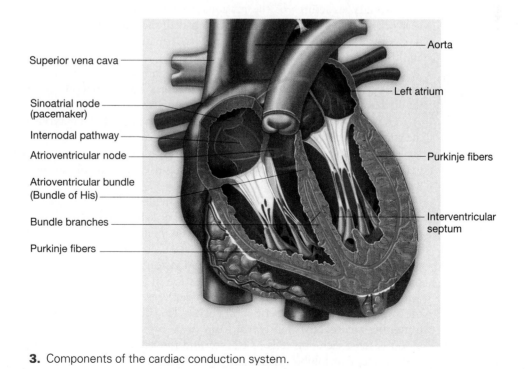

Superior vena cava

Aorta

Left atrium

Sinoatrial node
(pacemaker)

Internodal pathway

Atrioventricular node

Purkinje fibers

Atrioventricular bundle
(Bundle of His)

Bundle branches

Interventricular
septum

Purkinje fibers

3. Components of the cardiac conduction system.

Chapter 4 Introduction to Medical Terminology, Human Anatomy, and Lifespan Development **71**

Arteries are blood vessels that carry blood away from the heart. Arteries have strong muscular walls and are very elastic. They are able to change their diameter depending on the circumstances. The smallest arteries are called arterioles.

Veins are blood vessels that carry blood back to the heart. The walls of veins are not as thick or elastic as those of arteries. Some veins have valves to prevent the backward flow of blood. The smallest veins are called venules.

Musculoskeletal System

LO8 | Describe the major anatomical structures and function of the musculoskeletal system.

The primary structures of the musculoskeletal system are bones, muscles, tendons, and ligaments (Key Skills 4.4 and 4.5). The main function of this system is to provide structure, support, and protection for the body and internal organs and allow for body movement. In addition, the bone marrow of the skeletal system is responsible for producing stem cells that become blood cells and platelets.

There are 206 bones in the adult body. Our skeletal system is divided into the axial and appendicular sections. The axial skeleton comprises the skull, vertebrae, rib cage, and sternum. The appendicular skeleton is made up of the upper and lower extremities and the shoulder and pelvic girdles. A joint is the junction of two or more bones. Ligaments are tough, fibrous tissues that surround a joint to provide support and connect bone to bone.

The tissues of the muscular system constitute 40 to 50 percent of our body's weight. The skeletal muscles of the body are voluntary muscles, subject to conscious control. They exhibit the properties of excitability, that is, they react to nerve stimulus. Once stimulated, skeletal muscles are quick to contract and relax and can instantaneously be ready for another contraction. There are approximately 650 separate skeletal muscles, which provide contractions for movement, coordinated support for posture, and heat production. Muscles connect to bones by way of tendons. Common injuries to muscles include strains, sprains, and tears. We will talk more about these injuries in Chapter 20.

Nervous System

LO9 | Describe the major anatomical structures and function of the nervous system.

The primary structures of the nervous system include the brain, spinal cord, and the network of nerves that extend out to all parts of the body (Key Skill 4.6). Its main function is to control movement, interpret sensations, regulate body activities, and generate memory and thought.

The nervous system is divided into two sections: central and peripheral. The central nervous system includes the brain and spinal cord. The peripheral nervous system includes the sensory (incoming) and motor (outgoing) nerves.

The autonomic nervous system is the part of the peripheral nervous system that acts as the control system for most of the involuntary processes such as heart rate, respiratory rate, digestion, perspiration, and salivation. You can think of the autonomic nervous system as the "automatic" system. It does not require conscious control but instead is designed to work alone or autonomously.

The autonomic nervous system is further divided into the sympathetic (quick response) and parasympathetic (slow control) systems. The sympathetic division is responsible for the fight-or-flight response that releases adrenalin (epinephrine) for sudden survival responses such as increased heart and respiratory rates, improved near vision, and sweating to promote heat loss. The parasympathetic division works to maintain the body's normal status and controls functions such as digestion of food and elimination of waste.

The autonomic nervous system has structures that parallel the spinal cord and share the same pathways as the peripheral nerves. This division is involved with motor impulses (outgoing commands) that travel from the central nervous system to the heart muscle, blood vessels, secreting cells of glands, and the smooth muscles of organs. The impulses will stimulate or inhibit certain activities. Damage to the spinal cord or nerves can affect the transmission of these impulses and disrupt normal body functions.

Understanding the Skeletal System

Skeletal System

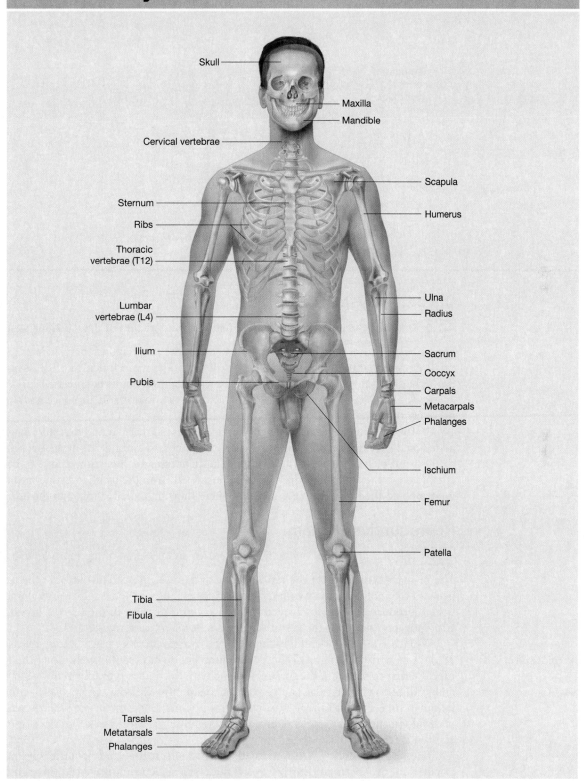

Skull

Maxilla

Mandible

Cervical vertebrae

Scapula

Sternum

Humerus

Ribs

Thoracic vertebrae (T12)

Ulna

Radius

Lumbar vertebrae (L4)

Ilium

Sacrum

Coccyx

Pubis

Carpals

Metacarpals

Phalanges

Ischium

Femur

Patella

Tibia

Fibula

Tarsals

Metatarsals

Phalanges

1. Major structures of the skeletal system.

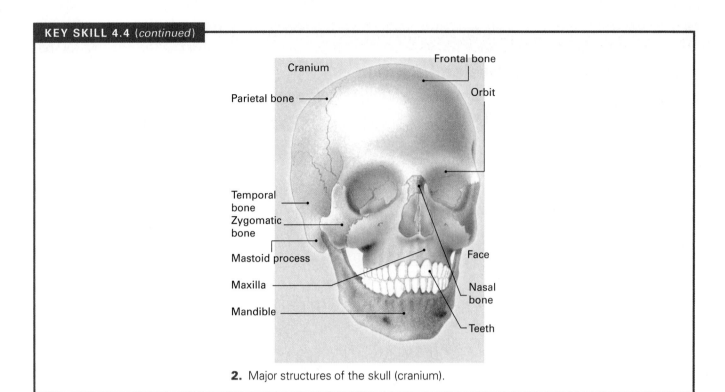

2. Major structures of the skull (cranium).

Digestive System

LO10 Describe the major anatomical structures and function of the digestive system.

The primary structures of the digestive system are the esophagus, stomach, liver, pancreas, small intestine, and large intestine (Key Skill 4.7). The main function of this system is to properly digest the food we eat so it can be absorbed through the intestines and used for energy for our cells. The digestive system also plays a major role in the removal of waste products from the body.

As food begins to travel through the digestive system, acid and digestive enzymes are added to the food. Digestive enzymes from the pancreas and bile from the liver are added as the food passes through the system. The processes of digestion and absorption are completed in the small intestine. Wastes are carried from the small intestine into the large intestine and then moved to the rectum, where they are expelled through the anus.

Reproductive System

LO11 Describe the major anatomical structures and function of the reproductive system.

The primary structures of the reproductive system (Key Skill 4.8) include the testes and penis in the male and the ovaries, fallopian tubes, uterus, and vagina in the female. This system produces hormones needed for sexual reproduction. In the female, it contains the structures necessary for the gestation and development of a fetus.

ovulation ▶ discharge of eggs from an ovary.

When a female is of childbearing age, the ovaries produce eggs that are released every 28 days as part of a process called **ovulation.** The ovum (egg) travels along the fallopian tube. During conception, the sperm meets up with the ovum, typically in the fallopian tube, and fertilization occurs. Once fertilized, the ovum, now called a zygote, travels through the fallopian tube and into the uterus, where it implants along the inside wall. After 2 weeks of development, the zygote is referred to as an embryo. After week 9 of development, the embryo is referred to as a fetus.

The testes (testicles) are contained within the scrotum and produce sperm. During ejaculation, the sperm are carried in a fluid called semen that is ejected through the erect penis during intercourse. Eventually, the sperm meet up with the ovum and fertilization may take place.

Understanding the Muscular System

Muscular System

- Masseter
- Sternocleidomastoid
- Deltoid
- Pectoralis major
- Triceps
- Biceps
- Rectus abdominis
- External oblique
- Sartorius
- Adductor femoris
- Quadriceps femoris
- Vastus medialis
- Gastrocnemius
- Tibialis anterior

1. The muscular system.

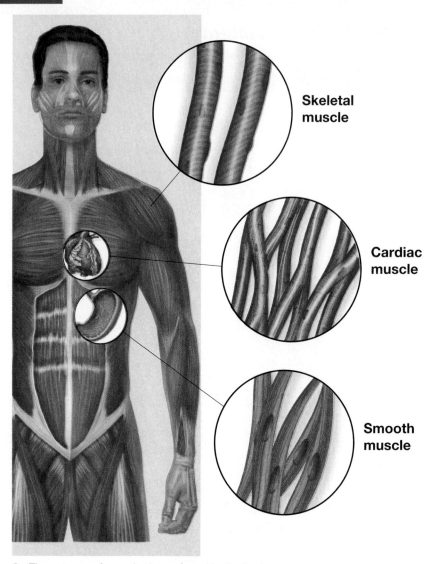

2. Three types of muscle tissue found in the body.

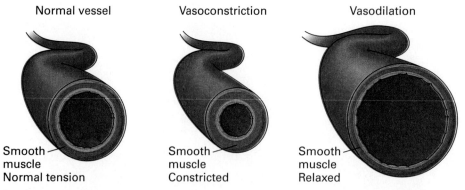

Normal vessel   Vasoconstriction   Vasodilation

Smooth
muscle
Normal tension

Smooth
muscle
Constricted

Smooth
muscle
Relaxed

3. Blood vessels are constructed of smooth muscle, which is capable of constricting
(getting smaller) and dilating (getting larger).

Understanding the Nervous System

Nervous System

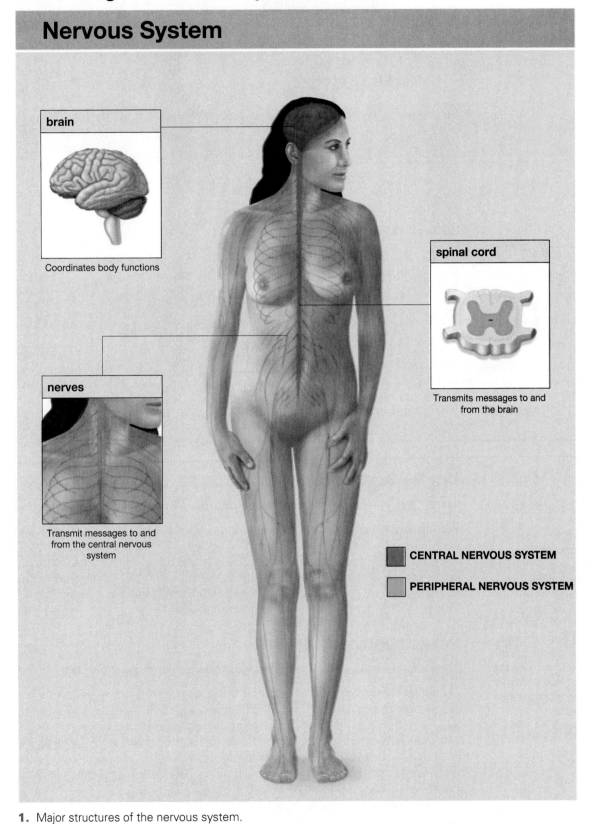

brain

Coordinates body functions

spinal cord

Transmits messages to and from the brain

nerves

Transmit messages to and from the central nervous system

■ CENTRAL NERVOUS SYSTEM

□ PERIPHERAL NERVOUS SYSTEM

1. Major structures of the nervous system.

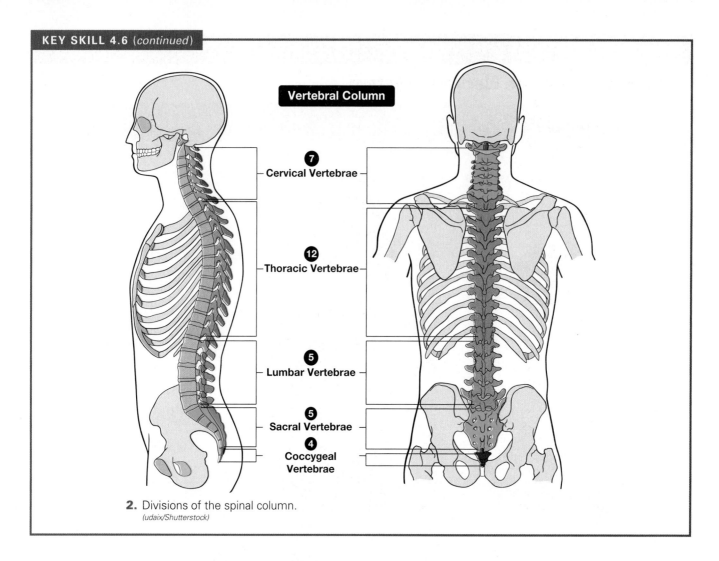

Vertebral Column

7 Cervical Vertebrae

12 Thoracic Vertebrae

5 Lumbar Vertebrae

5 Sacral Vertebrae

4 Coccygeal Vertebrae

2. Divisions of the spinal column.
(udaix/Shutterstock)

Urinary System

LO12 Describe the major anatomical structures and function of the urinary system.

The primary structures of the urinary system are the kidneys, ureters, bladder, and urethra (Key Skill 4.9). The main function of this system is to remove chemical wastes from the body and help balance water and salt levels in the blood. This waste is moved from the kidneys to the urinary bladder by way of a pair of small tube-like structures called ureters. A similar structure called a urethra extends from the bladder to the outside of the body. This allows for the removal of the urine from the body.

Integumentary System

LO13 Describe the major anatomical structures and function of the skin.

The integumentary system includes all the layers of the skin, nails, hair, sweat glands, oil glands, and mammary glands. The skin (Key Skill 4.10) is the largest organ of the body. In the average adult, the skin covers more than 22 square feet and weighs approximately 8 pounds. It protects the body from heat and cold as well as from toxins in the environment, such as bacteria and other foreign organisms. It regulates body temperature and senses heat, cold, touch, pain, and pressure. It also regulates body fluids and chemical balance.

The skin is composed of three layers:

- *Epidermis.* This is the outermost layer of skin where most of the nerve sensors are located.

JEDI

A thorough physical exam should be completed on every patient, regardless of their presenting gender. There are many nonbinary and transgender individuals whose anatomy and gender expression may differ from the descriptions and images presented in this textbook. To provide the best and most inclusive patient care, all patients should receive a full physical exam.

Understanding the Digestive System

Digestive System

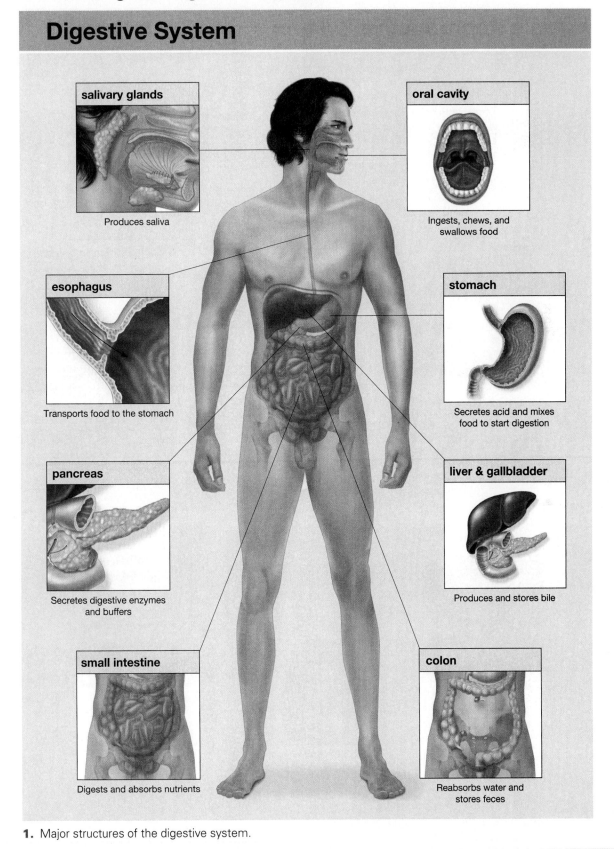

salivary glands
Produces saliva

oral cavity
Ingests, chews, and swallows food

esophagus
Transports food to the stomach

stomach
Secretes acid and mixes food to start digestion

pancreas
Secretes digestive enzymes and buffers

liver & gallbladder
Produces and stores bile

small intestine
Digests and absorbs nutrients

colon
Reabsorbs water and stores feces

1. Major structures of the digestive system.

Understanding the Reproductive System

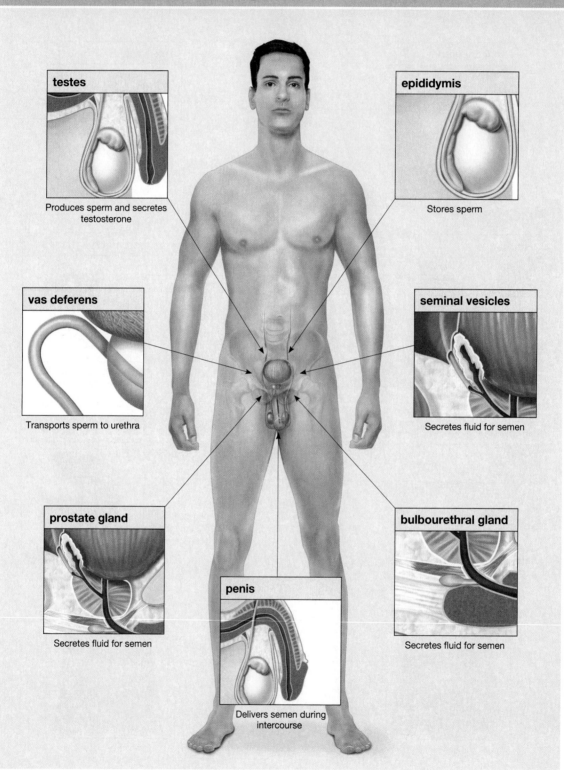

Male Reproductive System

testes
Produces sperm and secretes testosterone

epididymis
Stores sperm

vas deferens
Transports sperm to urethra

seminal vesicles
Secretes fluid for semen

prostate gland
Secretes fluid for semen

penis
Delivers semen during intercourse

bulbourethral gland
Secretes fluid for semen

1. Major structures of the male reproductive system.

Female Reproductive System

breast

Produces milk

uterus

Site of development of fetus

fallopian tube

Transports ovum to uterus

ovary

Produces ova and secretes estrogen and progesterone

vagina

Receives semen during intercourse; birth canal

vulva

Protects vaginal orifice and urinary meatus

2. Major structures of the female reproductive system.

Understanding the Urinary System

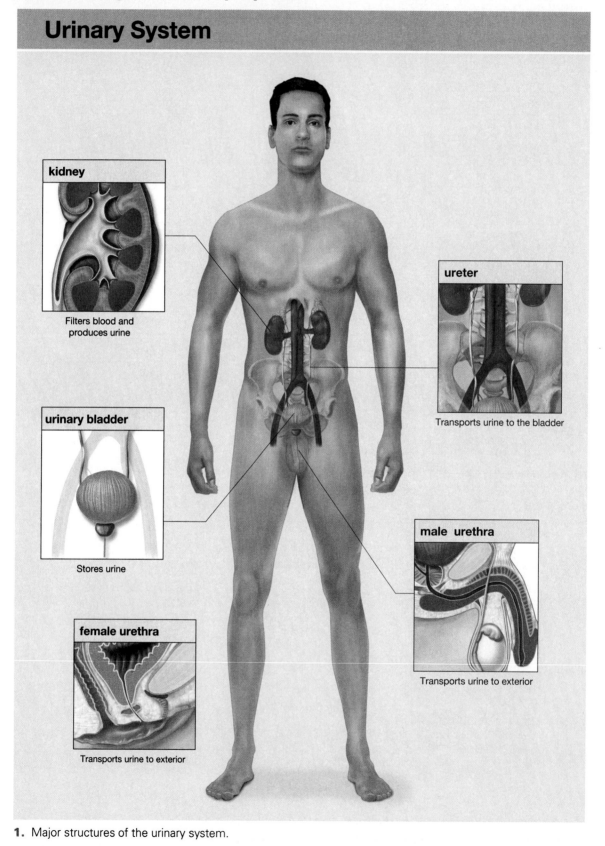

Urinary System

kidney

Filters blood and produces urine

ureter

Transports urine to the bladder

urinary bladder

Stores urine

male urethra

Transports urine to exterior

female urethra

Transports urine to exterior

1. Major structures of the urinary system.

Understanding the Integumentary System

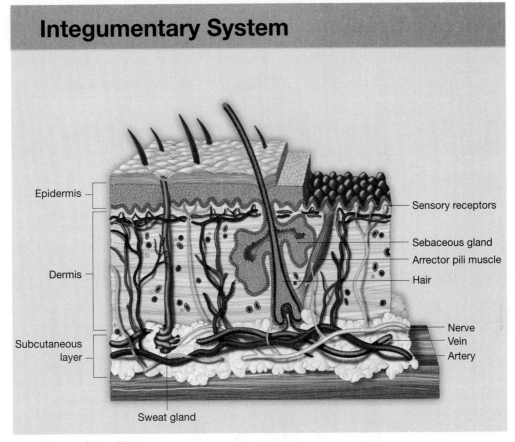

Integumentary System

Epidermis

Dermis

Subcutaneous layer

Sensory receptors

Sebaceous gland

Arrector pili muscle

Hair

Nerve
Vein
Artery

Sweat gland

1. Anatomy of the skin.

- *Dermis.* This is a thick layer that lies below the epidermis and gives skin its strength and elasticity. It contains blood vessels as well as hair follicles, sweat and oil glands, and sensory nerves.
- *Subcutaneous layer.* This layer is mostly connective tissue and fat that varies in thickness, depending on where it is located. The subcutaneous layer on the backs of the hands and tops of the feet is often quite thin. In contrast, it is often much thicker over areas such as the abdomen and buttocks.

Endocrine System

LO14 Describe the major anatomical structures and function of the endocrine system.

The endocrine system is made up of many hormone-producing glands and is responsible for regulating many processes within the human body (Key Skill 4.11). Some of the glands that make up the endocrine system include the thyroid, pituitary, adrenal, pancreas, and gonads. Some of the processes that the endocrine system regulates are metabolism, physical growth, hair growth, and reproduction. This is accomplished primarily through the production and release of specialized chemicals called hormones.

The hormone insulin is produced by the pancreas. Insulin is responsible for the regulation of glucose (sugar) levels in the blood. Epinephrine is a hormone produced by the adrenal gland that is responsible for stimulating the nervous system by causing increased heart rate, heart contractions, constriction of the blood vessels, and dilation of the airways.

Understanding the Endocrine System

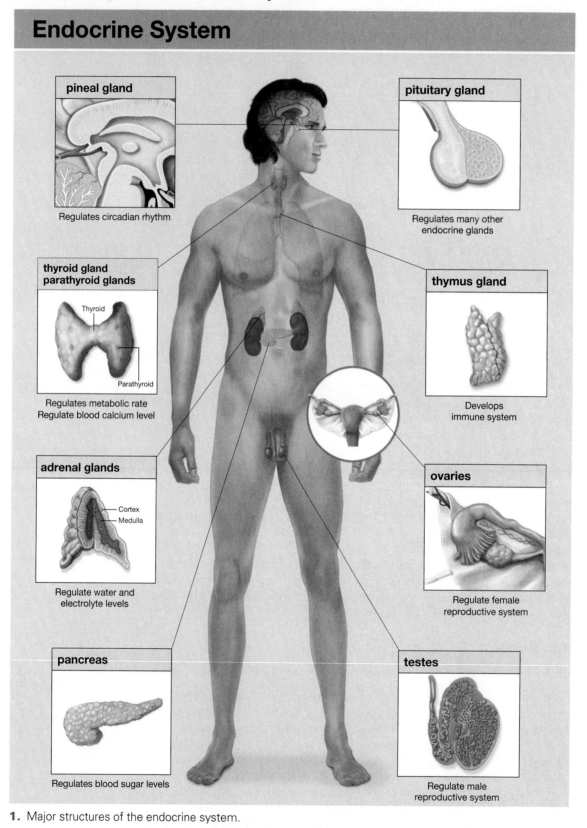

Endocrine System

pineal gland

Regulates circadian rhythm

pituitary gland

Regulates many other endocrine glands

**thyroid gland
parathyroid glands**

Thyroid

Parathyroid

Regulates metabolic rate
Regulate blood calcium level

thymus gland

Develops immune system

adrenal glands

Cortex
Medulla

Regulate water and electrolyte levels

ovaries

Regulate female reproductive system

pancreas

Regulates blood sugar levels

testes

Regulate male reproductive system

1. Major structures of the endocrine system.

Lifespan Development

LO15 Describe the major phases of lifespan development.

Throughout our lifespan, our body undergoes significant changes as it grows, develops, ages, and matures (Figure 4.7). These changes occur in three primary areas: biological (the physical body), cognitive (the mind), and psychosocial (how the individual interacts with their surroundings). Each phase of development has unique characteristics. As an Emergency Medical Responder, you must become familiar with these changes to provide the best care possible.

Lifespan development ranges from birth through death and can be divided into the following phases:

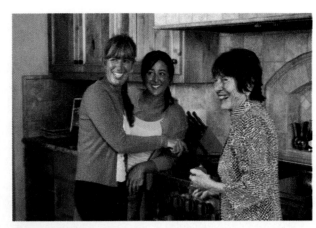

Figure 4.7 It is common for a single family to extend to several generations of living members.

- Neonate (birth to 28 days)
- Infant (birth to 1 year old)
- Toddler (1–3 years old)
- Early childhood (3–6 years old)
- Middle childhood (6–12 years old)
- Adolescence (12–18 years old)
- Early, middle, and late adulthood (18 to end of life)

The specific definition of an infant or child will vary depending on the context in which you are providing care. This is the case in the context of cardiopulmonary resuscitation and the use of the automated external defibrillator (AED). Some procedures will change according to the child's physical size more so than the exact age.

The body weight used for calculating the size of equipment to be used and medication doses for children is always given in kilograms. You must learn to estimate the weight of any patient you encounter and be able to convert pounds into kilograms.

- 1 kilogram = 2.2 pounds
- 1 pound = 0.45 kilograms

Developmental Characteristics

Because of the different behavioral characteristics of children at various ages, it is useful to become familiar with characteristics associated with each stage of child development and how they will affect your assessment of the patient.

Neonates and Infants (Birth to 1 Year)   When caring for and interacting with newborns or infants (Figure 4.8), it is important to keep in mind two important ideas: They will not like to be cold, and they do not like to be separated from their parents or primary caregivers. Once infants are crying from discomfort or anxiety, your assessment will become much more difficult to perform. A good part of the assessment exam can be done visually while you are taking the history from the parent or caregiver.

Toddlers (1–3 Years)   The toddler (Figure 4.9) has developed a sense of independence through walking and talking but is unable to reason well or communicate complex ideas. The toddler does not like to be touched by strangers or separated from primary caregivers. Like the infant, a good part of the assessment exam can be done visually while you are taking the history from the parent or caregiver. The alert toddler will be watching you closely. Even when speaking to the adults, use a calm, quiet voice. This may help to calm the toddler. Toddlers may interpret injury, illness, or separation from family as punishment, so they need lots of reassurance that they are not to blame and that their parents or caregivers are with them or know where they are.

Early Childhood (3–6 Years)   Children at this stage (Figure 4.10) have developed concrete thinking skills that allow them to understand and follow instructions. It is important to ask them for their version of how they feel and what happened.

> **REMEMBER**
>
> When beginning your assessment, use a quiet, confident, soothing voice, and allow the child to hold a toy or favorite object while being examined. When using a stethoscope, it may be helpful to first place it on a parent or favorite stuffed animal to show the child that it does not hurt.

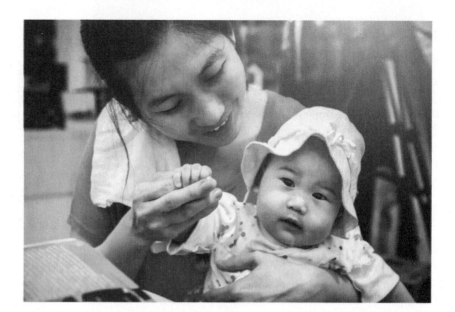

Figure 4.8 Infants prefer to be warm and favor their primary caregiver.
(kdshutterman/Shutterstock)

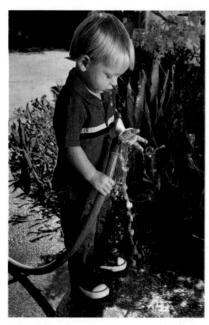

Figure 4.9 Toddlers are curious and often fearful of strangers.

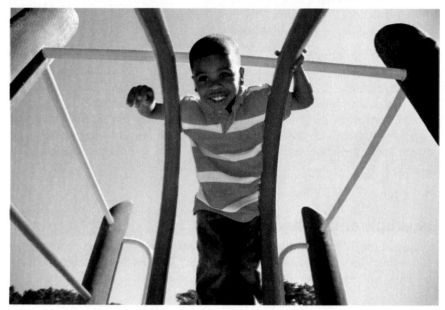

Figure 4.10 Children in early childhood are adventurous and need lots of reassurance.
(Fuse/Corbis/Getty Images)

REMEMBER

Whenever you approach a child, remember to "Get low and go slow." You must gain their confidence even if you know that you may have to cause them some pain as you help them. If there is no clear life-threatening condition, you should first engage the parents. Once the child feels you are trusted by their parents, they are more likely to trust you as well.

Like toddlers, children at this stage may believe they are being punished by an illness or injury for wrongdoing. They are very frightened of potential pain and the sight of blood. They need lots of reassurance and respond well to simple explanations that avoid medical or complicated terminology.

Separation causes them anxiety, so allow the parent or caregiver to hold or sit near the child as you begin your examination. In an effort to build trust, begin your examination with the extremities then move to the trunk, followed by the head. The child is typically quite modest, so replace items of clothing after taking them off, or allow the child to help you by pulling up their shirt or exposing the area of injury.

Middle Childhood (6–12 Years) By the time children reach this stage (Figure 4.11), they have a basic understanding of the body and its functions, and they usually try to cooperate with the physical exam. They are able to communicate and understand more complex ideas. Be careful what you say as children at this stage will often take what is said literally. Be aware that they are listening to every word you say, even if you are not talking

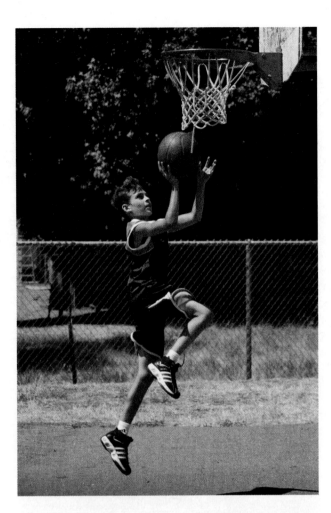

Figure 4.11 Children in middle childhood are more likely to understand what you are doing and cooperate with your exam.

to them. These children are aware of and afraid of death and dying. They also fear pain, deformity, blood, and permanent injury. They benefit from reassurance as well as inclusion in discussions involving their care.

Adolescence (12–18 Years) The adolescent (Figure 4.12) has a more thorough understanding of anatomy and physiology and is able to process and express complex ideas. Adolescents are frequent risk takers but are often poor judges of consequence.

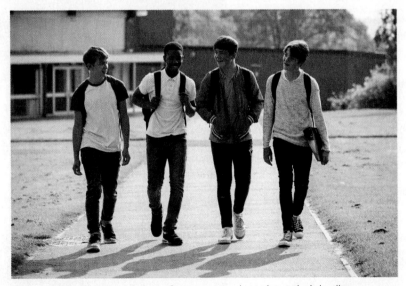

Figure 4.12 Adolescents are often very modest about their bodies.
(MBI/Shutterstock)

They are afraid of disfigurement and permanent injury yet often believe they are immortal or indestructible. They want to be treated as adults, but they may need the same level of support and reassurance as a younger child. Speaking to the adolescent respectfully and nonjudgmentally will improve your ability to obtain an accurate history. Protecting adolescents' privacy and modesty may gain their trust. It may be helpful to interview or examine them away from parents or caregivers.

Early Adulthood (18–30 Years Old)   It is during early adulthood (Figure 4.13) when many people complete their formal education and begin to consider finding a partner and starting a family. During this time, we are at the peak of health and are often very active. Adults at this stage make up a large number of those involved in traumatic injuries and accidents.

Middle Adulthood (30–60 Years)   It is during middle adulthood (Figure 4.14) that many develop routines that become well established, and the focus of life often shifts to the rearing of children. It is also a time in life during which many physiological changes occur, including a decrease in the ability to see and hear well. During this time, many people notice changes such as graying hair and the appearance of more permanent wrinkles in the skin.

Late Adulthood (60 to End of Life)   For many, late adulthood (Figure 4.15) represents a period in life when they experience more pronounced physical changes. These changes can be

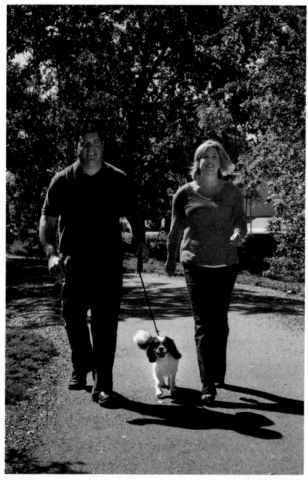

Figure 4.13 Individuals in early adulthood are most at risk for injuries from trauma.

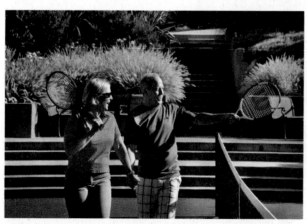

Figure 4.14 A couple in middle adulthood.

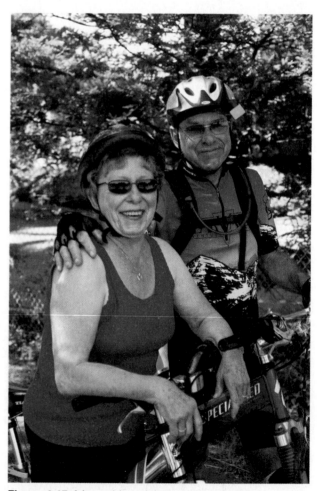

Figure 4.15 Many older adults remain very active.

greatly influenced by lifestyle and can include continued decline in the ability to see, hear, taste, and smell. Mobility can become difficult for some, and the awareness of one's own mortality is ever present. One of the characteristics common to late adulthood is a decrease in the ability to perceive pain. This can make it difficult for the Emergency Medical Responder to accurately assess illness and injury during the patient assessment. It is also common for people in this age group to have more than one disease or medical condition for which they are taking multiple medications.

FIRST ON SCENE WRAP-UP

It seems like forever before Marnie hears sirens approaching. Eric has yet to do anything except flutter his eyelids and groan. Although the direct pressure seems to have stopped most of the bleeding, Eric appears to be struggling more to breathe. Thankfully, Marnie hears vehicles rolling to a stop nearby, and the screaming sirens are quickly replaced by a multitude of slamming doors and running feet.

"Okay, we're here now," a woman says and puts her hand on Marnie's shoulder. She lets go of Eric and stands up. He is immediately surrounded by firefighters and paramedics who are tearing open packages and giving orders to each other. She takes a few steps back and sees her shift supervisor arrive on scene. "Great job, Marnie," he says. "How are you holding up? Is there anything you need right now?"

Summary

- The medical profession has a unique language all its own. To become a valuable participant in this new world, you must learn common word roots, suffixes, and prefixes specific to medical terminology.
- All descriptions relating to illness, injury, and patient care must refer to the patient in the anatomical position. This is a standardized position used by all medical professionals that allows descriptions to be standardized and consistent. The patient is the point of reference for all directional terms such as patient's left or patient's right.
- The four major body cavities are the cranial, thoracic, abdominal, and pelvic. These are areas that contain major organs and can hide significant blood loss.
- The cranium contains the brain and soft tissues surrounding the brain.
- The thorax contains the heart, lungs, and major vessels.
- The abdomen contains many of the vital organs, such as the liver, spleen, pancreas, gallbladder, and intestines.
- The pelvic cavity contains the bladder and intestines as well as the uterus, fallopian tubes, and ovaries of the female.
- The respiratory system comprises the upper airway, larynx, trachea, and the bronchi, bronchioles, and alveoli of the lungs. It is responsible for the movement of air into and out of the body and the exchange of oxygen and carbon dioxide. The primary muscle of respiration is the diaphragm.
- The cardiovascular system comprises the heart, vessels, and blood. It is responsible for the transportation of blood and nutrients throughout the body.
- The musculoskeletal system comprises the muscles, bones, and connective tissues such as ligaments and tendons. It provides structure and support for the body and allows mobility. It also provides protection against injury and helps support the immune system.
- The nervous system comprises the brain, spinal cord, and nerves. It is divided into the central nervous system (brain and spinal cord) and the peripheral nervous system (nerves).
- The autonomic nervous system is part of the peripheral nervous system and is divided into the sympathetic and parasympathetic systems. The autonomic nervous system controls the function of many vital systems throughout the body, such as heart rate and breathing rate.
- The digestive system comprises the esophagus, stomach, and intestines. The primary function of the digestive system is to break down food so it can be properly metabolized by the cells of the body. It also serves as a means to eliminate solid waste from the body.
- The reproductive system comprises the testes and penis in the male and the ovaries, fallopian tubes, uterus, and vagina in the female. This system is responsible for producing the hormones necessary for reproduction as well as maintaining the structures to support gestation of the fetus in the female.
- The urinary system comprises the kidneys, ureters, bladder, and urethra. It is responsible for the filtration and removal of waste from the blood as well as helping to maintain proper water and salt levels in the blood.
- The integumentary system includes the skin, hair, nails, sweat glands, and oil glands. The skin is made up of three layers: the epidermis, dermis, and subcutaneous. The skin helps protect us from harmful pathogens as well as maintain a stable body temperature.
- The endocrine system comprises many hormone-producing glands such as the thyroid, pituitary, and adrenal glands and is responsible regulating many important processes.
- As the human body grows and develops from a newborn infant into an adult, it passes through various developmental stages. There are significant biological, cognitive, and psychosocial changes at each stage of development. The better you understand these changes, the better you will be at assessing your patients and providing the proper care.

Take Action

"Where Do I Hurt?"

Being able to accurately describe the location of a sign or symptom is an important skill that you must learn to become an effective member of the EMS team. This activity will help you learn to properly describe the anatomical location of a series of random injuries or symptoms. Using a fellow classmate and a roll of masking tape, one of you will place small pieces of tape at various locations on your body. Begin with only two or three pieces of tape and keep them on the anterior side of the body. Next, the individual with the tape will stand before the other individual in the anatomical position. Using proper anatomical terms, your partner must describe in writing the location of the imaginary injuries or symptoms represented by the tape. To make the activity more challenging, place the pieces of tape in various locations on the body and have the "patient" lie on the floor in different positions.

Virtual Anatomy Tour

This activity will help you learn the location of the various organs in the abdominal cavity. You will need a fellow classmate, and one of you will play the role of patient while the other plays the role of student. With the patient lying supine on the floor, the student carefully palpates the four quadrants of the abdomen while describing the anatomy located in each quadrant. You may refer to your book as necessary until you have memorized the location of all the major organs.

First on Scene Patient Handoff

We have a 44-year-old male who appears to have been shot. I found an open wound to the right anterior chest, just below the nipple, and another open wound on his back right side, just below the scapula. His airway appears patent, and his respirations are rapid and shallow. I placed a sterile dressing over both wounds for bleeding control and have been monitoring his pulse and breathing until EMS arrived.

First on Scene Run Review

Recall the events of the First on Scene scenario in this chapter and answer the following questions related to the call. Rationales are offered in the Answer Key at the back of the book.

1. Describe the safety concerns that Marnie is facing on this call.
2. What did Marnie accomplish by placing her hand over the wound?
3. Which organs could be damaged with a gunshot to the chest?

Quick Quiz

To check your understanding of the chapter, answer the following questions. Then compare your answers to those in the Answer Key at the back of the book.

1. Which of the following best describes the anatomical position?
   a. Standing upright with arms at the sides
   b. Lying supine with arms outstretched and palms up
   c. Standing with hands at the sides and palms forward
   d. Lying prone with arms held straight out and palms down

2. The navel is on the ____ aspect of the body.
   a. posterior
   b. anterior
   c. inferior
   d. superior

3. The spine can be palpated (felt) on the ____ aspect of the body.
   a. posterior
   b. anterior
   c. inferior
   d. superior

4. The imaginary line that bisects the body into two halves (left and right) is known as the:
   a. proximal break.
   b. inferior aspect.
   c. recumbent line.
   d. midline.

5. Any location on the body that is closer to the midline is referred to as:
   a. medial.
   b. recumbent.
   c. lateral.
   d. inferior.

6. The thumb is considered ____ to the palm.
   a. distal
   b. proximal
   c. lateral
   d. medial

7. The lower airway includes all of the following EXCEPT the:
   a. bronchi.
   b. epiglottis.
   c. alveoli.
   d. trachea.

8. Which of the following is NOT a function of the circulatory system?
   a. Delivering blood to vital organs
   b. Removing waste products from the cells
   c. Breaking down food into nutrients
   d. Carrying oxygen throughout the body

9. A patient with a dislocated shoulder has sustained an injury to which body system?

    a. Digestive

    b. Musculoskeletal

    c. Integumentary

    d. Nervous

10. The central nervous system is made up of the:

    a. sensory nerves.

    b. brain and cervical spine.

    c. nerves in the hands and feet.

    d. brain and spinal cord.

11. The period of time from birth to 28 days is referred to as:

    a. the neonatal period.

    b. infancy.

    c. childhood.

    d. adolescence.

12. The recovery position is also known as the ____ position.

    a. lateral recumbent

    b. lateral

    c. superior

    d. stroke

13. The bladder is located in which body cavity?

    a. Cranial

    b. Thoracic

    c. Abdominal

    d. Pelvic

14. The ____ cavity is also known as the thoracic cavity.

    a. pelvic

    b. chest

    c. abdominal

    d. cranial

15. The ____ separates the thoracic cavity from the abdominal cavity.

    a. pelvic wall

    b. midline

    c. diaphragm

    d. stomach

16. Which of the following is TRUE of children in middle childhood?

    a. They are aware of death and dying.

    b. They do not understand simple concepts.

    c. They need to be with their parents at all times.

    d. They are not at risk for choking.

17. The ____ cavity contains the liver and part of the large intestine.

    a. pelvic

    b. abdominal

    c. thoracic

    d. cranial

18. The ____ is found in the upper left quadrant of the abdomen.

    a. appendix

    b. liver

    c. kidney

    d. spleen

19. The endocrine system includes the:

    a. glands and hormones.

    b. ovaries and uterus.

    c. liver and bile ducts.

    d. small and large intestines.

20. The ____ is/are found in an area behind the abdominal cavity.

    a. kidneys

    b. bladder

    c. small intestine

    d. gall bladder

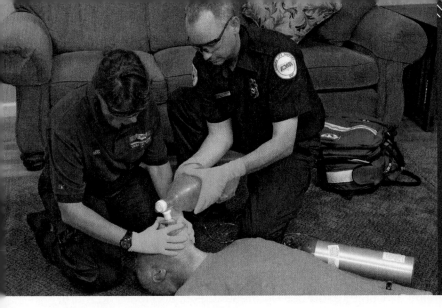

5

Introduction to Pathophysiology

Education Standards

Pathophysiology

Competencies

Uses knowledge of shock and respiratory compromise to respond to life threats.

LEARNING OBJECTIVES

Upon successful completion of this chapter, the student should be able to:

Cognitive

1 Define the chapter key terms.

2 Explain the importance of understanding basic pathophysiology.

3 Explain the concept of perfusion, including the components necessary to maintain perfusion.

4 Describe the composition of ambient air.

5 Describe the transport of oxygen and carbon dioxide in the blood.

6 Differentiate between the processes of aerobic and anaerobic cellular metabolism.

7 Explain how changes in respiratory system function can affect ventilation.

8 List factors that affect cardiac output.

9 Describe the two ways the heart can fail, resulting in decreased cardiac output.

10 List the responses by the body when the sympathetic nervous system is stimulated.

Psychomotor

There are no psychomotor objectives for this chapter.

Affective

11 Value the importance of developing a basic understanding of pathophysiology.

KEY TERMS

aerobic metabolism (*p. 95*)

anaerobic metabolism (*p. 95*)

cardiac output (CO) (*p. 99*)

heart rate (*p. 99*)

hypoperfusion (*p. 95*)

metabolism (*p. 95*)

patent (*p. 96*)

pathophysiology (*p. 94*)

shock (*p. 95*)

stroke volume (SV) (*p. 99*)

This chapter provides a very basic description of how the body responds when things do not function properly. A basic understanding of human anatomy and physiology creates the baseline for how the body should behave when its functions and processes are working normally. Understanding pathophysiology helps you recognize when things are not working so well. Being able to recognize abnormal signs and having even a basic understanding of what these signs mean will help you provide the best possible care for your patient.

It is possible to dedicate an entire lifetime to the study of pathophysiology, and this chapter will provide a very brief overview of some of the major concepts. Your continued study of anatomy, physiology, and pathophysiology can further broaden your spectrum of knowledge long after your EMR course ends. There are many available resources on these topics, and learning more will only make you a better provider.

FIRST ON SCENE

EMS dispatcher Brooke stretches her back, glances at her watch, and leans forward to scan the night's call log. "It's been pretty quiet tonight," she says to fellow dispatcher Jordan. "I thought it was going to be busier."

Chris looks around the side of his computer monitor and frowns. "You realize that you just jinxed us, right? And with only an hour to go before shift change!"

Brooke's laugh is cut short by a ringing on the emergency line. She answers, "Nine–one–one, what is your emergency?" Brooke has to strain to hear the gasping voice on the other end of the line. Initially she can only make out the words,

"Can't breathe." She mutes her phone and leans over to Chris. "I need you to send the rescue unit to this address for difficulty breathing. Code three!"

As Brooke returns to the caller, Chris keys the radio. "Six fifty-three, six five three, control, respond code three to 4512 Berry Lane for a difficulty breathing. Showing you dispatched at 0612 hours."

In a gas station parking lot across town, firefighters Case and Darin secure their seat belts and, as Darin shifts the idling truck into drive, Case acknowledges the dispatch and sees the address come up on the GPS.

Understanding Pathophysiology

LO2 Explain the importance of understanding basic pathophysiology.

pathophysiology ▶ study of how disease processes affect the function of the body.

Pathophysiology is the study of how disease processes affect the functions of the body. As an Emergency Medical Responder, you will encounter many people whose bodies are functioning abnormally due to illness or injury. Your understanding of how the body responds and the signs and symptoms it displays when things are wrong will help you identify issues and provide the proper care more promptly. Your knowledge may allow you to anticipate what the body needs sooner rather than later.

Cardiopulmonary System and Perfusion

LO3 Explain the concept of perfusion, including the components necessary to maintain perfusion.

LO4 Describe the composition of ambient air.

LO5 Describe the transport of oxygen and carbon dioxide in the blood.

Every cell, organ, and tissue in the body requires regular delivery of oxygen and nutrients (primarily glucose) and the removal of waste products. Recall from Chapter 4 that *perfusion* is the circulation of blood through tissues. This process relies on the interrelated function of the respiratory and cardiovascular systems. These two systems working together are called the cardiopulmonary system.

For oxygen to be delivered and waste products to be removed, all components of the cardiopulmonary system must be functioning together. First, there must be adequate oxygen in the ambient air (atmospheric air) we breathe. Ambient air, often referred to as "room air," typically contains 21 percent oxygen. Many things can affect the oxygen concentration in the air we breathe, including altitude, confined spaces, toxic vapors, and the presence of the products of combustion. The entire cardiopulmonary system can be functioning normally, but if there is not enough oxygen in the air we breathe, perfusion will be compromised.

In the respiratory system, air movement must bring oxygen all the way to the alveoli of the lungs and move carbon dioxide all the way out. There must be a significant quantity of air moving, and the alveoli must be capable of exchanging gas.

In the cardiovascular system, there must be enough blood, the heart must effectively pump that blood, and the system must contain enough pressure to move the blood between the body cells and the alveoli. The blood must also be capable of carrying oxygen and carbon dioxide. All of these individual components must be present and functioning for normal perfusion to occur.

Shock occurs when perfusion fails. In other words, shock occurs when the delivery of oxygen and nutrients to cells and removal of their waste products are inadequate to support cell function. This failure is referred to as **hypoperfusion**. The lungs, heart, blood vessels, and the blood itself must all work in concert to successfully deliver oxygen and nutrients to the cells and remove waste products. Interruption of any part of this process results in a failure of the cardiopulmonary system. Without a regular supply of oxygen and nutrients, cells cannot function normally and waste products begin to accumulate. Unless reversed, shock will kill cells, then organs, and eventually the patient.

shock ▸ life-threatening condition in which there is insufficient blood flow to tissues.

hypoperfusion ▸ decreased blood flow to an organ or tissues.

Aerobic and Anaerobic Metabolism

LO6 Differentiate between the processes of aerobic and anaerobic cellular metabolism.

The physical and chemical processes that are necessary for maintaining the life of a cell or organism are collectively called **metabolism**. Normal metabolism requires oxygen and fuel in the form of a simple sugar called glucose.

Metabolism that uses oxygen is called **aerobic metabolism** (Figure 5.1A). Cells utilize aerobic metabolism to generate the energy required to keep the body functioning. After oxygen and glucose are used for aerobic metabolism, waste products, including carbon dioxide, are left over and are subsequently removed from the body through circulation and breathing.

If injury or illness causes cells to be starved of oxygen or glucose, normal metabolism cannot occur. Instead, the cells must use less effective means of producing energy. The abnormal metabolism that occurs without oxygen is called **anaerobic metabolism** (Figure 5.1B). Anaerobic metabolism is much less efficient because, without oxygen or glucose, the cell is unable to generate the large amounts of energy required to keep the body alive. More waste is generated, including lactic acid, and cells may become damaged due to waste products accumulating.

Anaerobic metabolism can cause life-threatening problems in small areas of tissue or in entire body systems. During a heart attack, an area of heart tissue is deprived of oxygen and is subsequently damaged. Although a heart attack affects a relatively small area of tissue, it is nevertheless life threatening. A patient who is losing large amounts of blood due to trauma will be unable to deliver oxygen and glucose to much of the body. In this situation, it is possible for the majority of cells in the body to resort to anaerobic metabolism, overwhelming the body with waste products and potentially leading to death.

As you read through the descriptions of body system function and dysfunction in this chapter, consider how illness or injury affects normal metabolism. Think about how your actions as an Emergency Medical Responder can help support a patient who is ill or injured.

metabolism ▸ chemical reactions within each cell that provide energy for vital processes.

aerobic metabolism ▸ cellular process by which oxygen is used to metabolize glucose and energy is produced in an efficient manner with minimal waste products.

anaerobic metabolism ▸ cellular process by which glucose is metabolized without oxygen and energy is produced in an inefficient manner with many waste products.

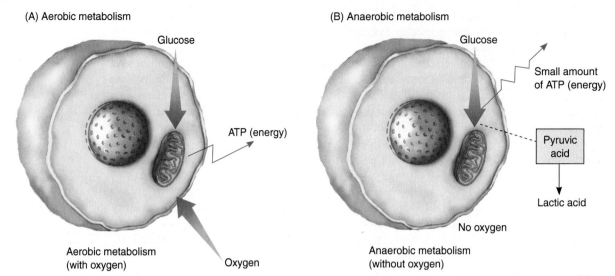

Figure 5.1 (A) Aerobic metabolism requires an adequate supply of glucose and oxygen. (B) Anaerobic metabolism occurs when there is not enough oxygen.

The Respiratory System

LO7 Explain how changes in respiratory system function can affect ventilation.

patent ▶ open and clear; free from obstruction.

The respiratory system includes structures of the airways, lungs, and muscles of respiration. Movement of air in and out of the body requires **patent** airways, meaning the pathways are open and clear. There are a number of potential challenges to maintaining patent airways when disease is present or trauma occurs. They include:

- *Upper respiratory tract obstructions.* Upper respiratory tract obstructions occur above the trachea and prevent air from entering the lower respiratory tract. One common cause of upper airway obstruction is a blockage caused by the tongue. Loss of muscle control can occur as a result of a decrease in mental status; this causes the tongue and soft tissues to block the movement of air. Obstructions are also frequently caused by foreign bodies (as when a person chokes on a piece of food) or by swelling. Trauma, burns, infection, or an allergic reaction can cause the soft tissues of the larynx to swell. Any of these obstructions can significantly impact the movement of air in and out of the lungs.
- *Lower respiratory tract obstructions.* The most common lower respiratory tract obstruction, called bronchoconstriction, occurs when the muscles around the bronchioles (small tubes in the lungs) spasm and reduce airflow in and out of the alveoli (Figure 5.2A and B). Common causes of bronchoconstriction include asthma and allergic reactions, during which the bronchioles spasm and become narrower than normal. This prevents oxygen-rich air from getting into the alveoli and slows the exhalation of carbon dioxide out of the lungs.

The lungs are the organs of breathing and are filled and emptied by changing pressure within the chest cavity. When an individual inhales through the nose and/or mouth, the diaphragm contracts, moving downward, and the chest wall lifts up and out, lowering the pressure inside the chest and pulling air into the lungs. During exhalation, the diaphragm and chest muscles relax, and air is exhaled as the chest cavity returns to its normal size.

Recall from Chapter 4 that *tidal volume* is the volume of air moved in and out in one breathing cycle (one inhalation and one exhalation). Tidal volume for the average adult is 500 mL of air with each breath. The typical adult will breathe between 12 and 20 times per minute while at rest. Respiration rates for infants and children are faster.

Adequate ventilation occurs when enough air is moved in and out of the lungs to meet the oxygen demand of the body. Changes in respiration rate or tidal volume can greatly

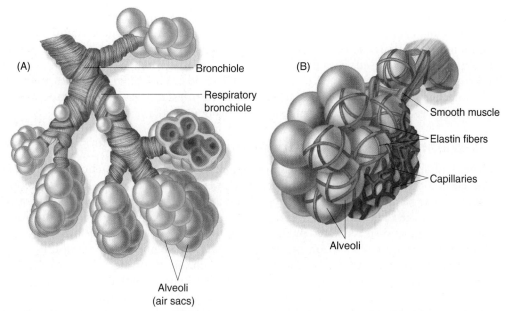

Figure 5.2 (A) The alveoli are where the exchange of oxygen and carbon dioxide takes place. (B) Alveoli are surrounded by capillaries that bring in oxygen and venules that carry away carbon dioxide.

affect the adequacy of ventilation. A patient must have a good balance between volume and rate to ensure adequate oxygen intake and removal of carbon dioxide. Breathing that is too slow will result in an excess buildup of carbon dioxide. Breathing that is too fast may lead to abnormally low levels of carbon dioxide. Neither situation is good for the patient long term.

Respiratory System Dysfunction

There are many causes of respiratory system dysfunction. In general, normal function is interrupted any time rate or volume becomes inadequate. Common causes of respiratory dysfunction include disruption of respiratory control, disruption of pressure, and damage to lung tissue.

Disruption of Respiratory Control   Breathing is controlled by an area of the brain called the medulla oblongata. The medulla oblongata communicates with the diaphragm and initiates inhalation. Disorders that affect this area of the brain can interfere with respiratory function. Medical conditions such as stroke, brain tumors, and infection can disrupt the medulla's function and alter the stimulus to breathe. Toxins and drugs can also affect the medulla's ability to regulate breathing by slowing respirations. Brain trauma can physically harm the medulla and impair its function.

Disruption of Pressure   When the chest expands, negative pressure is created inside the chest, which pulls air through the nose and mouth and into the lungs. When the chest relaxes and becomes smaller, positive pressure is created inside the chest, and air is pushed out. Changing pressures within the chest cavity rely on an intact chest compartment. If a hole is created in the chest wall, such as by a gunshot wound, air will be drawn in through this opening. This allows air to enter the pleural space, the space between the outer layer of lung tissue and the chest wall. When air is trapped in the pleural space, the lung may collapse and breathing becomes impaired. This is called a pneumothorax, which can be caused by a hole in the chest wall, the lung, or both. Furthermore, if bleeding develops within the chest, blood can accumulate in the pleural space. This is called a hemothorax, and it forces a lung to collapse away from the chest wall.

> **REMEMBER**
>
> During your primary assessment, you will assess a patient's breathing rate by counting the number of respirations per minute. Then, you must do your best to assess the adequacy of tidal volume, which is a bit more subjective. The best way to assess tidal volume is by observing chest rise and fall.

Damage to Lung Tissue When the lung tissue itself is damaged, breathing is impaired. Damage to lung tissue occurs when the tissue is physically injured, or when the alveoli are clogged and cannot function. The primary cause of physical damage is traumatic injury, although conditions such as emphysema and cancer can also damage lung tissue. When lung tissue is destroyed, it cannot exchange gas. In other situations, destruction of lung tissue occurs when the lungs become clogged with fluid or mucus. For example, pneumonia or infection can reduce the ability of the alveoli to transfer gases. The result of any such challenges is hypoxia (low oxygen) and high carbon dioxide.

Respiratory System Compensation

The respiratory system is very good at responding to challenges. When normal respiratory function is disrupted, the body attempts to compensate in other ways. For instance, if an area of lung tissue is disrupted due to pneumonia, the body will not be able to transfer as much oxygen and carbon dioxide into and out of the blood. As stated previously, respiratory function is regulated by the medulla oblongata in the brain. When a disruption in normal respiratory function occurs, the medulla recognizes the increase in carbon dioxide and attempts to correct the problem by altering respiratory rate and depth. By breathing faster and/or deeper, the body attempts to correct imbalances in oxygen and carbon dioxide. These changes in respiratory patterns are predictable, and identifying them can help Emergency Medical Responders recognize when a patient is experiencing a serious respiratory emergency.

The Cardiovascular System

Proper gas exchange occurs only when the respiratory system works in conjunction with appropriate cardiovascular function. But just as there can be many challenges to normal respiratory function, there can be many threats to normal circulation in the cardiovascular system.

Blood

Oxygen, nutrients, and waste products are transported throughout the body by the blood that circulates through the cardiovascular system. For the cardiovascular system to function properly, there must be sufficient blood volume to fill the blood vessels throughout the system. If the blood volume is inadequate, cells and tissues become starved of oxygen and nutrients, and waste products begin to accumulate. Insufficient blood volume is commonly caused by direct blood loss from major bleeding. Severe dehydration and burns can also affect blood volume. In these instances, fluid loss affects the amount of blood plasma and decreases the total amount of blood in the system.

Blood Vessels

The blood vessels are the pathways in which blood travels. Arteries, veins, and capillaries form this distribution network (see Key Skill 4.3). Arteries carry blood away from the heart. They are composed of three tunics (layers) and can change diameter by contracting their middle layer of smooth muscle. Veins carry blood back to the heart and can also change diameter due to a layer of smooth muscle. As blood leaves the heart, it first travels through arteries, which decrease in size as they move away from the heart and become arterioles. Arterioles then feed the oxygenated blood to tiny vessels called capillaries.

Capillaries have thin walls which, like cell membranes, allow for movement of substances into and out of the bloodstream. It is through these thin walls that oxygen is off-loaded and carbon dioxide is picked up from the cells of the body. Capillaries then connect to the smallest veins, called venules. As they grow larger, venules become veins and transport blood back to the heart.

Deoxygenated blood that has been returned to the right side of the heart is transferred to the lungs by way of the pulmonary arteries and arterioles. The pulmonary arterioles connect with pulmonary capillaries surrounding the alveoli. Oxygen is transferred from the air in the alveoli across the alveolar membrane to the surrounding capillaries. Carbon dioxide is off-loaded across the alveolar membrane from the bloodstream to the air in the alveoli. The newly oxygenated blood then continues from the pulmonary capillaries to the pulmonary venules and into the pulmonary veins. The pulmonary veins then return the oxygenated blood to the left side of the heart to be pumped to the body.

Blood moves through the cardiovascular system through a combination of pressure generated by the heart and blood vessels. When the heart contracts, a wave of blood leaves the left ventricle and enters the arterial system. While that initial "push" from the heart starts the blood moving through the system, the blood vessels themselves also help keep blood moving by controlling the overall pressure in the vascular system. If blood vessels are too relaxed, the diameter of arteries and veins will become larger. This lowers the overall pressure in the system, and blood will move more slowly. If the vessels constrict, the diameter of arteries and veins will become more narrow. This causes an increase in pressure in the system and causes blood to move faster.

Normal function of blood vessels is critical to maintaining circulatory system function. A variety of dysfunctions can interfere with the normal operation of blood vessels, including:

- *Loss of blood vessel tone.* Blood vessels are not able to control their own size (more specifically, their own internal diameter). If blood vessels are unable to constrict when necessary or they are allowed to dilate without control, blood pressure can drop significantly. Many conditions can cause this loss of tone. Injuries to the brain and spinal cord, uncontrolled infections that cause sepsis, and severe allergic reactions can all cause uncontrolled dilation of the vessels.
- *Permeability problems.* Certain conditions cause capillaries to leak fluid. In this case, fluid passes through the capillary walls too easily, and the fluid portion of blood leaves the intravascular space too readily. Severe infection (sepsis) and certain diseases are frequently responsible for these problems.
- *Hypertension.* Commonly called high blood pressure, hypertension can cause pressure-related problems such as stroke and kidney failure. Chronic smoking, certain drugs, and even genetics can cause abnormal constriction of the peripheral blood vessels, resulting in an abnormally high level of pressure. This increased pressure can be a major risk factor in heart disease and stroke.

The Heart

LO8 List factors that affect cardiac output.

LO9 Describe the two ways the heart can fail, resulting in decreased cardiac output.

The heart is often described as a simple four-chambered pump. Although its role is fairly simple, the pressure it creates by pumping is critical to the success of the cardiovascular system. The movement of blood and subsequently the transportation of oxygen and carbon dioxide are all dependent on the heart working properly.

The job of the heart is very straightforward: to move blood. To do this, it mechanically contracts and ejects blood. The volume of blood ejected in one contraction of the heart is known as **stroke volume (SV)**.

Cardiac output (CO) is the amount of blood ejected from the heart in 1 minute. Cardiac output is a function of both stroke volume and **heart rate** (number of heartbeats per minute). Cardiac output can be changed by altering either heart rate or stroke volume. Cardiac output is measured in liters per minute. An adult weighing approximately 160 pounds would have an average cardiac output of 5 liters per minute.

Cardiac output can also be affected by heart rates that are too fast. Normally, increasing heart rate would increase cardiac output. However, very fast rates (usually >180 in adults) limit the filling time of the heart and can *decrease* stroke volume. Some examples of impaired cardiac output include:

- A 33-year-old woman has tachycardia (fast heart rate) at a rate of 220. This does not give her ventricles enough time to fill between contractions. As a result, her stroke volume (and overall cardiac output) has dropped.

stroke volume ▶ volume of blood ejected from the heart in one contraction. Abbrev: SV.

cardiac output ▶ amount of blood ejected from the heart in 1 minute. Abbrev: CO.

heart rate ▶ number of heartbeats in 1 minute.

- A 67-year-old man has bradycardia (slow heart rate) at a rate of 40. His heart rate has decreased, along with his cardiac output.
- A 19-year-old has been stabbed in the abdomen. Because he has severe internal bleeding, not as much blood is returning to his heart, and stroke volume is therefore decreased. Cardiac output drops as a result.
- A 90-year-old woman is having her fourth heart attack. In this case, the wall of the left ventricle is no longer working. Because her heart has difficulty squeezing out blood, her cardiac output drops.

The autonomic nervous system also plays a large role in adjusting cardiac output. The sympathetic (fight-or-flight) response increases heart rate and the strength of contractions. The parasympathetic nervous system slows the heart rate and decreases contractility.

The heart can fail in two different ways—mechanically or electrically. Failure can result from a muscle (structural) problem or due to a problem with electrical stimulation of that muscle. Mechanical failure can be caused by a number of factors, including trauma, such as gunshot and stab wounds; squeezing forces, such as bleeding inside the heart's protective sac; or loss of function of cardiac muscle due to cell death, as in a heart attack. Electrical failure can result from problems in the heart's conduction system, which include tachycardia, bradycardia, and disorganized conduction, such as ventricular fibrillation. More information on cardiac dysfunction is discussed in later chapters.

FIRST ON SCENE (continued)

Pulling up to the address, Case and Darin are met at the curb by a man who identifies himself as the building landlord. "Please hurry," the man says, sounding winded. "He's up on the second floor, and he looks real bad. He's having a hard time breathing." Case and Darin grab their jump bag, oxygen, and AED, and follow the man up two flights of stairs. As they enter the cluttered apartment, they find a thin, frail, older man gasping for each breath.

"We are with the fire department, sir, and we are here to help. Can you tell me when you started having trouble breathing?" Darin asks. He notes that the man is very pale and is able to speak in only three- and four-word sentences. "Quick, give me a nonrebreather at 15 liters," Darin directs Case.

Cardiovascular System Compensation

LO10 List the responses by the body when the sympathetic nervous system is stimulated.

Just as the respiratory system predictably responds to a gas-exchange problem, the cardiovascular system causes predictable changes to compensate for poor perfusion. In most cases of hypoperfusion, the sympathetic nervous system causes blood vessels to constrict and the heart to beat faster and stronger. The ability to change the diameter of blood vessels is critical to the body's ability to compensate for problems in the circulatory system. For example, if an individual is bleeding, their overall blood volume will drop, causing a drop in blood pressure. The nervous system detects this drop in pressure and compensates by constricting (narrowing) the blood vessels. This allows the body to maintain a normal blood pressure even when there is less overall blood volume.

The nervous system also causes pupils to dilate and the skin to sweat. Receptors in the brain and blood vessels sense an increase in carbon dioxide and low levels of oxygen and stimulate the respiratory system to breathe faster and deeper. These signs of compensation can be seen during patient assessment. A patient in shock will have an increased pulse and respiratory rate. They may also have delayed capillary refill and pale skin resulting from constriction of the peripheral vessels. Pupils may be dilated, and the patient may be sweaty, even in cool environments.

As an Emergency Medical Responder, you should learn to recognize these findings as an indication that shock is present. Understanding compensation is a critical component in predicting more serious potential changes to come.

Children's cardiovascular systems compensate differently than those of adults. Children rely more on heart rate to overcome problems with cardiac output. Because of this, fast heart rates in children should always be considered to indicate shock until proven otherwise. Children also rely heavily on vasoconstriction to compensate for volume loss. As a result, they can maintain pressure in the cardiovascular system with relatively less blood than an adult. For this reason, blood pressure is a fairly unreliable indicator of shock in children. Children also have a higher metabolic rate than adults do. That means they burn more oxygen and require a more regular supply via perfusion to sustain normal function.

Shock is among the leading killers of pediatric patients. As an Emergency Medical Responder, you must learn to recognize the specific signs of hypoperfusion and compensation in children and adolescents. This will be discussed further in Chapter 24.

FIRST ON SCENE WRAP-UP

Later that day, Case and Darin run into the ambulance crew at the hospital. "Nice job, guys," one of the paramedics comments as they pass in the ambulance bay. "Your guy was just minutes away from going into respiratory arrest, and the oxygen really helped. He has a long history of emphysema and had run out of oxygen in his home tank."

"Thanks for the follow-up, guys," Case says. "It's good to hear a patient's outcome once in a while."

Summary

- Understanding pathophysiology helps you understand the basic and most important functions of the body and their critical dysfunctions.
- Aerobic metabolism (energy production using oxygen) is the normal way the body converts glucose into energy. Anaerobic metabolism (energy production without oxygen) can be used but is not as efficient, and it creates significantly more waste products.
- Cellular metabolism relies on a constant supply of glucose and oxygen.
- Perfusion requires the combined function of the respiratory and cardiovascular systems (cardiopulmonary system).

All functions must be operating correctly to deliver oxygenated blood to the cells and remove cellular waste.
- Oxygen is introduced into the body from the ambient air. This process requires a functioning respiratory system and the ability to move air in and out of the lungs.
- The cardiovascular system is the transport mechanism that delivers oxygen and nutrients to cells and removes carbon dioxide. Proper transport requires adequate blood volume, appropriate pressure within the system, and a functioning pump.

Take Action

Ask About Diabetes

Diabetes is a disease that results when the pancreas does not produce adequate amounts of the hormone insulin or when the body does not use insulin properly. The CDC estimates that as of 2021, more than 37 million people in the United States had diabetes. With so many living with diabetes, there is a good chance you know someone who has this disease. When you discover someone you know has diabetes, let them know you are training as an Emergency Medical Responder and ask if they would be willing to share their experiences as a person with this disease. Use the following suggested questions to guide your exploration:

1. How long have you been living with diabetes?
2. Do you have type 1 or type 2 diabetes?
3. Do you take medication to control the disease? If so, what do you take and how often?
4. Do you have limitations because of the disease?
5. How do you know when your blood sugar is out of balance (too high or too low)? How does it make you feel?
6. How do you monitor your blood sugar level?

First on Scene Patient Handoff

Carl is a 76-year-old male with a chief complaint of severe respiratory distress, which came on gradually over the past 30 minutes. He has a long history of emphysema and is on home oxygen. When we arrived, his respirations were 30 shallow and labored, pulse 124 weak and irregular, and we were not able to obtain a blood pressure due to his shaking so much. We placed him on a nonrebreather at 15 LPM, which seemed to help just a little.

First on Scene Run Review

Recall the events of the First on Scene scenario in this chapter and answer the following questions related to the call. Rationales are offered in the Answer Key at the back of the book.

1. How would you describe the patient's level of distress related to his difficulty breathing (mild, moderate, or severe) and why?
2. Why is this patient presenting with pale skin?
3. How is supplemental oxygen going to help this patient?

Quick Quiz

To check your understanding of the chapter, answer the following questions. Then compare your answers to those in the Answer Key at the back of the book.

1. The most basic unit of the human body is the:
   a. cell.
   b. organ.
   c. organ system.
   d. quadrant.

2. All cells require a constant supply of glucose, water, and:
   a. carbon dioxide.
   b. ATC.
   c. glycogen.
   d. oxygen.

3. Anaerobic metabolism in a cell produces carbon dioxide and:
   a. lactic acid.
   b. carbon monoxide.
   c. insulin.
   d. hemoglobin.

4. A breathing rate that is too slow will result in an excess buildup of ___ in the blood.
   a. electrolytes
   b. carbon dioxide
   c. oxygen
   d. carbon monoxide

5. Which of the following would be a predictable physical response to hypoperfusion (shock)?
   a. Decreased respiratory rate
   b. Increased heart rate
   c. Vasodilation
   d. Pupil constriction

6. A 4-year-old male patient suspected of being in shock has delayed capillary refill time. This is most likely caused by:
   a. vasodilation.
   b. cold ambient temperature.
   c. medicine he has been given.
   d. vasoconstriction.

7. During normal metabolism, what does the cell convert into energy?
   a. Glucose
   b. Water
   c. Oxygen
   d. Lactic acid

8. The process of using oxygen to fuel the creation of energy is called ___ metabolism.
   a. aerobic
   b. anaerobic
   c. inaerobic
   d. lactic

9. The regulation of breathing is controlled by the:
   a. lungs.
   b. diaphragm.
   c. medulla.
   d. peripheral nervous system.

10. The problem that can result when a patient does not get an adequate supply of oxygen is:
    a. hypoxia.
    b. pneumothorax.
    c. stroke.
    d. anoxia.

11. The smallest vessel that carries deoxygenated blood is a(n):
    a. artery.
    b. arteriole.
    c. venule.
    d. vein.

12. Stimulation of the sympathetic nervous system will result in all of the following EXCEPT:
    a. increased heart rate.
    b. increased respiratory rate.
    c. constriction of vessels.
    d. decreased heart rate.

13. The volume of blood ejected from the left ventricle with each contraction of the heart is known as:
    a. cardiac output.
    b. respiratory volume.
    c. stroke volume.
    d. minute volume.

6

Principles of Lifting, Moving, and Positioning of Patients

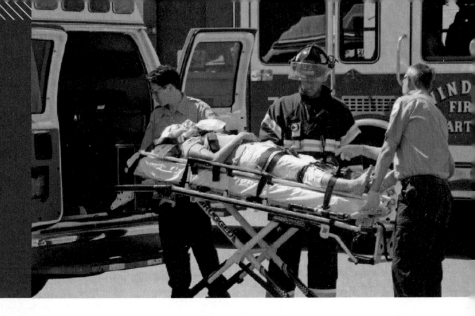

Education Standards

Preparatory—Workforce Safety and Wellness

Competencies

Uses knowledge of the EMS system, safety/well-being of the Emergency Medical Responder, and medical, legal, and ethical issues at the scene of an emergency while awaiting a higher level of care.

LEARNING OBJECTIVES

Upon successful completion of this chapter, the student should be able to:

Cognitive

1. Define the chapter key terms.
2. Explain the importance of active communication during patient lifts and moves.
3. Explain the characteristics of proper body mechanics.
4. Explain the importance of using proper body mechanics.
5. Explain the hazards of not using proper body mechanics when lifting and moving patients.
6. Differentiate between an emergent move and a standard move, and state when each should be used.
7. Identify common devices used for transporting patients.
8. Explain the purpose of the recovery position, and state when it should be used.
9. Describe the Fowler's, semi-Fowler's, and shock positions, and state when each should be used.
10. Explain the criteria for using patient restraints.
11. Identify the various types of patient restraints.
12. Explain the technique for the proper restraint of a patient.
13. Explain the complications associated with restraining a patient.

Psychomotor

14. Demonstrate the use of proper body mechanics while performing various patient moves and lifts.
15. Demonstrate the proper technique for standard moves, urgent moves, and emergent moves.
16. Demonstrate the proper use of equipment used to transport patients.
17. Demonstrate the proper technique for placing a supine patient into the recovery position.
18. Demonstrate the proper technique for log-rolling a patient.

Affective

19. Value the importance of proper body mechanics when participating in simulated patient moves and lifts.

KEY TERMS

blanket drag (*p. 108*)
body mechanics (*p. 106*)
clothing drag (*p. 108*)
direct carry (*p. 112*)
direct ground lift (*p. 110*)

draw sheet method (*p. 112*)
emergent move (*p. 108*)
extremity lift (*p. 111*)
Fowler's position (*p. 120*)
log roll (*p. 120*)

M any Emergency Medical Responders are injured every year because
they attempt to lift or move a patient or piece of equipment improperly.
Recent research found that among EMTs and paramedics, the annual
prevalence of back pain ranged from 30 to 66 percent, and the prevalence of
back injuries and contusions ranged from 4 to 43 percent. Falls, slips, trips,
and overexertion while lifting or carrying patients or equipment ranged from
10 to 56 percent, with overexertion being the most common type of injury.
Risk factors were predominantly lifting, working in awkward postures, loading
patients into the ambulance, and cardiopulmonary resuscitation procedures[1]

One of the most important things that you can do for yourself, your
coworkers, and your patients is to learn how to lift and move patients and
objects using proper body mechanics. Just as critical as knowing *how* to move
patients properly is knowing *when* they should be moved. There are many
factors you must consider before moving a patient, such as the safety of the
scene, the patient's condition, what care they may need, and the number of
rescuers available to assist.

This chapter discusses common situations in which an Emergency
Medical Responder may be required to move or reposition a patient. It also
describes moving and lifting techniques that use proper body mechanics
that make it possible for you to be a safe and healthy Emergency Medical
Responder for many years to come.

FIRST ON SCENE

Jesse had just changed the station on his satellite radio when
the front right tire on his car explodes, sending pieces of rubber
in all directions. He grabs the steering wheel with both hands
and eases the small car completely off the road and onto the
shoulder. He gets out, swearing under his breath, and walks
around to the front of the car to inspect the damage. The tire
isn't just flat. It is gone. A bare, bent wheel is the only thing that
remains.

A man driving a pickup stops in the roadway next to
Jesse's car and shouts through the open passenger window,
"Is everything okay?"

"Yeah. I just have to put the spare on," Jesse shouts back,
knowing that he is definitely going to be late for his Emergency
Medical Responder class at the community college.

"I'll pull over and help!" the man yells back. Jesse smiles
and starts to say, "Thanks!" but the man and his pickup truck
are suddenly gone in a deafening explosion of twisting metal,
rushing air, and spinning chrome wheels. Jesse stumbles
backward and falls to the ground. He watches in horror
as a speeding semi flashes larger than life just beyond him as
he hears the sound of locked-up tires roaring across the
pavement.

Principles of Moving Patients Safely

LO2 Explain the importance of active communication during patient lifts and moves.

With the proper technique, moving and lifting patients and objects can be done safely. Before you lift or move a patient or an object, it is important to first plan what you will do and how you will do it. Estimate the weight of the patient or object and, if needed, request additional help. Also consider any physical limitations that may make lifting difficult or unsafe for you and those assisting you. Whenever possible, lift with a partner whose strength and height are similar to your own. Clearly communicate with your partner and with the patient when you are ready to lift, and continue to communicate throughout the process. Eye contact is important when coordinating a lift. Make sure you and your partner make eye contact before initiating any lift.

When to Move a Patient

In general, an Emergency Medical Responder should move a patient only when absolutely necessary. Your primary role is to assess the patient, provide basic emergency care, and continue to monitor the patient's condition until personnel with more advanced training arrive. Emergency situations in which it may be necessary to move a patient include the presence of a dangerous environment where the patient is at risk for further injury; when you cannot adequately assess airway, breathing, circulation (ABCs) or bleeding; or when you are unable to gain access to other patients who need lifesaving care. You also may be called on to assist other EMS responders with performing certain types of patient moves.

Whenever possible, encourage the patient to remain at rest, even when the patient appears to be able to move. Remember that not all signs of illness or injury show themselves immediately, and sometimes patients do not realize how sick or injured they really are.

Body Mechanics

LO3 Describe the characteristics of proper body mechanics.

LO4 Explain the importance of using proper body mechanics.

LO5 Explain the hazards of not using proper body mechanics when lifting and moving patients.

Good **body mechanics** involve the proper and efficient use of your body to facilitate lifting and moving. Using proper body mechanics when moving and lifting patients will greatly increase safety for the patient and reduce the chances of injury for you and others who are assisting the patient. Proper body mechanics include the following principles:

- Position your feet properly. They should be on a firm, level surface and positioned about shoulder width apart. Take extra care if the surface is slippery or unstable. It may be necessary to postpone the move until more help or equipment is on hand.
- Lift using your legs, not your back. Keep your back as straight as possible, and bend your knees. Try not to bend at the waist any more than you absolutely must. This technique is known as a **power lift** (Key Skill 6.1).
- When lifting an object with one hand, avoid leaning to either side. Bend your knees to grasp the object and keep your back straight.
- Minimize twisting during a lift. Turning or twisting while lifting can result in serious injury.
- Keep the weight as close to your body as possible. The farther the weight is from your body, the greater your chance of injury.
- When carrying a patient on stairs, use a chair or commercial stair chair instead of a wheeled stretcher whenever possible. Keep your back straight, and let your legs do the lifting. If you are walking backward down stairs, ask someone to spot you by walking behind you and placing a hand on your back to help guide and steady you (Figure 6.1).

<aside>

SCENE SAFETY

Sometimes the best decision is to *not* move the patient. If the patient is too heavy, in an awkward position, or you simply do not have enough people to help, consider a new plan or call for additional help.

body mechanics ▶ how we hold our body when we sit, stand, and move; proper body mechanics minimize the risk of injury.

power lift ▶ technique used to lift a patient who is on a stretcher or cot.

SCENE SAFETY

Whenever walking backward down stairs to move a patient, it is best to have a second individual walk behind you and act as a spotter. Have your spotter place a hand on your back and guide you down the stairs.

</aside>

Power Lift

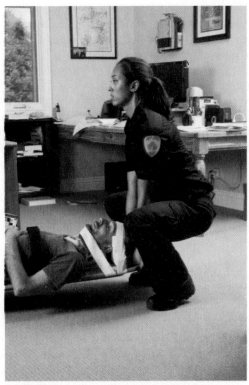

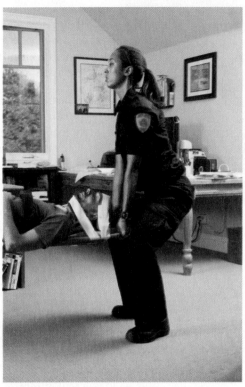

1. To begin the power lift, keep your back straight and eyes on your partner.

2. Lift using your legs, keeping your back straight.

3. While moving, keep the weight as close to your body as possible.

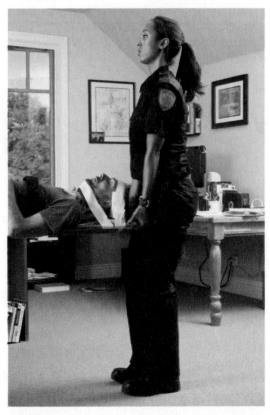

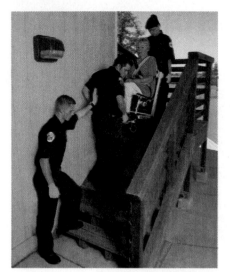

Figure 6.1 When using a stair chair, transport the patient face-first, and use a spotter as you walk backward down the stairs.

emergent move ▶ patient move carried out quickly when the scene is hazardous, care of the patient requires immediate repositioning, or you must reach another patient who needs lifesaving care; also called *emergency move*.

clothing drag ▶ emergent move in which the rescuer pulls the patient by their clothing, usually holding on near the shoulders.

blanket drag ▶ method used to move a patient by placing them on a blanket or sheet and pulling it across the floor or ground.

standard move ▶ preferred choice when the situation is not urgent, the patient is stable, and you have adequate time and personnel for a move.

Emergent Moves

LO6 Differentiate between an emergent move and a standard move, and state when each should be used.

There are times when a patient must be moved immediately, even if you do not have enough people or the appropriate equipment to do so. Such situations call for an **emergent move**, sometimes referred to as an *emergency move*. An emergent move should be considered in the following situations:

- The patient and/or the rescuers are in immediate danger. Situations that involve uncontrolled traffic, fire or threat of fire, possible explosions, impending structural collapse, electrical hazards, toxic gases, and other such dangers may make it necessary to move a patient quickly.
- Lifesaving care cannot be given because of the patient's location or position. The inability to properly assess and care for problems with a patient's breathing and/or circulation, including the inability to properly manage uncontrolled bleeding, makes it necessary to move a patient quickly.
- A patient must be moved to gain access to other patients who need lifesaving care. This is seen most often in motor vehicle crashes.

Emergent moves rarely provide complete protection for a patient's injuries, and they may even cause the patient additional pain. Still, the need to move a patient to ensure their safety or to provide lifesaving care sometimes outweighs the risks associated with moving the patient quickly.

One of the greatest dangers in moving a patient quickly is the possibility of making spinal injuries worse. If the patient is on the floor or ground, it is important to make every effort to pull the patient in the direction of the long axis of the body. This is the line that runs down the center of the body from the top of the head and along the spine. By pulling this way, you will minimize side-to-side movement of the spine as much as possible.

One of the most common types of emergent moves is the drag (Key Skill 6.2). Patients may be dragged with the rescuer holding them by their feet or shoulders. In a **clothing drag**, the rescuer grabs the patient's clothing, usually near the shoulders, and pulls the patient to safety. In a **blanket drag**, the patient is placed on a blanket, and the blanket is pulled across the floor or ground. Note that drags provide little if any protection for the neck and spine.

In most cases, drags are initiated from the shoulders by pulling along the long axis of the body. This causes the remainder of the body to fall into its natural anatomical position, with the spine and all limbs in normal alignment. Avoid dragging a patient sideways or by one arm or one leg unless absolutely necessary. A sideways drag can cause twisting motions of the spine that could aggravate existing injuries.

When using a drag to move a patient down stairs or down an incline, grab the patient under the shoulders and pull them headfirst as you walk backward. If possible, try to cradle the patient's head in your forearms as you drag.

Standard Moves

LO6 Differentiate between an emergent move and a standard move, and state when each should be used.

A **standard move** is the preferred choice when the situation is not urgent, the patient is stable, and you have adequate time and personnel to plan for a coordinated move. Standard moves should be carried out with the help of other trained personnel or bystanders. Take care to prevent causing the patient discomfort, pain, or additional injury. The following are situations in which a standard move may be appropriate:

- The patient is uncomfortable or their position is aggravating an injury.
- Indicated care requires moving the patient.
- In cases of serious chemical burns, getting the patient closer to a source of water for washing may be a reason to move them.
- The patient insists on being moved. If a patient will not listen to reasons they should not be moved and tries to move on their own, you may have to assist.

Jesse climbs to his feet and watches the big rig slow to a crawl and pull off onto the shoulder several hundred feet down the highway. The twisted heap that was the pickup truck sits smoking in the middle of the road just beyond it, the bed curled up over the top of the cab like a huge metal scorpion. Jesse looks back up the highway and sees a car and another semi bearing down on the scene, heading right into the setting sun. He turns and sprints as fast as he can down the shoulder of the road, past the parked semi, and up to a point where he is even with the wrecked pickup.

"Help me!" Incredibly, the man in the pickup is alive and seems fully conscious. Jesse can clearly see him in the still intact cab of the truck. "My legs are ... uh ... I think they're gone. What do I do?" The man keeps looking over at Jesse then back down into his lap.

Jesse sees other vehicles approaching at high speed. He begins to yell and wave his arms, trying to get the drivers' attention. Seconds later, a car swerves around the wreckage and continues on without braking, throwing up bits of broken glass and metal as it speeds by.

"Help me, please!" The man is now screaming over the deafening rumble of a rapidly approaching semi.

KEY SKILL 6.2

Emergent Moves: One-Rescuer Drags

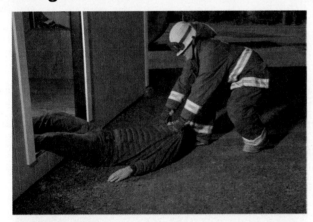

1. Clothing drag.

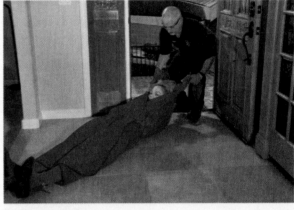

2. Blanket drag.

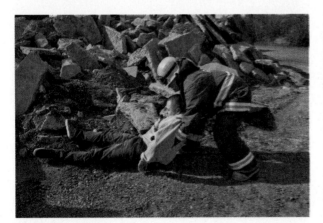

3. Shoulder drag.

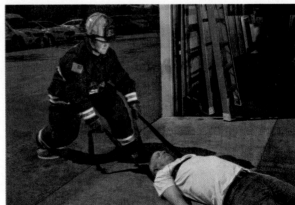

4. Strap drag.

Note: Always pull in the direction of the long axis of the patient's body. Do not pull a patient sideways.

Follow these rules when preparing to use a standard move:

- Complete a primary assessment.
- Be sure that you have a good reason to move the patient.
- Choose an appropriate number of rescuers for the specific type of move.
- Take care to avoid compromising a possible neck or spinal injury.
- Consider splinting suspected fractures, depending on the patient's condition.

Direct Ground Lift

The direct ground lift is a standard move that can be used to move a patient from the ground or floor to a bed or stretcher. This move is not recommended for use on patients with possible neck or spinal injuries. Depending on the size of the patient, two or three rescuers can accomplish this move.

direct ground lift ▶ standard lift in which three rescuers move a patient from the ground or floor to a bed or stretcher.

To perform a **direct ground lift** (Key Skill 6.3), the patient should be lying supine (face up), with their arms placed over their chest. You and your helpers should line up on one side of the patient. One rescuer should be at the patient's head, another at their hips and thighs. Each rescuer drops one knee to the ground and keeps the other foot planted on the floor.

KEY SKILL 6.3

Direct Ground Lift

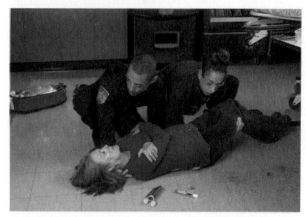

1. Position your arms under the patient. Be sure to cradle the head.

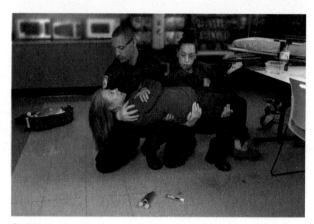

2. Lift the patient to your knees and roll them toward your chest.

3. Stand together and place the patient on the stretcher.

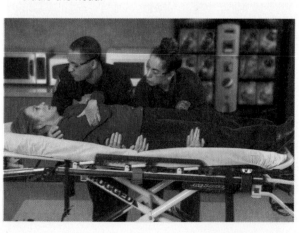

The rescuer at the patient's head places one arm under the patient's neck and grasps the far shoulder to cradle the head. The other arm is placed under the patient's back, just above the waist. The second rescuer places one arm above and one arm below the patient's thighs. On the signal of the rescuer at the head, both rescuers lift the patient up to the level of their knees. Then, on signal, the rescuers roll the patient toward their chests. Finally, on signal, everyone stands, lifting the patient onto a bed or stretcher. The patient can now be moved, reversing the process when it is time to place them in a supine position.

Extremity Lift

An **extremity lift** requires two people (Key Skill 6.4). This lift is ideal for moving a patient from the ground to a chair or a stretcher. It also can be used to move a patient from a chair to a stretcher. However, it should not be performed if there is a possibility of head, neck, spine, shoulder, hip, or knee injury or any suspected fractures to extremities that have not been immobilized.

The patient is placed face up with knees flexed. You kneel at the head of the patient, placing your hands under their shoulders. Have your helper stand at the patient's feet and grasp their wrists. Direct your helper to pull the patient into a sitting position while you push the patient from the shoulders. (Do not have your helper pull the patient by the arms if there are any signs of suspected fractures.) Slip your arms under the patient's armpits and grasp the wrists. Once the patient is in a semi-sitting position, have your helper crouch down and grasp the patient's legs behind the knees.

extremity lift ▶ standard move performed by two rescuers, one lifting the patient's arms and one lifting the patient's legs.

KEY SKILL 6.4

Extremity Lift

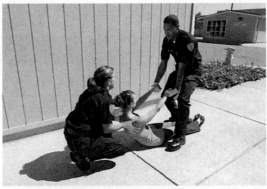

1. To get the patient into a sitting position, one rescuer pushes from behind while the other pulls from the wrists.

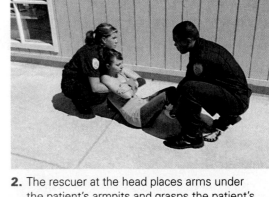

2. The rescuer at the head places arms under the patient's armpits and grasps the patient's wrists. While facing the patient, the rescuer at the feet grasps the patient's legs behind the knees.

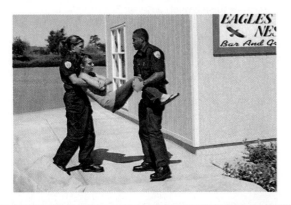

3. The rescuers stand together and carry the patient as needed.

Signal your helper so you both stand at the same time. For example, "Ready? Lift on three. One, two, three." Then move as a unit when carrying the patient. Try to walk out of step with your partner to avoid swinging the patient. The rescuer at the head should direct the rescuer at the feet when to stop the carry and when to place the patient down in a supine or seated position.

Direct Carry Method

direct carry ▶ carry performed to move a patient with no suspected spinal injury from a bed or from a bed-level position to a stretcher.

The **direct carry** is performed to move a patient with no suspected spine injury from a bed or from a bed-level position to a stretcher (Key Skill 6.5). First, position the stretcher perpendicular to the bed, with the head of the stretcher at the foot of the bed. Prepare the stretcher by unbuckling the straps and removing other items. Two rescuers stand between the bed and the stretcher, facing the patient. The first rescuer slides an arm under the patient's neck and cups the shoulder, while the second rescuer slides a hand under the patient's hip and lifts slightly. The first rescuer then slides their other arm under the patient's back, while the second rescuer places their arms underneath the patient's hips and calves. Finally, both rescuers slide the patient to the edge of the bed, lifting or rolling them toward their chests, and rotate and place the patient gently onto the stretcher.

Draw Sheet Method

draw sheet method ▶ method for moving a patient from a bed to a stretcher.

An additional way of moving a patient with no suspected spine injury from a bed to a stretcher is the **draw sheet method**. This move may be performed from the side, head, or foot of the bed, whichever gives you best access to the patient. Figure 6.2 illustrates this move from the side of the bed.

To perform the draw sheet method from the side of the bed, first loosen the bottom sheet under the patient and position the stretcher next to the bed. Be sure to secure the stretcher so it does not move while transferring the patient from the bed to the stretcher.

KEY SKILL 6.5

Direct Carry

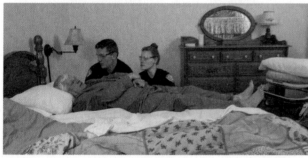

1. Position your arms under the patient and slide the patient to the edge of the bed.
(Maria Lyle/Pearson Education, Inc.)

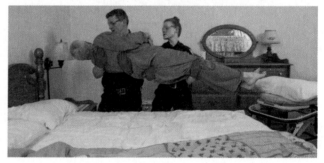

2. Lift the patient and curl them toward your chest.
(Maria Lyle/Pearson Education, Inc.)

3. Stand together and place the patient on the stretcher.
(Maria Lyle/Pearson Education, Inc.)

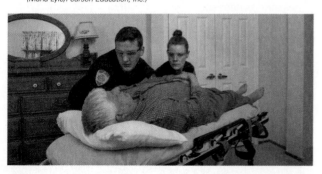

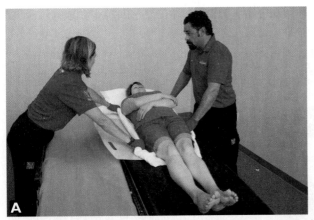 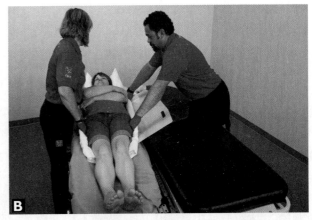

Figure 6.2 Using a slider board with the draw sheet method to transfer a patient from (A) a bed to (B) a stretcher.

Next, adjust the height of the stretcher to match the level of the bed, lower the rails, and unbuckle the straps. Both rescuers should reach across the stretcher and roll the sheet against the patient. Grasp the sheet firmly at the patient's head, chest, hips, and knees. Finally, draw the patient onto the stretcher, sliding them in one smooth motion.

Several devices make the task of moving patients from stretcher to bed easier and safer. Devices such as slider boards and slide bags (Figure 6.3A and B) are in use in many hospitals and nursing homes. Become familiar with the use of these devices before you attempt to use them for the first time.

Equipment for Transporting Patients

LO7 | Identify common devices used for transporting patients.

EMTs and advanced life support (ALS) personnel often ask Emergency Medical Responders to assist with preparing the patient for transport and with lifting, moving, and loading patients into the ambulance. To help with those tasks, you must be familiar with the various carrying and "packaging" devices used by EMS personnel.

Typical equipment used for packaging and loading a patient into an ambulance includes a wheeled stretcher. This device has many names depending on the area of the country. Common names include gurney, stretcher, cot, and pram. It is used to transport a patient from the scene of the emergency to the ambulance and from the ambulance to a hospital bed. It is secured in the back of an ambulance by way of a simple locking mechanism. In addition, the head and the foot ends of many stretchers can be elevated to make the patient comfortable or to assist in caring for certain conditions such as difficulty breathing.

JEDI

When moving a patient, be very aware of how and where you touch them. Appropriate touch is touch with a deliberate purpose by the rescuer that is related to overall patient care. When possible, you'll ask the patient to consent to being touched and moved. Always inform the patient if you will be touching them in or near sensitive areas. This prevents them from reacting in surprise and potentially making an illness or injury worse. When possible, use a closed-hand method in which all fingers are together.

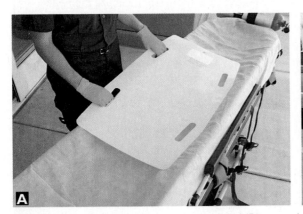 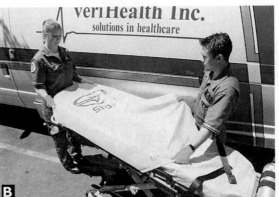

Figure 6.3 (A) Example of a slider board and (B) example of a slide bag.

There are many brands and types of wheeled stretchers (Key Skill 6.6). Common types include:

- *Single-operator stretcher.* This type allows one person to load the stretcher into the ambulance without the assistance of a second individual. The undercarriage is designed to collapse and fold up as the stretcher is pushed into the ambulance.

KEY SKILL 6.6

Using Wheeled Stretchers

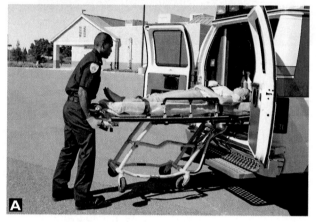

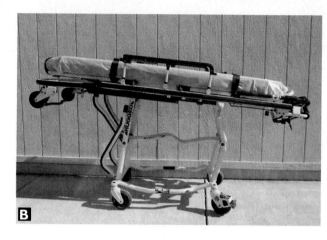

1. Single-operator stretcher (A and B)

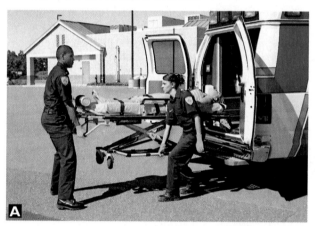

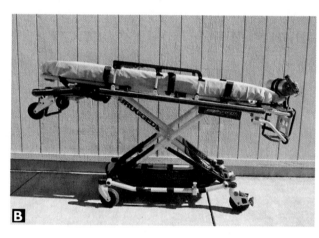

2. Dual-operator stretcher (A and B).

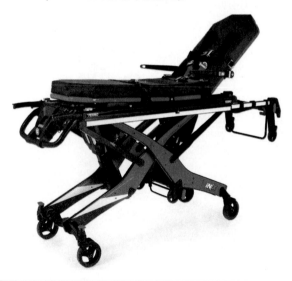

3. iN∫X™ Integrated Patient Transport and Loading System. Power-assisted stretchers minimize the need for heavy lifting by rescue personnel.
(© Ferno-Washington, Inc.)

- *Dual-operator stretcher.* This type requires two operators because a second individual must lift the undercarriage prior to pushing it into the ambulance.
- *Power stretcher.* This type is equipped with an electric or pneumatic mechanism that lifts and lowers the stretcher at the touch of a button. It minimizes the need for rescuers to lift a stretcher with a patient on it, thereby significantly reducing the risk of back injury.
- *Bariatric stretcher.* This type is designed to accommodate oversized patients up to a maximum of 1,600 pounds. It is wider and stronger and can be loaded into the ambulance with a specialized winch system.

Other types of equipment used for moving patients include the following (Key Skills 6.7 and 6.8):

- *Portable stretcher.* This type of stretcher is also known as a *folding stretcher* or *flat stretcher*. It is lighter than a standard wheeled stretcher and makes the task of moving a patient down stairs or out of tight spaces much easier. Portable stretchers are typically a combination of canvas and aluminum, and they usually fold or collapse for easy storage.
- *Flexible stretcher.* This stretcher is made of rubberized canvas or other flexible material such as heavy plastic, often with wooden slats sewn into pockets. The flexible stretcher usually has three carrying handles on each side. Because of its flexibility, it can be useful in restricted areas or narrow hallways.
- *Stair chair.* The stair chair helps rescuers move seated patients down stairways and through tight places where a traditional stretcher will not fit. Most stair chairs are made of sturdy folding frames with canvas or hard plastic seats and are easy to store. They have wheels that allow rescuers to roll them over flat surfaces. Some models have a tractor-tread mechanism that allows them to easily slide down stairways just by tilting them.
- *Basket stretcher.* This stretcher is sometimes referred to as a *Stokes basket*. It is most commonly used for wilderness or cliff rescue situations.
- *Scoop stretcher.* This stretcher is typically made of hard plastic or aluminum. It is called a scoop stretcher because it splits vertically into two pieces, which can be used to "scoop up" the patient.
- *Long spine board.* Spine boards are also known as *backboards*. The long spine board is used for patients who are suspected of having a significant spinal injury. Backboards have been proven to cause pain, agitation, and respiratory compromise in some patients. Current research suggests more discretion with the use of long backboards, with their use reserved for patients with the following conditions:[2]
  - Blunt trauma and altered level of consciousness
  - Spinal pain or tenderness
  - Neurologic complaint (such as numbness or motor weakness)
  - Anatomic deformity of the spine
  - High-energy mechanism of injury and any of the following: drug or alcohol intoxication, inability to communicate, or a distracting injury. A distracting injury is one that prevents the patient from realizing pain in the neck or spine, such as a significant injury to the forearm or chest.
- *Extrication vest.* The extrication vest is used to help immobilize and remove patients found in a seated position in a vehicle. It wraps around the patient's torso to stabilize the spine and has an extended section above the vest with side flaps for stabilizing the patient's head and neck. Rescuers secure the patient's head, neck, and torso with straps and padding. The vest has handles that aid in lifting the patient out of the vehicle and onto a long spine board.
- *Full-body immobilization device.* The most common type is the full-body vacuum splint. It consists of a large airtight bag filled with tiny beads. As the patient is placed on the device, it can be molded to fit the shape and contours of the patient's

SCENE SAFETY

Scoop stretchers might not be appropriate for immobilization of the spine. The authors of this textbook have contacted several manufacturers of scoop stretchers, and all have indicated that the scoop stretcher is not recommended for use as a primary spinal immobilization device. However, it may be appropriate to place the patient on a scoop stretcher and then secure the scoop to a long spine board for additional support. Consult your local protocols for the proper use of the scoop stretcher.

body. Once it is in place, a portable vacuum is activated to remove the air from the bag. The result is a hard, cast-like splint that immobilizes the patient.

- *Pedi-board.* Special spinal immobilization boards are made to fit infants and children. The back of a child's head is larger proportionately than an adult's, so boards have a depression in the head end to fit. However, it is still necessary to pad the child's body from the shoulders to the heels to ensure the airway is in a neutral position while the child is secured on the board.

KEY SKILL 6.7

Using Various Types of Stretchers

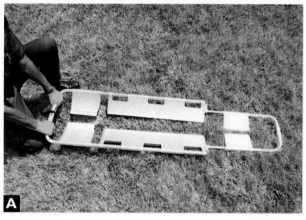
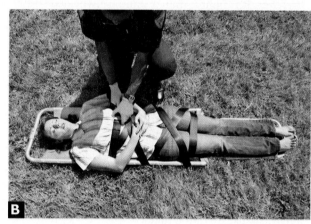

1. Scoop stretchers. (A) These stretchers are ideal for moving patients in the position in which they are found. (B) Once in place, the patient must be properly secured to the device before moving.

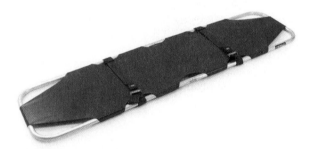

2. Portable stretcher. These are beneficial for carrying supine patients down stairs.
(© Ferno-Washington, Inc.)

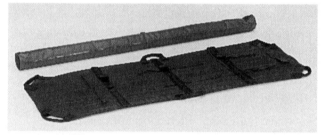

3. Flexible stretcher, commonly used in restricted areas or narrow hallways.

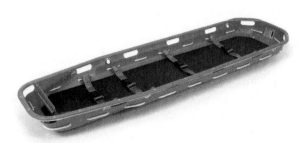

4. Basket stretcher. These are used in rescue situations and to transport over rough terrain.
(© Ferno-Washington, Inc.)

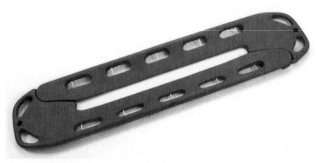

5. Combi-Board. This hard plastic board splits into two halves, much like the standard scoop stretcher.

Using Backboards

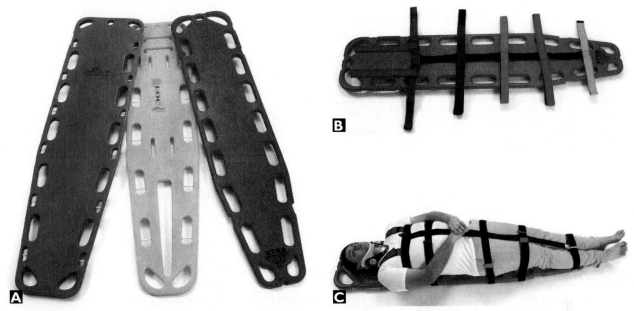

A

B

C

1. Long board. (A) Long backboards come in a variety of shapes and colors. (B) Spider straps are an excellent tool for securing a patient to a long board. (C) Patient secured to long board with spider straps.
(Maria Lyle/Pearson Education, Inc.)

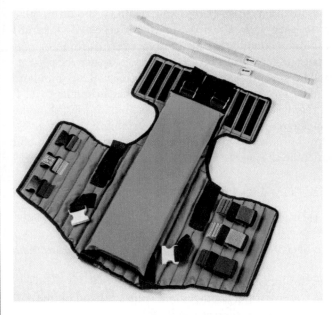

2. The Kendrick Extrication Device is a tool used to immobilize a seated patient.
(Maria Lyle/Pearson Education, Inc.)

In addition, research has shown that cooperative patients who are alert and oriented and who do not show signs of neurologic deficit may benefit from a soft cervical collar and placement in a position of comfort directly on the stretcher mattress, rather than receiving a hard collar and being placed on a backboard.[3]

Jesse can see the driver of the oncoming semi, immersed in a conversation on his cell phone, as he moves the steering wheel to the left, guiding the huge truck onto the grassy center divide of the highway, where it passes the collision scene without so much as downshifting. Once the truck's flatbed trailer clears the wreckage, it returns to the roadway and continues off into the distance.

"Please, please, help me!" the man screams at Jesse, his face contorted with pain and terror.

There are more oncoming vehicles but, at the moment, they are nothing more than colorful specks on the distant horizon.

Jesse runs to the pickup and is able to force the passenger side door open, breaking it back onto the hinges. He reaches over and releases the driver's seat belt and finds that the bench seat of the truck is covered with blood.

The man falls over onto the passenger side, grabbing for Jesse's arm. Jesse can see that both of his legs are injured and bleeding severely, pinched between the truck's displaced engine and the now raised floor of the cab. He quickly glances down the highway, sees the glint of the sun on a windshield, slides his hands under the man's arms, and begins moving backward as fast as he can.

Patient Positioning

Proper positioning of patients is one of the most important skills an Emergency Medical Responder can learn. Proper positioning is important for many reasons, including patient comfort and proper airway maintenance.

Recovery Position

| LO8 | Explain the purpose of the recovery position, and state when it should be used.

A patient with altered mental status and no suspected spinal injury should be placed on their side to help maintain an open and clear airway. This is especially helpful for unresponsive patients. This position is commonly called the **recovery position** or *lateral recumbent position*. Unless the patient's condition suggests otherwise, place the patient on their left side. Because most stretchers secure against the driver's side wall in ambulances, this positioning will have the patient face the EMT for the ride to the hospital.

Remember that patients with injuries, especially suspected spinal injuries, should not be moved until additional EMS resources arrive to evaluate and stabilize them.

Always position yourself appropriately to manage the patient's airway and monitor their mental status. Place the patient in the recovery position at the first sign of a decreased level of responsiveness.

To place a patient in the recovery position, perform the following steps (Key Skill 6.9):

recovery position ▶ position in which a patient with no suspected spinal injuries may be placed, usually on their left side; also called the *lateral recumbent position*.

1. Kneel beside the patient on their left side. Raise the patient's left arm straight out above their head.
2. Cross the patient's right arm over their chest, placing their right hand next to their left cheek.
3. Raise the patient's right knee until it is completely flexed.
4. Place your right hand on the patient's right shoulder and your left hand on the patient's flexed right knee. Using the flexed knee as a lever, pull toward you, guiding the patient's torso in a smooth, rolling motion onto their left side. The patient's head will rest on their left arm.
5. As best you can, position the patient's right elbow and right knee on the floor so they act like a kickstand, preventing the patient from rolling completely onto their stomach. Place the patient's right hand under the side of their face. The arm will support the patient in this position. The hand will cushion the patient's face and allow the head to angle slightly downward for airway drainage.

Placing the Patient in the Recovery Position

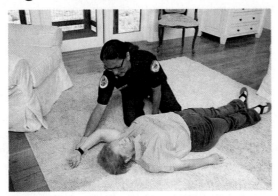

1. Move the patient's closest hand above their head.

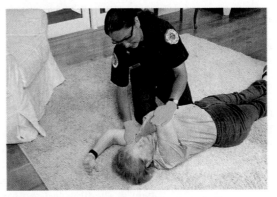

2. Move the patient's far hand across to the opposite shoulder, next to their cheek.

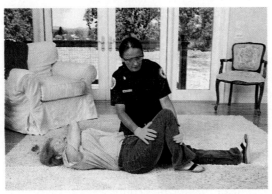

3. Bring the patient's far leg to the flexed position.

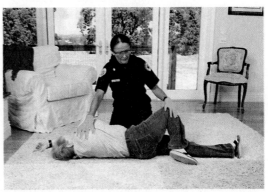

4. Using the knee and shoulder, carefully pull the patient onto their side.

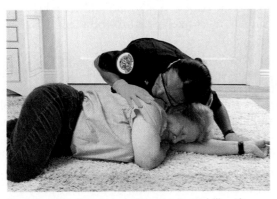

5. Adjust the knee and shoulder to stabilize the patient. Then recheck the patient's ABCs.

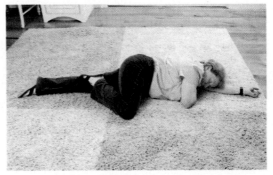

6. Once properly positioned, the knee and elbow will support the patient.

Fowler's and Semi-Fowler's Positions

LO9 Describe the Fowler's, semi-Fowler's, and shock positions, and state when each should be used.

Many patients may be placed in either a position of comfort or specific positions that allow for more effective care of particular conditions. These may include patients with complaints

Fowler's position ▶ patient is placed fully upright in a seated position, creating a 90-degree angle.

semi-Fowler's position ▶ patient is placed in a semi-seated position, reclining at a 45-degree angle.

such as chest pain, nausea, or difficulty breathing. For example, someone with difficulty breathing can be aided by placing them in either a **Fowler's position** (full sitting) or a **semi-Fowler's position** (semi-sitting). This will make it easier for them to breathe.

A trauma patient with no significant signs of spinal injury may be allowed to remain in a semi-Fowler's position and transported on the stretcher with a cervical collar in place as a precaution.

Shock Position

shock position ▶ elevation of the feet of a supine patient 6 to 12 inches; recommended for shock not caused by injury.

> **LO9** Describe the Fowler's, semi-Fowler's, and shock positions, and state when each should be used.

The **shock position** is an option that may be helpful for the patient who could potentially be in shock. This position should be used only for patients exhibiting signs of shock but who have no evidence of injury.[4] This position is achieved by placing the patient in a supine position and raising the legs 6 to 12 inches. In the shock position, the patient's legs are bent at the hips and the torso remains flat. Raising the legs helps promote venous blood return to the heart.

There may be times when a patient is in shock and one or more of these positions are not recommended, such as a patient with a significant head or chest injury. Always follow local protocols when positioning patients.

Log Roll

log roll ▶ method used to move a patient from the prone position to the supine position.

To move a prone patient to a supine position and ensure stability of the head and spine where an injury is suspected, perform a **log roll**. A log roll can also be used for transferring a supine patient onto a long backboard when there is a likelihood of neck or back injury. However, the lift-and-slide technique (described in the following section) has been shown to cause less movement of the neck and spine during transfer to a long backboard.[5]

A log roll can be accomplished with as few as two rescuers, but three is ideal to minimize twisting of the patient's spine during the procedure. Perform the following steps (Key Skill 6.10):

1. One rescuer should kneel at the top of the patient's head and hold or stabilize the head and neck in the position the patient was found. Notice which way the patient's head is facing, as you will most likely want to roll them in the opposite direction.
2. A second rescuer should kneel at the patient's side opposite the direction the head is facing. Quickly assess the patient's arms to ensure that there are no obvious injuries. Raise and extend the patient's arm that is opposite the direction the head is facing. Position that arm straight up above the head. This allows for easy rolling and provides support for the head during the roll. This is especially helpful if you must do the log roll alone.
3. A third rescuer should kneel at the patient's hips.
4. Rescuers should grasp the patient's shoulders, hips, knees, and ankles. If only one rescuer is available to roll the patient, they should grasp the heavy parts of the torso—the shoulders and hips.
5. The rescuer at the patient's head should signal and give directions: "On three, slowly roll. One, two, three." All rescuers should slowly roll the patient toward the rescuers in a coordinated move, keeping the spine in a neutral, in-line position. It is important to note that the rescuer holding the head should not initially try to turn the head with the body. Because the head is already facing sideways, allow the body to come into alignment with the head. Once the body and head are aligned, approximately halfway through the roll, the rescuer at the head will then move it with the body, keeping the head and body aligned until the patient is in the supine position.

Log Roll

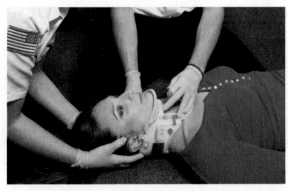

1. Manually stabilize the patient's head and neck as you place the board parallel to the patient. Maintain manual stabilization throughout the roll.

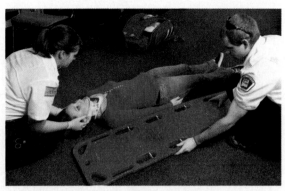

2. Kneel at the patient's side opposite the board. Reach across the patient and position your hands. Inspect the patient's back.

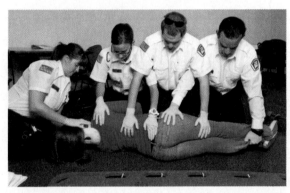

3. At the command from the rescuer at the head, roll the patient toward you. Then move the spine board into place.

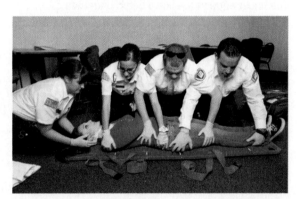

4. At the command of the rescuer at the head, lower the patient onto the spine board. Center the patient on the board.

Sometimes the patient is already supine but must be placed on a blanket or spine board. If this is the case, perform steps 1 through 5 as previously described. Without removing their hands, the rescuers continue with the following steps:

1. The rescuer at the patient's head should continue stabilization of the patient's head and neck until other rescuers position a blanket or long spine board (backboard) behind the patient.
2. At a signal from the rescuer at the head, the rescuers should slowly roll the patient in a coordinated move onto the blanket or spine board.
3. The rescuers should make sure the patient is positioned on the center of the spine board. If an adjustment is necessary, the spine is kept in neutral alignment.

Lift-and-Slide Technique

In studies published in the *Journal of Athletic Training*, the lift-and-slide technique was shown to result in less movement of the head and spine during transfer onto a long backboard.[6] Performing this maneuver requires a minimum of five and often six rescuers (Key Skill 6.11).

One rescuer maintains manual stabilization of the head while a cervical collar is placed. The other four rescuers position themselves on either side of the patient and, on the count of the rescuer at the head, lift the patient a few inches off the ground. An additional rescuer

SCENE SAFETY

The most important individual involved in performing a log roll is the individual at the patient's head. They must think ahead and position their hands in anticipation of the movement of the patient from face down to face up. Positioning the hands incorrectly will result in an awkward hand and body position of the rescuer and may result in excessive movement of the patient's neck.

Lift-and-Slide onto Long Board

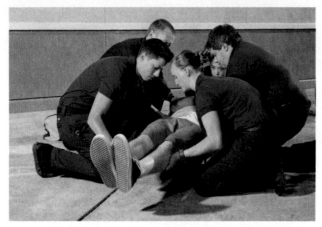

1. A minimum of five rescuers are required to lift the patient just enough to slide a board underneath.

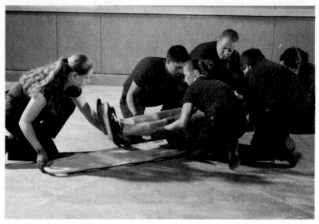

2. A sixth individual must carefully slide the board under the patient.

or bystander may be necessary to carefully position the backboard or stretcher beneath the patient. On the count of the rescuer at the head, everyone carefully lowers the patient down onto the backboard. The patient is then secured to the backboard.

Restraining Patients

LO10 Explain the criteria for using patient restraints.

restraint ▶ process of securing a combative patient's body and/or extremities to prevent injury to themselves or others.

It may become necessary to use a method of **restraint** on a patient when they become a danger to themselves or to others. Patients who have an illness or injury can suddenly become combative and begin lashing out at those around them. Patients who have a behavioral problem or psychiatric emergency may also suddenly refuse care and may attempt to leave the scene. Depending on the situation, it may be necessary to restrain the patient to protect yourself or them from further harm (Figure 6.4). In a perfect world, you would leave the job of restraining a patient to law enforcement personnel, but this is not always possible. Whenever possible, be sure to have law enforcement present when attempting to restrain a patient. It is very important to follow local protocol.

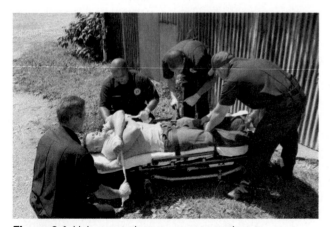

Figure 6.4 Using restraints to secure a patient to a stretcher.

Types of Restraints

LO11 Identify the various types of patient restraints.

Patients can be either physically or mechanically restrained. Physical restraint refers to the rescuer physically holding the patient so they cannot move. Mechanical restraint refers to the application of some sort of device to the patient to restrict their movements. Restraining a patient with your body is not ideal because it does not allow you to provide medical care. The use of mechanical restraints is a better option for a patient with an altered mental status (Figure 6.5A and B).

Handcuffs, shackles, plastic zip ties, and belly chains (a chain that is wrapped around an individual's waist with handcuffs attached) are examples of hard restraints.

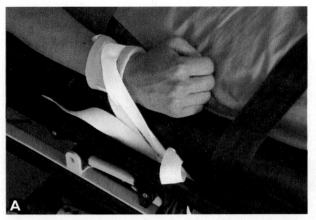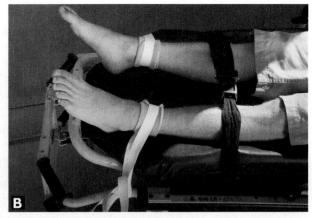

Figure 6.5 Examples of soft restraints. A soft restraint applied (A) to the wrist and (B) to the ankles.

These devices are used primarily by law enforcement and will rarely, if ever, be used by EMS personnel.

Leather or fabric cuffs, cloth straps, rolls of gauze, and cravats (triangular-shaped cloth folded into a strap similar to a bandana) are examples of soft restraints. You will find these items effective and more suited to properly restraining most patients without causing further injury.

Patient Restraint

LO12 Explain the technique for the proper restraint of a patient.

Attempting to restrain a patient is dangerous and can place you, your fellow rescuers, and the patient at risk for injury. Consider all your options such as verbal de-escalation or waiting for law enforcement to arrive before attempting restraint, and always follow local protocols. Follow these guidelines when restraining a patient:

- Ensure that you have adequate assistance—at least four people, including yourself.
- Plan the action and communicate so all those assisting clearly understand their responsibilities.
- Stay outside of the patient's range of motion until ready to act.
- Once the plan is clear, act immediately.
- Approach the patient all at once, with each person assigned to control a particular limb.
- Talk to the patient calmly during the restraining process.
- Secure all limbs with appropriate restraining equipment.
- *Do not* secure the patient face down.
- Following restraint, check the patient's airway, breathing, and circulation often.
- Clearly document the reason for restraining the patient as well as the procedure and equipment used.
- Ensure that the group uses only the force required to effectively restrain the patient.

> **SCENE SAFETY**
>
> It is not always a good idea to attempt to restrain a combative patient. If the patient is armed, too physically strong, potentially under the influence of drugs, in an unsafe area, or you do not have enough assistance, you should maintain your distance and attempt to keep the patient engaged until adequate assistance arrives.

Positional Asphyxia

LO13 Explain the complications associated with restraining a patient.

The most serious complication associated with improperly restraining uncooperative or combative patients is **positional asphyxia**, also called *restraint asphyxia*. This occurs when an individual is restrained in the prone position that either blocks the airway (such as with the chin held tightly to the chest) or in a manner that does not allow full expansion of the chest and lungs. Either can rapidly lead to death, and both are completely avoidable if proper technique is used and the restrained patient is continually assessed.

positional asphyxia ▶ potentially life-threatening lack of oxygen that results from securing an individual in the prone position, limiting their ability to breathe adequately; also called *restraint asphyxia*.

Restraint Injuries

Another complication—one that is much more common than positional asphyxia—is the injury of the patient, the rescuers, or both during the restraint process. Effective planning and communication among the rescuers and rapid, decisive action will go a long way toward preventing injuries while restraining a combative patient. Proper training in the application of restraint devices will also help to prevent injury to the patient once they are restrained.

FIRST ON SCENE WRAP-UP

By the time the emergency crews arrive, summoned by the driver of the semi that initially hit the pickup, several more cars and big rigs have sped through the collision scene. One even clipped the demolished pickup with its bumper, sending the vehicle skittering off the highway and into a ditch.

Jesse had pulled the injured man onto the side of the road. The semi driver who hit the pickup comes running up to the scene.

Shaken and winded, he asks, "Can I help?" Grateful, Jesse shows him how to hold the man's head in a neutral, in-line position while Jesse uses his jacket to apply pressure to the man's bleeding legs.

Later, the paramedic who arrives with the ambulance credits Jesse's quick thinking and actions with ultimately saving the patient's life.

Summary

- It is critical to understand and apply proper body mechanics when lifting patients and objects. Failure to use appropriate techniques can cause career-ending injuries.
- When lifting, always keep the weight as close to your body as possible, avoiding leaning or twisting, and use your leg muscles to lift the weight.
- When two or more rescuers are preparing to move a patient, eye contact and effective communication are very important to ensure a smooth process and to minimize the risk of injury to the rescuers and the patient.
- Although Emergency Medical Responders should ideally provide care for patients where they find them and provide comfort until more advanced help arrives, it is sometimes necessary for the patient to be moved from the immediate area for their own safety or to provide care. The emergent move technique most appropriate to the situation should be used.

- The recovery (lateral recumbent) position is effective to care for an unresponsive patient's airway when a spinal injury is not suspected.
- The lift-and-slide technique and the log-roll technique may be used to position a patient or transition them to a backboard. The lift-and-slide technique has been shown to cause less movement of the patient's head and spine during transfer onto a long backboard when there are at least five rescuers available to perform it.
- Patients can be uncooperative or even combative for a wide range of reasons. If a patient needs to be restrained for their own safety or the safety of others, it is important to use only the force necessary to apply proper restraints.
- Never restrain a patient in the prone position as this can lead to death from positional asphyxia, in which lack of oxygen occurs when the patient cannot breathe due to the way they have been restrained.

Take Action

Instant Replay

It is very common for athletes to watch videos of themselves to identify how they can improve their techniques, and Emergency Medical Responders can use the same process for developing better body mechanics. First, obtain a digital video camera and assemble a group of four or more students: one to act as the patient, two to be EMRs, and one to film the exercise. You should then record yourselves performing the different patient moves detailed in this chapter, immediately reviewing each video and critiquing it from the standpoint of proper body mechanics. Rotate roles so everyone has the opportunity to see and improve their technique. Consider creating a before-and-after compilation highlighting the initial techniques and the revised techniques following the critiquing process.

First on Scene Patient Handoff

Juan is 42 years old and was the driver of a pickup that was rear ended at high speed by a semi-truck. He has been conscious the entire time and complaining of severe pain in both legs. There is obvious injury and deformity to both legs. I placed him supine and applied direct pressure to the wounds on both legs. We have been keeping him still and monitoring his airway and breathing until EMS arrived. His pulse is 116 strong and regular, respirations 24 with good tidal volume.

First on Scene Run Review

Recall the events of the First on Scene scenario in this chapter, and answer the following questions related to the call. Rationales are offered in the Answer Key at the back of the book.

1. How could Jesse make the scene safe prior to entering?
2. How could Jesse help the driver of the pickup that was hit by the semi?
3. What would be the proper way to remove the patient from the pickup?

Quick Quiz

To check your understanding of the chapter, answer the following questions. Then compare your answers to those in the Answer Key at the back of the book.

1. *Proper body mechanics* are best defined as:
   a. properly using your body to facilitate a lift or move.
   b. using a minimum of three people for any lift.
   c. contracting the body's muscles to lift and move things.
   d. lifting with your back and not your legs.

2. Which of the following conditions would least likely require an emergent move?
   a. A blocked airway
   b. Severe bleeding
   c. Mild shortness of breath
   d. Cardiac arrest

3. When lifting a patient, your feet should be placed:
   a. one in front of the other.
   b. shoulder-width apart.
   c. as wide as possible.
   d. as close together as possible.

4. Good body mechanics means keeping your back ____ and bending at the knees when lifting a patient or large object.
   a. at a 45-degree angle
   b. straight
   c. curved
   d. slightly twisted

5. The load on your back is minimized if you can keep the weight you are carrying:
   a. as close to your body as possible.
   b. at least six inches in front of you.
   c. at least 18 inches in front of you.
   d. as low as possible.

6. What type of move is used when there is no immediate threat to the patient's life?
   a. Emergent
   b. Standard
   c. Rapid
   d. Nonrapid

7. When restraining a patient, it is important to remember that:
   a. the patient should be placed in the prone position.
   b. the restraints should be as tight as possible.
   c. the patient should be kept supine at all times.
   d. handcuffs should be used whenever possible.

8. Which of the following patients would best be served by being placed in the recovery position?
   a. A child who is unresponsive following a seizure
   b. An adult in cardiac arrest and in need of CPR
   c. A child who is face down and unresponsive in a pool
   d. An adult victim of a vehicle collision

9. Before restraining a combative patient, the Emergency Medical Responder should obtain ____ assistance.
   a. law enforcement
   b. medical direction
   c. ALS
   d. supervisor

10. Which of the following devices is best suited to carry a responsive patient with no suspected spinal injury down a flight of stairs?
    a. Flexible stretcher
    b. Wheeled stretcher
    c. Scoop stretcher
    d. Stair chair

Endnotes

1. Friedenberg R., Kalichman L., Ezra D., Wacht O., Alperovitch-Najenson D. "Work-Related Musculoskeletal Disorders and Injuries among Emergency Medical Technicians and Paramedics: A Comprehensive Narrative Review." *Arch Environ Occup Health.* Vol. 77, No. 1 (2022): 9–17.

2. Fischer P.E., Perina D.G., Delbridge T.R., Fallat M.E., Salomone J.P., Dodd J., Bulger E.M., Gestring M.L. "Spinal Motion Restriction in the Trauma Patient—A Joint Position Statement." *Prehosp Emerg Care.* Vol. 22, No. 6 (Nov-Dec 2018): 659–661.

3. White C.C., Domeier R.M., Millin M.G. "Standards and Clinical Practice Committee, National Association of EMS Physicians EMS Spinal Precautions and the Use of the Long Backboard—Resource Document to the Position Statement of the National Association of EMS Physicians and the American College of Surgeons Committee on Trauma." *Prehosp Emerg Care.* Vol. 18, No. 2 (Apr-Jun 2014): 306–314.

4. Ibid.

5. Del Rossi, Gianluca et al. "The 6-Plus–Person Lift Transfer Technique Compared with Other Methods of Spine Boarding." *Journal of Athletic Training* 43.1 (2008): 6–13. Print.

6. Ibid.

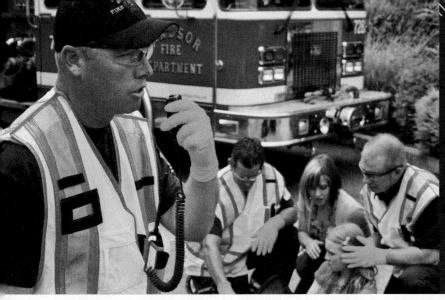

7

Principles of Effective Communication

Education Standards

Preparatory—EMS System Communication, Therapeutic Communication

Competencies

Uses knowledge of the EMS system, safety/well-being of the Emergency Medical Responder, and medical, legal, and ethical issues at the scene of an emergency while awaiting a higher level of care.

LEARNING OBJECTIVES

Upon successful completion of this chapter, the student should be able to:

Cognitive

1. Define the chapter key terms.
2. State the four types of communication.
3. Describe the characteristics of therapeutic communication.
4. Describe the components of effective communication.
5. List common barriers to effective communication.
6. Explain strategies for effective communication.
7. Explain strategies for successful interviewing.
8. Explain strategies for successful communication specific to pediatric and geriatric populations.
9. Describe the elements of an appropriate verbal transfer of care.
10. Identify common communication devices used in EMS.

11. Describe the proper technique for communicating via radio.

Psychomotor

12. Demonstrate effective communication strategies when dealing with instructional staff, classmates, and simulated patients.
13. Use therapeutic communication strategies to establish effective relationships with classmates and simulated patients.
14. Deliver an appropriate verbal transfer of care following a simulated patient encounter.
15. Demonstrate proper technique when communicating via radio.

Affective

16. Model sensitivity to cultural and age differences in all communications.

KEY TERMS

base station radio (*p. 136*)
body language (*p. 129*)
communication (*p. 128*)
interpersonal communication (*p. 129*)
health care literacy (*p. 134*)
message (*p. 130*)

portable radio (*p. 136*)
receiver (*p. 130*)
repeater (*p. 136*)
sender (*p. 130*)
therapeutic communication (*p. 129*)
transfer of care (*p. 135*)

In Chapter 4, we introduced you to basic medical terminology and the importance of learning the language of medicine. Without a clear understanding of this unique language, it would be very difficult to function in EMS in any meaningful way. Learning the words, phrases, and jargon that are unique to EMS is only half of the equation. You must also be able to communicate in ways that others will understand. You will need to communicate effectively with other EMS professionals and with ill and injured patients of all ages and cultural backgrounds. Your ability to communicate clearly, confidently, and in a manner that all parties understand will be key to your success. This chapter introduces common elements of effective communication and strategies to improve communication with diverse groups of people. It also introduces communication technology and devices commonly used in EMS.

FIRST ON SCENE

"Dispatch, Engine 86 en route to medical aid at 144 Paradise Way." Kaitlyn sets down the radio mic as she and her firefighter partner Jonie head toward their destination.

As they pull up to the coffee shop on the corner of Main Street and 4th Avenue, they see that a small crowd has gathered. They waste no time grabbing their jump bags and getting to the scene.

As they weave through the bystanders, they see a woman who appears to be in her early twenties propped against the side of the building in a seated position. Kaitlyn approaches

the woman and kneels beside her. She introduces herself and asks what happened. The woman shakes her head, her eyes watering; she looks embarrassed and scared. Kaitlyn repeats her question, and the woman holds up her hand indicating for her to stop. She is growing more agitated by the moment, nervously glancing at the crowd, back at Kaitlyn, and into her lap. Unclear what's going on, Kaitlyn looks at the bystanders and asks, "Did anyone see what happened?"

No one offers an answer. Why won't this young woman respond?

---

communication ▸ sharing or exchanging of information or news.

REMEMBER

Poor, incomplete, or wrong information has been the cause of many unsafe and dangerous situations. When the stakes are high, be sure to use clear and concise communication. Always ask clarifying questions when you don't understand something. It is also good practice to provide written documentation of patient demographics, signs and symptoms, and vital signs to the transporting crew.

What Is Communication?

Merriam-Webster's Collegiate Dictionary defines the word *communicate* as: "to have an interchange of ideas or information, to express oneself effectively." Sounds simple enough, doesn't it? While we may agree on what the word means, things begin to quickly break down when we attempt to make this simple act happen. Consider this example of one individual's attempt to communicate: "I know you believe you understand what you think I said, but I'm not sure that what you heard is not what I meant." This may have made perfect sense to the individual who said it, but to anyone who heard it, it's confusing and not clear.

As an Emergency Medical Responder, it is extremely important that you understand the characteristics of good **communication**. You will communicate with a wide variety of individuals during the course of a typical emergency call or duty shift. Individuals you are likely to communicate with on a regular basis include:

- Patients
- Your partner
- Other EMS personnel
- Fire personnel
- Law enforcement personnel

- Hospital personnel
- Family members of patients
- Friends of patients
- Bystanders

This list represents a wide variety of people, many of whom may speak a unique language for their specific profession or due to their cultural background, thus making the task of effective communication more challenging.

Types of Communication

LO2 | State the four types of communication.

All communication can be placed into one of four broad categories:

- *Verbal.* Words and sounds that make up spoken language. Verbal communication can be further broken down into types, such as interpersonal and therapeutic.
- *Nonverbal.* Communication that doesn't involve words, such as **body language**, eye contact, and gestures
- *Written.* Letters and words that are read (versus spoken)
- *Visual.* Signs, symbols, and other graphic depictions

body language ▶ communication using body movements and position.

Interpersonal Communication

One of the most important forms of verbal communication is **interpersonal communication**. Interpersonal communication refers to communication between three or fewer participants who are in close proximity to one another. This is often the case when two or three Emergency Medical Responders are working a shift together or when the communication occurs between caregivers and a patient. A key characteristic of good interpersonal communication is the immediate feedback between the sender and receiver.

interpersonal communication ▶ communication between three or fewer participants who are in close proximity to one another.

Therapeutic Communication

LO3 | Describe the characteristics of therapeutic communication.

We are familiar with the old saying, "Sticks and stones may break my bones, but words will never hurt me." We have also experienced the effects of a verbal attack and know that words can, indeed, hurt. Research has proven beyond a doubt that what you say to your patients can make a big difference in their ability to manage their illnesses and injuries: *"What we say to our patients can relieve pain and anxiety, speed up the healing process, shorten recovery time, and in many cases, save a life."*[1]

Therapeutic communication can be defined as the face-to-face communication process that focuses on advancing the physical and emotional well-being of a patient. How you talk to your patients makes a difference in how they respond to the illness or injury and to you.

You must be aware of the three objectives of therapeutic communication to maximize the results for you and the patient:

therapeutic communication ▶ face-to-face communication process that focuses on advancing the physical and emotional well-being of a patient.

- *Collecting information.* This is referred to as the patient history. The more information you can gather about the current situation as well as all prior medical history, the easier it will be to properly care for the patient.
- *Assessing behavior.* Here you are carefully observing the patient's behavior, looking for subtle signs that may offer clues to their condition.
- *Educating.* One of your responsibilities as a patient advocate is to inform and educate patients about their conditions. The hope is that, with proper education, patients will make optimal decisions regarding their medical care.

A key component of successful therapeutic communication is trust. You will have only a few moments at the beginning of your encounter with the patient to establish trust. Without trust, the patient may withhold important information about their condition or history or, in the worst case, they may refuse care altogether.

The Communication Process

LO4 Describe the components of effective communication.

If you were told to communicate, what is the first thing that comes to mind? For most of us, it might be the word *talk*. While talking is clearly a way to communicate, it represents only half of the total equation. The other half of an effective communication model involves *listening*.

Communication involves the following components:

- The **sender** is the person who introduces a new thought or concept or initiates the communication process.
- The **message** is the thought, concept, or idea being transmitted.
- The **receiver** is the person for whom the message is intended.

Figure 7.1 illustrates the many steps a message must go through to be effective, regardless of its simplicity or complexity. If the message gets blocked or misinterpreted at any one of the steps, the meaning of the message may get changed or, worse, lost. When dealing with issues related to safety and patient care, poor communication can be dangerous and even deadly.

Transmitting the Message

Now that you know the mechanics of how messages are processed, it will be helpful to have a basic understanding of how most messages are transmitted. Take a look at Figure 7.2 to see how messages are communicated to the receiver.

Research suggests that 55 percent of communication is delivered by way of body language, which includes gestures, expressions, posture, and many other physical manifestations. About 38 percent is transmitted by way of the voice—its quality, tone, and inflections, which all express important pieces of the message. Only 7 percent of any given message is transmitted by the specific words used.[2] You can see how this might work well when you are physically located next to or in front of the individual with whom you are communicating. However, a significant amount of communication in EMS occurs by way of the radio or a computer screen. Knowing this, you can begin to understand how not being able to see the person you are talking to can create many barriers to effective communication.

Barriers to Communication

LO5 List common barriers to effective communication.

There are many reasons a message might get blocked or misinterpreted. The first step in becoming a better communicator is to gain an awareness of the many barriers that can interfere with communication. Dr. Eric Garner, a leading communication researcher and educator, identified seven barriers to effective communication. They are[3]:

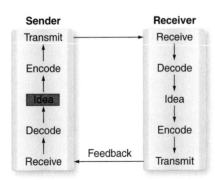

Figure 7.1 A message must pass through many steps in the communication process.

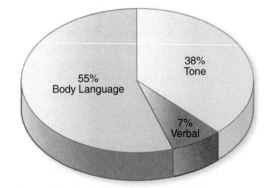

Figure 7.2 The majority of communication is delivered through body language.

- *Physical.* A physical barrier is any barrier, either real or perceived, that separates the sender and the receiver. Examples of physical barriers include walls, doors, distance, and territories or zones.
- *Perceptual.* Everyone brings different experiences to the table. People see things differently and have unique perspectives that can differ in so many ways.
- *Emotional.* This can be one of the biggest barriers when dealing with ill and injured patients. Emotional barriers include fear, mistrust, and suspicion. These can be difficult to overcome in the short time we have with our patients.
- *Cultural.* Each year the United States becomes more culturally diverse. Not understanding some of the basic cultural differences that exist among individuals can cause significant barriers that will prevent you from delivering the best care possible.
- *Language.* Not being able to communicate with your patient due to language differences can be an overwhelming barrier for many novice EMS personnel. While no one expects you to learn several languages, it will be very beneficial to learn some common words and phrases related to patient care if you live in a culturally diverse environment.
- *Gender.* A responder's perceptions or beliefs about gender may make it challenging to communicate with certain patients. Gender can also play a role culturally. It is important to provide care according to your training and local protocols and to communicate in a way that is respectful of each patient's unique needs.
- *Interpersonal.* An individual's attitudes and beliefs or like or dislike for the sender or receiver can interfere with the message being communicated.

JEDI

If your patient is alert and oriented, it is critical to establish rapport by asking them what form of communication works best for them. You may encounter individuals who are Deaf or hard of hearing or have vision loss. These situations may require you to be creative in how you communicate. All patients deserve the same amount of respectful communication. Be aware of your patient's needs and, whenever possible, explain to them what is going on so they can cooperate and allow you to provide optimal care.

FIRST ON SCENE (continued)

Kaitlyn bends over so she is face to face with the woman. "My name is Kaitlyn," she says, "I am here to help you. Can you tell me your name and what happened?"

"Talitha," the young woman says, glancing between her legs. Kaitlyn looks down and notices dark red blood flowing down the woman's legs. Kaitlyn continues, "Can I check the bleeding to see how I can help you?" Talitha nods. Kaitlyn lifts Talitha's dress, gasping at the sight of the blood covering both legs.

"We are going to need a medic here," Kaitlyn says as she turns to Jonie. "I've got a lot of bleeding and no injury I can see."

Jonie can see that Talitha is clearly nervous about the crowd surrounding them. Her eyes and those of the man beside her dart from the blood on the ground to the bystanders watching. "I'm going to need everyone to step back," says Jonie firmly. "We need some privacy, please."

Jonie rushes back to the engine, grabs a sheet and some bandages, and returns to Kaitlyn and Talitha.

Communication Strategies and Considerations

Some simple ideas and strategies can be used to enhance communication with patients, coworkers, and all those you will encounter while on the job.

Strategies for Effective Communication

LO6 Explain strategies for effective communication.

Following are some strategies that will help you become a better communicator:

- Speak clearly and use words and terminology that the receiver will understand. You should not use medical jargon when speaking to a patient. However, you should use proper medical terminology when speaking to another medical professional.

- Keep an open mind, and resist the urge to be defensive or accusatory. It is natural to respond defensively when another person is uncooperative or exhibits unpleasant or aggressive behavior. In some cases, you may be tempted to sound as if you think the patient's condition is a result of their own negligence. When this happens, both parties tend to shut down, and any chance of good communication is seriously jeopardized.
- Become an active listener. Active listening is more than just paying attention. It means putting your biases aside and making every effort to understand what the other individual is saying. Active listening includes using eye contact when appropriate and asking clarifying questions to further clarify the message.
- Be assertive when appropriate, especially when safety is at stake. Do not passively accept what the other individual is saying if you see things differently. Respectfully state your point in a manner that will ensure that you are understood.
- Remain aware of the role that body language plays in effective communication. Pay attention to your own body language, and ensure that it shows you are listening and attentive.
- Accept the reality of miscommunication. Even the best communicators fail at times. Do not allow yourself to get frustrated, but instead view the miscommunication as a lesson and use it to improve future communication.

REMEMBER

Be sure you know who all the players are at the scene. Introduce yourself to each of them, and verify their relationships to the patient. This practice avoids embarrassing mistakes such as misidentifying a woman holding a baby as the mother when, in fact, she is the grandmother.

Strategies for Successful Interviewing

LO7 Explain strategies for successful interviewing.

LO8 Explain strategies for successful communication specific to pediatric and geriatric populations.

When you think of a good interviewer, who comes to mind? Jimmy Fallon, Jimmy Kimmel, Oprah Winfrey? Those well-known interviewers are very skilled at interpersonal communications and the art of the interview. They can make guests feel comfortable enough to reveal very personal information and to do so while being observed by millions of viewers.

As an Emergency Medical Responder, you must develop excellent interviewing skills. But the interview you will be conducting is one in which you gather the patient's medical history. To provide the best care possible, you must learn as much as possible about the patient, their current condition, and any pertinent prior medical history in a very short period of time.

The following strategies will help you establish a good rapport with your patient and maximize your ability to obtain a good medical history:

- Immediately introduce yourself and your level of training.
- Obtain the patient's preferred name early on, and use it frequently during your interview.
- Position yourself at or below the patient's eye level whenever possible (Figure 7.3).
- Ask one question at a time, and allow the patient ample time to respond.
- Listen carefully to everything the patient tells you.
- Restate the patient's answers when necessary for clarification.

Developing your interviewing skills will take some time. Whenever possible, listen in when others with more experience interview patients, and pay attention to their techniques. Notice what works and what does not work, and use those lessons to your advantage.

Your interviewing strategies may need to be modified, depending on the age of your patient (Figure 7.4). For instance, obtaining a thorough medical history from a child may be

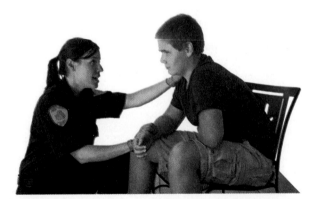

Figure 7.3 Positioning yourself at or below eye level with the patient demonstrates caring and compassion.

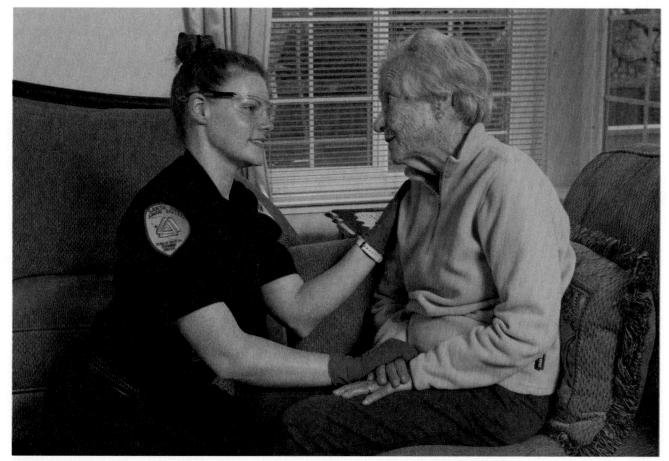

Figure 7.4 You may have to alter your approach with older patients, depending on their physical condition.

impossible if the child is too young or does not trust you. In this instance, you will need to rely on parents or other caregivers who know the child's history.

Cultural Considerations

The area where you live and work determines how likely it is that you will encounter patients from differing cultures. Although large cities are certainly full of people representing a variety of cultures, many smaller towns and rural areas are also home to people with differing cultural backgrounds. Be aware that each culture has specific expectations regarding verbal and nonverbal communication, personal space, and physical touch.

Although it is difficult to identify the cultural norms for all the potential patients you may encounter, the following guidelines will be helpful in making an encounter with a patient from a culture that is unfamiliar to you a little more successful:

- Demonstrate a healthy respect for different cultures and beliefs.
- Take time to carefully observe the surroundings as you enter the scene. Observe how others in the room are engaging with the patient and/or reacting to what is happening.
- Introduce yourself to each individual as appropriate. You may encounter someone at the door, another person with the patient, and, of course, the patient.
- If language is a barrier, immediately try to identify someone who may be able to translate for you.
- When using an interpreter, speak directly to the patient and not to the interpreter.
- Carefully manage your proximity to the patient, and avoid getting too close too soon.
- Speak slowly and clearly, and use language that is easy to understand. Avoid using medical jargon.
- Carefully explain your every move before reaching for or touching the patient, even for a simple pulse check. Be sure to obtain proper consent first.

If you are unfamiliar with the various cultural groups that may reside in your response area, speak with your instructor. They should be able to tell you which cultural groups have populations in the area. Take the time to learn some of the more common cultural norms of these groups in advance of a response. It will make your first encounter a more successful one.

Translation Services

Several U.S. companies offer translation services via telephone. Most hospitals and 911 dispatch centers subscribe to such services. Even though your agency may not use such a service, you may have access to one by contacting your local 911 dispatch center. Another option is one of the many translation apps for mobile phones. Google Translate is widely used.

Patients with Disabilities

Approximately 15 percent of adults in the United States report some degree of hearing loss. There is also a direct connection between age and reported hearing loss: About 14 percent of adults aged 20 to 69 have hearing loss, with the greatest amount of hearing loss reported in people between the ages of 60 and 69. Nearly 25 percent of adults aged 65 to 74 and 50 percent of those aged 75 and older report disabling hearing loss.[5]

You will need to demonstrate patience when communicating with someone who has hearing loss. Get down at eye level and speak slowly and directly to the individual. Expect to have to repeat yourself because the patient may not understand the first time. In some instances, communicating through written words may be a good option.

Many individuals with hearing loss are able to read lips, but you will need to speak slowly while facing them. Shouting will not help. Inquire if there is someone with the patient who may be able to interpret with sign language. It is highly recommended that you learn some simple words and phrases in American Sign Language (ASL). This will greatly improve the likelihood of developing a good rapport with patients who communicate using ASL.

Patients who have visual impairment will need you to explain what is going on before you begin to touch or move them.

Individuals with cognitive disabilities present their own set of challenges. Do your best to be patient and compassionate. You may have to rely on the caregiver to help with communication.

Some patients with disabilities and/or certain medical conditions such as diabetes, epilepsy, anxiety, and post-traumatic stress disorder (PTSD) may utilize a service animal to help manage their conditions. These animals should be accommodated whenever possible and allowed to accompany a patient who is transported.

Health Care Literacy

health care literacy ▸ degree to which an individual has the ability to obtain, understand, and use health information and services to make appropriate health-related decisions.

Navigating our health care system and its many rules, regulations, and obstacles can be overwhelming, to say the least. **Health care literacy** is the degree to which a person has the capacity to obtain, process, and understand basic health information and services needed to make appropriate health decisions. The vast majority of patients are novices when it comes to understanding and navigating the complex U.S. health care system. Understanding things like the difference between an urgent care clinic and an Emergency Department, how consent works, and instructions such as those for prescription drugs and those given upon discharge from an ER visit can be challenging, especially when faced with a health emergency. It is important to understand that your patients are likely not experts at the health care "game." They will need you to demonstrate patience as you care for them.

It will help to calm your patient and earn their trust if you explain everything you are doing. You also need to explain that they have a right to decline any care you might offer. Use clear and simple terms and explanations, and always ask for permission first. It is one of our responsibilities to educate and inform our patients so they can make the best decisions for their own health care.

Family-Centered Care

Family-centered care is an approach to the planning, delivery, and evaluation of health care that is grounded in mutually beneficial partnerships among health care professionals, patients, and families. As an Emergency Medical Responder at the scene of an emergency, you must do your best to be aware of family and/or friends who may be present with the patient. It is important to acknowledge them and include them in conversations about the care being provided, if the patient wants them to be included. Family members and friends can often provide helpful insights about the patient's current problem and previous medical history. If the patient has given permission, it is important to engage family and/or friends appropriately and keep them informed about what you are doing to help their loved one.

FIRST ON SCENE (continued)

An ambulance has arrived and Talitha has been loaded onto the gurney and into the unit by two female EMTs. The bleeding controlled, Kaitlyn makes eye contact with Talitha and tells her that one EMT will ride with her in the back and that Jonie has called ahead to make sure that a female doctor meets them at the hospital. She adds, "Your husband will be riding up front in the ambulance and will go to the hospital with you." Talitha visibly relaxes and smiles weakly. She is pleased that she is receiving the care and privacy she needs.

Transfer of Care

LO9 Describe the elements of an appropriate verbal transfer of care.

The verbal **transfer of care** happens at the scene when care of the patient is transferred from one care provider, the Emergency Medical Responder, to the next care provider, the ambulance crew. Another verbal transfer of care will occur when the ambulance crew turns care of the patient over to staff at the hospital. This is a very important component of the *continuum of care*, and it helps to ensure that the care is consistent and appropriate as the patient moves from one care provider to another.

transfer of care ▶ physical and verbal handing off of care from one health care provider to another.

The verbal transfer of care may be modified based on the patient's condition. If the patient is critical, the transfer of care may be very short and to the point. Do not be offended if the ambulance crew does not want to take time for a complete report when the patient is in need of immediate attention.

A good transfer of care should contain all of the following elements, regardless of whether the transfer happens at the scene or at the hospital:

- Patient's name and age
- Chief complaint
- Brief account of the patient's current condition
- Past pertinent medical history
- Vital signs
- Pertinent findings from the physical exam
- Overview of care provided and the patient's response to that care

Keep in mind that you may have to obtain some of this information from anyone who arrived on scene before you did, such as bystanders, family members, and law enforcement officers. Do not expect them to be able to provide a thorough verbal handoff. You will need to ask specific questions to obtain the information you require.

Radio Communications

LO10 Identify common communication devices used in EMS.

LO11 Describe the proper technique for communicating via radio.

Emergency Medical Responders use specific tools and technology to facilitate communication; these include cell phones, radios, laptops, and tablets. All EMS systems are connected by a very sophisticated arrangement of hardware and software designed to allow all the resources in the structure to communicate with one another. At the heart of the systems are the radios, pagers, antennae, repeaters, and specific frequencies that connect every vehicle and individual in the system. EMS is set in motion when someone initiates an emergency response by calling 911.

A typical radio system is made up of a combination of transmitters, receivers, **repeaters**, and antennae. Dispatch centers use powerful **base station radios** that can transmit over a wide area. When terrain is a factor and hills or mountains obstruct radio signals, specialized mountaintop repeaters are used to capture the signal and redirect it to the appropriate receiver.

EMS personnel often carry both pagers and **portable radios** that allow them to communicate with the dispatch center and each other (Figure 7.5). Pagers are used to notify response personnel of an emergency call, and portable radios are used to communicate directly with the dispatch center before, during, and after a call.

The use of radios requires a specific protocol when communicating with others within the system. For instance, you cannot simply push the button and speak any time you feel like it. Doing so might interrupt another individual using the same frequency. Instead, you should listen first and begin your transmission when there is a break in the traffic on your frequency. The term *radio traffic* refers to the verbal communication that takes place over a radio.

Imagine that you are Rescue One and you want to ask your dispatch center (Central Dispatch) to repeat the address where the emergency call is located. The conversation might go something like this:

RESCUE ONE: Central Dispatch, this is Rescue One with a request.

CENTRAL DISPATCH: Rescue One, Central Dispatch, go ahead with your request.

RESCUE ONE: Central Dispatch, Rescue One, can you repeat the address for our call?

CENTRAL DISPATCH: Rescue One, Central Dispatch, you are responding to 2700 Woolsey Road. That's two seven zero zero Woolsey Road. Do you copy?

RESCUE ONE: Central Dispatch, Rescue One, confirming two seven zero zero Woolsey Road.

CENTRAL DISPATCH: Rescue One, Central Dispatch, that's affirmative.

repeater ▶ fixed antenna that is used to boost a radio signal.

base station radio ▶ high-powered two-way radio located at a dispatch center or hospital.

portable radio ▶ handheld device used to transmit and receive verbal communications.

Figure 7.5 Portable radios are the most common communication tool used in EMS.

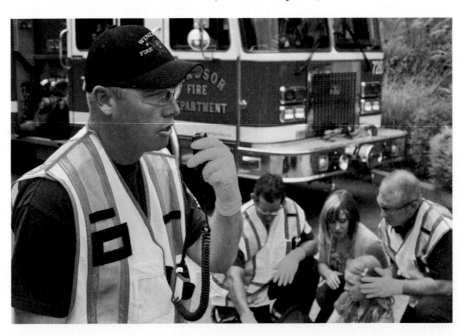

Do you see the pattern there? When you wish to contact another resource in the system, it is standard protocol to state the radio identifier (specified name) of the resource you are calling first. In this case, it was Central Dispatch. Follow that with your radio identifier, Rescue One. This is especially important when there are several resources using the same frequency, also known as a channel.

In the beginning, it is normal to be somewhat shy or intimidated by the prospect of talking on the radio. Not to worry. It quickly becomes second nature, and you will soon learn to enjoy talking with others on the radio.

It is important that your radio communications are clear and concise because others may need to use the same frequency to communicate. You will have time to convey longer explanations in person.

One way to become more familiar with radio protocol is to listen to a scanner. A scanner is a specialized radio that only receives radio traffic. Most scanners today can be programmed to receive just about any frequency, so you should be able to program it to the frequencies of the EMS system in your area. If you do not want to purchase a scanner, you also can listen to live radio traffic on the internet. A simple web search should turn up live radio traffic in your area.

Avoid the use of 10-codes often heard on TV and over citizen band radios, such as 10-4, 10-6, and so on. While some emergency response and public safety systems may use such codes, most EMS systems do not.

FIRST ON SCENE WRAP-UP

"That was different," Jonie says as he and Kaitlyn make their way to the engine. "Thank you for thinking on your feet and taking Talitha's modesty into account."

"I could tell from their body language that they were both really concerned about the crowd," Kaitlyn says. "I wanted them to trust us so we could address Talitha's bleeding as soon as possible.

Jonie nods and says, "It was good that you thought to involve her husband in her care. And I'm glad we were able to request a female doctor and a private room for Talitha."

Kaitlyn replies, "Me, too. We did good work today."

Summary

- Communication is a complex process that involves the interchange of ideas or information. It requires a sender, a receiver, and a message.
- There are four types of communication: verbal, nonverbal, written, and visual.
- Common barriers to effective communication include physical, perceptual, emotional, cultural, language, gender, and interpersonal. All these factors can interfere with the communication process.
- Therapeutic communication focuses on advancing the physical and emotional well-being of a patient. The objectives of therapeutic communication include collecting information, assessing behavior, and providing education.
- You must do your part to help your patients develop health care literacy by clearly explaining everything that you are doing and what is likely to happen when they are transported to the hospital.
- Family-centered care is an approach to health care that includes the patient, their family, and health care professionals. With the patient's permission, it is often appropriate to communicate with a patient's family and/or friends to ensure that the best care is provided for their loved one.
- Strategies for effective communication include speaking slowly and clearly, resisting the urge to be defensive, using active listening techniques, and being aware of body language.
- Strategies for successful interviewing include immediately introducing yourself and your level of training, obtaining the patient's name early on and using it frequently during your interview, positioning yourself at or below the patient's eye level whenever possible, asking one question at a time and allowing the patient ample time to respond, listening carefully to everything the patient tells you, and restating the patient's answers when necessary for clarification.
- As an Emergency Medical Responder, your skill of verbal transfer of care (handoff) is an important one. The elements of an appropriate verbal transfer of care include patient's name and age, chief complaint, brief account of the patient's current condition, past pertinent medical history, vital signs, pertinent findings from the physical exam, overview of care provided, and the patient's response to that care.
- You may have to modify your communication approach depending on the age of the patient. This is especially true when communicating with young children and elderly patients.
- Various types of communication technology are used by EMS professionals. Radios and pagers are a primary source of communication between dispatch centers and field personnel and hospitals. Base station radios are high-powered transmitters that broadcast a signal over a large area. Sometimes repeaters are used to boost the signal when distance and terrain are a factor.
- There is a common protocol for how to communicate using a radio. Each transmission should begin with the identifier (name) of the individual or agency you are calling followed by your identifier (name).

Take Action

Practice by Listening

One of the best ways to begin learning proper radio protocol is to listen to live radio traffic. You can do this in a couple of ways. The first is to borrow or purchase a radio scanner. This is a small handheld device that can be programmed to receive local radio traffic from just about any source—fire, police, or EMS. Another way to listen to live radio traffic is to use the internet. Go to www.radioreference.com. This website will allow you to listen in on thousands of different frequencies across the nation. In many instances, you will be able to listen in on local police, fire, or EMS frequencies in your area.

First on Scene Patient Handoff

Talitha is a 27-year-old female with a chief complaint of vaginal bleeding. Patient did not show signs of or share details of trauma. Per the patient, the bleeding began at approximately 3 p.m. and increased rapidly at 4 p.m. At that point, her husband called 911. We placed bandages and gauze over the vaginal area to absorb the bleeding. Patient's heart rate was 130 strong and regular, respirations were 24 and shallow, skin was pale, cool, and slightly moist. When we arrived on scene, the patient indicated she felt like she was going to faint.

First on Scene Run Review

Recall the events of the First on Scene scenario in this chapter and answer the following questions related to the call. Rationales are offered in the Answer Key at the back of the book.

1. Did Kaitlyn and Jonie check to see if the scene was safe? What would you do differently to ensure that the scene was safe?
2. How would you work with someone who had a cultural background and/or belief system that differs from your own?
3. What role does communication play in this situation?

Quick Quiz

To check your understanding of the chapter, answer the following questions. Then compare your answers to those in the Answer Key at the back of the book.

1. The word *communicate* is best defined as:
   a. delivering a message.
   b. talking to another individual verbally.
   c. an interchange of ideas or information.
   d. understanding what another individual is saying.

2. The words and sounds that make up a language describes which type of communication?
   a. Verbal
   b. Nonverbal
   c. Written
   d. Visual

3. Nonverbal communication is best characterized by:
   a. written words.
   b. spoken words.
   c. body language.
   d. signs and symbols.

4. All of the following are components of the communication process EXCEPT:
   a. sender.
   b. receiver.
   c. message.
   d. frequency.

5. Research suggests that the majority of a message is delivered by way of:
   a. body language.
   b. voice (tone).
   c. word use.
   d. eye contact.

6. The distance that exists between two parties who are communicating by radio is an example of which type of barrier?
   a. Perceptual
   b. Language
   c. Physical
   d. Interpersonal

7. While interviewing a patient, you ask questions about their medical history and reassure them that you will take care of them. This is an example of which type of communication?
   a. Therapeutic
   b. Direct
   c. Visual
   d. Interpersonal

8. All of the following are goals of therapeutic communication EXCEPT:
   a. pain management.
   b. collecting information.
   c. assessing behavior.
   d. providing education.

9. A good transfer of care should contain all of the following EXCEPT:
   a. patient's name and age.
   b. patient's address.
   c. chief complaint.
   d. vital signs.

10. Which of the following is the best example of an appropriate radio call?
    a. Engine 6, this is MedCom. Respond to 1111 Sonoma Ave.
    b. Engine 6, respond to 1111 Sonoma Ave.
    c. This is MedCom, calling Engine 6.
    d. MedCom, come in Engine 6.

Endnotes

1. Judith Acosta and Judith Simon Prager, *The Worst Is Over: What to Say When Every Moment Counts—Verbal First Aid to Calm, Relieve Pain, Promote Healing, and Save Lives* (San Diego, CA: Jodere Group, 2002): p. 5.
2. Jeff Thompson, "Is Nonverbal Communication a Numbers Game?" Beyond Words (blog), *Psychology Today*, September 30, 2011. Accessed January 30, 2018, at http://www.psychologytoday.com/blog/beyond-words/201109/is-nonverbal-communication-numbers-game
3. Eric Garner, "The 7 Barriers to Great Communications," Ezinearticles.com, February 28, 2006 (© Eric Garner, ManageTrainLearn.com). Accessed June 9, 2014, at http://ezinearticles.com/?The-7-Barriers-To-Great-Communications-&id=153524
4. World Health Organization, "Health Topics: Gender and Health," Accessed November 30, 2022, at https://www.who.int/health-topics/gender#tab=tab_1
5. National Institute on Deafness and Other Communication Disorders, "Quick Statistics," U.S. Department of Health and Human Services National Institutes of Health website, last updated December 15, 2016. Accessed February 6, 2018, at https://www.nidcd.nih.gov/health/statistics/Pages/quick.aspx

8

Principles of Effective Documentation

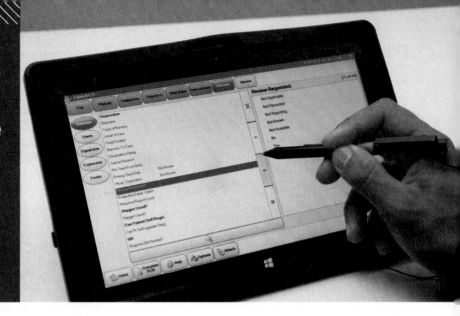

Education Standards

Preparatory—
Documentation

Competencies

Uses knowledge of the EMS system, safety/well-being of the Emergency Medical Responder, and medical, legal, and ethical issues at the scene of an emergency while awaiting a higher level of care.

LEARNING OBJECTIVES

Upon successful completion of this chapter, the student should be able to:

Cognitive

1. Define the chapter key terms.
2. Explain the purposes of the patient care report.
3. Describe the elements of a typical patient care report.
4. Describe the minimum data set required for documentation of patient care.
5. Explain the procedure for correcting errors made during documentation.
6. List various tools used to document patient care in the field setting.

Psychomotor

7. Demonstrate the ability to accurately document a simulated patient encounter.
8. Properly correct an error made during documentation.

Affective

9. Value the importance of complete and accurate documentation.

KEY TERMS

continuity of care (*p. 143*)
electronic documentation (*p. 146*)

minimum data set (*p. 144*)
patient care report (PCR) (*p. 141*)

Properly documenting the assessment and care of patients is a vitally important part of what you will be doing as an Emergency Medical Responder. You should take pride in everything you do, which includes how effectively you document your assessment and care of each patient. Your written reports—usually called run reports or patient care reports—will follow a patient through the health care system as the only lasting record of the care you provided.

Documentation has many other uses as well. It is used in the short term by emergency department personnel to get a clear picture of the patient's situation when first encountered by EMS responders, the illness or injuries discovered, and exactly what care was given prior to arrival at the hospital.

Documentation can also play an important role in minimizing your liability as an Emergency Medical Responder. If someone questions the care you provided, thorough, clear, and accurate documentation is the best way to address those concerns.[1]

FIRST ON SCENE

Battalion Chief Don leans back in his chair and rubs the bridge of his nose before setting his glasses back into place.

"So," he says, seeing that the young firefighter across the desk from him has finished reading the patient care report. "I'll ask you again. At what point during that call did you realize that the patient had stopped breathing? And what, exactly, did you do about it?"

Debra looks at him pleadingly, glancing from the piece of paper in her hands and back to the steady gaze of the chief several times before speaking.

"I can't imagine that I didn't start rescue breathing," is all she can say.

"You know what?" The chief leans forward and taps his index finger on the desk to accentuate his words. "I believe you, Debra. You're a solid firefighter and a good Emergency Medical Responder—one who would start rescue breathing immediately for a patient who had stopped breathing. But the lawyer representing that patient in his lawsuit against the city knows nothing about you except what you wrote in that patient care report. And based on that narrative, you look like a pretty negligent Emergency Medical Responder."

Patient Care Reports

LO2 Explain the purposes of the patient care report.

The documentation you provide is a permanent record of the patient care you performed. When you provide excellent, patient-centered prehospital care, you may be proud of your abilities. However, poor documentation after the fact will tarnish the record of what you have done.

The reporting done by Emergency Medical Responders can take on many names, depending on your region or service. The report is often called a **patient care report (PCR)**, run report, or prehospital care report. Some PCRs are written by hand (Figure 8.1), but many agencies have adopted electronic documentation methods (Figure 8.2).

Regardless of how the reports are completed, there are many reasons for accurate and complete documentation. These include:

- *Continuity of care.* Your report may be referenced by other care providers on the EMS team or at the hospital. They may look for the vital signs you obtained,

patient care report ▶ document that provides details about a patient's condition, history, and care, along with information about the event that caused the illness or injury. Abbrev: PCR.

Figure 8.1 Example of a paper version of a patient care report (PCR) form.

DATE	TRIP #	UNIT	CALL RECEIVED	DISPATCHED	EN ROUTE	ON SCENE

TRANSPORTING	ARRIVAL	TOTAL MLG	SERVICE PROVIDER	(For Billing Use Only)
BEG MILEAGE	END MILEAGE			

☐ INITIAL TRANSPORT   ☐ ADMITTED TO HOSPITAL   ☐ DISCHARGED FROM FIRST FACILITY   ☐ DISCHARGED
☐ RETURN TRIP   ☐ OUTPATIENT (I.E. RADIATION THERAPY, DR. APPOINTMENT)   ☐ ADMITTED TO SECOND FACILITY   ☐ NON-MEDICAL

SENDING FACILITY/SCENE LOCATION   RECEIVING FACILITY

PATIENT NAME (LAST, FIRST)	PHONE #	AGE	☐ MO ☐ YR	SEX ☐ M ☐ F	DOB	WEIGHT (kg)

PATIENT ADDRESS (STREET)   (CITY)   (STATE)   (ZIP)   SSN

ALTERNATE CONTACT (NAME)   (PHONE #)   (RELATION)

PRIMARY INSURANCE

COMPANY NAME	SUBSCRIBER NAME	POLICY # / GROUP #
ADDRESS (STREET)	(CITY) (STATE) (ZIP)	PHONE #

SECONDARY INSURANCE

COMPANY NAME	SUBSCRIBER NAME	POLICY # / GROUP #
ADDRESS (STREET)	(CITY) (STATE) (ZIP)	PHONE #

MED HX

MEDICAL HX

CURRENT MEDICATIONS   ALLERGIES

MENTAL STATUS	AIRWAY	BREATHING	PULSE	SKIN COLOR	SKIN MOISTURE	SKIN TEMP
☐ ALERT	☐ PATIENT	☐ NORMAL	☐ REGULAR	☐ NORMAL	☐ DRY	☐ NORMAL
☐ ORIENTED X____	☐ ASPIRATION RISK	☐ DYSPNEA	☐ IRREGULAR	☐ PALE	☐ MOIST	☐ COOL
☐ RESPONDS / VERBAL	☐ SECRETIONS	☐ RETRACTIONS	☐ STRONG	☐ FLUSHED	☐ DIAPHORETIC	☐ HOT
☐ RESPONDS / PAIN	☐ SUCTIONING REQ.	☐ ACC. MUSCLE	☐ WEAK	☐ CYANOTIC		
☐ UNRESPONSIVE				☐ MOTTLED		

IV

LOCATION   ☐ N/A ☐ SALINE / HEPARIN LOCK ☐ MONITORED GTT: RATE:_____ CC / HR, FLUID TYPE:_____
☐ NARCOTIC INFUSION (LOCKED) DRUG:_____   RATE:_____

ASSESSMENT

CHECK ALL THAT APPLY AND EXPLAIN WHY AND HOW IN THE NARRATIVE
☐ PATIENT BED CONFINED AT TIME OF SERVICE DUE TO:
  ☐ MOTOR CONTROL / MUSCLE TONE PRECLUDES SITTING UP
  ☐ DECUB. ULCERS / WOUNDS REQ. POSITIONING & CAREFUL HANDLING
  ☐ SEVERE CONTRACTURES
  ☐ PAIN INCREASES WITH SITTING / MOVEMENT
  ☐ SPECIAL ORTHOPEDIC DEVICE IN PLACE
  ☐ FRACTURE OR POSSIBILITY OF FRACTURE
  ☐ POST SPINAL INJURY
  ☐ OBESITY (WEIGHT MUST BE NOTED ABOVE)
  ☐ SUPPORTIVE DEVICES REQUIRED (I.E. WEDGE / PILLOWS)
  ☐ REQUIRES MULTIPLE ATTENDANTS
  ☐ PATIENT IN PAIN (SEE DESCRIPTION IN NARRATIVE)
  ☐ REQUIRES OXYGEN DURING TRANSPORT
  ☐ PATIENT SEDATED AT TIME OF SERVICE

RESTRAINTS
☐ CHEMICAL   (CIRCLE ALL THAT APPLY)
☐ PHYSICAL: POSEY VEST   WRIST   ANKLE   BELTS
OBSERVATION / SUPERVISION
☐ 5150 – DOCUMENTATION ATTACHED
☐ SEVERE DEMENTIA
☐ FLIGHT RISK
☐ PROTECT MEDICAL MODALITIES
AIRWAY MONITORING
☐ REQUIRED SECONDARY TO CONDITION
☐ UNABLE TO CONTROL SECRETIONS (ASPIRATION RISK)
☐ POOR MUSCLE TONE / CONTROL (QUADRIPLEGIC)
OTHER
☐ ISOLATION PRECAUTIONS DUE TO (POSS) INFECTIOUS DISEASE
☐ REQUIRED MONITORING BY OTHER LICENSED MEDICAL PROFESSIONAL ACCOMPANYING TRANSPORT
☐ TRANSFER TO HIGHER LEVEL OF CARE
☐ TRANSFER TO LOCKDOWN FACILITY / WARD

O₂ DELIVERY	CAPILLARY REFILL
____LPM ☐ NC ☐ NRB	☐ < 2 SEC ☐ > 2 SEC

VITALS

TIME	BP	PULSE	RR	TIME	BP	PULSE	RR	TIME	BP	PULSE	RR	TIME	BP	PULSE	RR

NARRATIVE

☐ PATIENT SECURED TO GURNEY USING ALL SECURING STRAPS AND GURNEY LOCKED INTO PLACE IN BACK OF AMBULANCE.   CARE TRANSFERRED TO (NAME / TITLE)

MED TEAM

ATTENDANT _____ (SIGNATURE) _____ EMP # ____   DRIVER _____ (SIGNATURE) _____ EMP # ____
_____ (PRINT)   _____ (PRINT)

medications or treatments you administered, and your observations at the scene. The information you record will help ensure that the patient receives thorough and consistent care by all providers. This is known as **continuity of care**. Each provider who assumes care for a patient must be properly informed of the patient's progression, so they can watch for trends and continue effective treatments.

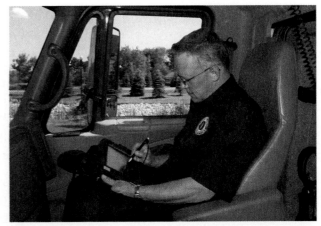

Figure 8.2 Electronic documentation of an emergency call is becoming more common.

- *Education.* Your written report may be used as an example for others of proper (or not so proper) documentation. If you respond to an unusual or challenging call, it may be used as a basis for training other providers who may encounter similar patients or situations.
- *Administration.* The report will be used in compiling statistical analysis on issues that affect your agency or community. Most states collect data on EMS calls from local providers and send that data to the federal government for analysis and system improvement.
- *Quality assurance.* Reports created by you and others in your agency may be reviewed as part of a structured process to improve the overall quality of the care your agency provides as well as that of the EMS system as a whole.
- *Legal.* The report you create is a legal document. It may be used in a civil or criminal court for any number of reasons.

continuity of care ▶ thorough and consistent delivery of care among all providers involved in caring for an individual patient.

REMEMBER

The old saying, "If you didn't document it, you didn't do it," is true when it comes to PCRs. If the actions you took and the treatment you provided are not included in your documentation, the only conclusion an individual reading your report can reach is that you simply did not do it.

It should be noted that the use of 24-hour (military) time is the standard for the medical profession. You will need to begin learning 24-hour time for documentation purposes.

You need to be aware that all patient information must be considered private and confidential, and you may not share it with anyone outside the chain of direct patient care. One exception to this is when a patient's information is requested by a law enforcement officer. A patient's health information is also protected by federal laws that govern how this information is both stored and shared. Many of these restrictions and regulations are contained in the Health Information Portability and Accountability Act (HIPAA) of 1996.

Elements of the PCR

LO3 Describe the elements of a typical patient care report.

Standard PCRs used throughout the EMS profession share several specific sections:

- *Run data.* This section includes information about the call itself, such as the names of the Emergency Medical Responders providing care, the agency they work for, and the date, time, and location of the incident. This section may also include the final outcome of the call, such as a patient's refusal to be treated or the name of the person who assumed patient care from you. Remember, all names, times, and locations recorded on your PCRs must be accurate because continued care, billing, and statistical information will all depend on the information you provide.
- *Patient data.* This section includes all the information about the patient, such as:
  - Name, address, date of birth, gender
  - Nature of the call
  - Detailed notes on the patient's complaint
  - Mechanism of injury
  - Assessment findings
  - Care administered prior to arrival of Emergency Medical Responders
  - Vital signs
  - Past medical history
  - Changes in the patient's condition
  - Treatment provided and the patient's response to that treatment

The information in each section of the report can be entered in various ways:

- *Fill-in.* Data is placed in specifically labeled spaces.
- *Check boxes.* Some PCRs have boxes that can be checked for information such as patient history, nature of illness, and care provided.
- *Narrative.* Space is provided for you to write the "story" documenting the patient's history, assessment, and care information that does not otherwise fit in check boxes or that requires expansion on the details.

Often the narrative will contain a blend of both objective information (based on facts and observations) and subjective information (based on feelings, thoughts, or opinions). The information you write in the narrative should be as objective as possible but may also contain subjective findings, such as what the patient describes they are feeling. Objective information comprises straightforward facts. Subjective information comprises personal opinions, judgments, points of view, and other details that are not easily measured. Subjective information is subject to interpretation. The statement, "The patient's right forearm was swollen and angulated," is objective, whereas the statement, "I believe the patient was attempting to perform a dangerous trick on his skateboard," is subjective.

FIRST ON SCENE *(continued)*

Debra closes her eyes and tries to remember the details of the call that occurred nearly 8 months earlier. She had been working out of Station 4, covering the eastern edge of the city, a sprawling industrial area known for manufacturing-related trauma calls during the day and fights and overdoses at night. She can remember the fire engine rolling to a stop at the abandoned warehouse. She also remembers a beige sedan parked haphazardly among toppled garbage cans, the sun glinting off the haze of cracks on the car's windshield.

She opens her eyes and looks at the on-scene time on the PCR in her hands: 2357.

"Wait a minute." She slides the document back onto the chief's desk and shakes her head wearily. "This call happened at night, and I'm remembering one that happened during the day. I'm getting calls all mixed up. It's just too long ago."

"Debra." The chief slides the PCR back into a red folder. "Except for an occasional one that really sticks with you, all of your calls will eventually blend together in your memory. That's why proper documentation and complete, accurate narratives are so critical. You never know when questions will come up about a particular situation long after you've forgotten that it ever even happened."

Minimum Data Set

LO4 Describe the minimum data set required for documentation of patient care.

In an effort to standardize the information collected from EMS calls around the nation, the U.S. Department of Transportation (DOT) has defined what it calls a **minimum data set**. Regardless of how much information any single agency collects on each call, the data must include all items that make up the minimum data set, which are:

minimum data set ▸ minimum information required by U.S. Department of Transportation standards for data collection on each patient; typically, applies only to 911 calls.

- Time the incident was reported to 911
- Time of dispatch
- Time of arrival at the patient's location
- Time the patient was transported from the incident location
- Time the patient arrived at the destination (hospital, aid station, etc.)
- Time the patient care was transferred to more advanced providers
- Patient's chief complaint
- Patient's approximate weight and vital signs
- Patient's demographics (age, gender, race)

The Narrative

A complete, thorough PCR should contain a narrative that tells a brief story about the patient and their chief complaint. This is often the most difficult part of the PCR for providers. The story you tell through the narrative should be clear, concise, and as objective as possible.

The use of nonstandard abbreviations should be avoided. However, if you do use abbreviations, make sure that you use those that are common to EMS. Do not simply make up your own abbreviations, as that will make it very difficult for others to interpret your exact meaning.

Objective Information   Some of the information you gather will be objective in nature. Objective information is impartial and unbiased. You can think of objective information as related to something you can see, hear, feel (palpate), or measure. Much of the objective information about a patient is documented in other sections of the PCR, but key objective information should be included in the narrative. For example, the following is a list of signs that you might observe during your care of a patient:

- Pulse rate
- Skin color
- Breathing rate
- Blood pressure
- Obvious swelling
- Obvious bruising
- The fact that the patient vomited

Subjective Information   Some of the information you will gather during your assessment will be subjective in nature. Subjective information is often the opinion of the EMR and is influenced by perception, personal feelings, and prior experience. Symptoms—things that a patient describes such as pain, discomfort, feeling nauseated, or feeling light-headed—are all subjective findings.

Sample Narrative   The following is a sample narrative about a patient who was experiencing chest pain:

> *Arrived on scene of a residence to find a 56-year-old man in moderate distress sitting on a couch. Patient described a chief complaint of pain in the center of his chest that began while mowing his yard. Patient stated that the pain radiated to his neck and both shoulders. He stated the pain was a 7 out of 10. Patient denied any previous medical history and denied taking any medications other than a daily 81 mg aspirin. Patient stated he felt short of breath, and he appeared to be pale and sweaty. We obtained baseline vital signs and provided supplemental O_2 at 4 LPM by cannula. Patient was then turned over to the care of the ambulance personnel.*

Correcting Errors

LO5   Explain the procedure for correcting errors made during documentation.

At times, when completing a PCR, you may document something incorrectly. For example, you might record that the patient's heart rate was 68 instead of 86. In this case, if you are using a paper form, you would cross out the incorrect item with a single line, initial it, and write the correct number beside or above it (Figure 8.3). Never completely cover the incorrect information because it may appear that you are attempting to hide something.

Errors made while using an electronic PCR program typically require that you submit an electronic addendum to the original report.

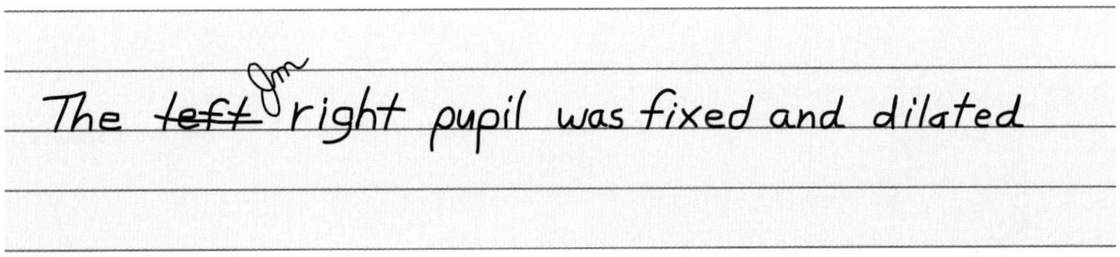

The ~~left~~ ^{Jm} right pupil was fixed and dilated

Figure 8.3 An example of how to properly document an error in documentation.

REMEMBER

Your documentation will likely become a part of the patient's permanent medical record. It will inform other health care providers how the patient first presented at the scene. It will also inform them of the care you provided. This is very important to ensure consistent and safe patient care.

SCENE SAFETY

Do not get distracted by trying to document everything while you are caring for your patient. You must focus on providing the best patient care first and document afterward.

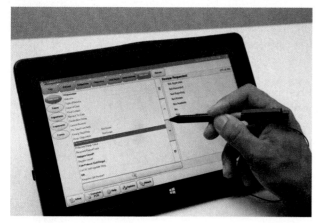

Figure 8.4 A typical electronic tablet used for documenting patient care.

electronic documentation ▶ refers to using technology such as laptop or tablet computers and cell phones to document patient condition and care.

Methods of Documentation

LO6 List various tools used to document patient care in the field setting.

An increasing number of EMS agencies are moving toward **electronic documentation**, but not all services are going down the same path. It is important for Emergency Medical Responders to have a general understanding of the various types of patient care documentation tools, which include:

- *Paper forms.* These traditional PCR forms are filled out by hand and are very common among EMS agencies because they can be easily shared with the transporting crew. In many cases, the form that the EMR completes may be abbreviated and shorter compared to the form that the transporting agency might use.
- *Computer-scan forms.* These PCR forms are completed by hand, but they use a fill-in-the-bubble format so they can be scanned into a computer for easy information management and data collection.
- *Laptop/tablet computers.* Software available for laptop and tablet computers allows responders to complete a PCR electronically and either print it from a docking station or send it wirelessly to a hospital or central database (Figure 8.4).
- *Smartphone applications.* There are smartphone apps that allow responders to complete and send documentation quickly and easily from their cell phones.

FIRST ON SCENE WRAP-UP

Following several months of litigation and three uncomfortable depositions in which Debra had to continually explain that she couldn't recall with any certainty what she had or had not done for the patient those many months ago, the city finally settled the case for an undisclosed amount.

Debra has since gained a reputation for completing the most clear and concise PCRs in the entire department and for keeping meticulous records about each call in which she participates.

Summary

- Patient care documentation is important for many reasons, including continuity of medical care, billing, legal proceedings, and quality assurance. It becomes a permanent part of a patient's medical record and can be used by EMS organizations to improve the overall quality of local emergency services.
- Patient care reports (PCRs) usually consist of two main categories of information: run data and patient data. They are usually completed using a combination of fill-ins, check boxes, and narrative.
- Each PCR has a minimum data set, which is the absolute minimum information that must be documented for each emergency response as defined by the U.S. Department of Transportation.

- Documentation errors should be corrected without trying to obscure the erroneous information because this could lead to speculation about dishonesty. A single line should be drawn through the mistake, the correct information entered above or beside it, and the change should be initialed. Electronic PCRs are corrected using an electronic addendum.
- Patient care documentation can be completed in numerous ways: via traditional paper-based forms, laptop and tablet computers, and smartphone applications. Regardless of the method, Emergency Medical Responders must ensure accuracy and completeness when documenting what happened on each response.

Take Action

Please Correct Me

You will need several blank paper PCR forms and a partner for this activity. Each individual should complete a blank PCR form for an imagined emergency scenario while intentionally making as many documentation mistakes as possible. Leave some areas blank, put incorrect information in other areas, and generally do a less-than-thorough job of completing the form.

Once you are both finished, exchange PCRs and attempt to find as many mistakes and inaccuracies as possible. Rewrite the narrative in a way that would be acceptable.

Do the activity a second time, using two new blank PCR forms. This time, make your errors less obvious and more difficult to find. You will find that it is not as easy as you might think to make intentional errors! Practice using the appropriate technique for correcting mistakes by crossing out and initialing the errors.

Understand that looking at someone else's PCR with a critical eye will help you become more critical of your own documentation, which will make you better at completing PCRs.

First on Scene Run Review

Recall the events of the First on Scene scenario in this chapter, and answer the following questions related to the call. Then decide why proper documentation on all PCRs is important. Rationales are offered in the Answer Key at the back of the book.

1. Could you add more info to the PCR after you turn in the report?
2. How would you go about adding information or correcting an error discovered in your documentation?

Quick Quiz

To check your understanding of the chapter, answer the following questions. Then compare your answers to those in the Answer Key at the back of the book.

1. PCRs are used for all of the following EXCEPT:
   a. billing.
   b. press releases.
   c. quality improvement.
   d. lawsuits.

2. Continuity of care is best described as:
   a. ensuring that the same care provider is responsible for treating a patient until admission to the hospital.
   b. ensuring that once a particular treatment is started it is not stopped.
   c. the thorough and consistent delivery of care among all providers.
   d. the proper documentation of the care provided to a patient.

3. You are writing the patient's history on a PCR and inadvertently document an incorrect medication. You should:
   a. discard the document and begin again.
   b. completely mark out the incorrect medication name with your pen so no one will be able to see it and become confused.
   c. not worry about it because Emergency Medical Responders do not administer medications.
   d. draw a single line through the error, write the correct medication, and initial the change.

4. After caring for a patient, you document the details of the call on the company-provided tablet, uploading the information into the company database. This is an example of which type of documentation?
   a. Paper PCR
   b. Internal PCR
   c. Electronic PCR
   d. Archival documentation

5. Which of the following would NOT be appropriate to include in a standard Emergency Medical Responder PCR?
   a. The exact location where the patient was initially contacted
   b. That the patient was having chest pain
   c. The names of the ambulance personnel who assumed care of the patient
   d. The cause of the injury

Endnotes

1. Short M., Goldstein S. EMS Documentation. 2021 Sep 28. In: StatPearls [Internet]. Treasure Island (FL): StatPearls Publishing; 2022 Jan–. PMID: 28846322.

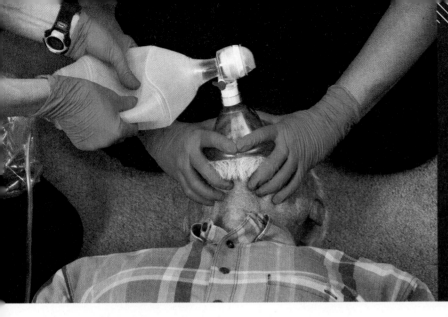

9

Principles of Airway Management and Ventilation

LEARNING OBJECTIVES

Upon successful completion of this chapter, the student should be able to:

Cognitive

1 Define the chapter key terms.

2 State the oxygen concentration of room air.

3 Describe common causes of respiratory compromise.

4 Differentiate between clinical and biological death.

5 Identify the anatomy of the respiratory system and describe basic respiratory physiology.

6 Describe the signs of a patent airway.

7 Differentiate the signs and symptoms of adequate and inadequate breathing.

8 Explain the benefits, indications, and contraindications of positive pressure ventilation.

9 Describe the management of a patient's airway when there is a suspected spine injury.

10 Explain the appropriate steps for rescue breathing with a barrier device.

11 Differentiate the signs of adequate versus inadequate ventilations.

12 Differentiate the airway management of pediatric, adult, and geriatric patients.

13 Describe common causes of airway obstruction.

14 Differentiate between anatomical and mechanical airway obstruction.

15 Differentiate the signs and symptoms of partial and complete airway obstruction.

16 Describe the care for a patient with partial and complete airway obstruction (adult, child, infant).

17 Explain the indications and contraindications for the insertion of an oropharyngeal airway.

18 Explain the indications and contraindications for the insertion of a nasopharyngeal airway.

19 Describe the proper use of the bag-mask device for a nonbreathing patient.

20 Explain the indications for oral and nasal suctioning.

21 Differentiate between manual, electric, and oxygen-powered suction devices.

Psychomotor

22 Demonstrate the proper technique for the head-tilt/chin-lift maneuver.

23 Demonstrate the proper technique for the jaw-thrust maneuver with and without a pocket mask.

24 Demonstrate the proper technique for the insertion of an oropharyngeal airway.

25 Demonstrate the proper technique for the insertion of a nasopharyngeal airway.

26 Demonstrate the proper technique for oral suctioning using both an electric and hand-operated suction device.

27 Demonstrate the proper technique for nasal suctioning using both an electric and hand-operated suction device.

28 Demonstrate the proper technique for the use of a bag-mask device for a nonbreathing patient (adult, child, infant).

29 Demonstrate the proper technique for providing positive pressure ventilations for a patient with inadequate respirations (adult, child, infant).

30 Demonstrate the proper technique for removal of a foreign body airway obstruction (adult, child, infant).

Affective

31 Value the priority of airway management in the overall assessment and care of the patient.

32 Explain the rationale for using a barrier device when ventilating a patient.

KEY TERMS

In this chapter, we will review the anatomy of the respiratory system and explain the process of ventilation (breathing) and the importance of an open and clear airway. We'll also address how to recognize patients who are not breathing adequately or may not be breathing at all and how to provide emergency care for these patients.

FIRST ON SCENE

"Lindsey!" The neighbor's voice is full of panic. "Lindsey, are you home?"

Lindsey is a full-time mother and part-time EMT. She had been dozing in the backyard with a paperback novel shielding her eyes from the sun. "Yeah, Kayla, I'm back here," she says, lifting the book and squinting toward the back fence and her neighbor's red face.

"Lindsey! Quick! It's Camille!" the neighbor stammers. "She fell off the pool slide onto the cement and she's not moving."

Lindsey jumps up from her lounge chair and races into her neighbor's yard. Frank, Kayla's husband and Camille's stepfather, is kneeling over the motionless girl.

"Nobody move her!" he says, probably louder than he intended. "I think her neck might be hurt."

Lindsey looks past Frank and sees the girl lying awkwardly semi-prone on the concrete with her chin propped against her chest.

"Kayla, I need you to call 911 right now," she says. Lindsey kneels next to the girl. "And, Frank, we need to gently roll her over."

Breathing and Ventilation

LO2 State the oxygen concentration of room air.

The air we breathe comprises a mixture of gases. It is made up of approximately 78 percent nitrogen and 21 percent oxygen. The act of breathing is commonly referred to by medical professionals as **ventilation** or respiration. Ventilation is the process by which air and oxygen are brought into the body.

ventilation ▶ process of breathing in and out; also called *respiration*.

How Breathing Works

LO3 Describe common causes of respiratory compromise.

LO4 Differentiate between clinical and biological death.

The body's cells, tissues, and organs need oxygen to function. The body uses oxygen to produce the energy needed to contract muscles, send nerve impulses, digest food, and build new tissues. In addition, the ventilation process allows for the removal of carbon dioxide, which is the waste byproduct of cells. The term **respiration** is used to describe the process that involves the exchange of oxygen and carbon dioxide within the cells (cellular respiration).

The normal range for ventilations per minute is between 10 and 29 for an adult[1], 18 to 34 for children between the ages of 1 and 18[2], and 30 to 60 for an infant younger than 1 year of age.[3] Respiration rates vary by individual, but each age group generally shares a normal range (Table 9.1).

The process of breathing maintains a constant exchange of carbon dioxide and oxygen. If breathing is not adequate or if it stops, cells can become starved for oxygen—a condition known as **hypoxia**. If breathing remains inadequate for too long, carbon dioxide accumulates in the body's cells, becoming a deadly poison. A patient who is not breathing adequately is said to be experiencing **respiratory compromise**. An early sign of respiratory compromise is **respiratory distress**. Respiratory distress is usually obvious because the patient's **work of breathing** increases. If adequate breathing is not restored quickly, the patient may progress to **respiratory failure**. Respiratory failure is characterized by an altered mental status. If respiratory distress is not adequately addressed, the patient will stop breathing altogether. This is a life-threatening condition known as **respiratory arrest**.

Respiratory compromise has many causes, including medical conditions such as asthma, bronchitis, heart attack, and severe allergic reactions. Other factors can also cause difficulty breathing, such as exposure to toxic substances or inhalation of super-heated air, as from a fire in an enclosed building.

The absence of breathing is called **apnea**. Once apnea sets in, the heart will soon stop. This is known as **cardiac arrest**. The heart requires a continuous supply of oxygen to function.

respiration ▶ exchange of oxygen and carbon dioxide within tissues and cells; sometimes used to describe the process of breathing.

hypoxia ▶ insufficient supply of oxygen in the blood and tissues.

respiratory compromise ▶ general term used to describe when a patient is not breathing adequately.

respiratory distress ▶ refers to breathing that becomes difficult or labored.

work of breathing ▶ increase in the effort it takes to breathe.

respiratory failure ▶ inadequate respiratory rate and volume secondary to poor oxygenation.

respiratory arrest ▶ absence of breathing.

apnea ▶ absence of breaths. See also *respiratory arrest*.

cardiac arrest ▶ absence of a heartbeat.

TABLE 9.1	Normal Respiration Rates by Age Group
Age Group	**Normal Range: Breaths per Minute**
Newborn (less than 1 month)	30 to 60
Infant (1 to 12 months)	30 to 60
Toddler (1 to 3 years)	24 to 40
Early childhood (3 to 6 years)	22 to 34
Middle childhood (6 to 12 years)	18 to 30
Adolescent (12 to 18 years)	12 to 16
Adult (18 to 64 years)	12 to 20
Older adult (65 to 80 years)	12 to 25
Elderly adult (81+ years)	10 to 30

clinical death ▶ moment when breathing and heart actions stop.

biological death ▶ occurs approximately 4 to 6 minutes after onset of clinical death and results when there is an excessive amount of brain cell death.

REMEMBER

When you deliver chest compressions during CPR, blood is pumped from the heart to the brain and to the arteries supplying the heart. When starting CPR on a witnessed cardiac arrest, you do not need to give oxygen yet because there is a reserve of oxygen in the blood that can be extracted simply by providing high-quality chest compressions.

---

diaphragm ▶ dome-shaped muscle that separates the chest and abdominal cavities. It is the primary muscle used in breathing.

inhalation ▶ process of breathing in.

exhalation ▶ process of breathing out.

The moment both heartbeat and ventilations stop, **clinical death** occurs. About 4 to 6 minutes after clinical death, oxygen is depleted and cells begin to die. This is the time period when it is most critical for the patient to receive CPR. If the patient's cells do not receive oxygen within 10 minutes, irreversible death may occur. The organ affected first, and the most critical one, is the brain. **Biological death** occurs when too many brain cells die. Clinical death can be reversed; biological death cannot (Figure 9.1).

The Mechanics of Breathing

LO5 | Identify the anatomy of the respiratory system and describe basic respiratory physiology.

Under normal circumstances, breathing is a process that occurs automatically and without any effort. Even though you can temporarily control the rate and depth of your breathing, that control is short term and is soon taken over by involuntary orders from the respiratory centers of the brain located in the medulla and pons. If you try to hold your breath, these centers will first urge you to breathe and then take over and force you to breathe. If you try to breathe slow, shallow breaths while running, those brain centers will automatically adjust the rate and depth of breathing to suit the needs of your body. The needs of your cells, not your will, are the determining factors in the control of breathing.

The volume of the chest cavity is increased by muscle contraction. This may sound backward because contractions usually make things smaller. However, as the muscles between the ribs contract, they pull the front of the ribs up and out. The primary muscle of breathing is the **diaphragm**. When the diaphragm contracts, it moves downward. Both actions result in an increase in the size and volume of the chest cavity.

With each **inhalation** (breath taken in), the size of the chest cavity increases, causing a decrease in the pressure within the lungs (Figure 9.2). When this occurs, the lungs expand automatically. As the lungs expand, the volume inside each lung increases. This means that the pressure inside each lung will decrease. As you may know, air moves from high pressure to low pressure. (A punctured automobile tire demonstrates this principle.) So, when the pressure inside the lungs becomes less than the pressure in the atmosphere, air rushes into the lungs. It moves from high pressure (atmosphere) to low pressure (lungs). It will continue to do so until the pressure in the lungs equals the pressure in the atmosphere.

For **exhalation** (breathing out), the process is reversed. The diaphragm and the muscles between the ribs relax, making the chest cavity smaller. As the chest cavity gets smaller, pressure builds in the lungs until it becomes greater than the pressure in the atmosphere, and we must exhale. Air flows from high pressure (full lungs) to low pressure (atmosphere).

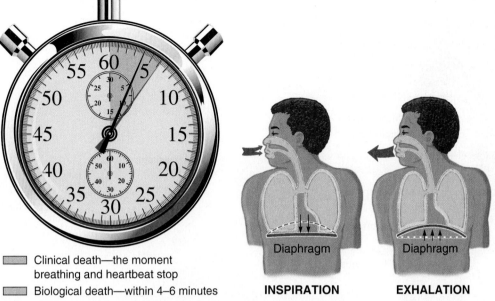

Clinical death—the moment breathing and heartbeat stop

Biological death—within 4–6 minutes

Figure 9.1 Without oxygen, brain cells begin to die within 4 to 6 minutes. Irreversible death may occur in as little as 10 minutes.

INSPIRATION   **EXHALATION**

Figure 9.2 The diaphragm contracts and moves downward on inspiration and relaxes and moves back up on exhalation.

Respiratory System Anatomy

LO5 Identify the anatomy of the respiratory system and describe basic respiratory physiology.

Several important parts of the respiratory system have been discussed: the respiratory centers in the brain and the muscles of respiration. Other major structures of the respiratory system include the upper and lower airways (Figure 9.3):

- *Nose.* The nose is the primary path for air to enter and leave the system. As air enters, the nose filters and helps to moisten it.
- *Mouth.* The mouth is the secondary path for air to enter and leave the system.
- *Pharynx.* The muscular tube that extends from the nasal cavity to the esophagus is the **pharynx**, commonly called the throat. The pharynx consists of the nasopharynx (behind the nose), the oropharynx (behind the mouth), and the hypopharynx, the lower section that ends at the top of the trachea and esophagus.
- *Larynx.* The **larynx** is a structure located at the top of the trachea. It contains the vocal cords and is also called the *voice box.*
- *Epiglottis.* A leaf-shaped structure, the **epiglottis** covers the opening of the larynx when we swallow, which prevents food and fluids from entering the trachea.
- *Trachea.* The **trachea** is the air passage to the lungs. It is located below the larynx and is sometimes called the *windpipe.*
- *Bronchial tree.* This is the structure formed by tubes that branch from the trachea. Its two main branches are the right main bronchus and left main bronchus. They branch into secondary bronchi in the lobes of the lungs. The secondary bronchi branch into still smaller bronchioles and eventually into alveoli, the microscopic air sacs where the exchange of gases takes place.
- *Lungs.* The lungs are the elastic organs that contain parts of the bronchi, the bronchioles, and the alveoli.
- *Alveoli.* These are the small air sacs at the end of the bronchioles where blood cells replenish their oxygen supply and release their accumulated carbon dioxide.

pharynx ▶ the throat.

larynx ▶ section of the airway between the throat and the trachea that contains the vocal cords.

epiglottis ▶ flap of cartilage and other tissues located above the larynx; helps close off the airway when a person swallows.

trachea ▶ tubelike structure that carries air into and out of the lungs.

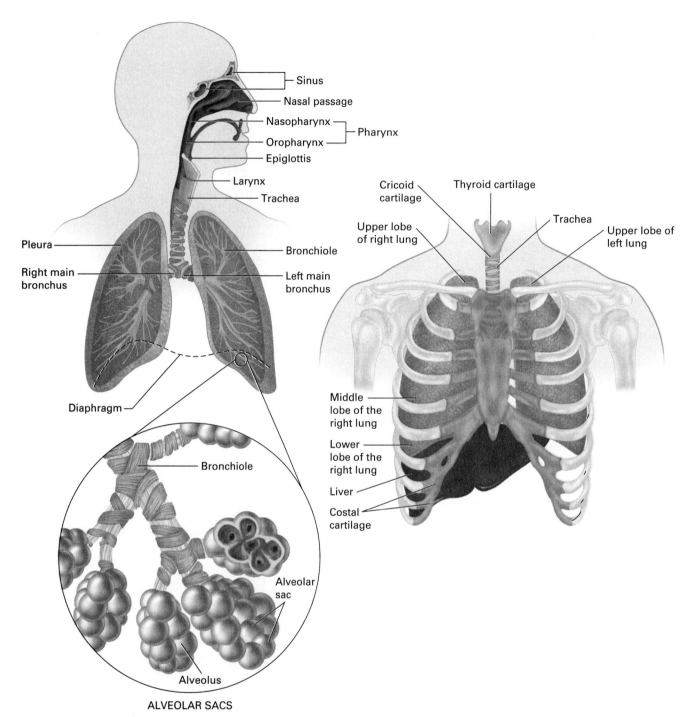

Figure 9.3 Major components of the respiratory system.

Ventilation Cycle

When the muscles responsible for breathing (the diaphragm and the intercostal muscles) contract and enlarge the chest cavity, air flows through the mouth and nose, into the throat, past the epiglottis, and into the trachea. Air then flows into the left and right main bronchi and through the smaller bronchioles to the clusters of alveoli. The alveoli are surrounded by tiny blood vessels called *capillaries*. It is here in the alveoli that oxygen and carbon dioxide exchange takes place. Oxygen travels through the walls of the alveoli and into the blood, which delivers it to the cells. Carbon dioxide travels from the blood through the alveoli walls, where it is eliminated when we exhale. This process of gas exchange is called respiration.

An Open and Clear Airway

LO6 Describe the signs of a patent airway.

Before a breath can be taken, there must be an open and clear pathway into the lungs. This path is commonly called the *airway* and consists of the passages from the nose and mouth to the pharynx and trachea. When an airway is open and clear, it is said to be *patent*. Assessing for and ensuring a **patent airway** will be one of the very first steps in the assessment of any patient you encounter.

In most situations, it will be obvious that the patient has a patent airway because they will be awake, sitting up, and talking normally. When the patient is unresponsive assessing the airway can become a bit more challenging. An airway can become blocked by anything small enough to get caught in the airway. Common causes of airway obstruction include the patient's tongue, secretions, vomit, a foreign object such as a piece of food or a small toy, and swelling of the tissues that form the airway. How to manage an airway that has become blocked is discussed later in this chapter. For now, just know that without a patent airway, there is no way a patient can breathe adequately.

patent airway ▶ open and clear airway.

> **REMEMBER**
>
> Noisy breathing is always a sign of a partial airway obstruction. A patent airway is free of all obstructions and allows for the movement of air in and out of the lungs without difficulty.

Signs of Normal Breathing

LO7 Differentiate the signs and symptoms of adequate and inadequate breathing.

As an Emergency Medical Responder, you must carefully assess the breathing of every patient you encounter. This will become one of the very first things you look for and evaluate as you approach your patient. When observing someone who is breathing normally, the process of breathing is almost invisible. When a patient is in respiratory distress, the most obvious sign is an increase in the effort it takes to breathe. This is called *work of breathing*. An increase in the amount of energy necessary to breathe is called *increased work of breathing*.

As you approach your patient, you must evaluate their breathing for the following characteristics:

- Look for adequate **tidal volume** (the amount of air being moved in and out of the lungs with each breath). Tidal volume can be assessed by observing the rise and fall of the chest with each breath. Normal tidal volume is present when the rise and fall of the chest is effortless and even. Decreased tidal volume is likely when chest rise and fall is too shallow, too rapid, or irregular.
- Listen for air entering and leaving the nose and mouth. The sounds should be quiet like a soft breeze (no gurgling, gasping, wheezing, or other unusual sounds). Noisy breathing indicates some form of partial airway obstruction.
- If the patient is unresponsive, you may need to place your ear and cheek next to their nose and mouth to feel and listen for air moving in and out. You also may observe the chest and abdomen or place a hand on the lower chest to feel for rise and fall.
- Observe skin color. Although skin color varies widely, the skin should not be extremely pale or show signs of **cyanosis** (bluish tint). Look for evidence of cyanosis around the lips and nail beds.
- Observe the patient's level of responsiveness. A responsive patient who is not having difficulty breathing is almost always breathing normally.

tidal volume ▶ amount of air being moved in and out of the lungs with each breath.

cyanosis ▶ bluish discoloration of the skin and mucous membranes; a sign that body tissues are not receiving enough oxygen.

> **JEDI**
>
> Although there is wide variation in skin color, a person's skin should never be extremely pale or have a bluish tint (a sign of cyanosis). Look for evidence of cyanosis by looking at mucous membranes, such as those around the lips and nail beds.

Signs of Abnormal Breathing

LO7 Differentiate the signs and symptoms of adequate and inadequate breathing.

A patient who is unable to breathe normally is said to have difficulty breathing or be in respiratory distress. The medical term for difficulty breathing or shortness of breath is **dyspnea**. The following are common signs and symptoms of abnormal or inadequate breathing:

- Increased work of breathing
- Shallow or absent rise and fall of the chest

dyspnea ▶ difficult or labored breathing, shortness of breath.

- Little or no air heard or felt at the nose or mouth
- Noisy breathing or gasping sounds
- Breathing that is irregular, too rapid, or too slow
- Breathing that is too deep or labored, especially in infants and children
- Use of **accessory muscles** in the chest, abdomen, and around the neck
- Nostrils that flare when breathing, especially in children
- Skin that is extremely pale or cyanotic (bluish tint)
- Sitting or leaning forward in a tripod position in an effort to make breathing easier

accessory muscles ▶ muscles of the neck, chest, and abdomen that can assist during respiratory difficulty.

Agonal respirations are a form of abnormal breathing that is common during cardiac arrest. Agonal respirations are characterized by slow, sporadic gasps of air from an unresponsive patient. Those gasping breaths should not be mistaken for normal breathing.

agonal respirations ▶ abnormal breathing pattern characterized by slow, shallow, gasping breaths that typically occur following cardiac arrest.

Rescue Breathing

LO8 Explain the benefits, indications, and contraindications of positive pressure ventilation.

Rescue breathing is the process of providing manual ventilations for a patient who is not breathing on their own or who is unable to breathe adequately. Another term for this process is **positive pressure ventilation**. Rescue breaths are indicated when a patient is unable to breathe with an adequate rate and volume to sustain life. Rescue breaths are not appropriate for a patient who is responsive or an unresponsive patient who is breathing with a normal rate and tidal volume.

rescue breathing ▶ act of providing manual ventilations for a patient who is not breathing or is unable to breathe adequately on their own.

positive pressure ventilation ▶ process of using external pressure to force air into a patient's lungs, such as with mouth-to-mask or bag-mask ventilations.

One type of rescue breathing is mouth-to-mask breathing. During mouth-to-mask breathing, you provide air that is coming from your lungs to the patient. For this reason, you might wonder if you are providing enough oxygen. The atmosphere contains about 21 percent oxygen. The air exhaled from your lungs can contain up to 16 percent oxygen. This is more than enough oxygen to keep most patients biologically alive until they can receive supplemental oxygen.

FIRST ON SCENE (continued)

"I don't think we should move her," Frank says, grabbing Lindsey's wrists as she touches the unresponsive girl's shoulder. "Shouldn't we wait for the ambulance?"

"Frank, she has no open airway right now. She's not breathing." Lindsey shakes her arms from Frank's grasp. "Now, unless we get her airway open, she's not going to last until the ambulance gets here."

Opening the Airway

Before a patient can breathe normally or before you can provide rescue breaths, the patient must have an open and clear airway. You must ensure that the nose, mouth, and back of the throat are clear of any obstructions. In an unresponsive patient, the tongue can relax and drop into the back of the throat, causing a partial or complete airway obstruction. This is referred to as an anatomical obstruction. The simple act of tilting the head and lifting the chin should correct this problem. If a responsive patient is showing signs of obstruction, such as choking, the problem is likely to be an object stuck in the throat. Immediately begin the steps for choke saving (described later in this chapter).

Repositioning the Head

In an unresponsive patient, simply repositioning the head may be enough to open the airway. If the patient is lying supine (on their back), tilt the head back slightly by removing pillows or by repositioning the patient so the head is not flexed forward. For infants and small children, you may place a flat pillow or folded towel beneath the shoulders to help maintain the head in a more neutral position.

There are two common methods of opening the airway of a supine patient. The **head-tilt/chin-lift maneuver** is used for patients with no suspected spine injury. The **jaw-thrust maneuver** is used for patients suspected of having an injury to the spine.

CREW RESOURCE MANAGEMENT

The proper management of a patient's airway is best performed with a minimum of two rescuers. One rescuer should focus on maintaining a patent airway, while the other focuses on providing ventilations as appropriate. Always anticipate the need for suction, as the patient may vomit at any time.

Head-Tilt/Chin-Lift Maneuver

LO9 | Describe the management of a patient's airway when there is a suspected spine injury.

To perform the head-tilt/chin-lift maneuver, place one hand on the patient's forehead and two fingers of your other hand on the bony part of the patient's chin. Gently tilt the head back while lifting the chin. Be careful not to compress the soft tissues under the jaw. Lift up the patient's chin so the lower teeth are almost touching the upper teeth (Figure 9.4A and B). This maneuver will lift the tongue away from the back of the throat and allow air to flow freely as the patient breathes. For patients with suspected spine injury, use the head-tilt/chin-lift maneuver only if the jaw-thrust maneuver is unsuccessful. This method can be used in conjunction with a **pocket face mask** when manual ventilations are required.

Jaw-Thrust Maneuver

LO9 | Describe the management of a patient's airway when there is a suspected spine injury.

The jaw-thrust maneuver is the recommended method for opening the airway of patients with possible neck or spine injuries (Figure 9.5A and B). Position yourself at the top of the patient's head. Reach forward and place the index and middle fingers of each hand on either side at the angles of the jaw. You may press your thumbs against the cheekbones for leverage. Lift the jaw forward. Do not tilt or rotate the patient's head. This method can be used in conjunction with a pocket face mask when manual ventilations are required.

Barrier Devices

All Emergency Medical Responders should use barrier devices, such as pocket face masks or face shields, when providing rescue breaths. When you perform rescue breathing, you can come into direct contact with the patient's body fluids such as respiratory secretions, saliva droplets, blood, or vomit. Take all steps necessary to ensure protection from infectious diseases.

head-tilt/chin-lift maneuver ▶ technique used to open the airway of a patient with no suspected neck or spine injury.

jaw-thrust maneuver ▶ technique used to open the airway of a trauma patient with possible neck or spine injury.

pocket face mask ▶ device used to help provide ventilations. Most have a one-way valve and HEPA filter. Some have an inlet for supplemental oxygen.

SCENE SAFETY

It is important to carefully consider the potential for spinal injury before opening the patient's airway. For example, the absence of an obvious mechanism of injury does not automatically rule out spinal injury. A patient found unresponsive in an alley could have been assaulted and therefore may have a neck or back injury. When in doubt, always take appropriate spinal precautions.

REMEMBER

If you are caring for a patient who has been injured and you are unable to effectively open the airway using the jaw-thrust maneuver, you must use the head-tilt/chin-lift maneuver instead. An open airway is always your first priority.

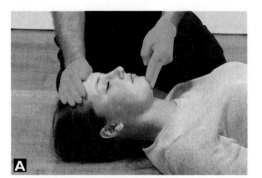 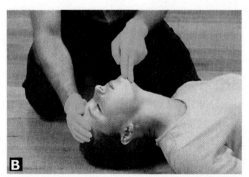

Figure 9.4 Use the head-tilt/chin-lift maneuver to open the airway if you do not suspect spinal injuries. (A) First, position your hands. (B) Then tilt the patient's head back as far as it will comfortably go.

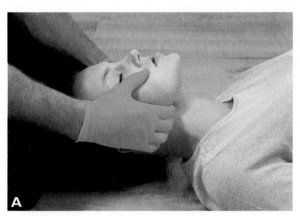
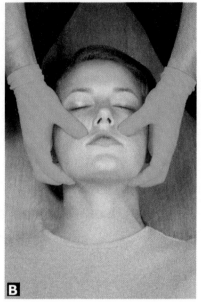

Figure 9.5 Use the jaw-thrust maneuver if there are possible neck or spine injuries. (A) Side view and (B) front view of proper hand position.

The pocket face mask is one example of a barrier device. These masks are available in many sizes and should fit the patient and seal easily to the facial contours of the adult, child, or infant. Pocket face masks are typically made of durable plastic and have a replaceable one-way valve and filter. Some masks have an oxygen inlet to allow for the administration of supplemental oxygen.

The face shield is another type of barrier device. It is a durable plastic sheet with a built-in one-way valve. When folded and stowed, it is small enough to be attached to a key ring; unfolded, it is large enough to cover the patient's lower face and act as a barrier to help minimize direct contact with body fluids.

Mouth-to-Mask Ventilation

LO10 Explain the appropriate steps for rescue breathing with a barrier device.

LO11 Differentiate the signs of adequate versus inadequate ventilations.

The mouth-to-mask technique of providing rescue breaths is the recommended method when only a single rescuer is present. It is quick to set up and relatively easy to facilitate. A pocket face mask allows you to provide ventilations without having to make direct skin-to-skin contact. The mask should have a one-way valve to minimize the chances of the rescuer breathing in exhaled air from the patient. The pocket face mask should also come with a disposable high-efficiency particulate air (HEPA) filter (Figure 9.6). The filter snaps inside the pocket face mask and traps air droplets and secretions that may contain dangerous pathogens.

The pocket face mask is made of soft plastic material that can be folded and carried in your pocket. It is available with or without an oxygen inlet. If the mask has a second port for oxygen, you can simultaneously ventilate the patient with air from your lungs and with additional oxygen from an oxygen source.

Another advantage of the pocket face mask is that it allows you to use both hands to maintain a proper head position and still hold the mask firmly in place. It is relatively easy to keep a good seal between the mask and a patient's face with this device (Figure 9.7A and B). The pocket face mask also can be used with or without an airway adjunct (discussed later in this chapter).

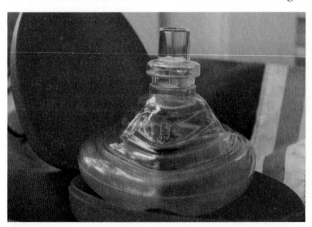

Figure 9.6 A typical pocket face mask with HEPA filter.

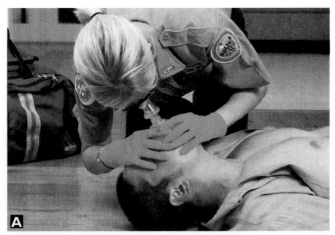 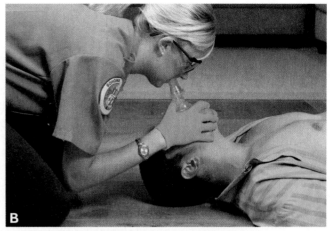

Figure 9.7 Providing ventilations with a pocket mask from the (A) lateral position or (B) the cephalic position.

To provide mouth-to-mask ventilations, make sure you are wearing appropriate PPE and follow these steps:

1. Kneel beside the patient (lateral position) and confirm unresponsiveness.
2. Open the airway using the most appropriate maneuver.
3. Firmly hold the mask in place while keeping the airway open. To accomplish this, place both thumbs and index fingers on the cone of the mask to form a C around both sides. Apply even pressure on both sides of the mask.
4. Take a normal breath and breathe slowly into the one-way valve, delivering each breath over 1 second.[4] Air will enter the airway through the patient's nose and mouth. Watch for the patient's chest to rise. Remember that there is no need to remove your mouth to allow the patient to exhale. The patient's exhaled air will escape through separate vents in the one-way valve. If air does not enter on the initial breath, reposition the patient's head and try again. If air still does not enter, perform the steps for clearing an obstructed airway (explained later in this chapter).
5. If the initial breath is successful but the patient does not begin breathing adequately on his own, assess for the presence of a pulse and begin CPR if indicated.

An alternative method for ventilating with a pocket mask is to kneel at the top of the patient's head (cephalic position). Place both thumbs and index fingers on the cone of the mask to form a C around both sides. Place the third, fourth, and fifth fingers of each hand under the jaw to form an E on both sides of the patient's jaw. Apply even pressure on both sides of the mask while maintaining a head tilt.

The best indication that you are providing good ventilations is obvious chest rise and fall with each ventilation. If you find that your efforts to ventilate the patient are not adequate, you must make adjustments such as repositioning the head, increasing the volume, changing the rate of ventilations, or adjusting the seal between the mask and the patient's face. It is common to see the patient's skin color improve with good ventilations.

Mouth-to-Shield Ventilation

LO10 Explain the appropriate steps for rescue breathing with a barrier device.

LO11 Differentiate the signs of adequate versus inadequate ventilations.

To provide mouth-to-shield ventilations, make sure you are wearing appropriate PPE and follow these steps:

1. Kneel beside the patient (lateral position) and confirm unresponsiveness.
2. Open the airway using the most appropriate maneuver.
3. Place the barrier over the patient's mouth. Keep the airway open as you pinch the nose closed.

SCENE SAFETY

The Occupational Safety and Health Administration (OSHA) and the Centers for Disease Control and Prevention (CDC) guidelines state that EMS personnel can reduce the risk of contracting infectious diseases by using pocket face masks with one-way valves and HEPA filter inserts when ventilating patients. Always have one on hand. Also wear protective gloves during assessment and care of all patients.

4. Open your mouth wide and take a normal breath.
5. Place your mouth over the face shield opening. Make a tight seal by pressing your lips against it.
6. Exhale slowly into the patient's mouth until you see the chest rise. If this first attempt to provide a breath fails, reposition the patient's head and try again.
7. If the patient has a pulse but is still not breathing, provide rescue breaths at a rate of 1 breath every 5 seconds.
8. If the patient does not have a pulse, begin CPR.

Continue CPR until the patient begins to breathe on their own, someone with equal or more training takes over, or you are too exhausted to continue. You must recheck for the presence of a pulse if the patient displays any signs of life such as breathing, coughing, moving, and so on.

If you are following the correct procedures and the patient's airway is not obstructed, you should be able to feel resistance to your ventilations as the patient's lungs expand. You should also be able to see the chest rise and fall, hear air leaving the patient's airway as the chest falls, and feel air leaving the patient's mouth as the lungs deflate. Constantly monitor the patient to determine if they have begun to breathe unassisted. Continue to monitor for the presence of a carotid pulse at the neck at least every minute.

The most common problems with the mouth-to-barrier technique are failure to:

- form a tight seal over the face shield opening and the patient's mouth (often caused by the rescuer failing to open their mouth wide enough to make an effective seal or pushing too hard in an effort to form a tight seal).
- pinch the patient's nose completely closed.
- tilt the patient's head back far enough to open the airway.
- open the patient's mouth wide enough to receive breaths.
- deliver enough air during a breath.
- provide breaths at the correct rate.
- clear the airway of obstructions.

Two additional problems—air in the patient's stomach and vomiting—are covered later in this chapter.

Special Patients

LO12 Differentiate the airway management of pediatric, adult, and geriatric patients.

Among your patients will be infants and children, older adult patients, and trauma patients (some with possible neck and spine injuries). You may also encounter patients with a **stoma**, which is a surgically created opening from inside the body to the outside, as in the anterior neck for breathing (tracheostomy) or in the abdomen for waste excretion.

Infants and Children

The airways of infants (birth to 1 year) and children (1 year to the onset of puberty) have several physical characteristics that differ from adults. In the infant and child:

- The mouth and nose are much smaller and more easily obstructed.
- The tongue takes up more space in the mouth and throat.
- The trachea is smaller and more easily obstructed by swelling. It is also softer and more flexible and can become obstructed by tilting the head back too far (hyperextension).
- The chest muscles are not as well developed, causing the infant and child to depend more on the diaphragm for breathing.
- The chest cavity and lung volumes are smaller, so **gastric distention** (air getting into the stomach, causing inflation of the stomach) occurs more commonly.

The airway of an infant or child can be occluded easily if the head is allowed to become too flexed or too extended. An infant's head should be placed in a neutral position and a child's head in a slightly extended position.

stoma ▸ surgically created opening from an area inside the body to the outside.

gastric distention ▸ inflation of the stomach.

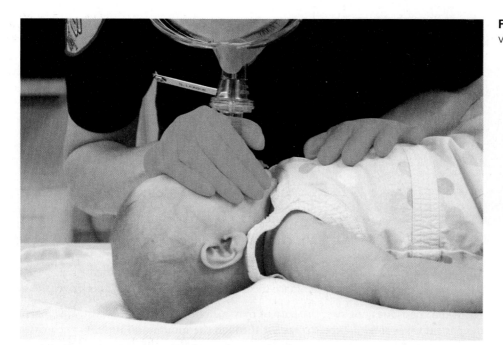

Figure 9.8 Mouth-to-mask ventilation of an infant.

You must recognize and aggressively care for airway and respiratory problems in infants and children. Respiratory distress can quickly lead to cardiac arrest in these patients.

When assisting ventilations for an infant (Figure 9.8) or a small child who has a pulse but is not breathing normally, make sure you take appropriate BSI precautions and follow these steps:

1. Kneel or stand beside the patient and confirm unresponsiveness.
2. Open the airway using the most appropriate maneuver.
3. Using an appropriate barrier device, give 1 breath every 2 to 3 seconds.[5] If air does not enter on the initial breath, reposition the head and try again. If air still does not enter, perform the steps for clearing an obstructed airway (explained later in this chapter).
4. Assist ventilations with gentle but adequate breaths. The volume of breath for the infant or child is determined by ventilating until you see the chest rise. Watch for the chest to rise with each breath.

If there is no reason to suspect spine injury, it is helpful to place a folded towel or similar object under an infant's shoulders to help maintain an open airway.

Terminally Ill Patients

Many terminally ill patients choose to spend their remaining time at home with family and friends. Hospice programs support and advise terminally ill patients and their family members. Many patients under hospice care have written orders regarding their care, which may not include rescue breaths or compressions. For guidelines on how to care for hospice patients and those who have do-not-resuscitate (DNR) orders in place, check your jurisdiction for training programs and follow your local protocols.

Stomas

Some people have had a surgical procedure called a **laryngectomy** or **tracheostomy**. A stoma is made from outside the neck to the trachea to create an airway for breathing. These patients breathe through that opening (Figure 9.9), not through the nose or the mouth.

Because the patient primarily takes air into the lungs by way of the stoma, you will have to use the mask-to-stoma technique to assist ventilations. Currently, there is no specific mask for ventilating these patients, but an infant-size mask often fits, allowing you to establish a seal around the stoma. You also may assist ventilations with a protective

> **REMEMBER**
>
> It may be difficult to get a good mask-to-face seal when dentures are loose or missing. Loose dentures can become an airway obstruction and interfere with your efforts to ventilate a patient. If dentures are secure, leave them in place. If they are loose, remove them.

laryngectomy ▶ total or partial removal of the larynx.

tracheostomy ▶ surgical opening on the anterior neck into the trachea to create an airway for breathing.

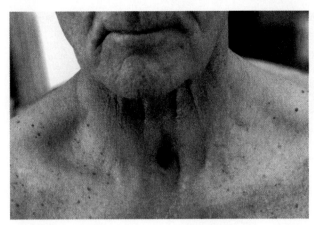

Figure 9.9 A surgical stoma on the anterior neck.
(Kevin Link/Pearson Education, Inc.)

bag-mask device ▶ device made up of a face mask, self-refilling bag, and one-way valve that is used to provide manual ventilations; also called a *bag-valve mask* or *BVM*.

face shield or by attaching a **bag-mask device** directly to the patient's stoma tube if one is in place in the stoma opening. Follow the protocols of your jurisdiction. If you don't see chest rise when attempting to ventilate through the stoma, cover the nose and mouth to block any escaping air during each rescue breath.

When ventilating a stoma patient, take appropriate BSI precautions and follow these steps:

1. Keep the patient's head in a neutral or normal position. Do not tilt the head.
2. Ensure that the stoma is free and clear of any obstructions such as mucus or vomit. Do not remove the breathing tube if one is in place.
3. Use the same procedures as you would for mouth-to-barrier resuscitation, *except:*
   • Do not pinch the patient's nose closed.
   • Place the mask or face shield on the neck over the stoma.

If the chest does not rise, the patient may be a partial neck breather. This means that the patient takes in and expels some air through the mouth and nose. In such cases, you will have to pinch the nose closed, seal the mouth with the palm of your hand, and ventilate through the stoma.

Trauma Patients

Opening the airway and assisting ventilations are easier for you to perform when the patient is lying supine. This means that a trauma patient who is not breathing but who is still in their vehicle must be repositioned. There is always a risk of causing further spine injury if you move the patient, but you must be realistic. If you wait for other EMS personnel to arrive or if you take time to put on a rigid cervical collar and secure the patient to a spine board, the patient will likely not survive due to a lack of oxygen to the brain. *Airway and breathing are always the first priorities of patient care.*

Without risking your own safety, take appropriate BSI precautions and reach the person as quickly as possible. Look, listen, and feel for breathing before moving them. If the patient is breathing, the airway is open and you do not have to move them. If you believe the mechanism of injury may have caused damage to the spine or neck and the patient is not breathing, stabilize the head and attempt to open the airway with the jaw-thrust maneuver. Then check again for breathing. If the patient is breathing, keep the airway open while maintaining the head and neck in a neutral position. Monitor breathing until assistance arrives. If the patient is not breathing and their position does not allow you to maintain an airway while you assist ventilations, you will have to reposition them.

Your instructor will show you methods to practice so you can reposition a patient with maximum head stabilization and as little spinal movement as possible.

REMEMBER

It is vital for you to first address any airway compromise in the trauma patient. While it is true that the trauma patient may also have a spine injury, restoring adequate perfusion is your first priority.

Air in the Stomach and Vomiting

A common side effect of rescue breathing is that it can cause air to enter the patient's stomach. This can be caused by forcing too much air into the lungs or delivering rescue breaths too quickly. Remember to carefully watch the chest rise as you ventilate. Provide only enough air to cause the chest to rise noticeably. Forcing more air than the lungs can hold during ventilation can cause or worsen gastric distention (inflation of the stomach). Air in the stomach will cause the abdomen to distend (get larger).

Watch for gastric distention when you ventilate a patient. Excessive gastric distention will reduce the lungs' ability to expand normally. Reduced lung capacity restricts ventilations and limits oxygen flow to the body. Gastric distention can also cause extra pressure in the stomach, which can result in the patient vomiting.

Do not worry about slight stomach bulging, but you will have to make adjustments if you notice excessive bulging. In cases of air in the stomach where you see a noticeable bulge, reduce the force of your ventilations and do the following:

- Reposition the patient's head to ensure an open airway.
- Be prepared for vomiting. If the patient begins to vomit, turn their whole body (not just the head) to one side so the vomit will flow out of the airway and not back into it. Have suction equipment on hand if you carry it in your unit.
- Do not push on the stomach to release the air. This may cause vomiting, which can block the airway or enter the lungs. Even if the patient is on their side when vomiting, the vomit will not simply flow out. With your gloved hand, clear the patient's mouth with gauze and finger sweeps, or use suctioning equipment.

CREW RESOURCE MANAGEMENT

Everyone on the team must be focused on the primary objective when managing a patient's airway. If anyone feels that you are not maintaining a patent airway or are unable to deliver adequate ventilations, they should speak up immediately and make sure everyone is aware of the situation so it can be fixed.

Airway Obstruction

The airway is divided into the upper and lower airways. The dividing line is the opening of the larynx. Lower airway obstructions are difficult to manage and often require advanced training. You will be able to assess and manage most upper airway obstructions.

Causes of Airway Obstruction

LO13 Describe common causes of airway obstruction.

LO14 Differentiate between anatomical and mechanical airway obstruction.

Many factors can cause the airway to become partially or completely obstructed, including a foreign object lodged in the airway or excess saliva or blood accumulating in the mouth.

The following are examples of upper airway obstructions that you may be able to relieve:

- *Obstruction by the tongue (anatomical obstruction).* This is one of the most common causes of airway obstruction in unresponsive patients; it is caused when the base of the tongue falls back in the pharynx and blocks the airway.
- *Foreign objects (mechanical obstruction).* Objects and other matter such as ice cubes or food can block the airway. Vomit or other liquids pooling in the back of the throat can also cause a blockage.

The following obstructions may be impossible for you to relieve, but you must still attempt to assist ventilations:

- *Tissue damage.* Tissue damage can be caused by trauma to the neck, upper airway burns from breathing super-heated air (from a fire or explosion), and poisons. The tissues of the throat and trachea become swollen and make it difficult for air to flow through the airway.
- *Allergic reactions.* The tissues of the mouth, tongue, throat, and/or the epiglottis become swollen in response to exposure to something a patient is allergic to, such as a bee sting or a certain food.
- *Infections.* The tissues of the throat and trachea can become infected and swollen and can produce airway obstruction.

Signs of Partial Airway Obstruction

LO15 Describe the signs and symptoms of partial and a complete airway obstruction.

A patient having difficulty breathing may have only a partial obstruction and may still be able to move some air. The signs of partial airway obstruction include:

- Noisy breathing, such as these symptoms:
  - *Snoring* is evidence of a partial obstruction usually caused by the tongue.
  - *Gurgling* is usually caused by fluids or blood in the oropharynx and/or upper airway.
  - *Stridor* is a high-pitched sound, typically on **inspiration** (inhalation), caused by swelling of the larynx; it is also called *crowing*.
  - *Wheezing* is a high-pitched whistling sound, usually due to swelling or spasms of the lower airway. It is more common during exhalation.
- Increased work of breathing, with skin that is very pale or blue at the lips or nail beds. The usual presentation in a responsive patient is fear, panic, or agitation. Very few things invoke terror in a person like a threatened airway or the inability to breathe.

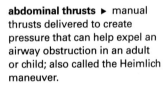
inspiration ▶ refers to the process of breathing in, or inhaling.

If a responsive patient is experiencing a partial airway obstruction, encourage them to cough. A forceful cough indicates that they have enough air exchange, and coughing may dislodge and expel foreign materials. Do not interfere with the patient's own efforts to clear the airway if they are able to produce repeated strong coughs.

If the patient has poor air exchange and cannot cough or coughs only weakly, begin care as if there were a complete airway obstruction (discussed later in this chapter).

Signs of Complete Airway Obstruction

When the airway is completely obstructed, the responsive patient will be unable to speak, breathe, or cough. The patient will often grasp their neck and open their mouth, which is the universal sign of choking (Figure 9.10). The unresponsive patient will not have any of the typical chest movements or the other signs of good air exchange.

Clearing a Foreign Body Airway Obstruction

abdominal thrusts ▶ manual thrusts delivered to create pressure that can help expel an airway obstruction in an adult or child; also called the Heimlich maneuver.

LO16 Describe the care for a patient with partial and complete airway obstruction (adult, child, infant).

The techniques for clearing foreign body obstructions vary based on whether the patient is responsive or unresponsive.

Responsive Adult or Child   Ongoing research conducted by the American Heart Association suggests that the use of **abdominal thrusts** is still the most effective method for clearing the airway of a responsive adult or child older than 1 year who is choking.[6] A slightly different technique is used to clear the airway of an infant.

For abdominal thrusts, the rescuer stands behind the patient, places one fist just above the navel, grasps that fist with the other hand, and provides inward and upward thrusts. These thrusts push up on the diaphragm muscle, creating pressure inside the chest cavity and forcing air out of the lungs. As the air is forced out of the lungs, it pushes the foreign object out ahead of it. This technique is known as the Heimlich maneuver.

Perform the following steps to remove a foreign body airway obstruction in a responsive adult or child (Key Skill 9.1):

1. Confirm that there is complete obstruction or a partial obstruction with poor air exchange. Ask, "Are you choking?" or "Can you speak?" Look and listen for signs of complete obstruction or poor air exchange. Tell the patient you will help.
2. Position yourself behind the patient and place one fist just above the patient's navel.

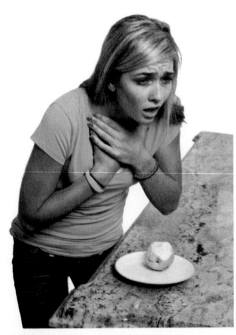
Figure 9.10 A patient displaying the universal sign of choking.

Abdominal Thrusts (Heimlich Maneuver)

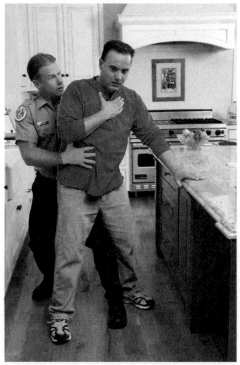

1. Stand behind the patient. Place one leg between the patient's legs to obtain a stable stance.

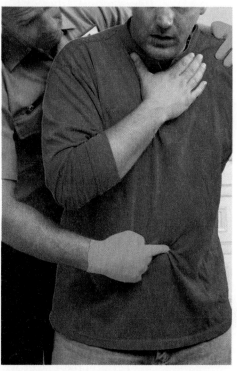

2. Reach around with one hand to locate the patient's navel.

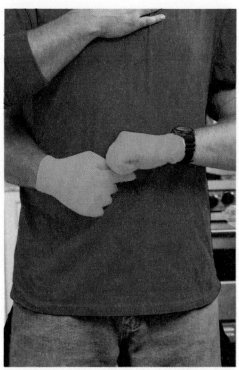

3. With the other hand, make a fist and place it just above the patient's navel.

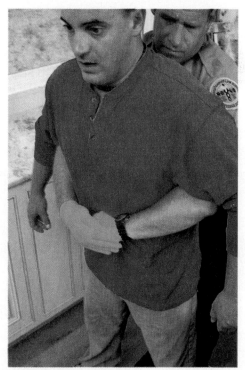

4. Grasp your fist with the first hand and pull in and up with swift, firm thrusts.

3. Grasp the fist with your other hand and perform up to 5 abdominal thrusts in rapid succession. Watch and listen for evidence that the object has been removed. The patient will begin to cough or speak if the object is removed.

Unresponsive Adult or Child   The following guidelines for the care of an unresponsive patient apply to adults and children (1 year of age and older). Act quickly to determine if you are able to provide adequate ventilations. Because the tongue is the most common cause of airway obstruction in unresponsive patients, make certain to open the airway using the most appropriate maneuver prior to attempting ventilation. Once you have confirmed that you are unable to ventilate, begin CPR. (Specific techniques for performing CPR are explained in Chapter 11.)

Perform the following steps when foreign body airway obstruction is suspected in an unresponsive adult or child:

1. Take the appropriate BSI precautions.
2. With the patient lying supine (face up) on a firm surface, tap and shout to assess responsiveness.
3. If unresponsive, direct someone to activate 911.
4. Begin CPR with chest compressions.
5. After each set of 30 compressions, open the airway and check for evidence of a foreign object and remove it if it is visible.
6. Attempt 2 rescue breaths. If breaths do not go in, continue CPR with chest compressions.

Responsive Infant   The steps for caring for an infant (younger than 1 year of age) are slightly different from those used for adults and children. For the responsive infant, a combination of back blows and **chest thrusts** is used to remove the foreign object.

Perform these steps when caring for a responsive infant with an airway obstruction:

1. Take appropriate BSI precautions.
2. Pick up the infant and support them between the forearms of both arms. Support the infant's head as you place them face down on your forearm. Use your thigh to support your forearm. Remember to keep the infant's head lower than the trunk (Figure 9.11).
3. Rapidly deliver 5 back blows between the shoulder blades. If this fails to expel the object, proceed to Step 4.
4. While supporting the infant between your arms, turn them over onto their back, again keeping the head lower than the trunk. Remember to support the infant's neck. Use your thigh to support your forearm (Figure 9.12).

chest thrusts ▶ manual thrusts delivered to create pressure that can help expel an airway obstruction in an infant or in pregnant or obese patients.

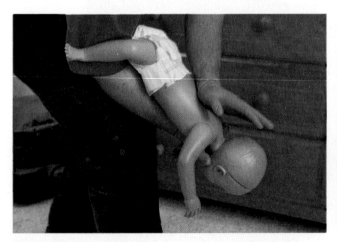

Figure 9.11 The proper positioning of an infant for back blows.

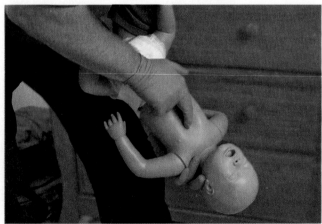

Figure 9.12 The proper positioning of an infant for chest thrusts.

5. Locate the compression site and deliver 5 chest thrusts with the tips of two or three fingers along the midline of the breastbone.

6. Continue with this sequence of back blows and chest thrusts until the object is expelled or the infant loses responsiveness.

7. If the infant becomes unresponsive before you can expel the object, perform 30 chest compressions.

Unresponsive Infant Perform these steps when caring for an unresponsive infant with a complete airway obstruction (Key Skill 9.2):

1. Take the appropriate BSI precautions.

2. With the infant lying face up (supine), tap and shout to assess responsiveness and check for signs of breathing.

3. If the infant is unresponsive and not breathing, direct someone to activate 911. Initiate chest compressions.

4. After each set of 30 compressions, open the airway and check for evidence of a foreign object. Remove it if it is visible.

5. Attempt 2 rescue breaths. If breaths do not go in, continue chest compressions and check the mouth for foreign bodies before giving rescue breaths.

> **REMEMBER**
>
> Back blows are recommended for conscious infants with complete airway obstructions. (Do not use back blows on children or adults.) Do not use abdominal thrusts on patients younger than 1 year of age because the risk of causing damage to the internal organs of infants is too great.

KEY SKILL 9.2

Caring for the Unresponsive Choking Infant

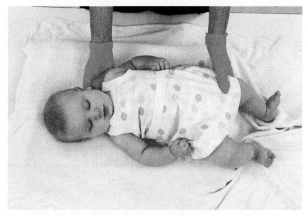

1. Place the infant supine on a firm surface.

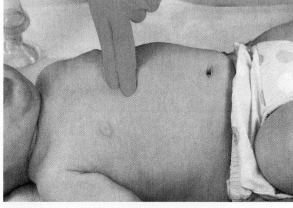

2. If unable to detect signs of breathing, start CPR beginning with chest compressions.

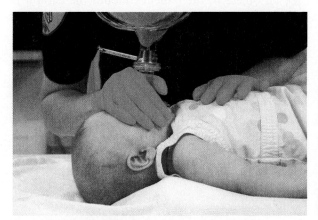

3. After 30 compressions, attempt 2 rescue breaths.

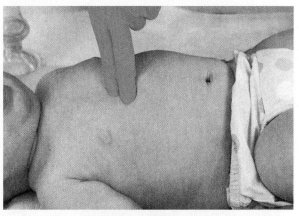

4. If unable to ventilate, continue with 30 compressions.

Obese and Pregnant Patients

Some choking patients present specific challenges that must be overcome if you are going to have any chance of clearing the airway. For example, a patient's large size may prevent you from getting your arms completely around them, making it impossible to provide adequate abdominal thrusts. Providing abdominal thrusts to a pregnant woman can cause serious injury to the developing fetus. For obese or pregnant patients who are responsive, attempt to provide chest thrusts as an alternative to abdominal thrusts (Figure 9.13A and B).

For the obese patient, the chest area is typically smaller in diameter than the abdomen, making it more likely that you can provide adequate and successful thrusts. An alternative for the obese patient is to have them stand against a sturdy wall and attempt abdominal thrusts from the front.

Perform the following steps to provide chest thrusts:

1. Confirm that there is complete obstruction or a partial obstruction with poor air exchange. Ask, "Are you choking?" or "Can you speak?" Tell the patient you will help.
2. Position yourself behind the patient and place the thumb side of one fist flat against the sternum.
3. Grasp the fist with the other hand and give up to 5 chest thrusts in rapid succession. Watch and listen for evidence that the object has been removed. If it has, the patient will begin to cough, speak, or breathe.
4. If the patient's airway remains obstructed, repeat the thrusts until the airway is cleared or until the patient loses responsiveness.
5. If the patient becomes unresponsive before you are able to clear the airway obstruction, direct someone to call 911 and begin CPR.

FIRST ON SCENE (continued)

Frank thinks for a second, his eyes moving from his unconscious stepdaughter to Lindsey's face. When he finally agrees to let Lindsey provide emergency care, Lindsey instructs him how to help her roll the girl over while keeping her head and neck in a neutral, in-line position.

As soon as Camille's chin moves from her chest, the child inhales noisily and begins breathing again. Frank closes his eyes and takes several deep breaths before opening them again. "Thank you," he says quietly.

Finger Sweeps

A finger sweep is the technique of using your finger to sweep through the patient's mouth in an attempt to remove a foreign object. It is important to know that you should perform finger sweeps only if you can see an object in the patient's mouth. Be careful not to accidentally force the object back down the patient's throat in your attempt to sweep it out.

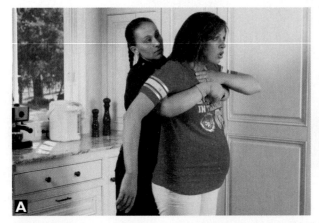
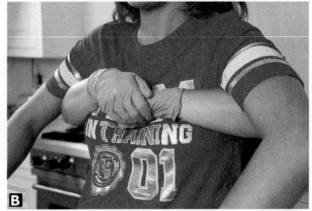

Figure 9.13 For a pregnant patient, (A) position yourself behind, then wrap your arms around the chest. (B) Place the fist of one hand flat against the sternum, grasp firmly with the other hand, and pull in sharply.

In most cases, a responsive patient has a **gag reflex**. Probing the mouth with your finger may stimulate the gag reflex and cause vomiting. If this occurs, the patient may inhale the vomit, resulting in the potential for serious illness later. Therefore, attempt finger sweeps only on unresponsive patients and only when you can actually see the object you are trying to remove.

Aids to Airway Management

The use of an appropriate airway adjunct can help provide more effective airway management. There are two types of airway adjuncts commonly used by Emergency Medical Responders: the **oropharyngeal airway (OPA)** and the **nasopharyngeal airway (NPA)**. As you learn to use these devices, it is important to understand that they are only tools that assist you in managing a patient's airway and breathing status—they do not guarantee an open airway.

The OPA and NPA help maintain an open airway for the patient, allowing more effective ventilations to be delivered. The bag-mask device allows the Emergency Medical Responder to deliver better ventilations for patients who are not breathing adequately on their own. The OPA and NPA are often used together with the bag-mask device to provide the best possible ventilations.

One disadvantage of all adjunct equipment is that it can delay the beginning of resuscitation if it is not readily available. Your pocket face mask and airway adjuncts should always be handy. Never delay the start of ventilations or CPR while you try to retrieve an airway adjunct.

Oropharyngeal Airway

LO17 Explain the indications and contraindications for the insertion of an oropharyngeal airway.

An oropharyngeal airway (OPA) is a device (usually made of plastic) that can be inserted into a patient's mouth. It has a flange that rests against the patient's lips. The lower portion curves back into the throat and rests against the patient's tongue, restricting its movement and minimizing the chance that it will block the airway. Once a patient's airway is opened manually—using the head-tilt/chin-lift or jaw-thrust maneuver—an OPA may be inserted to help keep the tongue away from the back of the throat (Figure 9.14).

OPAs should be used only in unresponsive patients who do not have a gag reflex. These devices can stimulate a patient's normal gag reflex, causing them to vomit. If the unresponsive patient vomits, they can aspirate (inhale) the vomit back into the airway and lungs, causing a blockage. If the patient is responsive (even if disoriented or confused) or unresponsive with a gag reflex, do not insert an OPA.

Do not continue to insert an OPA or leave it in the patient's mouth if you meet any resistance or if the patient begins to gag as you insert it. Immediately remove the OPA and prepare to suction if they vomit. Next, attempt to insert an NPA.

You may sense that the rules for deciding whether or not to use an OPA seem contradictory. You are not supposed to use an OPA on a patient with a gag reflex, yet you will not know if the patient has this reflex unless you attempt to insert the OPA. To resolve this dilemma, you must be very focused as you insert the OPA. Expect that they may have a gag reflex and, at the first indication that they do, remove the device. If you carry a suction unit and are trained to use it, have it ready for any patient who is unresponsive and may need an adjunct. You do not want to be caught unprepared should your patient vomit.

Measuring the Oropharyngeal Airway There are numerous sizes of OPAs designed to fit infants, children, and adults (Figure 9.15). To use an OPA effectively, you must select the correct size for the patient. Before inserting the device, hold it against the patient's face and measure to see if it extends from

gag reflex ▶ reflex spasm at the back of the throat caused by stimulation of the back of the tongue or the soft tissue near or around the oropharynx.

oropharyngeal airway ▶ curved plastic device inserted into the patient's mouth to minimize obstruction of the airway caused by the tongue; also called *oral airway*. Abbrev: OPA.

nasopharyngeal airway ▶ flexible tube inserted into a patient's nose to provide an open airway; also called *nasal airway*. Abbrev: NPA.

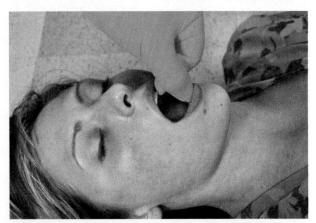

Figure 9.14 Prior to placing an OPA, open the mouth with the crossed-finger technique.

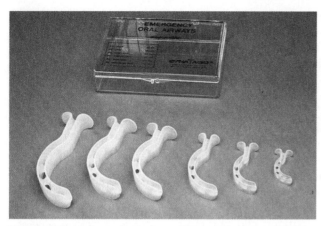

Figure 9.15 Various sizes of oropharyngeal airways (OPAs).

the corner of the patient's mouth to the tip of the earlobe on the same side of the face. An alternative method is to measure from the center of the mouth to the angle of the lower jaw. You may not find the exact size device for all patients. If this is the case, choose one that is slightly larger than your measurement.

An OPA that is the wrong size has the potential to cause more harm than good. If the device is too long, it might extend too far into the throat and block the airway. If it is too short, it will not restrict the movement of the tongue as it should, thus allowing the tongue to block the airway.

Inserting the Oropharyngeal Airway To insert an OPA, you should (Key Skill 9.3):

1. Take the appropriate BSI precautions.
2. With the patient on their back, manually open the airway using the head-tilt/chin-lift or jaw-thrust maneuver.
3. Select the appropriate-sized device by measuring from the corner of the mouth to the earlobe.
4. Insert the device by positioning it so its tip is pointing toward the roof of the patient's mouth.
5. Insert the device and slide it along the roof of the mouth, being certain not to push the tongue back into the throat.
6. Once the device is about halfway in, rotate it 180 degrees so the tip is positioned at the base of the tongue. Allow the top flange to rest against the outside of the lips.
7. Monitor the device constantly. Check to see that the flange of the OPA is against the patient's lips. If the device is too long, it will keep slipping out of the mouth and the flange will not rest on the lips. If it is too short, the patient's mouth may remain slightly open in an awkward position.
8. Ventilate the patient with the most appropriate technique.
9. Continue to closely monitor the patient's airway. If the patient becomes responsive, they may attempt to remove, displace, or cough up the device. You must be ready to assist or remove it for them.

An alternative method for inserting an OPA is to insert it sideways into the mouth until it is approximately halfway in. Then simply rotate it 90 degrees. Just as with the first method, make certain the tip of the airway is positioned at the base of the tongue. This method is less likely to cause trauma to the roof of the patient's mouth during insertion. As with all other skills, follow both your instructor's preference and local protocols.

Infants and Children The OPA is inserted in a specific way in infants and children because their mouth is smaller than that of an adult and the upper portion of the oral cavity is more easily injured. Rotating the airway can damage the soft palate or the uvula. To minimize injury to the roof of the mouth while inserting an OPA, the following method is recommended:

1. Use a tongue blade to gently place downward pressure on the tongue.
2. Insert the OPA with the tip pointing toward the tongue and throat, in the same position it will be in after insertion, rather than upside down.

Nasopharyngeal Airway

LO18 Explain the indications and contraindications for the insertion of a nasopharyngeal airway.

The nasopharyngeal airway (NPA) is a soft, flexible tube that is inserted into the nose to create a clear and open path for air. It is the preferred choice when the patient is not totally unresponsive or has a gag reflex.

REMEMBER

Proper measurement of an airway adjunct prior to insertion will help ensure that it performs as expected. An OPA or NPA that is too long or too short may obstruct the airway rather than help keep it open.

REMEMBER

An OPA or NPA should be used whenever you provide manual ventilations. When choosing which to use, you can safely assume that a patient who is totally unresponsive and not breathing will tolerate insertion of an OPA. The patient who is only somewhat unresponsive will more than likely have a gag reflex, which will prohibit the insertion of an OPA. In this case, the best choice may be an NPA.

REMEMBER

It is best to ensure that the flange of the OPA rests outside of the patient's lips instead of against the teeth. If you lose sight of the flange, the airway may have fallen back into the throat, becoming an airway obstruction.

Inserting an Oropharyngeal Airway

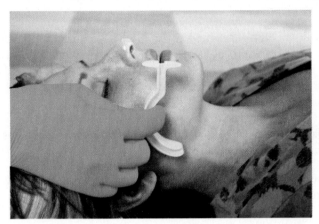

1. Properly measure the oropharyngeal airway (OPA) prior to insertion.

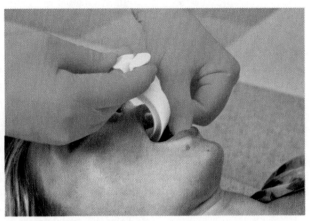

2. Insert the OPA with the tip pointing to the roof of the patient's mouth. When halfway in, rotate 180 degrees.

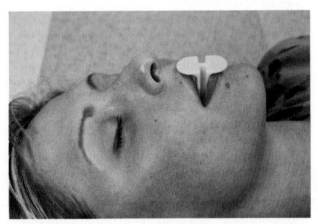

3. The flange should rest on the outside of the lips and never any farther than the teeth.

Alternative Insertion Methods

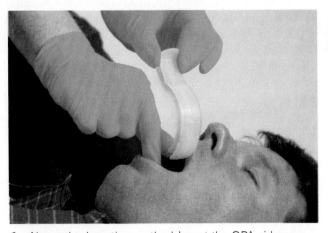

1. *Alternative insertion method*: Insert the OPA sideways and rotate 90 degrees.

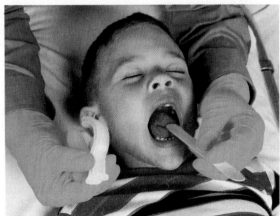

2. *Alternative insertion method*: Insert the OPA into a child's mouth using a tongue depressor.

Warning: Never practice the use of airways on anyone. Manikins should be used for developing airway skills.

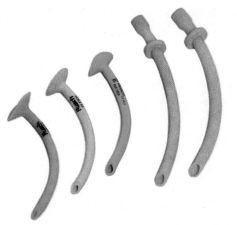

Figure 9.16 Various types and sizes of nasopharyngeal airways (NPAs).

An NPA is easy to insert because you do not have to reposition the patient's head or pry open the mouth. If there is any injury to the mouth, teeth, or oral cavity, the NPA will still provide an open airway for the patient.

Measuring the Nasopharyngeal Airway There are numerous sizes of NPAs designed to fit infants, children, and adults (Figure 9.16). To use an NPA effectively, you must select the correct size for the patient. The most widely used method for determining the correct size is to measure from the tip of the patient's nose to the tip of the earlobe.

If the device is not the correct size, do not use it on the patient. Instead, select another one and remeasure to ensure the correct size before inserting.

Inserting the Nasopharyngeal Airway Perform the following steps to insert an NPA (Key Skill 9.4):

1. Take the appropriate BSI precautions.
2. Select the appropriate-sized device by measuring from the tip of the patient's nose to the tip of the earlobe.
3. Use a water-based lubricant on the outside of the tube before you insert it.
4. Keep the patient's head in a neutral position while you gently push the tip of the nose upward. Insert the device straight back through the nostril. If the device has a beveled (angled) end, that end should point toward the septum (the midline of the nose). Gently advance the device until the flange rests firmly against the patient's nostril. Never force the device. If it will not advance into the nostril easily, remove it and try it in the other nostril. If the device will not advance into the other nostril, make another attempt with an NPA that is slightly smaller in diameter.

Note that it was once thought the presence of facial trauma was a contraindication for the placement of a nasopharyngeal airway. That is no longer the case. The benefits of a clear airway outweigh the risk that the NPA could accidentally enter the cranial space through a fracture site.

Bag-Mask Ventilation

LO19 Describe the proper use of the bag-mask device for a nonbreathing patient.

The bag-mask device is one of the most commonly used devices for ventilating a nonbreathing patient. Some EMS systems also use the bag-mask device to ventilate patients with inadequate respirations (such as with a drug overdose). It also acts as an effective infection-control barrier between you and your patient. The bag-mask device is available in sizes for infants, children, and adults.

The bag-mask device delivers room air (21 percent oxygen) to the patient when it is squeezed through the device to the patient's lungs. (In contrast, a pocket face mask will deliver up to 16 percent oxygen from your exhaled air.) The bag-mask device can be connected to an oxygen supply source to enrich room air and deliver a concentration of up to 100 percent oxygen.

There are many brands of bag-mask devices available, but all have the same basic parts: a self-refilling bag, one-way valve, and face mask. All bag-mask devices have a standard fitting that makes them compatible with most respiratory equipment and face masks. Most bag-mask devices used in the field today are disposable and intended for single use on one patient (Figure 9.17).

The principle behind the operation of the bag-mask device is simple. When you squeeze the bag, air is delivered to the patient through a one-way valve. When you release the bag, fresh air enters the bag from the rear while the exhaled air from the patient flows out near the mask. The exhaled air does not go back into the bag.

REMEMBER

OPAs and NPAs are only adjuncts, tools to help ensure an open airway. It does not maintain an open airway all by itself. You must still carefully monitor your patient's airway and manually maintain the appropriate head position at all times.

REMEMBER

If you meet resistance while inserting the NPA, attempt insertion in the other nostril.

REMEMBER

Most NPAs are made with the bevel facing to the left. Therefore, they are meant to fit into the right nostril. Before inserting the NPA into the left nostril, use a pair of scissors to carefully snip the end of the airway to change the bevel from the left to the right. Then lubricate and insert. It is not recommended to insert an NPA against its natural curvature because it is likely to rotate on its own after being inserted.

Inserting a Nasopharyngeal Airway

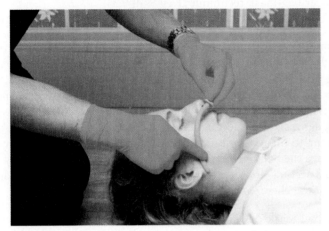

1. Select the appropriate-sized nasopharyngeal airway (NPA).

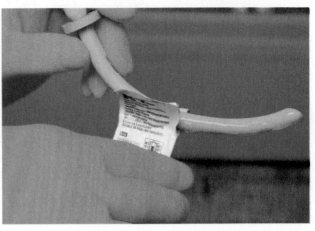

2. Apply a water-based lubricant before insertion.

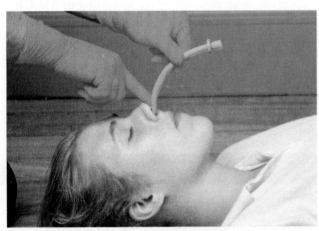

3. Gently insert the NPA, advancing it until the flange rests against the nostril.

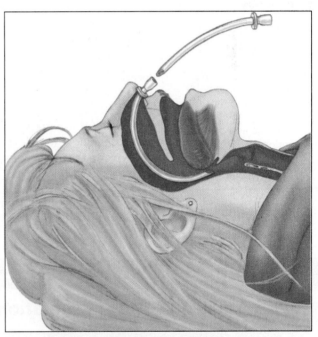

4. Illustration of a properly inserted NPA.

There are times when the bag-mask device will not deliver air to the patient's lungs. Sometimes the problem occurs because the patient has an airway obstruction that must be cleared. More often, the problem is caused by an improper seal between the patient's face and the mask. If this occurs, you should reposition your fingers and check placement of the mask.

Two-Rescuer Bag-Mask Ventilation

For the best possible results, the bag-mask device should be used with two rescuers.[7] Prior to using the bag-mask device, insert an appropriate airway adjunct. One rescuer must use two hands to maintain a good mask seal while the second rescuer squeezes the bag. Note that for trauma patients who must have their airway opened by the jaw-thrust

> **REMEMBER**
>
> It is commonly recommended that an OPA or NPA should be inserted before attempting to ventilate the patient with a bag-mask device.

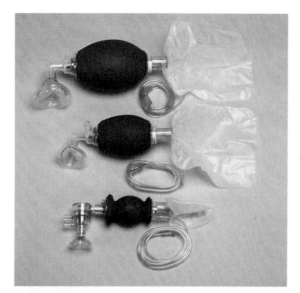

Figure 9.17 Bag-mask devices are available in several sizes.

maneuver, the two-rescuer method is more effective. The rescuer holding the mask in place can more easily perform the jaw-thrust while the other rescuer provides effective ventilations.

Perform the following steps to provide ventilations using the two-rescuer bag-mask technique (Key Skill 9.5):

1. Take the appropriate BSI precautions.
2. Ensure an open airway and position yourself at the patient's head. Clear the airway if necessary.
3. Insert an appropriate airway adjunct.
4. Rescuer 1 should kneel at the top of the patient's head, holding the mask firmly in place with both hands.
5. Rescuer 2 should kneel beside the patient's head and connect the bag to the mask (if not already done). They should then squeeze the bag once every 6 seconds for an adult (once every 2 to 3 seconds for a child or infant). Ensure adequate rise and fall of the chest each time the bag is squeezed.

The bag-mask device also can be used effectively during two-rescuer CPR. The first rescuer maintains both hands on the mask, ensuring a good mask seal. The second rescuer can squeeze the bag to provide two back-to-back ventilations following each cycle of compressions.

One-Rescuer Bag-Mask Ventilation

For a single rescuer working alone, the bag-mask device can be difficult and challenging to operate. The bag-mask device is not the recommended method for a single rescuer.[8] This is especially true if you have small hands or do not use a bag-mask device on a regular basis. The most difficult part is maintaining an adequate mask seal with one hand. If you are assigned a bag-mask device for use in the field, practice using it in the classroom until your technique is well developed.

Perform the following steps to ventilate a patient using the bag-mask device as a single rescuer (Key Skill 9.6):

1. Take the appropriate BSI precautions.
2. Ensure an open airway and position yourself at the patient's head. Clear the airway if necessary.

KEY SKILL 9.5

Two-Rescuer Bag-Mask Ventilation

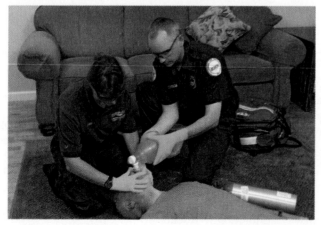

1. Proper technique for using the bag-mask device with two rescuers.

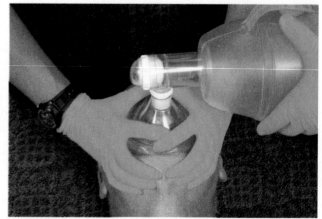

2. Proper hand position for bag-mask ventilation with two rescuers.

One-Rescuer Bag-Mask Ventilation

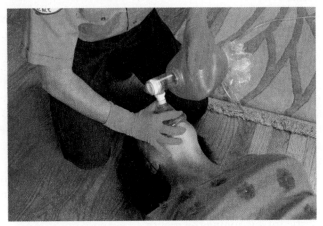

1. Suggested technique for using the bag-mask device with one rescuer.

Alternative Method

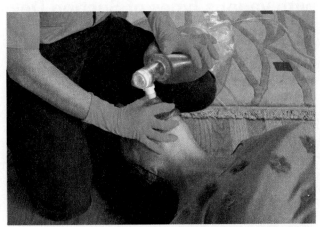

1. *Alternative method*: Press the bag against your leg with the palm of your hand.

3. Insert an appropriate airway adjunct.

4. Use the correct mask size for the patient. Place the apex (top) of the triangular mask over the bridge of the nose. Rest the base of the mask between the patient's lower lip and the projection of the chin.

5. With one hand, hold the mask firmly in position.

6. With your other hand, squeeze the bag at the appropriate rate, delivering each breath over approximately 1 second. Observe for adequate rise and fall of the patient's chest.

> **REMEMBER**
>
> In some instances, as a single rescuer, it may be more effective to provide assisted ventilations using the mouth-to-mask technique than to attempt to use a bag-mask device by yourself.

CREW RESOURCE MANAGEMENT

Bag-mask ventilation is best performed by two rescuers. One rescuer focuses on maintaining an open airway while the other focuses on providing good ventilations. Both rescuers should pay attention to chest rise with each ventilation and make adjustments as necessary if the patient vomits or ventilations become difficult.

Suction Devices

LO20 Explain the indications for oral and nasal suctioning.

LO21 Differentiate between manual, electric, and oxygen-powered suction devices.

It is quite common for an ill or injured patient to experience nausea in response to their condition. Sometimes, this nausea can lead to vomiting, putting the airway at risk for obstruction. Other times, trauma to the head, face, or mouth can lead to bleeding inside the nose, mouth, and airway

One of the simplest methods for clearing blood, mucus, and other body fluids from a patient's airway is to position the patient on their side (recovery position) and use finger sweeps appropriately. In addition to this manual method, the use of a mechanical suction device can be very helpful in clearing fluids. There are several types of portable suction devices available, including manually powered, oxygen- or air-powered, and electrically powered units (Key Skill 9.7).

All types of suction units must have specialized, noncollapsible tubing, a collection container, and an appropriate suction tip or catheter for inserting into the patient's mouth or nose. Catheters are available as a soft, flexible tube for suctioning the nose and as rigid plastic for suctioning the mouth.

KEY SKILL 9.7

Become Familiar with Various Types of Suction Devices

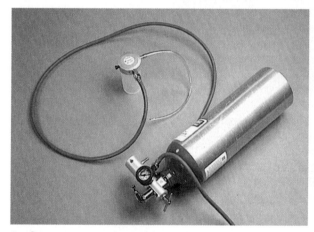

1. Oxygen-powered portable suction unit.

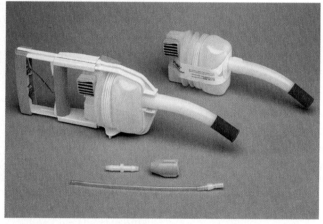

2. Manually operated suction device (V-VAC).

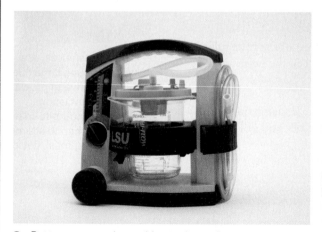

3. Battery-powered portable suction unit.

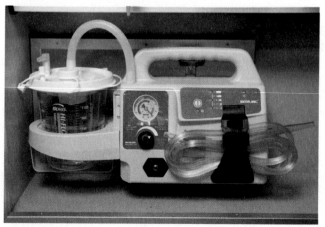

4. Suction unit installed in an ambulance patient compartment.

General Guidelines for Suctioning

Follow these guidelines when using any type of suctioning device:

- Always use appropriate BSI precautions, including a mouth and eye shield. The potential for being sprayed with body fluids such as vomit, blood, and saliva is high.
- Measure the suction catheter prior to insertion.
- Activate the suction unit only after it is completely inserted and as you withdraw the catheter.
- If there is a copious amount of fluid in the patient's airway, it may be helpful to roll them onto their side first and then suction. You may need to suction, ventilate, and suction again in a continuous sequence as long as necessary.
- Keep your suctioning time to a minimum. Remember that while you are suctioning, you are not ventilating. One suggested guideline is to suction for no more than 15 seconds for adults, 10 seconds for children, and 5 seconds for infants.
- Twist and turn the tip of the catheter as you remove it to minimize the chance it will become stuck on the soft tissue lining the mouth and nose.
- When suctioning the mouth, concentrate on the back corners of the mouth, where most fluids tend to accumulate. Do not place the tip directly over the back of the tongue because this will likely stimulate the gag reflex.

Measuring a Suction Catheter

It is important to measure the suction catheter prior to insertion.

Oral Suctioning   Two methods are commonly used to measure the appropriate length of insertion for oral suctioning. The first is to measure the catheter just as you would an OPA, from the corner of the mouth to the earlobe. The second method is to insert the catheter only as far as you can see. This method is easier said than done and is more practical when the patient is lying supine. It becomes much more difficult to maintain visualization of the tip of the catheter when the patient is on their side.

Nasal Suctioning   Soft suction catheters are always much longer than necessary for the typical shallow suctioning required. For this reason, it is essential that you measure the depth of insertion prior to suctioning. The most common method for determining the appropriate length of a soft catheter prior to nasal suctioning is to measure from the tip of the patient's nose to the earlobe.

Suctioning Techniques

There are many variations in the techniques used to suction the mouth, nose, or stoma. You must follow your local protocols. In general, you will follow these steps (Key Skill 9.8):

1. Before suctioning any patient, be sure to take the appropriate BSI precautions.
2. Attach the catheter and activate the unit to ensure that there is suction.
3. Position yourself at the patient's head. If possible, turn the patient onto their side. Follow guidelines for protection of the spine.
4. Measure the catheter prior to insertion.
5. Open the patient's mouth and clear obvious matter and fluid from the oral cavity by letting the mouth drain or by using finger sweeps with a gloved hand.
6. Insert the tip of the catheter to the appropriate depth.
7. Activate the suction only when the tip or catheter is fully inserted. Twist and turn it from side to side and sweep the mouth. This twisting action prevents the end of the catheter from grabbing the soft tissue inside the mouth.
8. Remain alert for signs of a gag reflex and/or vomiting.

Suctioning

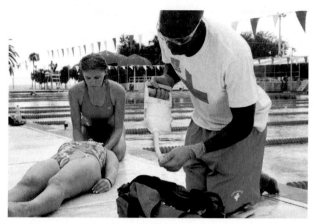

1. Check the function of the suction unit prior to using.

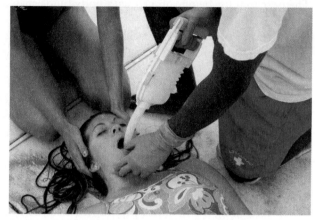

2. For oral suction, insert the tip of the device only as far as you can see. Then initiate suction.

FIRST ON SCENE WRAP-UP

A few minutes later, just as Camille is beginning to blink her eyes and look around, a team of firefighters appears in the backyard followed closely by an ambulance crew. The ambulance crew performs a primary assessment and begins oxygen therapy while the firefighters help secure the girl to a long spine board, move her to the wheeled stretcher, and get her into the ambulance.

"She has good sensation and motor function in her extremities," one of the EMTs says to Lindsey. "I think she probably just got a good bump on the head. It could have been a lot worse."

"Tell me about it," Lindsey says and waves reassuringly at Frank and Kayla as they get into their car to follow the ambulance.

Summary

- Being able to breathe adequately is essential to life. Conditions such as asthma and bronchitis and events such as drowning and choking can disrupt this essential process and cause respiratory compromise.
- A patent airway is one that is clear and open and allows for the effortless flow of air in and out of the lungs. The air that we breathe contains approximately 21 percent oxygen.
- Clinical death occurs when both breathing and heartbeats stop. Biological death occurs approximately 4 to 6 minutes following clinical death.
- When something disrupts the normal breathing process, breathing becomes inadequate and the patient is at risk of becoming hypoxic. Signs of inadequate breathing include increased work of breathing and shallow, rapid, noisy, or gasping breathing.
- To assist a patient who is not breathing adequately or at all, you must provide rescue breaths using an appropriate barrier device. Using a firm seal with the mask, you will breathe once every 6 seconds for adults and once every 2 to 3 seconds for children and infants.
- There are many causes of airway obstruction. Some of the most common are the patient's tongue, blood, or saliva (anatomical obstructions), and foreign objects such as food or small objects (mechanical obstructions).
- A responsive patient with a complete obstruction is unable to breathe, cough, or speak and will usually look panicked.

- You must provide abdominal and/or chest thrusts to remove the obstruction.
- The preferred method for opening the airway of an unresponsive patient who is uninjured is the head-tilt/chin-lift maneuver. The preferred method for an unresponsive patient with a suspected neck or spine injury is the jaw-thrust maneuver.
- If you are working with a patient with a suspected neck or spine injury and you are unable to open the airway using the jaw-thrust, you must attempt the head-tilt/chin-lift maneuver.
- Unresponsive patients with no gag reflex should receive an airway adjunct. The OPA helps keep the tongue from falling to the back of the throat and thus blocking the airway.
- For patients with a gag reflex or those who are somewhat responsive, the NPA may be the best choice as an airway adjunct.
- When a patient is not breathing adequately or at all, you must provide positive pressure ventilations or rescue breaths.
- The best sign that you are providing adequate rescue breaths is good chest rise and fall with each breath.
- To minimize the flow of air into the stomach during rescue breaths, you should provide slow, even breaths that do not overinflate the chest.
- If the patient's airway becomes obstructed with fluid such as saliva, blood, or vomit, it will be necessary to suction the mouth and/or nose to remove this fluid and clear the airway.

Take Action

Opening the Airway

You will have the opportunity to practice opening the airway of a manikin as well as practice giving rescue breaths using a barrier device. It is important to realize that practicing those skills on a manikin is often very different than on a real person. For this exercise, practice two specific skills using a real person.

The two skills are the head-tilt/chin-lift and the jaw-thrust maneuvers. First, you must locate a suitable person to serve as your patient. This is best if it is someone you know well, perhaps even a family member. Begin by clearly explaining the steps to your volunteer, and then ask the person to lie down on the floor, flat on their back. Kneeling at the side of the person's head, practice the head-tilt/chin lift by placing one hand on the forehead and two fingers of the other hand on the bony part of the chin. Now gently tilt the head as far back as it will comfortably go. Remind your patient to just relax and allow you to do the work. The first thing you will notice is that a real patient's head is significantly heavier than that of the manikin. It is good to get this experience before you are in an emergency situation.

Next, kneel at the top of the patient's head and practice the jaw-thrust maneuver. Remind your patient to relax and let you do the work. Begin by placing your thumbs directly on the cheekbones of your patient. Next, grasp the corners of the jaw with the index and middle finger of each hand. Using your thumbs as counter pressure, pull forward on the corners of the jaw and move the lower jaw upward, creating an exaggerated underbite. By lifting the jaw up, you will bring the tongue with it and keep the tongue from blocking the back of the throat.

First on Scene Patient Handoff

We have a 9-year-old female named Camille who fell approximately 8 feet from the top of a slide onto concrete. Witnesses state that she landed face down, was unresponsive, and did not appear to be breathing immediately after the fall. Bystanders rolled the patient face up and she immediately began breathing spontaneously. The patient had a strong and regular pulse the whole time and became responsive just prior to the arrival of EMS. Her parents state that she has no prior medical history.

First on Scene Run Review

Recall the events of the First on Scene scenario in this chapter and answer the following questions related to the call. Rationales are offered in the Answer Key at the back of the book.

1. Did Kayla make the right decision to roll Camille onto her back? What are some reasons you would want to roll someone quickly?
2. What was likely causing the obstruction of Camille's airway?
3. What is your priority when a patient has an obstructed airway as well as a possible neck injury? How do you manage both?

Quick Quiz

To check your understanding of the chapter, answer the following questions. Then compare your answers to those in the Answer Key at the back of the book.

1. Rescue breathing is:
   a. any effort to restart a normal heart rhythm.
   b. the application of manual ventilations.
   c. the use of oxygen to assist breathing.
   d. the ability to restore normal heart rhythm and breathing.

2. When performing the head-tilt/chin-lift maneuver on an adult, tilt the head:
   a. as far back as possible.
   b. into the sniffing position.
   c. to get the tongue to close the epiglottis.
   d. so that the upper and lower teeth are touching.

3. The recommended method for opening the airway of a patient with a possible neck or spine injury is the ____ maneuver.
   a. jaw-thrust
   b. mouth-to-nose
   c. abdominal-thrust
   d. head-tilt/chin-lift

4. Clinical death occurs when the patient's:
   a. brain cells begin to die.
   b. breathing has stopped for 4 minutes.
   c. pulse has been absent for 5 minutes.
   d. heartbeat and breathing have stopped.

5. A pocket face mask allows the rescuer to provide ventilations while minimizing:
   a. having to hold the mask firmly in place.
   b. delivering their own breaths to the patient.
   c. direct contact with the patient's mouth and nose.
   d. worrying about keeping the head and spine in-line.

6. During rescue breathing, you should check for the effectiveness of ventilations by:
   a. looking for chest rise and fall.
   b. listening for airflow from the mouth and nose.
   c. observing skin color, such as paleness or cyanosis.
   d. looking for chest rise and fall, listening for airflow, and observing skin color.

7. If an infant becomes unresponsive before you can clear an airway obstruction, you should first:
   a. place the infant face down and lift their chest with your hands.
   b. place them on a firm surface and begin chest compressions.
   c. hold them face up and deliver chest thrusts.
   d. turn them face down and deliver back slaps.

8. Which of the following is an indication for suctioning the upper airway?
   a. Snoring sounds during breathing
   b. Complete foreign body airway obstruction
   c. Gurgling sounds during breathing
   d. An unconscious patient

9. Which of the following improves ventilations delivered by way of a bag-mask device?
   a. Inserting an oropharyngeal airway
   b. Applying suction for 4 to 6 minutes
   c. Alternating chest thrusts and squeezing the bag
   d. Combining finger sweeps with a mouth-to-mouth technique

10. Which one of the following is recommended for clearing an airway obstruction in a conscious 10-month-old baby?
    a. Abdominal thrusts and chest thrusts
    b. Chest thrusts and back blows
    c. Back slaps and finger sweeps
    d. Abdominal thrusts and finger sweeps

11. The primary muscle of respiration is the:
   a. trachea.
   b. esophagus.
   c. diaphragm.
   d. pharynx.

12. The ____ prevents food and other material from entering the trachea.
   a. tongue
   b. alveoli
   c. pharynx
   d. epiglottis

13. Deep within the lungs, the ____ are the tiny balloon-like structures where gas exchange takes place.
   a. alveoli
   b. bronchioles
   c. trachea
   d. epiglottis

14. All of the following are signs of difficulty breathing EXCEPT:
   a. poor chest rise.
   b. pale or bluish skin color.
   c. use of accessory muscles.
   d. good chest rise and fall.

15. When caring for an unresponsive patient, tilting their head back improves the airway by:
   a. lifting their tongue from the back of the throat.
   b. shifting the epiglottis from front to back.
   c. allowing fluids to flow more easily.
   d. opening their mouth.

16. Which of the following is an example of a mechanical airway obstruction?
   a. Tongue
   b. Swollen trachea
   c. Foreign object
   d. Enlarged epiglottis

17. Noisy breathing is a sign of ____ airway obstruction.
   a. bilateral
   b. complete
   c. adequate
   d. partial

18. You have just made two attempts to ventilate an unresponsive child with an airway obstruction. Your next step is to:
   a. begin chest compressions.
   b. continue to ventilate.
   c. perform five chest thrusts.
   d. provide back slaps.

Endnotes

1. Rodríguez-Molinero, A., Narvaiza, L., Ruiz, J., & Gálvez-Barrón, C., "Normal Respiratory Rate and Peripheral Blood Oxygen Saturation in the Elderly Population," *J Am Geriatr Soc*, Vol. 61 (2013): 2238–2240. https://doi.org/10.1111/jgs.12580
2. Fleming, S., Thompson, M., Stevens, R., Heneghan, C., Plüddemann, A., Maconochie, I., Tarassenko, L., & Mant, D, "Normal Ranges of Heart Rate and Respiratory Rate in Children from Birth to 18 Years of Age: A Systematic Review of Observational Studies," *Lancet*, Vol. 377, No. 9770 (March 19, 2011): 1011–1018. doi: 10.1016/S0140-6736(10)62226-X. PMID: 21411136; PMCID: PMC3789232.
3. Ibid.
4. Panchal, A.R., Bartos, J.A., Cabañas, J.G., Donnino, M.W., Drennan, I.R., Hirsch, K.G., Kudenchuk, P.J., Kurz, M.C., Lavonas, E.J., Morley, P.T., O'Neil, B.J., Peberdy, M.A., Rittenberger, J.C., Rodriguez, A.J., Sawyer, K.N., & Berg, K.M., "Adult Basic and Advanced Life Support Writing Group. Part 3: Adult Basic and Advanced Life Support: 2020 American Heart Association Guidelines for Cardiopulmonary Resuscitation and Emergency Cardiovascular Care," *Circulation*, Vol. 142, No. 16_suppl_2 (October 20, 2020): S366–S468. doi: 10.1161/CIR.0000000000000916. Epub 2020 Oct 21. PMID: 33081529.
5. Ibid.
6. Ibid, S696.
7. Berg, R.A., Hemphill, R., Abella, B.S., Aufderheide, T.P., Cave, D.M., Hazinski, M.F., Lerner, E.B., Rea, T.D., Sayre, M.R., & Swor, R.A., "Part 5: Adult basic life support: 2010 American Heart Association Guidelines for Cardiopulmonary Resuscitation and Emergency Cardiovascular Care." *Circulation*, 2010; 122(suppl 3): S685–S705.
8. Ibid.

10

Principles of Oxygen Therapy

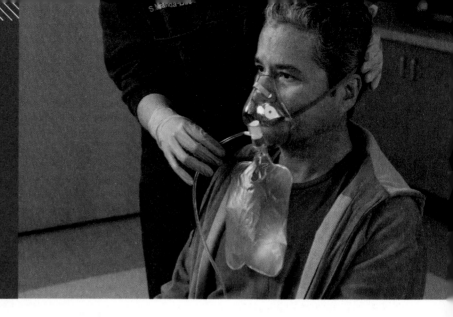

Education Standards

Airway Management—
Airway Management,
Respiration, and
Ventilation

Competencies

Applies knowledge of
anatomy and physiology
to ensure a patent
airway, adequate
mechanical ventilation,
and respiration

LEARNING OBJECTIVES

Upon successful completion of this chapter, the student should be able to:

Cognitive

1. Define the chapter key terms.
2. Explain the benefits of supplemental oxygen.
3. Explain the indications for supplemental oxygen.
4. Differentiate among common sizes of oxygen cylinders used in EMS.
5. Describe the potential hazards of working with high-pressure cylinders.
6. Explain the safe practices when working with high-pressure cylinders.
7. Describe the purpose and functions of an oxygen regulator.
8. Explain the indications for the use of a nasal cannula.
9. Explain the indications for the use of a nonrebreather mask.

Psychomotor

10. Demonstrate the proper use of a nonrebreather mask.
11. Demonstrate the proper use of a nasal cannula.
12. Demonstrate the ability to add supplemental oxygen to a pocket mask and/or bag-mask device.
13. Demonstrate the proper technique for attaching a regulator to a cylinder.
14. Demonstrate the ability to identify and troubleshoot a leaky oxygen cylinder/regulator.

Affective

15. Recognize the value that supplemental oxygen might offer for most ill and injured patients.

KEY TERMS

humidifier (*p. 184*)
hydrostatic test (*p. 187*)
liter flow (*p. 187*)
nasal cannula (*p. 188*)
nonrebreather mask (*p. 189*)
O-ring (*p. 186*)
oxygen concentration (*p. 184*)

oxygen saturation (*p. 184*)
oxygen supply tubing (*p. 191*)
pin index safety system (*p. 187*)
pressure gauge (*p. 184*)
pressure regulator (*p. 184*)
reservoir bag (*p. 189*)
supplemental oxygen (*p. 183*)

As you have already learned, a constant supply of oxygen to the body's cells is essential to keeping all body systems functioning properly. When an individual becomes ill or injured, the normal flow of oxygen into and throughout the body can become disrupted. In these instances, providing supplemental oxygen can help overcome this deficiency.

This chapter offers an overview of the proper equipment and techniques necessary to provide your patients with supplemental oxygen. It is important to point out that the U.S. Food and Drug Administration (FDA) considers supplemental oxygen a drug that requires a prescription from a health care provider. Not all EMS systems authorize Emergency Medical Responders to administer oxygen. Your instructor will inform you as to the protocols for oxygen administration in your area.

 FIRST ON SCENE

"Emergency Medical Responders," Bryn calls out as she makes her way through the open doorway of an aging townhome. "Someone called us for help?"

"In here!" responds a young woman from down the hallway.

Bryn and Thien bring their equipment into the kitchen, where a young woman is kneeling next to an older woman hunched over in her wheelchair.

"She's having trouble breathing! I've never seen Grandma this bad before. Mom's gonna kill me if something happens to Grandma. Please help us."

"What's her name?" Bryn asks as she reaches for her oxygen equipment. The rescuers notice the discolored and dirty cannula on the woman's face and the oxygen canister on the floor beside the wheelchair. The woman is clearly in distress. She is gasping for air, and her eyes look unfocused. She is clearly scared.

"It's Joanne Smith," the young girl answers. "Her name is Mrs. Joanne Smith. My name is Grace. Please, can you help her?"

Importance of Oxygen

LO2 Explain the benefits of supplemental oxygen.

LO3 Explain the indications of supplemental oxygen.

The air in our environment (room air) contains approximately 21 percent oxygen and 79 percent nitrogen. This concentration of oxygen is more than adequate when all body systems are working properly. When a patient becomes suddenly ill or injured, the demand for oxygen can increase.

A patient may need **supplemental oxygen** for many reasons, including breathing or heart problems, stroke, major blood loss, and shock, just to name a few. The most common signs that a patient may be in need of supplemental oxygen are:

supplemental oxygen ▶ supply of 100 percent oxygen for use with ill or injured patients.

- *Altered mental status.* The brain is one of the first organs to suffer when there is not enough oxygen. Changes in mental status such as anxiety, restlessness, drowsiness, confusion, and unresponsiveness are all indications of a serious underlying problem.
- *Abnormal vital signs.* Changes to what would otherwise be normal vital signs such as low blood pressure, rapid pulse, rapid breathing, and poor skin signs (pale, cool, moist) may indicate a lack of sufficient oxygen.

- *Significant mechanism of injury (MOI).* Any individual who has had a significant injury, regardless of an open wound or not, may have sustained damage to the circulatory system resulting in a disruption in normal blood flow to the vital organs.
- *Increased level of distress.* Patients may appear to be in significant distress, as indicated by difficulty breathing or significant pain.

Many ill or injured patients may benefit from supplemental oxygen. Supplemental oxygen is a source of 100 percent oxygen. It is typically stored in metal or composite cylinders produced in a variety of shapes and sizes. **Oxygen concentration** refers to the percentage of oxygen being delivered to the patient. Supplemental oxygen usually mixes with room air, which is 21 percent oxygen. So the actual oxygen concentration available to the patient will be somewhere between 21 and 100 percent depending on the delivery device used.

The air we exhale contains approximately 16 percent oxygen. Providing rescue breaths without supplemental oxygen provides the patient with only the minimum oxygen concentration required for short-term survival. By providing supplemental oxygen, you will be able to greatly increase the oxygen concentration delivered to your patient.

While many patients benefit from supplemental oxygen, too much oxygen may be harmful to some patients. Be sure to consult with your instructor and local protocols to confirm the standard of care for providing oxygen in your EMS system, area, or region.

Oxygen saturation is a measurement of how much oxygen is in the blood. For most healthy adults, normal oxygen saturation levels are between 95 and 100 percent. Current American Heart Association guidelines recommend that oxygen delivery be monitored and adjusted to obtain an oxygen saturation of greater than 94 percent.[1] The ability to monitor a patient's oxygen saturation is accomplished using a device called a pulse oximeter. Your agency or unit may not carry this device. For more information on pulse oximeters and what they do, see Appendix 1.

Oxygen Therapy Equipment

A typical oxygen delivery system includes an oxygen source (oxygen cylinder), a **pressure regulator** (also called an oxygen regulator), and a delivery device (Figure 10.1). Occasionally, a **humidifier** will be added to provide moisture to the oxygen if the patient will be receiving supplemental oxygen for an extended period of time.

Oxygen Cylinders

LO4 Differentiate among common sizes of oxygen cylinders used in EMS.

When providing oxygen in the field, the standard source of oxygen is a seamless steel or aluminum cylinder filled with pressurized oxygen. The maximum service pressure is equal to approximately 2,000 pounds per square inch (psi). Cylinders come in various sizes, each identified by a specific letter. The sizes commonly used by Emergency Medical Responders include (Figure 10.2):

- Jumbo D (contains about 640 L of oxygen)
- Standard D (contains about 425 L of oxygen)
- E (contains about 680 L of oxygen)

Part of your duty as an Emergency Medical Responder is to make certain that the oxygen cylinders are full and ready to use before they are needed for patient care. In most cases, you will use a **pressure gauge** to determine the pressure remaining in the tank. The pressure gauge is located on the pressure regulator and displays the actual pressure inside the tank. A cylinder is considered full at 2,000 psi, half full at 1,000 psi, and one-quarter full at 500 psi.

The length of time that you can use an oxygen cylinder depends on the pressure in the cylinder and the flow rate being delivered to the patient. Each size of cylinder has a

---

oxygen concentration ▶ percentage of oxygen being delivered to a patient.

oxygen saturation ▶ measurement of how much oxygen is in a patient's blood.

REMEMBER

Oxygen is considered a medication and must be prescribed by a health care provider. All EMS systems and agencies have a provider responsible for medical oversight who authorizes the use of oxygen by personnel within their system.

pressure regulator ▶ device used to lower the delivery pressure of oxygen from a cylinder; also called an *oxygen regulator.*

humidifier ▶ device used to increase the moisture content of supplemental oxygen.

pressure gauge ▶ device on a pressure regulator that displays the pressure inside an oxygen cylinder.

SCENE SAFETY

Oxygen is stored under very high pressure. When not in use, place the oxygen cylinder on its side to prevent it from falling over and becoming damaged.

REMEMBER

You cannot tell if an oxygen cylinder is full, partially full, or empty by lifting or moving it. You must always check the pressure in the cylinder by using the pressure gauge.

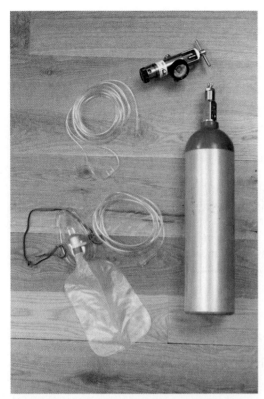

Figure 10.1 A typical oxygen delivery system consists of an oxygen cylinder, pressure regulator, mask, and cannula.

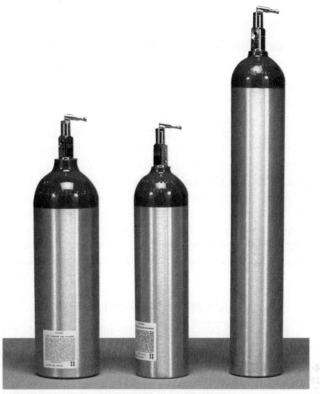

Figure 10.2 Commonly used sizes of portable oxygen cylinders. Left to right: Jumbo D, Standard D, and E.
(Michael Gallitelli/Pearson Education, Inc.)

predefined conversion factor that is used to help determine the duration of oxygen for a given situation (Table 10.1).

The method of calculating cylinder duration is called the duration of flow formula:

$$\frac{\text{Tank Pressure} \times \text{Conversion Factor}}{\text{Liters per Minute (LPM)}}$$

Example: To determine the duration of oxygen of a D cylinder with a pressure of 2,000 psi and a flow rate of 10 LPM.

$$\frac{2000 \text{ psi} \times 0.16}{10 \text{ LPM}} = \frac{320}{10} = 32 \text{ minutes}$$

Most EMS agencies keep a supply of full oxygen cylinders on hand. When a cylinder gets below a predetermined pressure, it should be replaced with a full tank or refilled depending on the procedure used by your system or agency. Many agencies consider 500 psi to be the minimum service pressure for an oxygen cylinder. Oxygen cylinders should never be allowed to go completely empty. If they do, moisture can accumulate inside the tank and cause oxidation or rust to develop. For this reason, never allow the pressure in an oxygen cylinder to fall below 200 psi.

TABLE 10.1	Oxygen Cylinder Conversion Factors
Cylinder Size	**Conversion Factor**
D	0.16
E	0.28
M	1.56
H	3.14

"It looks like her tank is empty," says Thien. "I'm going to transfer her to our tank and switch to a nonrebreather if that's good with you."

"Sounds like a plan. You do that while I try to get a respiratory rate," says Bryn.

Mrs. Smith's breathing is very labored. They can hear wheezing without a stethoscope. Her skin is cool and very pale. She is sitting in the tripod position, unable to speak but a few words at a time.

"Grace," Bryn says as she jots down Mrs. Smith's respiratory rate. "You said your grandma is on oxygen all the time, but when

we got here, her tank was empty. Do you have any idea how long she has been going without oxygen?"

"No," Grace admits sheepishly. "My brother and I have been helping take care of her since we had to cut down on the caretaker's hours. I don't even know how to turn on the oxygen or who to call to order it."

"Okay, Mrs. Smith," Thien says to the patient, as the reassuring hiss of oxygen fills the reservoir bag of the nonrebreather mask. "Just breathe as normally as you can. The oxygen is going to help you breathe easier. You're going to be fine. We have an ambulance on the way."

Oxygen System Safety

LO5 Describe the potential hazards of working with high-pressure cylinders.

LO6 Explain the safe practices when working with high-pressure cylinders.

Working with oxygen therapy equipment requires an awareness of its hazards, proficiency with proper techniques, and following protocols that ensure safety for patients and Emergency Medical Responders.

Hazards of Oxygen Cylinders   Certain hazards are associated with oxygen administration:

- Oxygen used in emergency care is stored under pressure (2,000 psi or greater). If the tank is punctured or if a valve breaks off, the supply tank and the valve can become projectiles, injuring anyone nearby.
- Oxygen supports combustion and causes fire to burn more rapidly.
- Oxygen and oil do not mix. When they come into contact with one another, there can be a severe reaction, which may cause an explosion.

Safe Practices for Oxygen Administration   While all oxygen systems are designed with safety in mind, there are tips to remember when working with them. Following are some general guidelines to keep in mind when working with high-pressure cylinders:

- Never allow smoking around oxygen equipment.
- Never use oxygen equipment around open flames or sparks.
- Never use grease or oil on devices that will be attached to an oxygen cylinder. Do not handle those devices when your hands are greasy.
- Never put tape on the cylinder outlet or use tape to mark or label any oxygen cylinder or oxygen delivery equipment. The oxygen can react with the adhesive left behind and produce a fire.
- Never store a cylinder near high heat or in a closed vehicle parked in the sun.
- Always keep portable oxygen cylinders lying flat. If you must stand a tank upright, keep your hand on the tank to prevent it from falling over.
- Always use the pressure gauges and regulators that are intended for use with oxygen and the equipment you are using.

O-ring ▶ gasket used to seal a regulator to the oxygen cylinder.

- Always ensure that the **O-ring** is in good condition and free of cracks. This will help prevent dangerous leaks.
- Tighten all valves and connections hand-tight only. Tightening too much may damage connections and make it difficult to remove.
- Open and close all valves slowly.

- Always store reserve oxygen cylinders in a cool, ventilated room as approved by your EMS system.
- Always have oxygen cylinders hydrostatically tested. This should be done every 5 years for steel tanks (3 years for aluminum cylinders). The date for retesting should be stamped on the top of the cylinder near the valve. This test is to ensure the integrity of the metal tank and prevent failure due to weak metal caused by corrosion on the inside.

The U.S. DOT requires that all compressed gas cylinders be inspected and pressure tested at specific intervals. The cylinders used in EMS that contain medical grade oxygen must be tested at least every 5 years. That test is commonly referred to as a **hydrostatic test**. It is used to confirm the integrity of the cylinder and that no leaks exist. For that test, a visual inspection of the tank must be performed first. Then the tank is filled with water and pressurized to five-thirds the service pressure, or approximately 3,360 psi. The most recent hydrostatic test date must be stamped into the crown of the cylinder and easily readable. Only specialized testing centers are authorized to perform this test.

hydrostatic test ▸ process of testing high-pressure cylinders.

CREW RESOURCE MANAGEMENT

Every member of the team is responsible for safety. All members should keep an eye out for where the oxygen cylinders are located and ensure that they are safe and secure throughout the call, especially during transport.

liter flow ▸ measure of the flow of oxygen being delivered through a mask or cannula.

pin index safety system ▸ safety system used to ensure that the proper regulator is used for a specific gas, such as oxygen.

Oxygen Regulators

LO7 | Describe the purpose and functions of an oxygen regulator.

The pressure in a full oxygen cylinder is approximately 2,000 psi. This is much too high of a pressure to be used directly from the cylinder. A pressure regulator (also called an oxygen regulator) must be connected to the oxygen cylinder before it may be used to deliver oxygen to a patient (Figure 10.3).

All oxygen regulators have a minimum of three functions:

- *Reduce tank pressure.* The regulator reduces the pressure of oxygen leaving the tank to allow for efficient delivery to the patient. It can reduce the pressure from 2,000 psi to between 30 psi and 70 psi.
- *Display tank pressure.* The regulator displays the pressure inside the cylinder via a pressure gauge. The gauge displays the actual (unregulated) pressure remaining inside the tank, which is a direct indication of how much oxygen you have left in the tank.
- *Control the delivery of oxygen.* Most regulators have a **liter flow** valve, sometimes called the *flow meter.* The liter flow valve is an adjustable dial on the regulator that allows you to select a specific flow of oxygen to the patient in liters per minute (LPM). An oxygen delivery device, such as a mask, can be connected to the liter flow valve. Then, when it is placed on the patient, it delivers the selected flow of supplemental oxygen.

Connecting the Regulator On portable oxygen cylinders, a yoke assembly is used to secure the regulator to the cylinder valve assembly. The yoke has pins that must mate with the corresponding holes in the valve assembly on the cylinder. This is called a **pin index safety system** (Figure 10.4). The position of the pins varies for different gases to prevent an oxygen delivery system from being connected to a cylinder containing another gas. There are three pins on the regulator that must be matched to

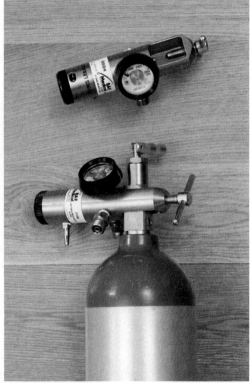

Figure 10.3 Pressure regulators: (top) off the tank and (bottom) attached to the tank.

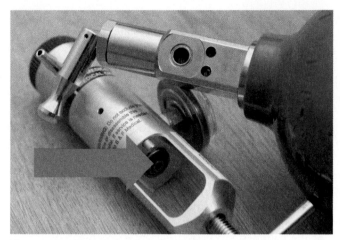

Figure 10.4 The pin index safety system and the presence of the O-ring as indicated by the blue arrow.

three holes on the tank valve. The largest pin is the oxygen port. This pin is the pathway through which oxygen flows from the cylinder to the regulator. The two other pins serve as a means to properly align the regulator onto the yoke. Before placing the regulator onto the yoke, you must ensure the presence of an O-ring. The O-ring sits over the oxygen port and serves as a gasket to ensure an airtight seal between the regulator and the cylinder valve.

Before connecting the regulator to an oxygen cylinder, open the cylinder valve slightly for just a second to clear dirt and dust out of the delivery port. This is called "cracking" the cylinder valve. Be sure that the open valve is facing away from you and that your hand or fingers are not blocking the escaping oxygen. There is enough pressure in the tank to eject dust and particles, which can cause injury to the eyes.

Humidifiers A humidifier is an unbreakable container of sterile water that can be placed in-line between the flow valve and the oxygen delivery device. As the oxygen from the cylinder passes through the water, it picks up moisture from the water. In turn, the oxygen becomes more comfortable for the patient to breathe. Nonhumidified oxygen delivered to a patient over a long period of time (more than 20 minutes) will dry out the mucous membranes and passages of the upper airway. For the short period of time in which the patient receives oxygen in the field, this is not usually a problem.

Oxygen Delivery Devices

LO8 Explain the indications for the use of a nasal cannula.

LO9 Explain the indications for the use of a nonrebreather mask.

You will encounter two types of patients who may need supplemental oxygen: those who are breathing on their own and moving air adequately, and those who are breathing inadequately or not at all. Two devices are commonly used by Emergency Medical Responders to deliver oxygen to patients who are breathing on their own: the nasal cannula and the nonrebreather mask.

Nasal Cannula The **nasal cannula** delivers oxygen into the patient's nostrils by way of two small plastic prongs (Figure 10.5A and B). Nasal injuries, colds, and other types of nasal airway obstruction greatly reduce its efficiency.

A nasal cannula has an effective flow rate of between 1 and 6 LPM (Table 10.2). These flow rates provide the patient with an increased oxygen concentration between 25 and 45 percent. The approximate relationship of oxygen concentration to LPM flow is 4 percent oxygen concentration per liter of flow:

Room air is 21% concentration
25% concentration with 1 LPM
29% concentration with 2 LPM
33% concentration with 3 LPM
37% concentration with 4 LPM
41% concentration with 5 LPM
45% concentration with 6 LPM

For every 1 LPM increase in oxygen flow, you deliver an approximately 4 percent increase in the concentration of oxygen. At 4 LPM and above, the patient's breathing patterns may prevent delivery of the stated percentages. At 5 LPM, drying of the nasal membranes is likely. Above 6 LPM, the device does not deliver any higher concentration of oxygen and may be uncomfortable for most patients.

nasal cannula ▶ device used to deliver low concentrations of supplemental oxygen to a breathing patient.

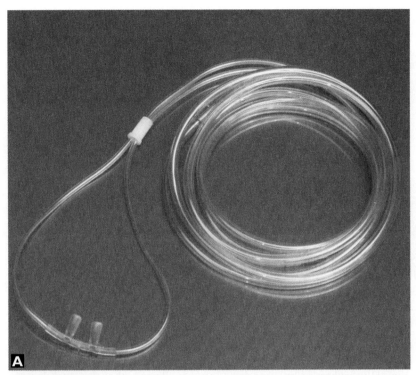
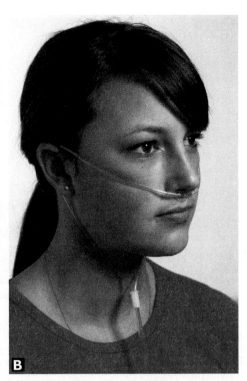

Figure 10.5 (A) Example of an adult nasal cannula and (B) a nasal cannula properly placed on the face of the patient.

TABLE 10.2	Oxygen Delivery Devices		
	Flow Rate	**% Oxygen Delivered**	**Special Use**
Nasal cannula	1 to 6 LPM	25% to 45%	Most medical patients in mild to moderate distress
Nonrebreather mask	10 to 15 LPM	80% to 95%	Most trauma patients and medical patients in moderate to severe distress

Nonrebreather Mask   A **nonrebreather mask** is used when the patient requires a higher concentration of oxygen than the nasal cannula can deliver. The nonrebreather mask consists of a face mask, a one-way valve, and a **reservoir bag**. The reservoir bag must remain full and will ensure that the patient receives the highest possible concentration of oxygen.

It is important that you inflate the reservoir bag *before* placing the mask on the patient's face (Figure 10.6A and B). A full reservoir bag will ensure that the patient receives the maximum concentration of oxygen directly from the reservoir with each breath. This is done by using your finger to cover the one-way valve inside the mask between the mask and the reservoir.

When placing the mask on the patient, take care to ensure a proper seal with the patient's face. The reservoir must not deflate by more than one-third when the patient takes their deepest breath. You can maintain the volume in the bag by adjusting the oxygen flow on the regulator. The patient's exhaled air does not return to the reservoir; instead, it is vented through the one-way flaps or portholes on the mask. The minimum flow rate when using this mask is typically 10 LPM, but a higher flow (12 to 15 LPM) may be required to keep the reservoir filled.

Venturi Mask   The Venturi mask is a variation of the nonrebreather mask. The key to the Venturi mask is its adjustable "jets" that allow the rescuer to more accurately determine the specific oxygen concentration delivered to the patient. Venturi masks are more commonly seen and used in the hospital setting.

Blow-by Delivery   Another technique for the delivery of supplemental oxygen to a breathing patient is called the blow-by method. It can be used for any patient who cannot

nonrebreather mask ▶ device used to deliver high concentrations of supplemental oxygen.

reservoir bag ▶ device attached to an oxygen delivery device that temporarily stores oxygen.

REMEMBER

The proper use of a nonrebreather mask is not dependent on any particular flow rate. The best way to determine proper flow rate is to choose a rate that allows the reservoir bag to deflate slightly when the patient takes a breath in and to completely reinflate before the next breath.

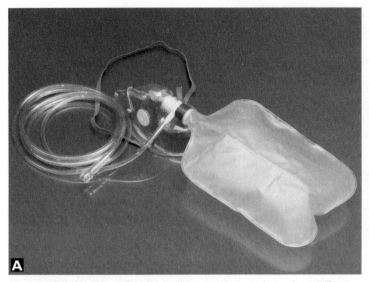

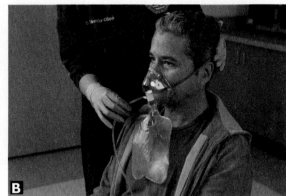

Figure 10.6 (A) Example of an adult nonrebreather mask and (B) a nonrebreather properly placed on the face of a patient.

tolerate having a traditional mask or cannula placed on their face. With the blow-by technique, you can use a nonrebreather mask set to 15 LPM and simply have the patient hold the mask as close to the face as comfortable. This technique is especially good for small children who are typically frightened by a mask or cannula. Be sure that the mask is held as close to the face as possible to ensure that a good supply of oxygen reaches the patient.

Administering Oxygen

Key Skills 10.1 and 10.2 will take you step-by-step through the process of preparing the oxygen delivery system and administering oxygen.

Administration of Oxygen to a Nonbreathing Patient

Three devices are commonly used in the EMS setting to provide high-concentration oxygen while providing rescue breaths for a nonbreathing patient: the pocket mask with oxygen inlet, the bag-mask device, and the demand-valve device. When using these devices, an appropriate airway adjunct should be inserted first. Always follow local protocols.

KEY SKILL 10.1

Administering Oxygen: Preparing the Oxygen Delivery System

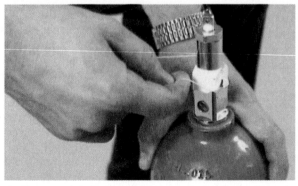

1. Remove the plastic wrapper or cap protecting the cylinder yoke.
(Michael Gallitelli/Pearson Education, Inc.)

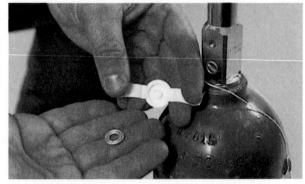

2. Keep the plastic washer that is available in some setups.
(Michael Gallitelli/Pearson Education, Inc.)

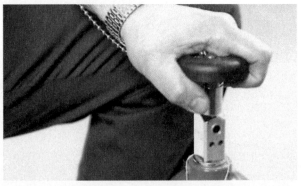

3. Quickly open the main valve for 1 second to remove any dust.
(Michael Gallitelli/Pearson Education, Inc.)

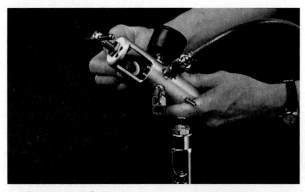

4. Ensure that O-ring is present on the regulator oxygen port.
(Michael Gallitelli/Pearson Education, Inc.)

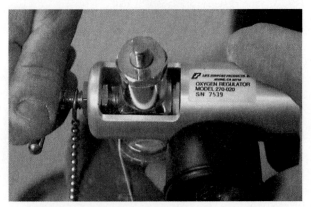

5. Place the regulator on the yoke, and tighten the T-screw hand-tight. Do not overtighten.
(Michael Gallitelli/Pearson Education, Inc.)

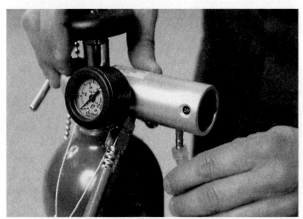

6. Attach tubing from the delivery device.
(Michael Gallitelli/Pearson Education, Inc.)

Pocket Mask with Oxygen Inlet The pocket face mask connected to an oxygen supply can deliver higher concentrations of oxygen than a pocket mask alone. Using **oxygen supply tubing**, connect one end to the liter flow valve of the regulator and the other end to the oxygen inlet on the pocket mask (Figure 10.7). Turn on the liter flow to 10 LPM, and use the mask as you normally would to provide rescue breaths.

oxygen supply tubing ▶ tubing used to connect a delivery device to an oxygen source.

Bag-Mask Device The bag-mask device is an efficient tool for providing manual ventilations for a nonbreathing patient or a patient who is breathing inadequately. It is best used with two rescuers. The first rescuer obtains a tight mask-to-face seal and keeps the airway open. The second rescuer squeezes the bag to achieve good chest rise and fall. Most bag-mask devices can accept supplemental oxygen; however, it is not required. When available, attach the bag-mask to an oxygen source and adjust the flow to no less than 15 LPM. Many bag-mask devices have an oxygen reservoir (long tube or bag) to increase the oxygen concentration delivered to the patient. Used without a reservoir, it will deliver approximately 50 percent oxygen. Used with a reservoir, it will deliver an oxygen concentration up to 100 percent.

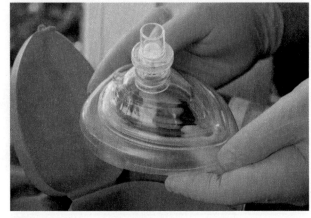

Figure 10.7 A typical pocket face mask with one-way valve.

Administering Oxygen

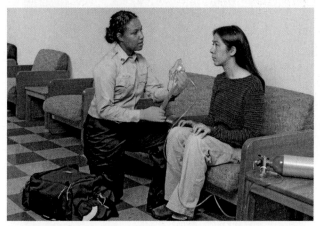

1. Explain the need for oxygen therapy.

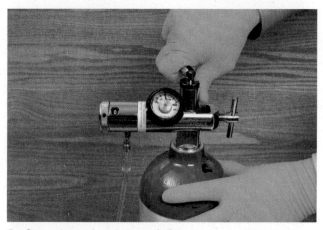

2. Open the main valve one full turn.

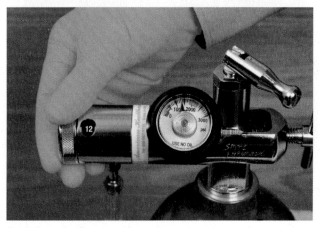

3. Adjust the flow to appropriate rate.

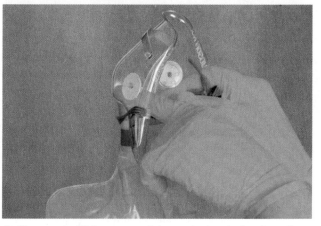

4. Be sure to fill the reservoir bag prior to placing it on the patient by turning on the flow and placing your finger over the valve inside the mask.

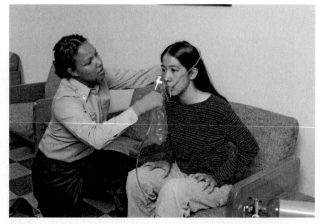

5. Position the oxygen delivery device on the patient.

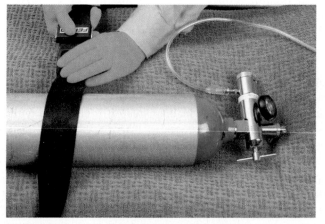

6. Secure the cylinder during patient transfer.

Maintain an open airway, hold a tight mask-to-face seal, squeeze the bag to deliver oxygen, and release the bag to allow for a passive exhalation (Figure 10.8). There is no need to remove the mask when the patient exhales. The bag mask also can be used to assist the breathing efforts of a patient who has inadequate respirations (as in a drug overdose).

Demand Valve Device   A demand valve device delivers oxygen through a specialized regulator. That regulator can deliver 100 percent oxygen "on demand" when the patient inhales. The rescuer can also activate the flow of oxygen by pressing a trigger on the device. Standard features of the demand valve device include a peak flow rate of 40 LPM, an inspiratory pressure-relief valve that opens at approximately 60 cm of water pressure, and a trigger that enables the rescuer to use both hands to maintain a mask seal while activating the device.

To operate a demand valve device, place an appropriate-sized mask on the demand valve. Follow the same procedures for placing and sealing the mask as you would for the bag-mask device. Then press the trigger to deliver oxygen until the patient's chest rises. Release the trigger after the chest inflates, and allow for passive exhalation. Repeat this step as often as necessary for the specific patient. If the chest does not rise, reposition the head or reopen the airway, check for obstructions, reposition the mask, check for a seal, and try again.

Monitor your patient carefully whenever you are providing assisted ventilations. High pressure caused by forcing air or oxygen into a patient's airway can cause air to enter the esophagus and fill the stomach. Air distends the stomach, which presses into the lung cavity and reduces expansion of the lungs. To minimize this problem, maintain a patent airway and mask-to-face seal, and ensure good chest rise and fall with each breath. Do not continue to provide ventilations after chest rise; allow passive exhalation after each breath.

If you suspect neck injury, have an assistant manually stabilize the patient's head or use your knees to prevent head movement. Bring the jaw to the mask without tilting the head or neck, and trigger the mask to ventilate the patient.

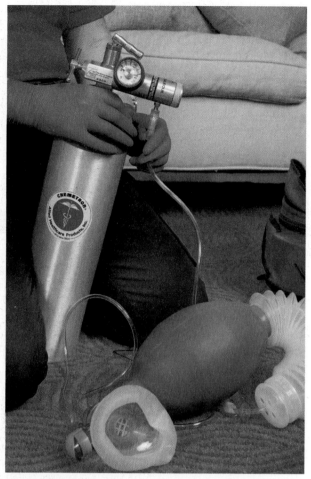

Figure 10.8 Example of an adult bag-mask device connected to an oxygen supply.

General Guidelines for Oxygen Therapy

Many patients may benefit from supplemental oxygen. However, there are some patients for which too much oxygen may be harmful. Be sure to consult with your instructor and local protocols to confirm the standard of care for providing oxygen in your system, area, or region.

Examples of situations when a patient may benefit from supplemental oxygen include:

- Cardiac arrest (during resuscitation)
- Respiratory distress
- Heart attack (depending on oxygen saturation)
- Shock
- Allergic reaction

It is always important to explain to your patient what you are doing when providing care. Attempting to place a cannula or mask on their face without explaining what you are doing can frighten a patient. Once frightened, they may have a hard time feeling comfortable with you or the care you are attempting to provide.

Before placing the device on the patient's face, explain that you would like to provide them with oxygen and that it will help them feel better. Show the patient the device and explain how it works and how it will fit on their face. Then gently place the device on their face, and confirm that they are comfortable with it. Adjust it as necessary to make it comfortable. Remind the patient to breathe as normally as possible.

If your patient is anxious and seems reluctant to accept the device, provide extra reassurance. In the case of a mask, allow them to hold the device and place it themselves. This will allow the patient to remove the device if they feel the need. Sometimes the mask can make a patient feel claustrophobic. Monitor the patient closely, and provide reassurance as necessary if their breathing does not improve.

FIRST ON SCENE WRAP-UP

"Mrs. Smith's respiratory rate has gone from 32 to 24, and it's a little easier for her to breathe now," Bryn reports to the arriving paramedics. Color has slowly returned to her cheeks, and she is sitting up a little straighter.

Mrs. Smith looks worried and reaches out for her granddaughter as the paramedics prepare to transfer the patient from her wheelchair.

"Grandma, it's okay," Grace says. "These people are here to help."

"Don't worry," Bryn tells Mrs. Smith as the paramedics connect the oxygen mask to their own cylinder. "The oxygen will help your breathing."

"Thank you," the patient mutters softly.

"Our pleasure," Bryn says, as she looks at Thien and smiles. "Though oxygen was the real hero here."

Summary

- A constant supply of oxygen is essential to keeping all body systems functioning properly. Sometimes an illness or injury can disrupt the normal flow of oxygen into the body. In those situations, many ill or injured patients will benefit from supplemental oxygen.
- Oxygen is stored and transported in portable containers called cylinders. The oxygen contained in these cylinders is stored under very high pressure (2,000 psi) and can pose a risk to those working around them if not handled properly.
- When working with high-pressure cylinders, it is important to keep the cylinders lying flat to minimize the risk of their falling over and getting damaged. All valves should be opened and closed slowly, and all cylinders should be stored in a cool environment and away from sources of flame or heat.
- There are many different sizes of oxygen cylinders, but the sizes most commonly used in EMS are the Standard D, Jumbo D, and E.
- A pressure regulator (also called oxygen regulator) reduces the pressure of the oxygen coming out of the cylinder, which makes

it usable for patients. The regulator has a pressure gauge that displays how much pressure is in the tank and a liter flow valve that allows for regulation of the flow of oxygen to the patient.
- The nasal cannula and the nonrebreather mask are two devices commonly used to provide supplemental oxygen for the breathing patient. The cannula can deliver oxygen concentrations up to 45 percent with normal flow rates of between 2 and 6 LPM. The nonrebreather mask can deliver oxygen concentrations up to approximately 95 percent with typical flow rates between 10 and 15 LPM.
- The amount of supplemental oxygen provided to a patient is determined based on factors such as mental status, vital signs, and mechanism of injury.
- When a patient is not breathing adequately on their own, you must provide positive pressure ventilations. This can be performed using a pocket mask, bag mask, or a demand valve device.
- If available, a pulse oximeter can be used to monitor oxygen saturation.

Take Action

In-Service or Expired?

One very important safety precaution that often gets overlooked is the check of the hydrostatic test date on each oxygen cylinder. Your agency or training institution probably has oxygen cylinders for patient care or training. Take some time to inspect each cylinder. Then, look for the hydrostatic test date stamped on the top side of the cylinder. Because this test must occur every 5 years, and a typical cylinder can last for decades, you may find a cylinder with multiple test stamps. Locate the most current date, and determine if the cylinder is expired. Should you find a cylinder that is out of date, be sure to let your instructor, supervisor, or equipment officer know immediately.

First on Scene Patient Handoff

Joanne Smith is an 87-year-old female with a chief complaint of difficulty breathing, increasing over the past several hours. Mrs. Smith has a history of emphysema and is on low-flow oxygen around the clock. Upon arrival we found her home oxygen supply was empty and immediately placed her on supplemental oxygen by nonrebreather mask. When we arrived, the patient was in moderate distress with a respiratory rate of 32, shallow and labored. Her skin was pale and cool. The oxygen seems to be helping quite a bit as her respiratory rate has come down to 24, good tidal volume, and unlabored.

First on Scene Run Review

Recall the events of the First on Scene scenario in this chapter, and answer the following questions related to the call. Rationales are offered in the Answer Key at the back of the book.

1. What kind of questions would you ask Grace about her grandma?
2. What kind of respiratory history would Mrs. Smith likely have to be on home oxygen?
3. What information should Bryn give the arriving paramedic?

Quick Quiz

To check your understanding of the chapter, answer the following questions. Then compare your answers to those in the Answer Key at the back of the book.

1. Supplemental oxygen can be helpful to ill or injured patients by:
   a. reducing the concentration of available oxygen.
   b. increasing the concentration of available oxygen.
   c. helping to eliminate carbon dioxide.
   d. increasing the concentration of carbon dioxide.

2. Which of the following best describes the oxygen consumption of a normally functioning human being?
   a. The body requires a constant supply of oxygen at 79 percent.
   b. The body needs a minimum of 10 percent oxygen to survive.
   c. The body exhales an average of 21 percent carbon dioxide with each breath.
   d. Each breath we exhale contains approximately 16 percent oxygen.

3. All of the following are reasons a patient might need supplemental oxygen EXCEPT:
   a. a significant mechanism of injury.
   b. being upset over the breakup with a boyfriend/girlfriend.
   c. a suspected heart attack.
   d. difficulty breathing.

4. Which one of the following best defines the term *oxygen concentration*?
   a. Percentage of carbon dioxide in room air
   b. Amount of oxygen remaining in one exhalation
   c. Ratio between oxygen and carbon dioxide
   d. Concentration of oxygen inspired by the patient

5. The pressure gauge of a full oxygen cylinder will display approximately ____ psi.
   a. 500
   b. 1,000
   c. 1,500
   d. 2,000

6. A typical oxygen regulator will NOT:
   a. display tank pressure.
   b. display ambient air pressure.
   c. control liter flow.
   d. regulate tank pressure.

7. You are caring for a patient complaining of mild shortness of breath and have them on a nasal cannula at 6 LPM. What oxygen concentration are you delivering to the patient?
   a. 25 percent
   b. 29 percent
   c. 33 percent
   d. 45 percent

8. You are caring for a victim of a motor vehicle crash and have placed them on a nonrebreather mask. Which of the following best describes how you know the liter flow has been adjusted properly?
   a. The patient is able to speak in complete sentences.
   b. The reservoir bag completely deflates with each breath.
   c. You see no movement of the reservoir bag with each breath.
   d. The reservoir bag refills completely between breaths.

9. You are caring for a patient who was ejected from a vehicle that rolled over. They are alert and responsive. Respirations are 20 times per minute, unlabored, and with good tidal volume. Which device is most appropriate to deliver oxygen to this patient?
   a. Nasal cannula
   b. Demand valve device
   c. Bag-mask device
   d. Nonrebreather mask

10. You are caring for a patient who was involved in a serious motor vehicle collision. They are conscious and alert and breathing 18 times per minute with good tidal volume. You would provide oxygen to this patient based on:
    a. the patient's level of distress.
    b. abnormal vital signs.
    c. the mechanism of injury.
    d. the respiratory rate.

11. You are a single rescuer caring for a patient in cardiac arrest. Your equipment bag and a supply of oxygen are within reach. Which of the following is the most appropriate choice for beginning rescue breaths on this patient?
    a. Pocket mask with supplemental oxygen
    b. Bag mask without supplemental oxygen
    c. Mouth-to-mouth
    d. Waiting for another rescuer before beginning rescue breaths

12. The proper placement of a(n) ____ will help ensure an airtight fit between the regulator and the tank valve.
    a. cannula
    b. Venturi
    c. O-ring
    d. demand valve

13. You are caring for a 12-year-old boy who is having severe difficulty breathing. His respirations are 22 per minute, and he is speaking in short sentences. The best choice for oxygen therapy for this patient is a:
    a. demand valve device.
    b. nasal cannula.
    c. nonrebreather mask.
    d. bag-mask device.

14. Your patient is a 54-year-old female experiencing mild shortness of breath after exertion. She is breathing about 14 times per minute with good tidal volume. What is the best choice for oxygen therapy for this patient?

    a. Bag-mask device

    b. Nasal cannula

    c. Venturi mask

    d. Pocket mask

15. The cylinders used in EMS that contain medical-grade oxygen must be tested at least every 5 years. That test is commonly referred to as a:

    a. hydrostatic test.

    b. pressure relief test.

    c. cylinder integrity test.

    d. tank test seal.

Endnote

1. Merchant, R. M., Topjian, A. A., Panchal, A. R, Cheng, A., Aziz, K., Berg, K. M., Lavonas, E. J., Magid, D. J., "Adult Basic and Advanced Life Support, Pediatric Basic and Advanced Life Support, Neonatal Life Support, Resuscitation Education Science, and Systems of Care Writing Groups. 2020 American Heart Association Guidelines for Cardiopulmonary Resuscitation and Emergency Cardiovascular Care," *Circulation*, Vol.142, No.16, Suppl. 2 (October 20, 2020):S337–S357. doi: 10.1161/CIR.0000000000000918. Epub 2020 Oct 21. PMID: 33081530.

11

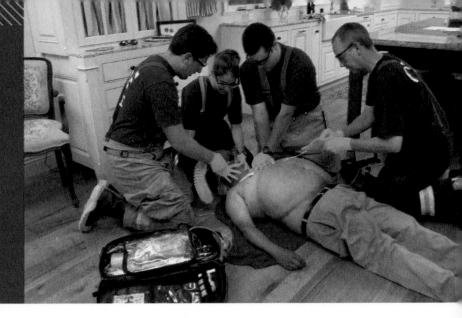

Principles of Resuscitation

Education Standards

Shock and Resuscitation

Competencies

Uses assessment information to recognize respiratory failure, respiratory arrest, and cardiac arrest based on assessment findings and manages the emergency while awaiting additional emergency response.

LEARNING OBJECTIVES

Upon successful completion of this chapter, the student should be able to:

Cognitive

1. Define the chapter key terms.
2. Review cardiovascular and respiratory anatomy and physiology (see Chapter 4).
3. Explain the components of the adult and pediatric prehospital chains of survival.
4. Explain the most common causes of cardiac arrest for adult and pediatric patients.
5. Explain the steps for performing single-rescuer CPR on an adult, child, and infant.
6. Describe the signs of cardiac arrest.
7. Explain the importance of minimizing interruptions during CPR.
8. Explain the steps for performing two-rescuer CPR on an adult, child, and infant.
9. Explain the purpose of an automated external defibrillator (AED).
10. Describe the indications and contraindications for the use of an AED.

Psychomotor

11. Demonstrate the proper technique for performing single-rescuer CPR on a simulated patient in cardiac arrest.
12. Demonstrate the proper technique for performing two-rescuer CPR on a simulated patient in cardiac arrest.
13. Demonstrate the proper use of an AED on a simulated patient in cardiac arrest.

Affective

14. Value the importance of prompt assessment and action for patients of cardiac arrest.
15. Demonstrate an understanding of the needs of family members of a cardiac arrest victim.

KEY TERMS

advanced life support (ALS) (*p. 199*)
agonal breaths (*p. 202*)
asystole (*p. 215*)
automated external defibrillator (AED) (*p. 200*)
cardiac arrest (*p. 199*)
cardiopulmonary resuscitation (CPR) (*p. 201*)
chain of survival (*p. 199*)
chest compressions (*p. 199*)

defibrillation (*p. 199*)
fibrillation (*p. 215*)
infant (*p. 211*)
myocardial infarction (MI) (*p. 200*)
neonate (*p. 211*)
pediatric patient (*p. 200*)
sniffing position (*p. 212*)
ventricular fibrillation (VF) (*p. 215*)
ventricular tachycardia (*p. 215*)

E ach year more than 135 million people worldwide die from cardiovascular disease with from 20 to 140 cardiac arrests per 100,000 population and survival rates ranging from 2 to 11 percent. In the United States, more than half a million children and adults suffer a cardiac arrest each year, with less than 15 percent surviving.[1]

Over the years, the techniques of cardiopulmonary resuscitation (CPR) have been refined to increase its effectiveness. It is important to make a point of practicing your CPR skills often and keeping up to date with the latest research findings.

This chapter presents the latest guidelines for CPR as well as the use of the automated external defibrillator (AED).

FIRST ON SCENE

"What do you think, Chris?" Maria, security manager for Western Legends Hotel and Casino, is examining a CCTV video screen closely. "Chris?" She turns to see why the hotel's lead security agent hasn't answered her.

Chris sits several feet from her, both hands on his chest. His face is ghostly pale. "What's wrong, Chris? Chris?"

Maria stands quickly, sending her chair crashing into a bookshelf. Chris looks up at her, his bulging eyes reflecting the wall of video monitors next to him. He tries to speak several times and then collapses into a heap on the floor.

"Chris!" Maria screams and drops to her knees next to him, shaking his shoulders. "Are you okay?"

There is no response, and his eyes, partially hidden behind half-closed lids, stare vacantly at her.

"Okay," Maria says to herself. "Okay, calm down. First things first." Maria searches her memory for the procedures that she learned in last spring's Emergency Medical Responder course. She takes a deep breath, rolls Chris onto his back, and checks for signs of breathing.

The Chain of Survival

LO3 | Explain the components of the adult and pediatric prehospital chains of survival.

The American Heart Association has identified specific elements for adult and pediatric patients that help improve outcomes in cases of cardiac arrest. These elements make up the **chain of survival** and are slightly different for patients in prehospital and hospital settings. For a patient to have the best chance of survival following **cardiac arrest**, each link in the chain of survival must be strong.

The six links in the adult chain of survival are:

- *Activation of emergency response system (911).*
- *High-quality CPR with an emphasis on chest compressions.* The sooner **chest compressions** are initiated, the sooner circulation can be restored to the patient's brain and vital organs.
- *Defibrillation.* **Defibrillation** is the application of an electric shock to a patient's heart in an attempt to convert a lethal rhythm into a normal one. The time from cardiac arrest to defibrillation is an essential factor in patients' survival rate. The shorter the time between collapse and defibrillation, the better.
- *Advanced resuscitation.* Also known as **advanced life support (ALS)**, this is the care provided by more highly trained EMS personnel such as advanced emergency medical technicians (AEMTs) and paramedics. In addition to using defibrillators,

chain of survival ▶ adult: activation of EMS, high-quality CPR, defibrillation, advanced resuscitation, post–cardiac arrest care, and recovery.

chain of survival ▶ pediatric: prevention, activation of EMS, high-quality CPR, advanced resuscitation, post–cardiac arrest care, and recovery.

cardiac arrest ▶ absence of a heartbeat.

chest compressions ▶ rapid, deep, regular compressions on the center of the chest in an attempt to circulate blood to the brain, lungs, and heart.

defibrillation ▶ application of an electric shock to a patient's heart in an attempt to convert a lethal rhythm to a normal one.

advanced life support ▶
prehospital emergency care that
involves the use of intravenous
fluids, drug infusions, cardiac
monitoring, defibrillation,
intubation, and other advanced
procedures. Abbrev: ALS.

they provide other interventions such as advanced airways, intravenous fluids, and administration of life-saving medications.

- *Post–cardiac arrest care.* A more formal and organized approach to post–cardiac arrest care occurs when the patient is delivered to a definitive care hospital with expert cardiovascular, neurological, and intensive care capabilities. These include cardiac catheterization facilities and the performance of therapeutic hypothermia.
- *Recovery.* Recovery following cardiac arrest continues long after the initial event. Recovery may involve interventions to address the initial cause of the arrest as well as rehabilitation focusing on neurological recovery.

The links in the pediatric chain of survival are:

- *Prevention.* Many of the causes of cardiac arrest in children can easily be prevented when adult caregivers are aware of the risks associated with the environment. Accidental drowning and choking are just a couple of causes that can be minimized with proper prevention.
- *Activation of emergency response system (911).*
- *High-quality CPR.*
- *Advanced resuscitation.*
- *Post–cardiac arrest care.*
- *Recovery.*

automated external
defibrillator ▶ electrical device
that, when applied to the chest,
can detect certain abnormal
heart rhythms and deliver a
shock to the patient's heart.
This shock may allow the heart
to resume a normal pattern of
beating. Abbrev: AED.

Each link in the chain of survival is essential to improving patient outcomes. In recent years, defibrillator technology has improved to the point that an **automated external defibrillator (AED)** can be operated with minimal training. Today, AEDs can be found in many locations such as fitness studios, airports, shopping malls, stadiums, and other public places.

To gain an idea of the number of people who die from cardiac arrest each year, imagine a fully loaded jetliner carrying more than 300 passengers crashing, with no survivors. Now imagine three of these fully loaded jetliners crashing every day, 365 days a year. Would that cause the public to question the safety of air travel? It most certainly would. That is the approximate number of people who die from cardiac arrest each year. Yet little attention is paid to this epidemic. Learning CPR and recognizing the signs of cardiac arrest allow Emergency Medical Responders to make a real and lasting difference in people's lives.

Circulation and CPR

LO2 Review cardiovascular and respiratory anatomy and physiology (see Chapter 4).

LO4 Explain the most common causes of cardiac arrest for adult and pediatric patients.

At the center of the circulatory system is the heart. When the heart beats, it acts as a pump. Blood from the body flows into the heart and is sent to the lungs. In the lungs, the blood releases carbon dioxide gathered while circulating through the body and exchanges it for oxygen. This oxygen-rich blood is then returned to the heart, where it is pumped back out to the body.

When everything is working properly, the circulatory system keeps oxygenated blood moving to all parts of the body (Figure 11.1). As blood flows through the body, it also gathers nutrients from the small intestines, picks up hormones from special glands, and releases wastes to the kidneys. This constant exchange is important for the proper functioning of the vital organs—and for life.

myocardial infarction ▶ when
areas of the heart muscle do not
get enough oxygen and cells
begin to die; commonly called a
heart attack. Abbrev: MI.

pediatric patient ▶ refers to an
infant or child. For the purposes
of CPR, patients from birth to
1 year of age are considered
infants. Patients from the age of
1 year to the onset of puberty
are considered children.

Many things can affect the proper function of the heart, including injury due to trauma. In adults, one of the most common causes of cardiac arrest is a **myocardial infarction (MI)**, commonly called a heart attack. The signs of cardiac arrest are unresponsiveness, no breathing, and no pulse. In **pediatric patients**, cardiac arrest is most often caused by a respiratory crisis such as choking or drowning, which leads to respiratory arrest. Untreated respiratory arrest results in cardiac arrest.

From body
Superior vena cava

To lung
Right pulmonary artery (branches)

Aorta

To lung
Left pulmonary artery

From lung
Right pulmonary vein (branches)

From lung
Left pulmonary vein

Right atrium

Left atrium

Left ventricle

Right ventricle

Inferior vena cava

Descending aorta

From body

To body

Cardiopulmonary Resuscitation

Cardiopulmonary resuscitation (CPR) is an emergency procedure that involves the application of both external chest compressions and ventilations to someone in cardiac arrest. *Cardio-* refers to the heart and *pulmonary* refers to the lungs. Resuscitation means to revive.

During CPR, you must:

- perform rapid, deep chest compressions to circulate the patient's blood.
- ensure and maintain an open airway.
- breathe for (ventilate) the patient.

CPR—How It Works

LO5 Explain the steps for performing single-rescuer CPR on an adult, child, and infant.

During the period between clinical death and biological death, brain cells begin to die. By performing CPR early, you can circulate oxygenated blood to the brain and help delay the onset of biological death.

Before you begin CPR, you must position the patient on their back on a firm surface. You will compress the patient's chest straight down over the sternum (breastbone) and between the nipples. Note that in patients where the sternum is not obvious, the proper location can be found by moving your hand from the patient's armpit until the heel of your hand reaches the center of the patient's chest.

This compresses the heart between the sternum and the back of the thoracic cavity. This squeezing of the heart causes an increase in pressure in the thoracic (chest) cavity

cardiopulmonary resuscitation ▶ combined chest compressions and rescue breaths that maintain circulation and breathing. Abbrev: CPR.

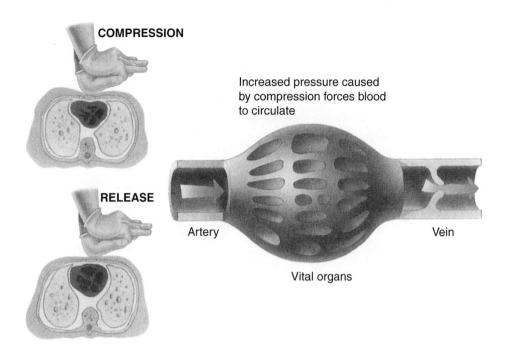

Figure 11.2 During CPR, pressure in the chest cavity caused by compressions forces blood to circulate.

COMPRESSION

Increased pressure caused by compression forces blood to circulate

RELEASE

Artery

Vein

Vital organs

and forces blood out of the heart and into the arteries to circulate to the brain, lungs, and throughout the body (Figure 11.2). When compression is relaxed and pressure is released, a vacuum is created inside the chest, causing blood to flow back into the heart. One-way valves in the patient's heart and veins keep the blood moving in the proper direction.

During CPR, your breath provides oxygen to the patient's blood, which is then circulated to the brain and other vital organs with each compression.

There may be times when no appropriate barrier device is available, and the rescuer does not want to take the risk of being exposed to the patient's bodily fluids via mouth-to-mouth contact. According to the American Heart Association, providing compressions only is significantly better than providing no assistance at all, and it minimizes the risk of the rescuer coming in contact with bodily fluids.[2] Studies have shown that there is some air movement in and out of the lungs with each chest compression.[3]

> **REMEMBER**
>
> The goal of CPR is to provide minimal circulation to the heart and brain until defibrillation can be performed to return the heart to a normal rhythm.

When to Begin CPR

LO6 Describe the signs of cardiac arrest.

As an Emergency Medical Responder, you must always perform a primary assessment of your patient. This assessment includes looking to see if the patient is responsive and for the presence and adequacy of circulation (a pulse) and breathing. The patient may appear to be gasping for air, but there is little, if any, air movement. These gasping breaths are called **agonal breaths** and should not be considered normal breathing.

agonal breaths ▶ abnormal breathing pattern characterized by slow, shallow, gasping breaths that typically occur following cardiac arrest; also called *agonal respirations*.

If the patient is unresponsive and not breathing, you must then confirm the absence of a pulse by locating the carotid pulse point in the neck. Always check for the carotid pulse on the side of the neck where you are kneeling. This will minimize the chances of putting pressure on the trachea and obstructing the airway. Check the pulse for no more than 10 seconds. If the patient is unresponsive, not breathing, and does not have a pulse, you must begin CPR with chest compressions.

> **REMEMBER**
>
> Oxygen remains in the blood even after the heart stops beating. The blood in the arteries contains oxygen, which can be delivered to the heart and brain by way of high-quality chest compressions.

While the steps to determine a patient's responsiveness, breathing, and circulation appear to be done in a particular order, the reality is that all three functions are performed simultaneously. This limits delays in starting CPR if it is indicated. Another concern many people have is, "What if I start CPR on someone who is not in cardiac arrest?" Studies have shown that CPR is unlikely to stop a patient's heart from beating.

Follow these steps when assessing a patient and performing CPR:

1. Form a general impression of the patient as you approach. Does the patient appear to be awake, or are they unresponsive? Start with a strong shake of the shoulder and shout, "Are you okay?"
2. Assess for a pulse and breathing at the same time; this should take no more than 10 seconds. Look for the absence of breathing (no chest rise and fall) or gasping breaths, which are not considered adequate. To assess for a pulse in an adult or child (1 year and older), check the carotid pulse in the neck (Figure 11.3). To assess the pulse of an infant (younger than 1 year), check the brachial pulse in the upper arm (Figure 11.4).
3. If a pulse and normal breathing are absent, begin high-quality CPR by first positioning the patient on their back on a firm surface.
4. If you are alone and the patient is a child or an infant, begin CPR immediately and continue for 2 minutes. Then, if 911 has not already been called, call 911 and get the AED.

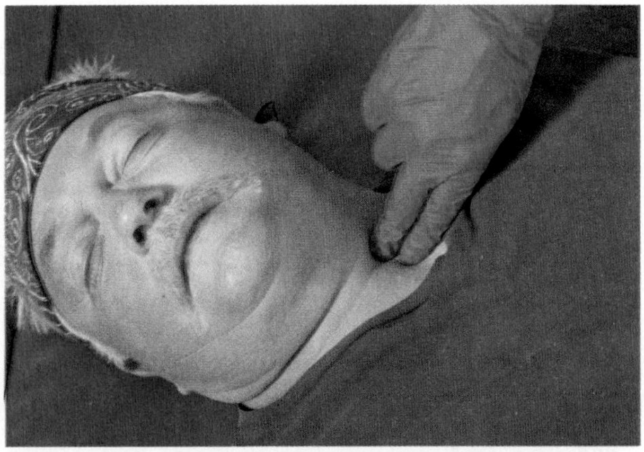

Note that from here on, the discussion will center on adult and child CPR unless otherwise noted. Infant CPR is addressed later in this chapter.

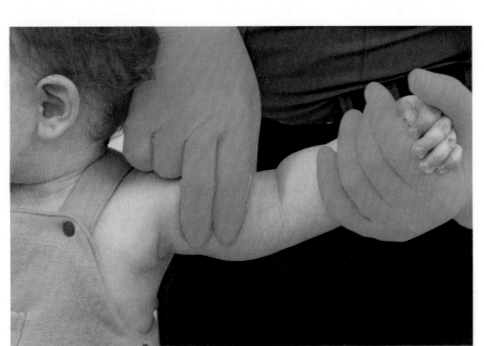

Figure 11.3 Use the carotid artery to assess for the presence of a pulse in an unresponsive adult or child.

Locating the CPR Compression Site

External chest compressions are not effective unless they are delivered to a specific site on the patient's chest (Key Skill 11.1). If you apply compressions to the wrong site, you may injure the patient or provide ineffective compressions. Follow these steps to locate the compression site on an adult patient:

1. After determining that the patient needs CPR, place the patient face-up on a firm surface, such as the ground or floor. This is necessary for compressions to be effective.
2. Kneel at the patient's side near their shoulder.
3. Quickly move or remove clothing that may be covering the patient's chest.

SCENE SAFETY

The American Heart Association strongly suggests the use of appropriate barrier devices when performing rescue breaths on any patient. If you do not have an appropriate barrier device, you may perform hands-only CPR (compressions are performed but not rescue breaths). Compressing the chest moves some air in and out of the lungs and is more beneficial than not doing CPR at all.

Figure 11.4 Use the brachial artery to assess for the presence of a pulse in an infant.

Locating CPR Compression Site on Adult and Child

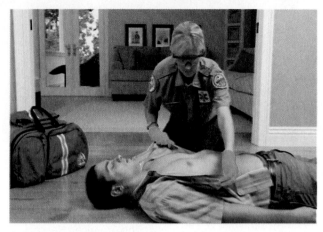

1. Quickly move or remove any clothing that is covering the patient's chest.

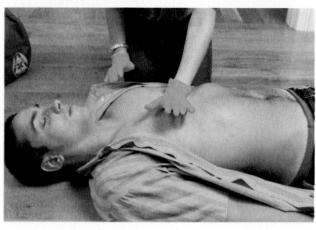

2. Place the heel of one hand on the center of the patient's bare chest, on the lower half of the sternum (breastbone).

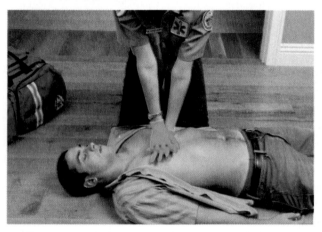

3. Place the heel of your other hand on top of the first. Either extend or interlace your fingers.

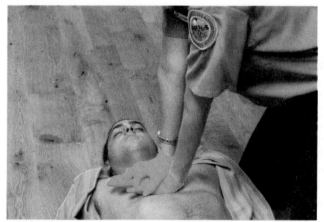

4. Make sure your elbows are locked and your shoulders are directly over your hands.

4. Place the heel of one hand on the center of the patient's bare chest, on the lower half of the sternum.

5. Put the heel of your other hand on top of the first. Either extend or interlace your fingers.

External Chest Compressions

The correct technique for external chest compressions is as follows:

1. Keep the heels of both hands parallel to each other—one on top of the other—with the fingers of both hands pointing away from you.

2. Either extend or interlace your fingers (Figure 11.5A and B). For some it may be easier to do compressions by grasping the wrist of the hand placed at the compression site. Practice different positions until you find one that is comfortable for you.

3. Keep your elbows straight and locked. Do not bend your elbows when delivering or releasing compressions.

4. Position your shoulders over your hands (Figure 11.6). Keep both your knees on the ground, about shoulder-width apart.

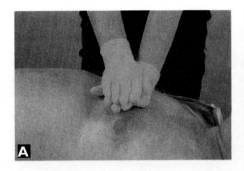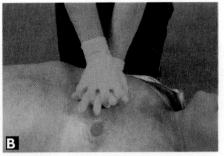

Figure 11.5 Hand positions at the CPR compression site: (A) extending fingers; (B) intertwining fingers.

5. Deliver compressions straight down and apply enough force to the adult or child patient to depress the sternum at least 2 inches, but no more than 2.4 inches. Compressions that are too deep may damage internal organs. For a child, compress the chest with the heel of one hand (Figure 11.7). The depth of compressions is assessed visually as best you can. Compressions will be effective for the patient and less tiring for you if you bend from the hips in a smooth up-and-down motion. Perform chest compressions hard and fast at a rate of 100 to 120 per minute.

6. Release pressure on the chest completely between compressions to allow the patient's heart to refill with blood.

7. Provide sets of 30 compressions and pause briefly between sets to provide 2 rescue breaths.

Providing Rescue Breaths During CPR

Follow these guidelines when providing rescue breaths during CPR:

- After each set of 30 compressions, provide 2 breaths. Allow the chest to deflate between breaths.
- Deliver each breath slowly over 1 second.
- Rescue breaths for an adult should be delivered at a rate of 1 breath every 6 seconds or about 10 breaths per minute.

Do not overventilate the patient. If you force too much air into the patient's lungs, the excess air may overflow from the lungs into the stomach and may eventually cause the stomach to distend (gastric distention). Provide breaths until you see the chest rise. Then stop and allow the chest to fall. Ventilations that are too fast could cause the patient to vomit and result in a compromised airway. Providing slow, steady breaths minimizes the chance that your breath will push air into the patient's stomach.

To provide effective mouth-to-mask ventilations, you may position yourself either at the top of the patient's head or at the patient's side (Figure 11.8A and B). The position at

> **REMEMBER**
>
> The four elements of high-quality compressions are: proper position of the hands, proper rate of compressions (100 to 200 per minute), proper depth of compressions (at least 2 inches or 5 cm), and full recoil of the patient's chest. It is important to minimize the interruption of compressions as much as possible.

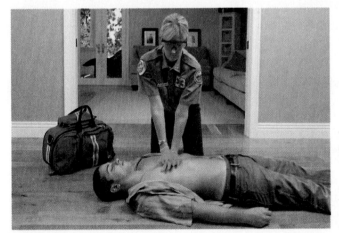

Figure 11.6 Position your shoulders directly over the compression site.

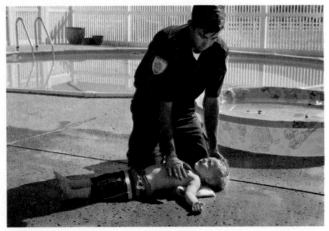

Figure 11.7 For chest compressions on a child, use the heel of one hand.

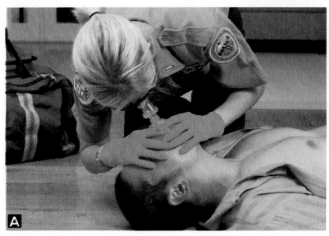
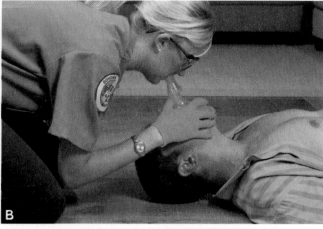

Figure 11.8 Deliver ventilations from (A) the side of the patient's head or (B) from the top of the patient's head (recommended only if the patient has a pulse but is not breathing and during two-rescuer CPR).

the top of the patient's head is preferred for patients with a pulse but no respirations and for two-rescuer CPR. The lateral (to-the side) position is required for one-rescuer CPR because you will need to alternate between compressions and ventilations seamlessly. Practice both positions on a manikin. Remember that good CPR delays the onset of biological death and increases the patient's chances for survival.

Rates and Ratios of Compressions and Ventilations

LO7 Explain the importance of minimizing interruptions during CPR.

Effective CPR depends on the correct rate and ratio of compressions and ventilations. For effective CPR, you must:

- deliver compressions at a rate of 100 to 120 per minute.
- provide ventilations at a ratio of 2 breaths for every 30 compressions. Deliver each breath over 1 second.
- avoid interrupting compressions for longer than 10 seconds once you have begun CPR. Interrupt compressions only for ventilations or for moving the patient.

The rate for chest compressions refers to the speed rather than the number of compressions the rescuer delivers in 1 minute. Because rescuers must interrupt chest compressions to deliver breaths, the actual number of compressions delivered in 1 minute will be less than 100. To be sure you provide compressions at the proper rate of 100 to 120 per minute, count out loud as you deliver compressions. Many EMS systems require crews to carry and use a metronome to ensure an accurate rate. You may also "hear" specific songs in your head that maintain an approximate 100-beat-per-minute rate. One such song is "Stayin' Alive" by the Bee Gees.

Effective CPR

LO7 Explain the importance of minimizing interruptions during CPR.

You will be performing CPR correctly if:

- your hands are in the center of the patient's chest over the lower half of the sternum.
- you are compressing the chest at least 2 inches hard and fast at a rate of 100 to 120 per minute.
- you are releasing all pressure off the chest between compressions.
- you see the chest rise and fall during ventilations.
- you interrupt compressions as little as possible.

If you are performing CPR correctly, you may notice the patient's skin color improve, but this does not always occur. Sometimes the patient may try to swallow, gasp, or move their limbs. Those actions do not necessarily mean that they are recovering. However, such movements are signs of life and do mean that you should stop CPR and check for the return of breathing and pulse.

If the patient regains a pulse but is not breathing, stop compressions and continue with ventilations only. If there is no pulse, continue CPR. Patients will usually require defibrillation and possibly other advanced medical procedures before they regain heart function.

Adult and Child CPR

LO5 Explain the steps for performing single-rescuer CPR on an adult, child, and infant.

LO8 Explain the steps for performing two-rescuer CPR on an adult, child, and infant.

In this section, we outline step-by-step procedures for performing one- and two-rescuer CPR. These procedures follow the American Heart Association (AHA) recommendations. The extensive research done by the AHA has found them to be most efficient in saving the lives of patients in cardiac arrest. Also, remember that the steps incorporate the primary assessment. Table 11.1 provides a summary of CPR techniques.

One-Rescuer CPR

LO5 Explain the steps for performing single-rescuer CPR on an adult, child, and infant.

To perform one-rescuer CPR on an adult or child (Key Skill 11.2):

1. Position the patient face up on a hard surface and check for responsiveness. Gently tap the patient's shoulder and ask, "Are you okay?" If you are alone with an unresponsive adult patient, call 911 immediately and get a defibrillator if one is available. If you are alone with an unresponsive child, provide 5 cycles of compressions and ventilations (approximately 2 minutes). Then call 911.
2. Check for pulse and breathing for no more than 10 seconds. If pulse and breathing are absent or agonal, begin CPR. Deliver 30 chest compressions. Keep your arms straight, elbows locked, and shoulders directly over the compression site.
   - Compress the adult patient's chest at least 2 inches. Compressions on a child should be about 2 inches.
   - Deliver compressions hard and fast at a rate of 100 to 120 per minute.
   - Release pressure completely to allow the heart to refill.

TABLE 11.1	Summary of CPR Techniques		
	Adult	**Child**	**Infant**
COMPRESSIONS			
Method	Heels of two hands	Heel of one hand or two thumbs	Two fingers or two thumbs with hands encircling chest
Depth	At least 2 inches (5 cm) but not more than 2.4 inches	At least 2 inches but no more than 2.4 inches	One-third the diameter of the chest or about 1.5 inches (4 cm)
Rate	100 to 120/minute	100 to 120/minute	100 to 120/minute
VENTILATIONS (patient with a pulse)			
Method	Barrier device	Barrier device	Barrier device
Rate	1 breath every 6 seconds	1 breath every 2 to 3 seconds	1 breath every 2 to 3 seconds
Ratio of Compressions to Breaths			
One Rescuer	30:2	30:2	30:2
Two Rescuers	30:2	15:2	15:2

One-Rescuer CPR for the Adult or Child

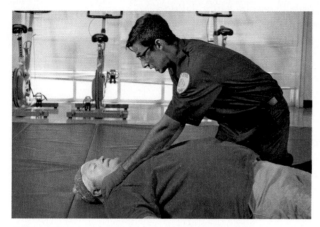

1. Establish responsiveness of patient. If unresponsive, activate 911 and get an AED, if available.

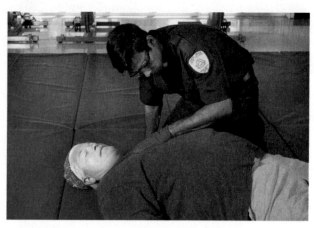

2. Look for signs of a pulse and breathing at the same time.

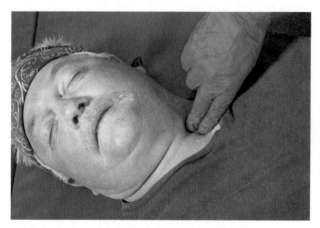

3. Check for a carotid pulse and signs of adequate breathing for no more than 10 seconds.

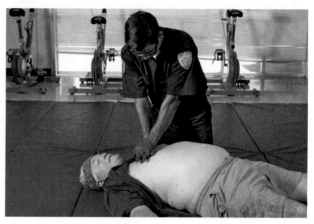

4. If no pulse, begin chest compressions.

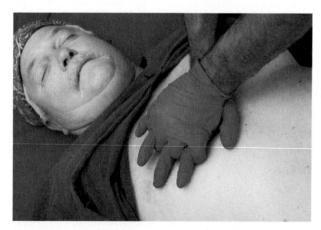

5. Provide 30 compressions at a depth of 2 inches and a rate of 100 to 120 compressions per minute.

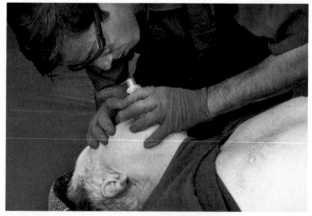

6. After 30 compressions, open the airway and provide 2 ventilations. Each breath should be delivered over 1 second. Look for chest rise and fall.

3. After 30 compressions, open the airway by using the head-tilt/chin-lift maneuver or, if you suspect a spine injury, by using the jaw-thrust maneuver. Provide 2 slow breaths. Allow the chest to fall between breaths. Watch for chest rise and fall with each breath.
4. Continue CPR. Deliver 30 compressions followed by 2 ventilations.
5. If the patient has a carotid pulse but no respirations, provide 1 breath every 6 seconds (10 breaths per minute).
6. Do not interrupt CPR for any longer than 10 seconds or longer than is absolutely necessary. If the patient regains a pulse and/or breathing, stop CPR.

Health care providers, such as Emergency Medical Responders, who have a duty to perform CPR should also be trained, equipped, and authorized to use an automated external defibrillator (AED).

FIRST ON SCENE (continued)

"Sydney, do you copy?" Maria grabs the portable radio after confirming that Chris is not breathing and doesn't have a pulse.

"Yeah, go ahead," comes a reply over the radio.

"I need you to get an ambulance here and bring an AED to the security office right now! Chris is in cardiac arrest!" Maria drops the radio onto the floor next to her and begins chest compressions.

As she counts out loud, she focuses on the hallway monitor to see when Sydney is coming with the AED.

Two-Rescuer CPR

LO8 | Explain the steps for performing two-rescuer CPR on an adult, child, and infant.

All EMS personnel should learn and remain proficient in both one- and two-rescuer CPR techniques. CPR performed by two trained rescuers is more efficient and less tiring for both rescuers (Figure 11.9). Two-rescuer CPR minimizes the transition time between ventilations and compressions and therefore maximizes the effectiveness of both. For the adult patient, the compression-ventilation ratio remains 30:2. When performing two-rescuer CPR on a child, the compression-ventilation ratio changes to 15:2.

Use of an AED is also more efficient with two rescuers. One rescuer can begin to set up the AED and attach the pads to the patient while the other begins a primary assessment of the patient. If you arrive on the scene and find that an AED is being used, ensure that the individuals are performing the steps properly and taking the necessary safety precautions. Offer to assist them and support their actions. You also may need to relieve or guide someone who is unsure of the procedure.

Changing from One- to Two-Rescuer CPR In many situations, a bystander may start one-rescuer CPR before Emergency Medical Responders arrive. Upon arrival, assess the patient's pulse before taking over and performing two-rescuer CPR with your partner.

If you arrive as a sole Emergency Medical Responder and determine that a bystander's CPR techniques are inadequate or incorrect, take over one-rescuer CPR. If the bystander is CPR trained but has no barrier device and is reluctant to ventilate a stranger, perform the ventilations yourself with your own pocket face mask. Have the bystander take over chest compressions. Monitor their effectiveness and provide any necessary coaching to ensure high-quality compressions.

SCENE SAFETY

To perform two-rescuer CPR safely, each rescuer should use their own barrier device with a one-way valve and HEPA filter insert.

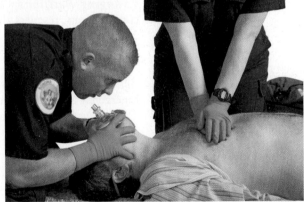

Figure 11.9 During two-rescuer CPR, compressions should be paused to allow for the delivery of ventilations.

CREW RESOURCE MANAGEMENT

Efficiency is especially important when working as a team to resuscitate a patient in cardiac arrest. Each team member should know their role and perform it in concert with other members of the team. This approach is often called "pit crew CPR" because it requires the same kind of synchronized activity that is characteristic of race car pit crews.

If a member of the EMS system is performing CPR when you arrive, begin two-rescuer CPR.

To make a smooth transition from one-rescuer to two-rescuer CPR, follow these steps:

1. If, upon arriving on the scene, you see a rescuer performing CPR, identify yourself. If not already done, activate the EMS system.
2. While the first rescuer is delivering 2 breaths, get in position next to the patient's chest.
3. After the 2 breaths, resume chest compressions. The first rescuer should then resume ventilations, providing 2 ventilations after every 30 of your compressions on an adult patient and after 15 compressions on a pediatric patient.
4. Provide compressions at the rate of 100 to 120 per minute with a pause after every 30 compressions to allow for 2 ventilations.
5. After 2 minutes or approximately 5 cycles of 30 compressions and 2 ventilations, you and the other rescuer change positions.

If the Emergency Medical Responder is equipped with an AED and arrives on the scene to see CPR being performed, they should immediately set it up, turn it on, and attach pads in preparation for early defibrillation. Do this without interrupting the CPR in progress. Stop CPR only when the AED begins to analyze. (Specifics on AED operation are discussed in a later section.)

Compressions and Ventilations During two-rescuer CPR, deliver 30 compressions at a rate of 100 to 120 compressions per minute. After every 30 compressions, deliver 2 ventilations. The compressor counts aloud so both rescuers are able to establish and maintain the correct rate. By hearing the count, the ventilator is prepared to provide a breath after every 30 compressions while the compressor pauses to allow for adequate ventilation.

CPR Procedure The complete sequence for two-rescuer CPR is illustrated in Key Skill 11.3. Your instructor will demonstrate how to ventilate a patient in both positions—top and lateral—using the barrier devices and oxygen-delivery equipment that your jurisdiction requires.

Changing Positions To minimize rescuer fatigue and ensure high-quality chest compressions, rescuers should change positions after every set of 5 cycles (approximately 2 minutes). At the end of 30 compressions, the ventilator provides 2 ventilations. Then the rescuers quickly change positions.

Activating the EMS System With pediatric patients, it is recommended that the solo Emergency Medical Responder provide 2 minutes of rescue support before activating EMS. This is due to the fact that most pediatric cardiac arrests are caused by respiratory arrest. You may be able to carry the child or infant and continue emergency care while calling EMS.

CREW RESOURCE MANAGEMENT

Changing positions during two-rescuer CPR maximizes its effectiveness by keeping the compressor from becoming fatigued. It is crucial to rotate positions every 2 minutes. Communication is key to making this change as seamlessly as possible, taking no more than 10 seconds to complete.

REMEMBER

Overinflation of the chest during ventilation increases the pressure in the chest. This reduces the amount of blood that returns to the heart, causing CPR to be less effective. Inflate the lungs just to the point when you notice chest rise but no farther.

Two-Rescuer CPR for the Adult or Child

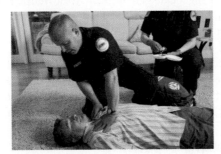

1. The first rescuer positions the patient and determines unresponsiveness. If the patient is unresponsive, activate 911 and obtain an AED.

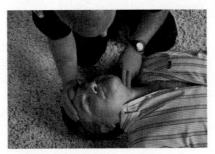

2. Assess for signs of a pulse and breathing for no more than 10 seconds.

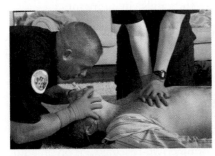

3. If no pulse, the second rescuer locates the compression site and begins compressions. Deliver 30 compressions at a rate of 100 to 120 per minute.

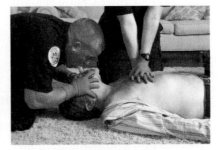

4. After each set of 30 compressions, the first rescuer provides 2 slow back-to-back breaths, each lasting 1 second, waiting for the chest to fall between breaths. The second rescuer should pause compressions to allow for adequate ventilations.

Infant and Neonatal CPR

LO5 Explain the steps for performing single-rescuer CPR on an adult, child, and infant.

LO8 Explain the steps for performing two-rescuer CPR on an adult, child, and infant.

For the purposes of field resuscitation, neonate and infant patients are defined as follows:

- A **neonate** is a baby less than 1 month of age.
- An **infant** is a child older than 1 month and less than 1 year of age.

neonate ▶ baby less than 1 month of age

infant ▶ child between 1 month and 1 year of age

Positioning the Infant

Just as you do for adults and children, place the infant patient face up on a hard, flat surface. Be aware that infant's heads are larger in proportion to their bodies than those of children and adults. When an infant is on their back, their neck may flex forward, potentially closing the airway. To help ensure an open airway, maintain the head in a neutral position.[4] It may be necessary to provide support under the shoulders with a folded blanket or towel (Figure 11.10).

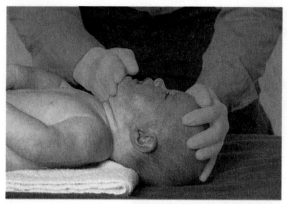
Figure 11.10 To help maintain airway alignment of an infant, place a folded towel or similar material beneath the shoulders. Note that head is in sniffing position.

Opening the Airway

It takes very little effort to open an infant's airway. For an infant with no spine injury, use the head-tilt/chin-lift maneuver. With one hand, tilt the head gently back to a neutral or slightly extended position. This is sometimes referred to as the **sniffing position**. Extending the neck of an infant too far can cause the airway to close off and keep air from entering the lungs.

Place your fingers under the bony part of the chin, and lift to finish the technique of opening the airway. Be careful not to compress the soft tissues of the neck because this may obstruct the airway. In cases of suspected spine injury, use the jaw-thrust maneuver.

Assessing Breathing

Assess for signs of breathing. Look for the rise and fall of the chest and abdomen. If there is no breathing, check for the presence of a pulse.

sniffing position ▶ slight extension of the neck and head

Checking for a Pulse

Follow these steps when assessing for a pulse in an infant:

1. Feel for a pulse at the brachial artery for no more than 10 seconds.
2. The brachial pulse point is located on the medial side of the arm between the elbow and armpit.

Infant CPR Techniques

LO5 Explain the steps for performing single-rescuer CPR on an adult, child, and infant.

LO8 Explain the steps for performing two-rescuer CPR on an adult, child, and infant.

Ventilations If your assessment finds the infant patient has a good pulse but is not breathing adequately or breathing is absent, provide rescue breaths (ventilations). With the airway open and using an appropriate barrier device, provide ventilations at a rate of 1 breath every 2 to 3 seconds. To ensure appropriate volume, look for chest rise. Be careful not to overinflate the lungs, which can cause air to enter the stomach (gastric distention) and vomiting.

You may find it easier to seal your mouth over the infant's mouth and nose. If the patient is a very large infant, seal your mouth over the patient's mouth and pinch the nostrils closed. If you do not see chest rise after repositioning the airway, begin chest compressions.

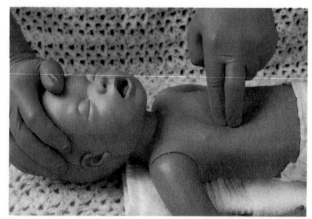
Figure 11.11 For compressions on an infant, place two fingers on the center of the chest just below the nipple line.

External Chest Compressions For infant CPR, external chest compressions and artificial ventilation can easily be performed by a single rescuer or shared between two trained rescuers, depending on available resources.

In infant CPR, apply compressions to the center of the chest. Place two fingers on the sternum, just below the nipple line (Figure 11.11). Compress the infant's sternum one-third the anterior-posterior diameter of the chest, or about 1.5 inches (4 cm). Compress at a rate of 100 to 120 per minute.

If possible, maintain an open airway with one hand while compressing the chest with two fingers of the other hand. Provide 2 rescue breaths after each set of 30 compressions. Watch carefully for the rise and fall of the infant's chest.

When there are two rescuers, the preferred method for chest compressions for the infant is the two-thumbs, encircling-hands technique. One rescuer (compressor) places both thumbs

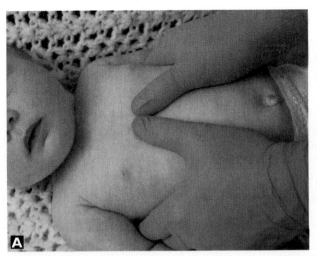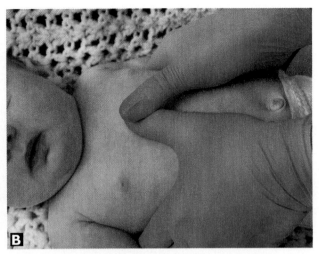

Figure 11.12 (A) For an infant, place two thumbs side-by-side on the center of the chest, just below the nipple line. (B) For a neonate, place two thumbs one on top of the other on the center of the chest, just below the nipple line.

side-by-side over the lower half of the infant's sternum or about one finger-width below the nipple line (Figure 11.12A and B). For very small infants or newborns, you may place one thumb on top of the other. The other rescuer provides ventilations.

Infant CPR Rates and Ratios   For infant CPR, deliver compressions at the rate of 100 to 120 per minute. For a single rescuer, perform compressions and ventilations at a ratio of 30:2. For two rescuers, perform compressions and ventilations at a ratio of 15:2.

The following steps outline key points for infant CPR:

1. Determine unresponsiveness by gently tapping the bottom of the infant's feet and shouting, "Are you all right?" If no response, then . . .
2. Direct someone to call EMS. If you are alone, provide 2 minutes of CPR before calling EMS. Most pediatric cardiac arrests are caused by respiratory arrest; therefore they are likely to respond to immediate CPR.
3. Position the infant in a supine (face-up) position on a flat, hard surface. You may support small infants on your forearm.
4. Check for signs of a pulse and breathing.
5. If there is a pulse but no respirations, provide ventilations at a rate of 1 breath every 2 to 3 seconds. If there is no pulse or there is a heart rate of less than 60 beats per minute, begin compressions.
6. Provide chest compressions. Place two fingers in the center of the chest just below the nipple line. Compress at a rate of 100 to 120 per minute. Provide ventilations at a 30:2 ratio if performed by one rescuer and 15:2 if performed by two rescuers.

Possible Complications

In some cases, damage to the chest may occur even when CPR is performed properly. Providing proper chest compressions on an adult will likely result in the separation of the cartilage where the ribs meet the sternum, which produces a cracking sound. During the first few compressions, you are likely to feel and hear a popping sound, much like when a person cracks their knuckles. Do not stop CPR. Instead, reconfirm proper hand position, and continue to provide compressions. This is an expected side effect of good chest compressions. A fractured rib will heal. But stopping CPR will result in death.

Another problem occurs when too much air is forced into the patient's lungs. The excess air overflows out of the lungs and enters the stomach by way of the esophagus. This can result in gastric distention. Do not try to force excess air out of the stomach. To do so might cause the patient to vomit, which could lead to airway obstruction. In some cases, the patient may aspirate (inhale) stomach contents, and if you try to provide breaths, you will force the vomit into the lungs.

Special CPR Situations

In some cases, depending on the patient's situation and condition, steps related to CPR may need to be modified to provide the best care. Always follow local protocols.

Moving the Patient

Usually, there are only two reasons for an Emergency Medical Responder to move a patient who is receiving CPR: transport and immediate danger at the scene. Most of the time, the patient is moved after the EMTs assume responsibility for care. In preparation for transport when the EMTs arrive, place the cardiac-arrest patient on a long spine board when available. This will allow for easy transfer to the stretcher and provide a firm surface when doing compressions.

Trauma

Many rescuers are unsure about starting CPR on trauma patients. When rescuers see indications of possible injuries to the neck or spine, they may feel it is more important to immobilize the spine before they start CPR. If rescuers find a patient with a crushed chest, they may be afraid of causing internal injuries if they perform chest compressions. Patient injuries should not prevent you from starting CPR. If you delay or do not start CPR, the patient will die.

Hypothermia

Patients who are victims of prolonged exposure to a cold environment (hypothermia) may have vital signs that are very difficult to assess. You should take extra time—at least a full minute—when assessing both pulse and breathing. No attempt should be made to rewarm the patient in the field. Resuscitation attempts should continue until the patient can be rewarmed by the receiving facility. In most cases, a patient is not considered dead until the core body temperature has been raised and they remain unresponsive to resuscitation efforts.

Stopping CPR

When caring for a patient in cardiac arrest, your duties are twofold: to have someone activate EMS and to start CPR immediately. Only a medical director or a health care provider at the scene who has accepted responsibility for the patient may order you not to begin CPR. You also may choose not to begin CPR if there are obvious signs of prolonged death, such as the presence of muscle rigidity (rigor mortis) and pooling of blood (lividity).

Patients who are elderly and/or who have terminal cancer or other medical conditions may have signed documents declaring their wishes as to whether they want CPR to be performed in the event of a cardiac arrest. These documents are referred to as advance directives and Do Not Resuscitate (DNR) orders. They may be a legal document or simply a statement signed by the patient and their health care provider. If it is unclear whether a DNR order exists for the patient, it is prudent to begin CPR while others look for the paperwork. If the proper DNR documentation is presented, it is appropriate to stop resuscitative efforts.

Bystanders and members of the patient's family may tell you that the patient would not want to be resuscitated. You are not to obey such requests without seeing proper documentation. Let the family know that you understand their feelings, but your duty as an Emergency Medical Responder is to begin CPR. If the family does not have the required documentation for the patient, you must begin CPR.

The longer a patient is in cardiac arrest before CPR is started, the less likely CPR will be effective. Once you have started CPR, continue to provide CPR until:

- the patient regains a pulse; then provide ventilations only.
- spontaneous pulse and breathing begin.
- equally or more highly trained members of the EMS system can continue in your place.
- you turn over responsibility for patient care to a physician.
- you are exhausted and no longer able to continue.

REMEMBER

In spite of a family member's request to not perform CPR on a patient, you must have appropriate legal documentation of the patient's wishes in the form of an advance directive or Do Not Resuscitate (DNR) order. If it is unclear whether or not a DNR order exists for the patient, begin CPR while others look for the documentation.

Automated External Defibrillation

LO9 Explain the purpose of an automated external defibrillator (AED).

EMS personnel and many laypeople are trained in the use of an automated external defibrillator (AED). AEDs can assess a heart's rhythm, determine if defibrillation is necessary, and deliver an electric shock when needed. Almost all jurisdictions have approved and adopted the use of AEDs.

External Defibrillation

The term **fibrillation** refers to disorganized electrical activity within the heart that renders it incapable of pumping blood. The most common cause of fibrillation in the adult patient is a heart attack, while the most common cause in the pediatric patient is respiratory arrest. Fibrillation results in a disorganized quivering of the heart muscle, much like a spasm or seizure.

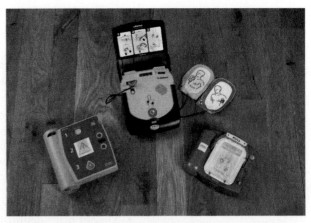

Figure 11.13 Examples of various AEDs on the market today.

Defibrillators are designed to deliver an electric shock that will convert an abnormal heart rhythm to a normal rhythm so the heart can begin beating normally. The shock does not start a heart that has stopped completely, but it will give the fibrillating heart a chance to spontaneously reestablish an effective rhythm on its own. The entire process is called defibrillation.[5]

Many kinds of defibrillators are available today. The two basic kinds are manual defibrillators and automated external defibrillators (AEDs). Most ALS providers carry manual defibrillators. They require the rescuer to interpret the patient's heart rhythm and then decide whether the patient should receive a shock. The skills needed to accomplish those tasks require significant training beyond the level of most Emergency Medical Responders and EMTs.

The AED (Figure 11.13) can be fully automated or semiautomated:

- The fully automated AED assesses the patient's heart rhythm, advises that a shock is necessary, and delivers the shock without any input from the rescuer.
- Semiautomated defibrillators analyze the patient's rhythm and simply advise the rescuer if a shock is needed. The rescuer must then push a button to deliver the shock.

AEDs can recognize two very specific abnormal heart rhythms: ventricular fibrillation and ventricular tachycardia. The most common type of fibrillation affects the lower half (ventricles) of the heart and is called **ventricular fibrillation (VF)**. When an individual's heart goes into VF, the brain and other vital organs no longer receive an adequate supply of oxygenated blood, and the patient becomes unresponsive. VF does not produce blood flow or a pulse, so the patient will be found unresponsive with no pulse and no breathing. The sooner VF can be defibrillated, the better the patient's chances for survival.

AEDs can also recognize the abnormal heart rhythm called **ventricular tachycardia**, V-tach for short. V-tach is a rapid rhythm that originates in the ventricles and rarely produces a pulse. It does not pump blood very efficiently. Less than 10 percent of the prehospital cardiac arrest cases have this problem. Defibrillation may help some of these patients.

When there is no electrical activity within the heart, the condition is called **asystole** or "flatline" because the lack of electrical activity would appear as a flat line on an electrocardiogram. In this situation, an AED would not be effective.

fibrillation ▶ disorganized electrical activity within the heart that renders the heart incapable of pumping blood.

ventricular fibrillation ▶ disorganized electrical activity, causing ineffective contractions of the lower heart chambers (ventricles). Abbrev: VF.

ventricular tachycardia ▶ abnormally rapid contraction of the heart's lower chambers, resulting in very poor circulation; also called *V-tach*.

asystole ▶ no electrical activity within the heart; also called *flatline*.

CREW RESOURCE MANAGEMENT

Once the AED is on scene, it is a good practice to dedicate one person on the crew to manage the device. This person can also keep an eye on the quality of compressions and ventilations and can provide feedback to the team as appropriate.

Using AEDs

LO10 Describe the indications and contraindications for the use of an AED.

A defibrillator must be ready for use at any given moment. Make certain you follow manufacturer guidelines to ensure that the defibrillators you use are in working order and prepared for use.

Basic Warnings   Emergency Medical Responders may be trained to use either fully automated or semiautomated defibrillators. The medical director for your EMS system may have approved one or both of these devices. Whichever your system uses, you are responsible for noting certain warnings when working with AEDs:

- Place the AED only on a patient who is in cardiac arrest.
- Do not place defibrillator patches over a patient's medication patch or implanted pacemaker. With gloved hands, remove the medication patch and wipe the chest dry.
- Make certain that no one is touching the patient during the "analyze" or "shock" phases.
- Do not attempt to assess or shock a patient who is moving or when the defibrillator or its leads are being moved.
- Do not attempt to defibrillate a patient who is lying in a puddle of water.
- Your medical director may have specific guidelines for defibrillating infants under 1 year of age. Follow your local protocols.

Protocols for the use of AEDs for trauma patients vary by state and jurisdiction. Follow your EMS system's protocols, and carefully assess the patient and mechanism of injury or the nature of the illness. Contact medical direction if you are not certain about what to do.

Patients with certain heart conditions may have a small internal defibrillator surgically implanted inside the chest or abdomen. This device, called an implantable cardioverter defibrillator (ICD) is very much like an external AED, only much smaller. It detects abnormal heart rhythms and delivers electric shocks when needed to restore a normal rhythm. You might not know the device is in place unless the patient or a family member tells you it is there. Your care of a patient in cardiac arrest will not change with the presence of an ICD.

When to Place an AED   The use of a defibrillator must follow specific procedures of assessment and care. You must determine if the patient is, indeed, a candidate for the placement of an AED. To be a candidate, the patient must:

- be unresponsive.
- have no carotid pulse.
- have no normal respirations.

All the criteria must be met before you can place an AED on a patient who is in suspected cardiac arrest.

Perform a primary assessment to confirm that the patient is, indeed, in cardiac arrest. If you are first on the scene and have confirmed the patient meets all the criteria, begin CPR and place the AED as soon as possible. If you do not have an AED, continue CPR.

If you arrive on scene with an AED and someone else is providing CPR, your job will be to prepare and attach the defibrillator. Make certain that both of you are clear of the patient before delivering a shock.

If a cardiac arrest is witnessed, you should begin CPR immediately and place an AED as soon as it is available. In the event of an unwitnessed cardiac arrest, some medical directors may recommend performing CPR for approximately 2 minutes before attempting to defibrillate. This will provide circulation to the heart muscle, which may increase the chances of successful defibrillation in some patients.

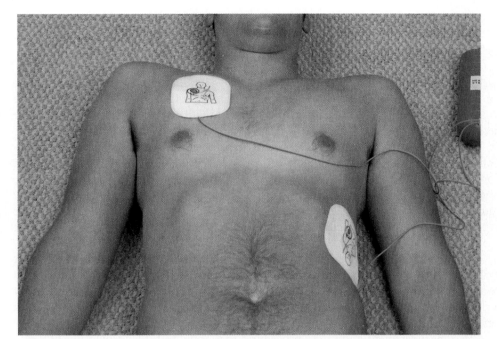

Figure 11.14 Correct placement of AED electrode pads on an adult chest.

Attaching the Defibrillator   While the first rescuer performs CPR, the rescuer operating the AED should perform the following steps:

1. Bare the patient's chest. If the patient's chest is wet, quickly wipe it dry. Make certain the patient is not lying in a puddle of standing water. Ground that is wet with no standing water is safe for defibrillation.
2. It is important that the surface of the patient's chest, where the pads are to be placed, is dry. Place pads on the patient's bare, dry chest one at a time. It may be necessary to shave the chest because hair can prevent the pads from sticking properly. Place one pad on the patient's upper right chest below the clavicle (collarbone) and next to the sternum (breastbone). Place the second pad on the patient's left side just below the nipple line. Most pads and devices have illustrations showing the correct placement of the pads (Figure 11.14).
3. Finally, make sure the pads are firmly plugged into the device. Some pads come preconnected, and others need to be plugged in after the pads have been placed. Follow the specific directions for your device.

FIRST ON SCENE (continued)

Maria's arms and lower back are beginning to ache when Sydney turns the corner at the end of the hall and sprints to the locked office door. The sound of footfalls grows louder until they slide to a halt, and she hears her fumble with a set of keys, find the right one, and push the door open.

Fluorescent lights flood the small office, making Maria squint and causing Chris to look hideously pale. "Quick!" Maria shouts. "Get the AED on him!"

Sydney pops the cover open, glancing at the large, illustrated directions as she turns on the unit and pulls out the electrode pads. The AED begins to provide audible verbal instructions as Maria grabs Chris's shirt and tears it open, sending buttons skittering in all directions.

Maria stretches her back, panting, as Sydney yanks the paper backing from each electrode and places them on Chris's motionless body.

AEDs will not function properly if the pads do not fully adhere to the patient's chest and/or the cables are not tightly inserted into the device. If either of these problems exist, the "No contact" or "Check pads" prompt will sound or appear on the AED.

Operating the Semiautomated Defibrillator The following is an example of the operational procedure for a semiautomatic AED. Several semiautomatic models are currently available. Follow the instructions given in the manufacturer's manual for your specific model.

The AED sequence presented here is a typical protocol programmed into many AEDs. Each EMS system has its own protocols for the use of AEDs, which may differ from what is presented here. Some jurisdictions may require Emergency Medical Responders to give a different number of shocks before transporting or continuing CPR, while others may require rescuers to perform CPR for 2 full minutes or perform some other step before preparing and attaching the defibrillator. Always know and follow local protocols before attempting to use an AED.

Once turned on and applied to the patient, semiautomatic AEDs will analyze the heart rhythm and advise if a shock is necessary. Some models require pushing a button to begin the analysis sequence. In either case, the AED will automatically charge to a preset energy level. At this point, it is necessary for the rescuer to push a button to deliver the shock (Key Skill 11.4).

The same assessment and safety procedures that apply to fully automatic AEDs also apply to the operation of semiautomatic AEDs. Some older models may not have a voice synthesizer. Regardless of the model, they all require the rescuer to push a button to deliver the shock.

KEY SKILL 11.4

Operating an AED

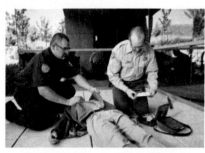

1. Once you have confirmed that the patient is unresponsive and has no pulse, turn on the AED and move or remove any clothing covering the patient's chest.

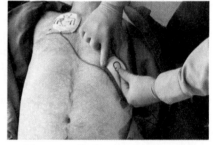

2. Place the pads and connect the cable to the device (if not already connected).

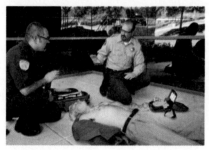

3. When prompted, clear the patient and press the "Shock" button.

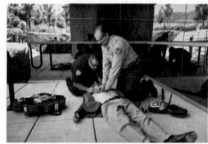

4. After delivery of the shock, immediately begin chest compressions.

To operate a semiautomatic AED, you should:

1. Assess the patient to confirm that they are in cardiac arrest.
2. Have your partner or someone else trained to perform CPR begin CPR while you set up the AED. If you are alone, make sure EMS has been called and immediately attach the AED.
3. Turn on the AED and attach the pads. Once the pads are in place, the AED will begin to analyze the patient's heart rhythm. Some devices may require you to press the "Analyze" button. Make certain that no one is touching the patient while the device analyzes.
4. If a shockable rhythm is detected, the AED will advise so and charge to the appropriate energy level. When needed, the AED will prompt you to push the "Shock" button.
5. After you push the "Shock" button, the AED will deliver one shock.
6. Following the shock, immediately begin CPR. (The most current AEDs are programmed to pause for 2 minutes after each shock to allow you to perform CPR.)
7. After 2 minutes, the AED will advise you to stop CPR. It will then reanalyze the heart rhythm and, if indicated, advise the rescuer to deliver another shock. This sequence of one shock followed by 2 minutes of CPR should continue until more highly trained providers arrive on scene.

Potential Problems

The majority of problems with AED operations can be easily corrected. Most problems involve poor attachment of the pads or cables. Ensuring that the pads are in full contact with the patient's chest and that the cables are tightly connected to the device is usually all that is needed.

Make sure the patient's chest is dry and free of anything that can prevent the pad from adhering well, such as hair or medication patches that occupy the pad placement sites. With gloved hands, remove any medication patches and wipe off any medication remaining on the patient's chest. If necessary, shave the pad placement areas of the patient's chest using the disposable safety razor provided in the AED kit for this purpose.

Most AEDs are programmed to run self-diagnostic checks every 24 hours. Should one of the self-checks detect a failure of any of the AED's internal systems, an error message or audible alarm will sound, alerting the rescuer to the failure. It is important to know the error messages that can be displayed by your specific device. Some errors are only advisory in nature and allow continued use of the device, while others indicate a failure of a major system, rendering the AED inoperable. Become familiar with all error messages and alarms.

Quality Assurance

To be effective, a prehospital AED program requires ongoing evaluation to identify and correct any problems. This process of assessment and quality assurance should focus on specific situations that involve standard operating procedures, equipment performance, routine maintenance, physician-directed standing orders, care delivered by rescuers, and the effectiveness of training programs. Changes in any aspect of the program must be the result of a medical director's evaluation and orders.

All AEDs have an internal recording device that can digitally record the patient's heart rhythm, including shocks delivered. This information can be downloaded to a computer so the medical director can evaluate the event. Evaluation is an important part of any AED program and serves to improve rescuer performance and ensure quality patient care.

Carefully document all incidents involving the use of an AED. Your notes should include the time you arrived on scene, your assessment findings, the number of shocks delivered, and the patient's response following each shock.

Part of your equipment inspection and assessment should include the operation of AED recording devices. Follow the manufacturer's instructions and your EMS system's

SCENE SAFETY

Make certain that no one is touching the patient when a shock is delivered. Before pressing the "Shock" button, check the patient from head to toe and verbally confirm that everyone is "all clear."

REMEMBER

Always follow the manufacturer's manual and your EMS system's guidelines for the AED you use.

recommendations to correct any problems before the unit is put into service. In addition, it is important to ensure that the AED kit always includes the necessary supplies, such as an extra set of electrode pads (adult and pediatric), razors, gloves, and towels.

FIRST ON SCENE WRAP-UP

The afternoon crowd in the casino is sparse, and not many people notice the ambulance crew pulling their gurney through the main doors and walking quickly to the bank of elevators. On the third floor, they meet a woman who directs them down a long hallway to the CCTV room. A woman in a disheveled business suit is sitting cross-legged on the floor next to an older man in the recovery position.

"It worked," she says with a huge, tired smile. The patient is breathing steadily and slowly running his fingers over the foam pads stuck to his chest.

"You're a very lucky man," one of the EMTs says as she places an oxygen mask on the patient's face. "It looks like this young lady over here saved your life."

Chris looks over at Maria, who is now blushing, and smiles weakly as he pats her hand. "Thank you," he mouths, the hissing oxygen louder than his quiet words.

Summary

- Like the chain of EMS resources, the chain of survival is also a linked system of patient-care events. These events include immediate recognition and activation of EMS, early CPR, rapid defibrillation, effective advanced life support (ALS), post-cardiac arrest care, and recovery care. In the case of pediatric cardiac arrest, prevention is also part of the chain.
- Survival of the brain depends on breathing and circulation. When the heart stops beating, a patient is in cardiac arrest and cannot circulate oxygenated blood to the brain. The major signs of cardiac arrest are unresponsiveness, no breathing, and no pulse.
- If a patient is unresponsive, call 911 and check for a pulse and breathing. If the patient is not breathing or has only gasping breaths, begin CPR immediately.
- If you are alone and caring for a pediatric patient, provide 2 minutes of CPR before leaving the child to activate EMS.
- To provide proper CPR, you will place the patient in a supine position on a hard surface. If the patient is unresponsive, check for signs of a pulse and breathing. If patient is not breathing or is showing only gasping breaths, begin CPR.
  - For an adult or child, provide compressions at a rate of 100 to 120 per minute and a depth of 2 inches (5 cm). Compressions that are too deep may damage internal organs.
  - For an infant (up to 1 year of age), provide compressions at a rate of 100 to 120 per minute and compress the chest one-third the depth of the infant's chest or about 1.5 inches.
  - After 30 compressions, provide 2 rescue breaths over 1 second each and begin compressions again. Do not stop CPR for more than 10 seconds other than to move the patient because of danger at the scene. Continue CPR until the patient regains a pulse and/or breathing or until you are relieved by an equally or more highly trained individual, care for the patient is accepted by a physician, or until you can no longer continue because of exhaustion.
- Automated external defibrillators (AEDs) are lifesaving units used by Emergency Medical Responders and are available in many public locations. AEDs are electrical devices that can convert certain abnormal heart rhythms to a normal cardiac rhythm; they must be used with caution and according to specific protocols.
- The general steps for the use of a typical AED are as follows:
  - Confirm the patient is unresponsive and has no breathing or pulse.
  - Turn on the AED, expose the patient's chest, and securely attach the pads. Wipe dry or shave hair if necessary.
  - Follow the AED's prompts to defibrillate and check breathing and pulse. Follow AED prompts to check a pulse or start CPR if there is no pulse.

Take Action

Local Resources

As more and more people become trained in their use, AEDs are becoming more widely available. It is quite common to find AEDs available for public access in airports, shopping malls, amusement parks, and any place that attracts the public in large numbers. In fact, there are probably at least several businesses in your own town or city that have an AED and personnel trained in its use.

For this activity, identify at least three public locations that have AEDs available. You will have to make some calls or talk to people who work in different locations. You may wish to contact the following agencies and locations to ask if they have AEDs available in the event of a cardiac arrest. Also ask which employees are trained in their use.

- *Large shopping malls.* Often it is the security staff that carries the AED and is trained in its use.
- *Large employers.* Many large employers have designated employees, often members of specialized teams or Security departments, who are trained to respond to medical emergencies.
- *Police agencies.* Some jurisdictions have police vehicles equipped with AEDs.
- *Public venues.* Often airports, fairgrounds, race tracks, zoos, museums, and amusement parks have AEDs available.

First on Scene Patient Handoff

We have a male, approximately 60 years of age, who experienced a witnessed cardiac arrest approximately 10 minutes ago. CPR was initiated immediately, and an AED was placed approximately 4 minutes following the arrest. The AED delivered one shock, and we have been continuing CPR since the last shock. It is unknown if the patient has any cardiac history.

First on Scene Run Review

Recall the events of the First on Scene scenario in this chapter, and answer the following questions. Rationales are offered in the Answer Key at the back of the book.

1. Did Maria respond appropriately following Chris's collapse to the floor? What should you look for when determining if your patient is breathing?
2. Was it the correct decision for Sydney to put the AED on Chris? What are the criteria for using an AED on a patient in cardiac arrest?
3. What information should Maria give the EMTs when they arrive?

Quick Quiz

To check your understanding of the chapter, answer the following questions. Then compare your answers to those in the Answer Key.

1. The appropriate rate of compressions during CPR is ____ per minute.
   a. 80 to 100
   b. no faster than 80
   c. 100 to 120
   d. no faster than 120

2. You are caring for an adult patient who was found unresponsive. You cannot locate a pulse and observe only gasping respirations. You should:
   a. open the airway and give a breath.
   b. attempt to locate a pulse for 30 seconds.
   c. begin chest compressions.
   d. look for signs of drug overdose.

3. The recommended location for assessing for the presence of a pulse on a child is at the ____ artery.
   a. brachial
   b. carotid
   c. radial
   d. femoral

4. What is the most common cause of pediatric cardiac arrest?
   a. Respiratory arrest
   b. Coronary artery disease
   c. Congenital heart defects
   d. Shaken baby syndrome

5. What is the recommended ratio of chest compressions to ventilations for an adult patient in cardiac arrest?
   a. 30 to 2
   b. 15 to 2
   c. 5 to 1
   d. 3 to 1

6. You are caring for an adult victim of sudden cardiac arrest. To give this patient the best chance for survival, you should provide immediate:
   a. CPR without defibrillation.
   b. defibrillation without CPR.
   c. CPR with supplemental oxygen.
   d. CPR with defibrillation as soon as possible.

7. What is the most common cause of cardiac arrest in the adult population?
   a. Stroke
   b. Diabetes
   c. Heart attack
   d. Drug overdose

8. You are caring for a child who has a good pulse but is not breathing on her own. You should provide rescue breaths for this patient once every ____ seconds.
   a. 2 to 3
   b. 5 to 6
   c. 6 to 7
   d. 10

9. Which of the following statements best describes the appropriate ventilation volume for a child who is not breathing?
   a. Twice that of an infant
   b. The weight minus the age
   c. Enough to cause the chest to rise
   d. Exactly half the volume of an adult

10. After assessing responsiveness, you must check for the presence of normal breathing. Do this by:
    a. shaking the patient.
    b. looking for chest rise.
    c. observing pupil response.
    d. sweeping the mouth for obstructions.

11. You have just delivered a shock with an automated external defibrillator (AED). You should:
    a. check for the presence of a pulse.
    b. begin chest compressions.
    c. check for breathing.
    d. press the "Analyse" button on the AED.

12. You are alone when you discover and remove an unresponsive 4-year-old child from a public pool. When should you call 911?
    a. After providing 2 minutes of CPR
    b. Immediately after removing him from the pool
    c. After 10 minutes of CPR with no response
    d. After rescue breaths but before compressions

13. Which of the following represents the most appropriate hand location for chest compressions on an adult?

   a. Over the lower half of the sternum
   b. Over the top of the sternum
   c. Over the left side of the chest
   d. On the very bottom of the sternum

14. Which of the following best describes the purpose of an automated external defibrillator?

   a. It restarts breathing in an apneic patient.
   b. It clears the blockage of the coronary arteries.
   c. It returns the patient to consciousness.
   d. It corrects an abnormal heart rhythm.

15. You are at a Little League baseball game and see a parent collapse to the ground. You are the first individual to reach the woman. You should first:

   a. place her in the recovery position.
   b. send someone to call 911.
   c. check for responsiveness.
   d. give 2 slow breaths.

Endnotes

1. "Cardiopulmonary Resuscitation Quality: [corrected] Improving Cardiac Resuscitation Outcomes Both Inside and Outside the Hospital: A Consensus Statement from the American Heart Association," *Circulation*, Vol. 128, No. 4 (July 23, 2013): 417–435.

2. Theresa M. Olasveengen, Mary E. Mancini, Gavin D. Perkins, Suzanne Avis, Steven Brooks, Maaret Castrén, Sung Phil Chung, Julie Considine, Keith Couper, Raffo Escalante, Tetsuo Hatanaka, Kevin K. C. Hung, Peter Kudenchuk, Swee Han Lim, Chika Nishiyama, Giuseppe Ristagno, Federico Semeraro, Christopher M. Smith, Michael A. Smyth, Christian Vaillancourt, Jerry P. Nolan, Mary Fran Hazinski, Peter T. Morley, Adult Basic Life Support Collaborators, "Adult Basic Life Support: 2020 International Consensus on Cardiopulmonary Resuscitation and Emergency Cardiovascular Care Science with Treatment Recommendations," *Circulation*, Vol. 142, No. 16, Suppl. 1 (October 20, 2020): S41–S91.

3. Lance B. Becker, Robert A. Berg, Paul E. Pepe, Ahamed H. Idris, Thomas P. Aufderheide, Thomas A. Barnes, Samuel J. Stratton, Nisha C. Chandra, "A Reappraisal of Mouth-to-Mouth Ventilation During Bystander-Initiated Cardiopulmonary Resuscitation. A Statement for Healthcare Professionals from the Ventilation Working Group of the Basic Life Support and Pediatric Life Support Subcommittees, American Heart Association," *Circulation*, Vol. 96 (1997): 2102–2112.

4. Nypaver, M. and Treloar, D., "Neutral Cervical Spine Positioning in Children," *Annals of Emergency Medicine*, Vol. 23, No. 2 (1994): 208–211.

5. "Defibrillation," American Heart Association website, updated February 21, 2012. Accessed June 3, 2014, at http://www.heart.org/HEARTORG/Conditions/Arrhythmia/PreventionTreatmentofArrhythmia/Defibrillation_UCM_305002_Article.jsp

12

Obtaining a Medical History and Vital Signs

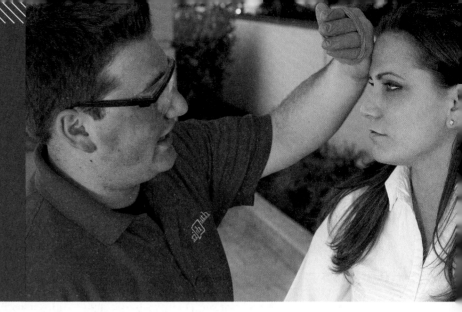

Education Standards

Assessment—Secondary Assessment, History Taking, Monitoring Devices

Competencies

Use scene information and patient assessment findings to identify and manage immediate life threats and injuries within the scope of practice of the EMR.

LEARNING OBJECTIVES

Upon successful completion of this chapter, the student should be able to:

Cognitive

1. Define the chapter key terms.

2. Explain the importance of a thorough medical history.

3. Explain the difference between a sign and a symptom.

4. Describe the components of the SAMPLE history tool.

5. Describe the components of the OPQRST assessment tool.

6. State the characteristics that are obtained and measured when assessing respirations, pulse, blood pressure, skin signs, and pupils.

7. Describe the methods used to assess each of the five primary vital signs.

8. Differentiate normal and abnormal vital sign values for the infant, child, and adult patient.

9. Explain the role that monitoring vital signs plays in the overall assessment and care of the patient.

10. Differentiate the techniques used to assess a pulse in an infant, child, and adult patient.

Psychomotor

11. Demonstrate the ability to properly obtain and accurately trend and document vital signs.

Affective

12. Demonstrate a caring and compassionate attitude with classmates and simulated patients.

KEY TERMS

auscultation (*p. 237*)
baseline vital signs (*p. 231*)
blood pressure (*p. 235*)
capillary refill (*p. 242*)
cyanotic (*p. 240*)
diaphoretic (*p. 241*)
diastolic (*p. 236*)
hypertension (*p. 236*)
jaundice (*p. 240*)
medical history (*p. 225*)
mental status (*p. 230*)

OPQRST assessment tool (*p. 228*)
palpation (*p. 237*)
pulse (*p. 233*)
SAMPLE history tool (*p. 227*)
sign (*p. 225*)
stethoscope (*p. 237*)
symptom (*p. 226*)
systolic (*p. 236*)
trending (*p. 231*)
vital signs (*p. 230*)

Two of the most powerful skills you must develop to properly care for ill or injured patients are asking good questions and accurately assessing a patient's vital signs. Together, they make up much of the assessment for every patient you encounter.

Obtaining a good medical history requires that you become comfortable asking very personal questions related to a patient's medical condition. You must learn the appropriate questions to ask for the specific situation, as well as those that will provide insight into pertinent past medical history.

In addition to developing your interviewing skills, you must learn to properly obtain complete and accurate vital signs. Obtaining vital signs requires several isolated skills that will enhance your ability to see, touch, and hear what is going on with your patient. This chapter introduces basic principles and offers many tips that will assist you in developing your proficiency in obtaining a medical history and vital signs.

FIRST ON SCENE

"Call an ambulance, Eduardo! I'm on my way over!" Morgan, a newly certified Emergency Medical Responder, slams down the phone and ducks under her desk to grab the first-aid bag. As she dashes down the entryway of the quiet, empty lodge, she begins to run the coming scenario through her mind. It will take EMS a good 15 minutes to reach the hotel on this side of the lake, so she knows she will have time to get a complete set of vitals.

"There you are, Morgan!" The young hotel employee seems shaken. "I called for an ambulance, but they said it is 20 minutes or so away."

"I figured as much," Morgan replies. She eyes the man lying on a poolside chaise. His breathing is rapid and watery sounding. His skin is pale and sweaty. "Hello, sir. My name is Morgan, and I'm a trained Emergency Medical Responder. What seems to be the problem?"

The man starts saying something in Spanish, but it is interrupted by gasps of breath. "Eduardo," Morgan says, pulling out her vitals kit. "I'll need your help interpreting what he's saying."

Obtaining a Medical History

LO2 Explain the importance of a thorough medical history.

LO3 Explain the difference between a sign and a symptom

It is safe to say that a good patient assessment is likely to result in good patient care. A good patient assessment includes knowing how to ask questions and discover information that is not immediately obvious. All the information you gather about the patient's current and previous medical conditions is referred to as the patient's **medical history.**

Much of what you learn about your patient during the assessment comes from what the patient tells you (Figure 12.1). When the patient is unresponsive and there is no one at the scene who can answer your questions, you are at a great disadvantage, and so is your patient.

The first thing you must know about obtaining a patient history is the difference between a sign and a symptom. A **sign** is something you can see and observe about your patient. Think of signs much like those along the road that tell you to stop or yield. If you are alert and paying attention, those signs tell you a lot about what is going on around you. The same applies to a patient's condition. A sign can be pale skin or a rapid pulse or an open wound to the chest. Most signs are obvious if you are alert and properly trained on how to look for them.

medical history ▶ previous medical conditions and events for a patient.

sign ▶ something that can be observed or measured when assessing a patient.

Common signs include:

- Blood pressure
- Pulse
- Respirations
- Skin color, temperature, moisture
- Pupil reaction
- Bleeding
- Bruising
- Unresponsiveness
- Confusion
- Deformity

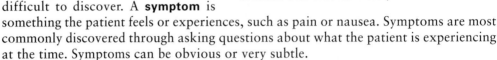

Figure 12.1 Get down at eye level with your patient and make good eye contact as you begin to obtain their medical history.

symptom ▶ something the patient complains of or describes during the secondary assessment.

Symptoms are different and more difficult to discover. A **symptom** is something the patient feels or experiences, such as pain or nausea. Symptoms are most commonly discovered through asking questions about what the patient is experiencing at the time. Symptoms can be obvious or very subtle.

Common symptoms include:

- Pain
- Nausea
- Shortness of breath
- Cough
- Chest discomfort
- Headache
- Dizziness
- Fatigue
- Blurred vision
- Anxiety

> **REMEMBER**
>
> Two of the most powerful skills you must develop to properly care for ill or injured patients are asking good questions and accurately assessing a patient's vital signs.

Your assessment must be focused on gathering and documenting as many pertinent signs and symptoms as possible to ensure that your care, and the care others provide after you, is appropriate.

Interviewing Your Patient

LO4 Describe the components of the SAMPLE history tool.

LO5 Describe the components of the OPQRST assessment tool.

In most situations, an alert patient is your best source of information. Nearly every encounter with an alert patient will begin with questioning the patient about what they are feeling or what happened that made them call for assistance. Recall from Chapter 1 that this is known as the patient's *chief complaint*. Whenever appropriate, it is best to direct your questions to the patient. In the case of a young child who is still nonverbal, it is appropriate to interview a parent, guardian, or caregiver. If the patient is unresponsive, you must look to other sources for information. Family members, bystanders, and first responders should all be questioned as appropriate to gather as much information about the patient as possible.

Ask questions slowly and clearly, using a caring tone of voice. Allow plenty of time for the patient to process and respond to your question before asking another one. Repeat or rephrase the question if necessary. Listen carefully to what the patient is telling you, and document important details as necessary. It can be very frustrating for the patient when the Emergency Medical Responder does not listen and the patient must repeat answers they have already given.

Be careful not to put words in the patient's mouth. Instead, provide them with choices, be patient, and allow the patient to choose. It is also important to use the patient's own words when documenting your assessment or handing the patient off to the next level of care. If the patient tells you they feel as though an anvil is sitting on their chest, use their words rather than paraphrasing.

The level of cooperation and quality of answers you receive from your patient can be greatly influenced by the rapport you establish early on. This can also be influenced by others on the scene. A simple sequence can be used for most situations and will work well for quickly establishing a rapport with your patient. Read the following dialogue, and see if you can identify the five components of the sequence:

EMERGENCY MEDICAL RESPONDER: "Hello, my name is Chris. I'm with the fire department. Would you mind if I ask you some questions?"
PATIENT: "Hi, Chris. Uh, no, I don't mind."
EMERGENCY MEDICAL RESPONDER: "What is your name?"
PATIENT: "Jordan."
EMERGENCY MEDICAL RESPONDER: "How old are you, Jordan?"
PATIENT: "I'm 48."
EMERGENCY MEDICAL RESPONDER: "Jordan, you look like you are in quite a bit of discomfort. Can you tell me what you are feeling right now?"
PATIENT: "I was out back cutting down weeds with the mower when I suddenly felt tightness in my chest."

Did you identify the five components of the sequence? They are:

- *Introduction.* "Hello, my name is Chris. I'm with the fire department." This is a courteous introduction that tells the patient the role you play in the team.
- *Consent.* "Would you mind if I ask you some questions?" Obtaining consent to care for the patient is not only good manners but is also a legal requirement.
- *Patient's name.* "What is your name?" Using a patient's name frequently is one of the most effective ways to establish a rapport and gain the confidence of your patient.
- *Patient's age.* While it is often easy to guess a patient's approximate age, it is just as easy to ask and get the actual age.
- *Chief complaint.* "Jordan, you look like you are in quite a bit of discomfort. Can you tell me what you are feeling right now?" Obtaining the chief complaint will guide your assessment.

This simple and respectful approach can be easily memorized and modified to meet the needs of just about any situation. It will go far in helping you establish a positive rapport with your patient.

Now that you have completed your introduction and obtained the chief complaint, what is next? What questions should you ask? How will you remember all that you should ask? Not to worry—there are tools for this purpose.

SAMPLE History Tool   One of the most common tools used for obtaining a patient's medical history is the **SAMPLE history tool**. It is a simple acronym that contains six key reminders. The acronym helps guide the flow of the interview and helps you keep in mind the most important questions to ask your patient. Each letter represents a specific element of your interview and should trigger specific questions related to the patient's medical history:

S — *Signs/symptoms.* This is a reminder to observe the patient for obvious signs of illness or injury and ask or clarify what they may be feeling. You might ask the patient, "So tell me again. What are you feeling?" or "Tell me again where you hurt the most." If the patient states that they have pain in the right shoulder (symptom), this should trigger you to quickly examine the shoulder, looking for any signs such as deformity or bleeding. Though you may already know the patient has shoulder pain, it is important to find out more. Are there any obvious signs of injury? Are there signs or symptoms other than those directly related to the chief complaint?

A — *Allergies.* Question the patient about any known allergies to things such as medications, food, or insect stings. More importantly, you want to know about allergies that may be related to the patient's current complaint. It is a good idea to ask if they have recently been exposed to anything to which they are allergic. Most patients have a pretty good idea what they are allergic to.

SAMPLE history tool ► acronym used as a reminder in obtaining a patient history during the secondary assessment; SAMPLE stands for signs/symptoms, allergies, medications, past pertinent medical history, last oral intake, and events leading to the problem today.

M — *Medications.* You will want to ask the patient if they are currently taking any medications, prescribed or over-the-counter. If the patient says yes, then you must ask if they are current with all their medications. In other words, have they been taking them as prescribed up to and including today? If the patient is at home or has their medications with them, ask to see all the medications the patient is taking and gather them together so they are easily accessible for the ambulance crew when they arrive. You aren't expected to memorize all medications and the purpose of each. It is perfectly appropriate to ask the patient why they are taking a particular medication.

P — *Past pertinent medical history.* You must also determine the medical history unrelated to the current emergency. You might ask, "Do you have any past history of medical conditions or issues such as heart problems, breathing problems, diabetes, or seizures?" Your job is to discover the history, document it thoroughly, and pass it along to the next level of care.

L — *Last oral intake.* For instance, "What have you eaten or had to drink today?" Document what the patient has taken in, when, and an approximate quantity. The primary purpose for this is to alert you to any connection to the current problem (e.g., food allergy) as well as to alert the next level of care to any stomach contents that may be an issue if the patient needs surgery. Many patients respond to general anesthesia with nausea and vomiting, and the surgical staff will take additional precautions as necessary.

E — *Events leading to the illness or injury.* You may ask, "What were you doing when this began?" The chain of events can often provide important clues to the patient's problem. For example, it is important for the doctor to know if a patient complaining of chest pain was at rest when the pain began or if it started as a result of exertion. **E** also stands for *else*, as in "Is there anything else I should know?"

CREW RESOURCE MANAGEMENT

It is typically best if only one member of the team asks the patient questions during the assessment. It can be confusing to the patient and important information can be missed if multiple members of the team are trying to obtain a medical history at the same time.

OPQRST assessment tool ▶ mnemonic used as a reminder during a secondary assessment to help assess the patient's chief complaint; the letters stand for onset, provocation, quality, region/radiate, severity, and time.

OPQRST Assessment Tool   Another tool used for obtaining a deeper patient history is the **OPQRST assessment tool.** Just like the SAMPLE history, each letter stands for a word designed to trigger more specific questions. The OPQRST assessment tool drives a more detailed assessment related to the chief complaint and can be very helpful in gathering additional information that the SAMPLE tool may miss.

OPQRST is most commonly used for the assessment of pain or discomfort, but it can be used for other problems as well. Those who use the OPQRST will slip it in immediately following the *S* in SAMPLE. The letters in OPQRST stand for onset, provocation, quality, region/radiate, severity, and time:

O — *Onset. Onset* triggers questions pertaining to what the patient was doing when the pain or symptoms began. For example, "What were you doing when the pain began?" or "What were you doing when you first began to feel short of breath?" The correct questions allow you to determine if the onset was sudden or gradual.

P — *Provocation. Provocation* triggers questions pertaining to what might make the pain or symptoms better or worse. For example, "Does anything you do make the pain better or worse?" or "Does it hurt to take a deep breath or when I push here?" or "Do you get dizzy when you stand up?".

Q — *Quality.* *Quality* triggers questions pertaining to what the pain or symptom actually feels like. For example, "Can you describe how your pain feels?" and "Is your pain sharp or dull?" and "Is it steady or does it come and go?".

R — *Region/Radiate.* *Region* and *radiate* trigger questions pertaining to where the pain is originating and where it may be moving or radiating to. For example, "Can you point with one finger to where your pain is the worst?" and "Does your pain move or radiate to any other part of your body?" and "Do you feel pain anywhere else other than your chest?".

S — *Severity.* *Severity* triggers questions pertaining to the severity of the pain or discomfort. A standard 1 to 10 scale is typically used like this: "On a scale of 1 to 10, with 10 being the worst pain you have ever felt, how would you rate your pain right now?" You can take this a step further by asking the patient to describe the severity of the pain when it first began using the same scale. Once you have been with the patient a while and provided care, you will want to ask the severity question again to see if the pain is getting better or worse.

T — *Time.* *Time* triggers questions pertaining to how long the patient may have been experiencing pain or discomfort. A simple question such as "When did you first begin having pain today?" or "How long have you had this pain?" will usually suffice.

It is important to point out that there are many different acronyms and memory tools that can be used to assist the Emergency Medical Responder in performing a more thorough assessment. Two of the more commonly used tools have been presented here. Your instructor or EMS system may have different or additional tools. Find the tool or tools that work best for you.

Additional Sources of Information

You may encounter a patient who is unresponsive or unable to answer your questions about their condition or history. If this is the case, you must depend on family members, bystanders, or first responders for information (Figure 12.2). Here are some examples of questions you may want to ask others at the scene if the patient is unable to provide meaningful information:

- *What is the patient's name?* If the patient is a minor, ask if the parents are present or if they have been contacted.
- *Did you see what happened?* For example, if the patient fell from a ladder, did they appear to faint or pass out first? Were they hit on the head by something?
- *Did the patient complain of anything before this happened?* You may learn of chest pain, nausea, shortness of breath, a strange odor where the patient was working, or other clues.
- *Does the patient have any known illnesses?* Family or friends may know the patient's medical history, such as heart problems, diabetes, allergies, or other problems that may cause a change in their condition.
- *Does the patient take any medications that you know of?* Often, knowing what medications a patient takes can tell us something about their medical history.

Medical identification jewelry can also provide important information if the patient is unresponsive and a history cannot be easily obtained from others at the scene. A special bracelet may be worn on the wrist or a medallion worn on a cord or chain around the neck. Information about the patient's medical condition is engraved on the reverse side of the bracelet or medallion, along with a phone number for additional information.

> **REMEMBER**
>
> One technique to consider when interviewing family members is to move them a small distance away from the patient so the patient's emergency care does not distract them. However, do not attempt to isolate them completely from their loved one.

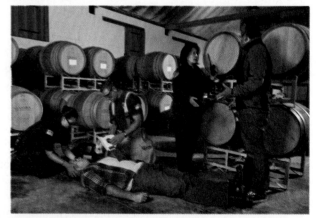

Figure 12.2 You must depend on bystanders or family members when your patient is unresponsive or unable to provide a medical history on their own.

"His name is Luis. He says he fell asleep out here and when he woke up, he felt like he was choking on water," Eduardo says, translating the man's short, gurgling words. "He says he doesn't have the strength to get up."

"Go ahead and raise the back of that lounge chair, but be careful," Morgan says. Glancing at her watch, she counts the rapid weak pulse in her patient's wrist. "Respirations are about 36, very shallow with a gurgling sound, and his pulse is 104 and regular, but it's pretty weak."

Morgan quickly jots down her findings, noting the time. She attaches the blood pressure cuff, and Luis pulls away, saying something she doesn't understand. Morgan looks Luis in the eye and says, "Luis, I'm going to help you as much as I can, okay? Can you help me by answering some questions, please?" Luis listens to the translation Eduardo gives and leans back, looking calmer.

CREW RESOURCE MANAGEMENT

To ensure the most efficient use of resources, it is usually best to dedicate one person to obtaining a medical history while another member of the team obtains vital signs. If you have more personnel at the scene, you can assign someone to act as the scribe by taking notes and recording key findings while others perform their assessments.

Vital Signs

LO6 State the characteristics that are obtained and measured when assessing respirations, pulse, blood pressure, skin signs, and pupils.

LO7 Describe the methods used to assess each of the five primary vital signs.

LO8 Differentiate normal and abnormal vital sign values for the infant, child, and adult patient.

LO9 Explain the role that monitoring vital signs plays in the overall assessment and care of the patient.

vital signs ▶ signs used to evaluate a patient's condition (respirations, pulse, blood pressure, skin, pupils, and mental status).

mental status ▶ general condition of a patient's level of consciousness and awareness.

In the context of medicine, the word *vital* refers to that which is required for the continuation of life. In EMS, several specific signs are commonly observed and measured. The list of signs may differ slightly from system to system, but most EMS systems include the following in their list of **vital signs**: respirations, pulse, blood pressure (BP), skin signs, pupils, and **mental status**. Though it can be argued that not all of these signs are truly "vital" to life, respirations, pulse, and blood pressure are truly necessary for someone to be considered living.

Overview

As you learn about the various vital signs, keep in mind that your goal is to paint as complete a picture of your patient as possible. No single vital sign should be used to drive the care you provide. Vital signs can alert you to problems that require immediate attention. Taken at regular intervals, they can help you determine if the patient's condition is getting better, getting worse, or staying the same.

Perfusion Recall from Chapter 4 that *perfusion* is the adequate delivery of well-oxygenated blood and nutrients to all parts of the body and the elimination of waste products. Each of the vital signs serves as a window into the patient's perfusion status. For instance, a patient with an abnormally slow pulse or low blood pressure may not be getting enough blood to all parts of the body, meaning that the flow of blood (perfusion) is compromised. Another example is a patient with breathing difficulty. They may not be getting enough air to adequately supply the blood with enough oxygen. In this case, the flow of blood may be adequate, but the blood itself is lacking sufficient oxygen. One more example is a patient with extremely pale skin; this may be a sign of shock.

Baseline Vital Signs   The first vital signs you obtain from your patient are referred to as the **baseline vital signs**. All subsequent vital signs are compared to the baseline set. This comparison helps determine if the patient is stable or unstable, improving or growing worse, and benefiting or not benefiting from the care you are providing. For example, comparing baseline vital signs before and after initiating an intervention, such as administering oxygen, can give clues as to whether the oxygen is helping the patient.

baseline vital signs ▶ first set of vital signs obtained on a patient.

Trending   One of the values of obtaining and documenting vital signs is that they can be trended. **Trending** is the process of comparing three or more sets of vital signs from the same patient over time. Vital signs can change for the better or for the worse, or they can remain generally the same. Each represents a trend and can provide valuable information about your patient.

A careful analysis of vital signs can alert you to current or developing problems. For example, the presence of cool, moist skin along with a rapid pulse and increased breathing rate can indicate possible shock in the presence of a significant mechanism of injury. Hot, dry skin with a rapid pulse could indicate a serious heat-related emergency. You can determine which patients are a high priority for immediate transport by taking and closely monitoring their vital signs. A patient with abnormal vital signs to begin with or a patient whose vital signs are getting worse would be high priority for rapid transport.

trending ▶ comparing three or more sets of signs and symptoms over time to determine if the patient's condition is worsening, improving, or remaining the same.

It's important to note that vital signs differ for everyone. What is normal for one patient may not be normal for another. Vital signs can change, and they are affected by factors other than the patient's medical condition. The temperature of the environment, exercise, and even emotions can all affect an individual's vital signs, moving them into what might be considered an abnormal range. Vital signs vary significantly by age and a person's physical condition, as well. Familiarize yourself with the normal ranges for different age groups.

The key for vital signs is to not rush to a conclusion too soon. Usually, it is better to gather as much information as possible before coming to a conclusion about how best to manage your patient. There are exceptions to this rule, though. For instance, if you cannot locate a pulse, you would not try to get a blood pressure before starting CPR. Without a pulse, the person will die, so time is of the essence.

Mental Status

A patient's mental status can provide valuable information about their condition. This assessment is typically done during the first minute with the patient and can be performed as you introduce yourself and begin asking questions about the illness or injury.

A patient with an altered mental status (AMS) should be considered unstable and in need of immediate AMS care. A patient's mental status, also referred to as level of consciousness (LOC), or level of responsiveness, is commonly evaluated using the AVPU scale:

A — *Alert.* The patient is alert and spontaneously interacting with the environment around them.

V — *Verbal.* The patient is responsive to verbal stimuli, which means they respond when you speak to them or ask a question. They may or may not provide any meaningful information.

P — *Pain.* The patient is responsive only to painful stimuli. This patient appears to be unconscious and does not respond to your verbal commands or questions. However, they respond by groaning or pulling away when you provide some type of painful stimulus, such as rubbing the sternum with your knuckles or pinching the muscle above the shoulder near the neck.

U — *Unresponsive.* The patient is unconscious or completely unresponsive. This patient does not offer any type of response to verbal or painful stimulus.

There can be many shades of gray for patients in the "alert" category. Patients can be awake and talking to you but present as very disoriented and confused. Simply calling them alert is often not descriptive enough. To further assess patients who fall into the "alert" category, an additional assessment tool can help define just how alert and oriented they actually are. It helps you find out if patients are aware of:

- who they are (person).
- where they are (place).
- time of day (time).
- their current situation (event).

A patient who is able to tell you only their name and where they are can be described as "alert and oriented ×2," or simply A&O × 2. The individual who knows who they are, where they are, the time of day, and what has happened to him or her would be described as A&O × 4.

Respirations

Respiration, also called ventilation, is the process of breathing in (inhaling) and out (exhaling). A single respiration is one entire cycle of breathing in and out. You will evaluate several characteristics when assessing a patient's respirations: rate, depth, ease, and sounds.

- The respiratory rate is a count of the patient's breaths—one inhalation plus one exhalation—and is classified as normal, rapid, or slow. The respiratory rate is documented as number of breaths per minute.
- While you are counting respirations, note if the depth is normal, shallow, or deep. Breathing depth that is normal is said to be a good tidal volume (GTV).
- Notice if the breathing is easy or whether it appears labored, or difficult, which may indicate an increased work of breathing.
- Listen for any abnormal sounds during breathing, such as snoring, gurgling, gasping, or wheezing.
- If the patient is responsive, ask if they are having any pain while they breathe. Normal breathing is quiet and effortless. A patient who requires effort to breathe is said to have an increased work of breathing.

Table 12.1 shows some problems that are associated with variations in respirations. To assess respirations, follow these steps:

1. Grasp the patient's wrist as if you were going to count the pulse rate. Hold their arm firmly against their upper abdomen (Figure 12.3A and B). Do this because many patients will unknowingly alter their respiratory rate when someone is watching them breathe.
2. Observe the patient's chest move in and out. Listen for abnormal sounds.

TABLE 12.1   **Assessment Signs: Respirations**

OBSERVATION	POSSIBLE PROBLEM
Rapid, shallow breaths	Shock, heart problems, heat emergency, diabetic emergency, heart failure, pneumonia
Deep, gasping, labored breaths	Airway obstruction, heart failure, lung disease, chest injury, diabetic emergency
Slowed breathing	Head injury, stroke, respiratory failure, narcotic overdose
Snoring	Stroke, fractured skull, drug or alcohol overdose, partial airway obstruction
Crowing	A high pitched sound often caused by a partial airway obstruction, swelling of the airway
Gurgling	Airway obstruction due to fluids, lung disease
Wheezing	Asthma, emphysema, airway obstruction, heart failure
Coughing blood	Chest trauma, lung infection, punctured lung, internal injuries

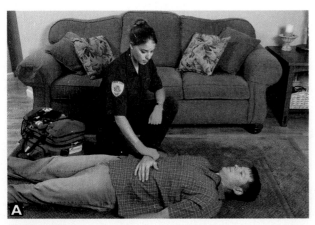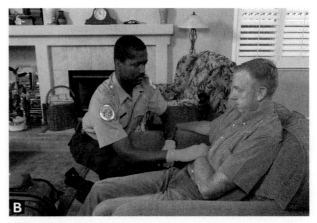

Figure 12.3 (A) Emergency Medical Responder assessing respirations on a supine patient. (B) Assessing respirations on a seated patient.

3. Count the number of breaths the patient takes in 15 or 30 seconds. (One breath equals one inspiration plus one expiration.) To obtain the respiratory rate (number of breaths per minute), multiply the number of breaths in 15 seconds by 4 or the number of breaths in 30 seconds by 2.
4. While counting respirations, note depth (normal, shallow, or deep) and ease of breathing (unlabored or labored).
5. Record your findings by documenting rate, depth, and ease.

Here are some examples of how you might document respirations:

- 16, GTV, and unlabored
- 32, shallow, and labored
- 8, shallow, and unlabored
- 36, deep, and labored

The average range for respirations for an adult at rest is 12 to 20 breaths per minute (Table 12.2). A respiratory rate higher than 30 or lower than 10 breaths per minute is considered abnormal and may require some intervention.

Pulse

LO10 Differentiate the techniques used to assess a pulse in an infant, child, and adult patient.

The presence of a **pulse** gives us insight into the circulatory status of the patient. A good pulse indicates that blood is moving well throughout the body. The pulse is caused when an artery that lies close to the skin pulsates as the pressure increases and decreases

pulse ▶ pulsation of the arteries felt with each heartbeat.

TABLE 12.2	**Respiration**
AVERAGE RESPIRATION RATE (BREATHS PER MINUTE) BY AGE	
Adult	12 to 20
Adolescent: 13–17 years	12 to 16
Child: 6–12 years	18 to 30
Young Child: 4–5 years	22 to 34
Toddler: 1–3 years	24 to 40
Infant: < 12 months	30 to 60

Source: The American Heart Association's Pediatric Advanced Life Support Provider Manual, American Heart Association, 2015.

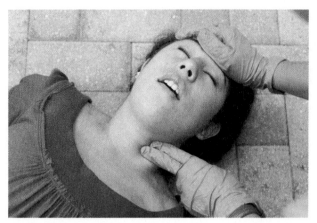

Figure 12.4 Locating the carotid pulse point in the neck.

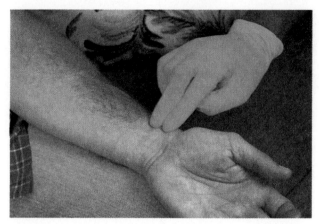

Figure 12.5 Locating the radial pulse point in the wrist.

with each heartbeat. Several pulse points can be used to evaluate heart rate as well as circulatory status in an extremity such as an arm or a leg. The carotid (neck) and femoral (groin) pulses are referred to as *central pulses* because they are in the torso of the body (groin), or just above it (neck, Figure 12.4). The brachial (upper arm), radial (wrist, Figure 12.5), and pedal (foot) pulses are referred to as *peripheral pulses* because they are in the extremities.

When assessing a patient's pulse, you must assess three characteristics: rate, strength, and rhythm.

- Pulse rate is the number of beats per minute. This measurement determines whether the patient's pulse is normal, rapid, or slow.
- Strength is the force of the pulse: strong or weak.
- Rhythm is the steadiness of the pulse: regular or irregular.

When caring for a responsive patient, you can check the radial pulse at the patient's wrist. For an unresponsive patient, the carotid pulse in the neck should be used.

Radial pulse refers to the radial artery found in the lateral portion of the forearm, on the thumb side of the wrist. If, for any reason, you are unable to feel the radial pulse, assess the carotid pulse. The absence of a radial pulse when there is a carotid pulse indicates an abnormally low blood pressure and possible shock. A radial pulse may not be detectable if the patient's blood pressure is too low or if there is an extremity injury that is interrupting blood flow to the distal arm.

To measure a radial pulse rate:

1. Use two or three fingers to locate the pulse. Do not use your thumb because it has its own pulse, which could be mistaken for the patient's.
2. Place your fingertips on the lateral side of the patient's anterior wrist, just above the crease between hand and wrist. Slide your fingers from this position toward the thumb side of the wrist (lateral side). Keeping the tip of the middle finger on the crease between wrist and hand will ensure that you are placing the fingertip over the site of the radial pulse.
3. Apply moderate pressure until you feel the pulse. If the pulse is weak, you may have to apply more pressure. Applying too much pressure can cause the pulse to fade. By having all three fingers in contact with the patient's wrist and hand, you should be able to judge how much pressure you are applying.
4. Once you feel the pulse, count the beats for either 15 or 30 seconds, depending on local protocols.
5. While counting, do your best to note the strength and rhythm of the pulse.
6. Multiply your 30-second count by 2 or your 15-second count by 4 to determine the number of beats per minute.
7. Record your findings by documenting the rate, strength, and rhythm.

TABLE 12.3 Pulse

AVERAGE PULSE RATES (BEATS PER MINUTE) BY AGE	
Adult	60 to 100
Child > 10 years	60 to 100
Child 2 to 10 years	60 to 140
Child 3 months to 2 years	100 to 190
Newborn to 3 months	85 to 205
PULSE QUALITY	**SIGNIFICANCE/POSSIBLE CAUSES**
Rapid	Exertion, anxiety, pain, fever, dehydration, blood loss, shock
Slow	Head injury, drugs, some poisons, some heart problems, lack of oxygen in children
Irregular	Abnormal electrical heart activity (arrhythmia)
Absent (no pulse)	Cardiac arrest

Note: In infants and children, a high pulse is not as great a concern as a low pulse. A low pulse may indicate imminent cardiac arrest.

Here are some examples of how you might document pulses:

- 72, strong, and regular
- 88, strong, and irregular
- 104, weak, and regular
- 120, weak, and irregular

Adults For an adult at rest, the normal pulse rate is 60 to 100 beats per minute (Table 12.3). Any rate above 100 for a resting patient is considered abnormally rapid (tachycardia). Any rate below 60 is usually considered abnormally slow (bradycardia). Some exceptions are a well-conditioned athlete whose normal resting pulse may be 50 beats per minute or less and a patient who is taking medications to slow their heart rate. In emergency situations, because of anxiety or excitement, it is not unusual for the pulse to be above 100 beats per minute.

Infants The primary pulse point for obtaining a pulse in infants under the age of 1 year is the brachial pulse in the upper arm. This is due to the difficulty in isolating the radial and carotid pulses given the anatomy of infants. To obtain a brachial pulse in an infant, place your index and middle fingers over the brachial artery on the inside of the baby's upper arm, between the elbow and armpit. Press gently with your fingers until you can feel the pulse. You may use the tip of your thumb on the opposite side of the arm to apply counterpressure. Be sure not to use the pad of your thumb because it may be possible to feel your own pulse there.

> **REMEMBER**
>
> Do not start CPR based only on the absence of a radial pulse. As the blood pressure drops, it becomes very difficult to feel a peripheral pulse such as the radial pulse. Before initiating CPR, *always* confirm the absence of a carotid pulse first.

Blood Pressure

Blood pressure is the measurement of the pressure of blood against the walls of the arteries, both when the heart beats and when it is at rest.[1] Blood pressure and perfusion are closely related in that good perfusion requires a good blood pressure. The lower the blood pressure drops below normal, the less effective perfusion is. A single blood pressure reading that is significantly above or below the normal range for a patient can be a valuable tool in determining the current state or condition of the patient. Repeated blood pressure measurements are valuable for trending the patient's condition and can also help identify changes in the patient's condition over time.

Blood pressure is determined by measuring the pressure changes in the arteries. The phase of the cardiac cycle during which the heart contracts and blood is forced out of the chambers is called *systole*. The pressure generated within the arteries during contraction is the

blood pressure ▶ measurement of the pressure inside the arteries, during and between contractions of the heart.

systolic ▶ pressure within the arteries when the heart beats; *systole* is the contraction phase of the cardiac cycle.

diastolic ▶ pressure within the arteries when the heart is at rest; *diastole* is the resting phase of the cardiac cycle.

REMEMBER

Certain conditions can result in significant differences in pulse and blood pressure between the right and left arms. If the pulse and/or blood pressure is abnormal the first time you take it, obtain it in the other arm, and give that information to the arriving EMTs. If pulse and blood pressure are normal and time permits, obtain another set of vital signs in the opposite arm for comparison.

hypertension ▶ high blood pressure.

systolic blood pressure. The systolic blood pressure is affected by many factors, such as the force of the heart's pumping action, the resistance and elasticity of the arteries, blood volume (blood loss means lower pressure), blood thickness or viscosity, and the amount of other fluids in the cells.

After the left ventricle of the heart contracts, it relaxes and refills. This relaxation phase is called *diastole*. During diastole, the pressure in the arteries falls. When measured, this pressure is the **diastolic** blood pressure.

Blood pressure is measured in units called *millimeters of mercury (mm Hg)*. These are the units on the blood pressure gauge. Because this system of measurement is standard for blood pressure readings, you will not have to say "millimeters of mercury" after each reading. Report the systolic pressure first, then the diastolic, as in 120 over 80 (120/80).

The reading of 120/80 is considered a normal blood pressure reading, which represents the average blood pressure obtained from a large sampling of healthy adults. There is a wide range of "normal" for adults and children.

Attempting to obtain blood pressure in young children can be challenging due to their small size and difficulty sitting still. It may not be practical to attempt to obtain a blood pressure in children under age 3. Blood pressure is not usually measured in the field for children under age 3 because it requires specialized equipment.

In 2017, the American Heart Association and the American College of Cardiologists released updated guidelines for the identification of high blood pressure, also called **hypertension**. Blood pressure categories in the new guidelines are:

- Normal: Less than 120/80 mm Hg
- Elevated: Systolic 120 to 129 *and* diastolic of 80 or less
- Stage 1: Systolic 130 to 139 *or* diastolic 80 to 89
- Stage 2: Systolic at least 140 *or* diastolic at least 90 mm Hg
- Any systolic reading greater than 180 *and/or* any diastolic reading greater than 120 is considered a medical emergency and requires immediate attention.

You will not know the normal blood pressure for a patient unless the individual is alert, knows the information, and can tell you what it is. Because you will not know the normal reading for a particular patient, you will take several readings to identify a trend in the patient's condition.

FIRST ON SCENE *(continued)*

"Now, Luis, you said you weren't allergic to anything, but are you taking any medications?" Morgan asks, focusing on his breathing. It seems that sitting him up has improved the ease and tidal volume of his breathing, as well as his color.

"He says yes, he takes medicine for his heart. He doesn't know the names, but he has them up in his room," Eduardo says, standing up. "Should I go grab them?"

"No. I need you here. Send one of the others to get them," Morgan says, reaching down to gently lift the towel covering Luis's legs. "Swollen ankles. This is making more sense of the high blood pressure I recorded a minute ago. Help me ask Luis about his medical history a bit more, and then I'll get another set of vitals."

An initial measurement may show that a patient has a blood pressure within normal limits, but the condition may worsen. For example, a patient going into shock may have a rapid pulse and a normal blood pressure reading when you first arrive at the scene. A few minutes later, the blood pressure may fall dramatically. Taking several readings while you are providing care is a way of identifying changes in the patient's status. Changes in blood pressure are significant and let you know that additional care is needed and transport is a priority.

For a typical adult, a systolic blood pressure reading below 100 mm Hg should be considered lower than normal unless the patient tells you otherwise (Table 12.4). Some small adult females and small-build athletes may have a normal systolic blood pressure of 90 mm Hg.

TABLE 12.4 Blood Pressure

AVERAGE BLOOD PRESSURE BY AGE		
PATIENT	**SYSTOLIC (MM HG)**	**DIASTOLIC (MM HG)**
Adult	≤ 120	≤ 80
Adolescent (13 to 17 years)	113 to 131	64 to 83
Child 6 to 12 years	96 to 115	57 to 76
Child 2 to 5 years	88 to 106	42 to 63

A systolic reading above 120 is typically considered high blood pressure.[2] Many patients will show an initial rise in blood pressure at the emergency scene. This is usually due to anxiety, fear, or stress caused by the incident and will return to normal once the situation or condition is under control. You will need more than one reading to confirm high blood pressure. High blood pressure readings are typical in individuals who are obese or who have a history of high cholesterol. There are many other underlying medical conditions that cause high blood pressure that you will be unable to determine at the emergency scene.

Determining Blood Pressure by Auscultation Two common techniques are used to measure blood pressure in emergency care. The first is by listening, which is called **auscultation** and requires the use of a **stethoscope**. The second is by feeling, which is called **palpation**. The palpation method will reveal only the systolic pressure.

The auscultation method requires the use of a stethoscope to hear the sound of the blood pulsating through the artery. You must begin by adjusting the earpieces so they fit properly in your ears. Hold the earpieces of the stethoscope between the thumb and index finger of each hand. Adjust the direction of the earpieces by gently turning them so each piece points slightly forward (Figure 12.6). This is to ensure that the openings of the earpieces point directly into your ear canals and will help ensure that you will hear the pulsations once the blood pressure cuff is inflated.

To determine blood pressure using a blood pressure cuff and a stethoscope, follow these steps:

1. Have the patient sit or lie down (Figure 12.7A and B). Cut away or remove clothing that is on the arm. Support the arm at the level of the heart. Do not use the arm if there is any possibility of injury.
2. Select the correct size blood pressure cuff. The average adult cuff can accommodate an arm that is up to 13 inches in circumference. A cuff that is too small will produce falsely high readings, and one that is too large will produce falsely low readings.
3. Wrap the cuff around the individual's upper arm. The lower border of the cuff should be about 1 inch above the crease in the elbow. The center of the bladder inside the cuff must be placed over the brachial artery in the upper arm (Figure 12.8 and Key Skill 12.1).
4. Apply the cuff securely but not too tightly. You should be able to place one finger under the bottom edge of the cuff (Figure 12.9).
5. Place the earpieces of the stethoscope in your ears. Be sure to adjust the earpieces so they face forward into your ear canals. If you are using a dual-head stethoscope, which has both a bell and a diaphragm, make certain to check that the appropriate side is activated before placing it on the patient.

auscultation ▶ listening to internal sounds of the body, typically with a stethoscope.

stethoscope ▶ device used to auscultate sounds within the body. Commonly used to obtain blood pressure.

palpation ▶ using one's hands to touch or feel the body.

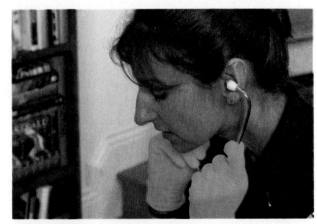

Figure 12.6 Adjust the earpieces of the stethoscope so they point forward slightly, into the ear canal.

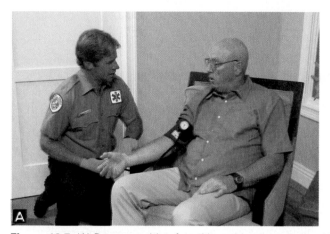
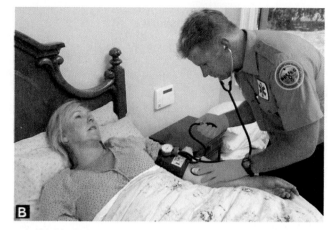

Figure 12.7 (A) Proper position for taking a blood pressure while seated. (B) Obtaining a blood pressure on a supine patient.

6. Use your fingertips to locate the brachial artery at the crease in the elbow.

7. Position the diaphragm of the stethoscope over the brachial artery pulse site. Do not let the head of the stethoscope touch the cuff. If it touches the cuff, the stethoscope will rub against it during inflation and deflation. You will hear the rubbing sounds, which may cause you to record a false reading.

8. Close the valve and inflate the cuff to approximately 180 mm Hg for an adult and 120 mm Hg for a child.

9. Once the cuff is inflated, open the valve slowly to release pressure from the cuff. It should fall at a smooth rate of 2 to 3 mm Hg per second, or a little faster than the second hand on a watch.

10. Listen carefully as you watch the needle move. Note when you hear the sound of the pulse (clicking or tapping). The first significant sound that you hear is the systolic pressure. Note that you will often notice the needle bouncing as you hear sounds via the stethoscope. The needle bounce is NOT a reliable way to determine the systolic pressure, as the movement does not always coincide with the actual sound you are hearing via the stethoscope.

11. Let the cuff continue to deflate. Listen for and note when the sound of the pulse fades (not when it stops). When the sound turns dull or soft, this is the diastolic pressure.

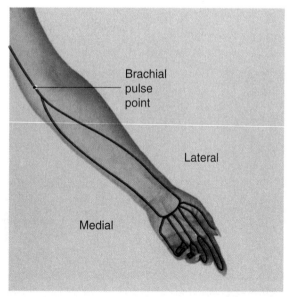

Figure 12.8 Location of the brachial artery pulse point.

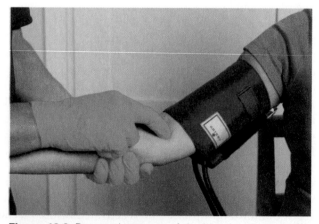

Figure 12.9 Proper placement of the blood pressure cuff.

Blood Pressure by Auscultation

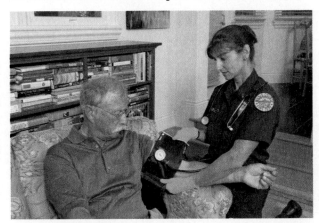

1. Place the cuff snugly around the upper arm.

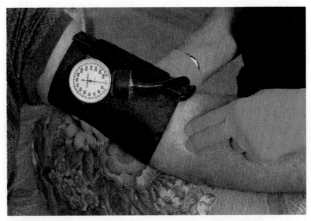

2. Palpate the brachial pulse point, and place the diaphragm of the stethoscope directly over the pulse point.

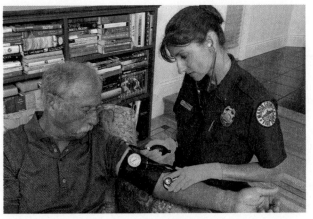

3. Quickly inflate the cuff then release the pressure to obtain the blood pressure readings.

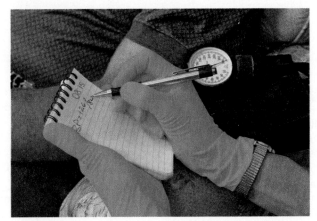

4. Document your readings, along with the time they were taken.

12. Let the rest of the air out of the cuff quickly. Be sure to squeeze the cuff to release all the air. If practical, leave the cuff in place so you can take additional readings.

13. Record the time, the arm used, the position of the patient (e.g., supine, sitting), and the pressure readings. Round off the readings to the next highest number. For example, 145 mm Hg should be recorded as 146 mm Hg. (The markings on the gauge are in even numbers. You may hear the first sound when the needle is between two markings and want to record it as an odd number, but all blood pressure readings are recorded as even numbers.)

If you are not certain of a reading, be sure the cuff is totally deflated, wait 1 or 2 minutes, and try again, or use the individual's other arm. Should you try the same arm too soon, you may get a false high reading.

Determining Blood Pressure by Palpation   Using the palpation method (feeling the radial pulse) tends not to be as accurate as the auscultation method. It will provide you with one reading: an approximate systolic pressure. This method is used when there is too much ambient noise, making it difficult to hear with a stethoscope.

Blood Pressure by Palpation

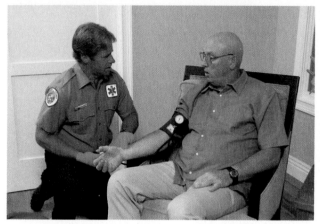

1. Place the cuff and locate the radial pulse prior to inflating the cuff.

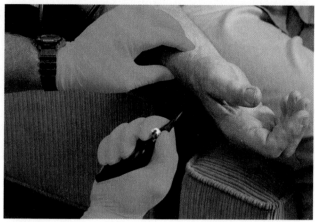

2. Inflate the cuff until you feel the radial pulse go away. Continue inflating the cuff to approximately 30 mm Hg beyond where the pulse went away. Release the pressure in the cuff and note the pressure on the gauge when the radial pulse returns. This will be the approximate systolic pressure.

REMEMBER

It is important to be familiar with the equipment you will be using. Some blood pressure cuffs have a marker to indicate how to line up the cuff over the brachial artery. Some cuffs have no markers, while others have inaccurate markers. It is best to locate the center of the bladder and line it up over the brachial artery on the inside of the arm.

cyanotic ▶ bluish coloration of the skin caused by an inadequate supply of oxygen. Typically seen at the mucous membranes and nail beds.

jaundice ▶ medical condition that causes yellowing of the skin and whites of the eyes. Typically caused by liver failure or obstruction of the bile duct.

To determine blood pressure by palpation, place the cuff in the same position on the arm as you would for auscultation. Then proceed with the following (Key Skill 12.2):

1. Find the radial pulse on the arm with the cuff.
2. Close the valve and inflate the cuff until you can no longer feel the pulse.
3. Continue to inflate the cuff to a point 30 mm Hg above the point where the pulse disappeared.
4. Slowly deflate the cuff, and note the reading when you feel the pulse return. This is the systolic blood pressure. You will not get a diastolic pressure reading by palpation.
5. Record the time, the arm used, the position of the patient, and the systolic pressure. Note that the reading was by palpation. If you give this information to someone orally, make sure you say the reading was by palpation, as in, "BP is 146 by palpation."

Skin Signs

Skin signs are often the easiest vital signs to assess because they do not require any special skill or equipment. The three characteristics you will be evaluating are color, temperature, and moisture. All three can be assessed by observing the patient's face and feeling the forehead.

When assessing skin color in light-skinned patients, observe the skin of the face, noting if it appears pink (normal) or if it is pale or flushed (reddish) or yellow. In dark-skinned patients, observe the palms, nail beds, and inside of the lips to look for pink appearance. Skin that is not being perfused well will appear pale or **cyanotic** (bluish). Skin that is receiving an abnormal amount of blood flow might appear flushed (red). Skin that is yellow in appearance is described as jaundiced, indicating **jaundice**, an underlying condition related to the liver.

Next, use the back of one hand to assess skin temperature (Figure 12.10). Pull the glove away from the back of your hand, and hold your hand skin-to-skin against the patient's forehead. Be sure that you do not expose your ungloved hand to any patient body fluids as you do this. Note if the skin appears warm (normal), cool, or hot. At the

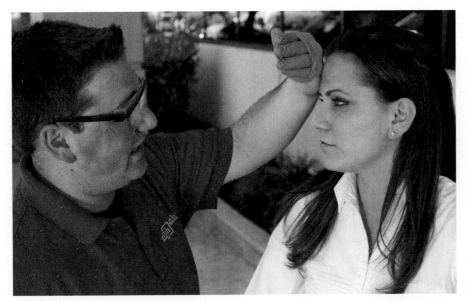

Figure 12.10 Use the back of an ungloved hand to assess skin temperature and moisture.

same time you are assessing color and temperature, you can assess for moisture. Note if the skin appears dry (normal) or moist (sweaty). Excessive sweating is called *diaphoresis*, and this condition can be classified as mild, moderate, or severe. Being excessively sweaty is described as **diaphoretic**.

Table 12.5 lists some of the problems associated with skin color, relative skin temperature, and moisture.

Here are some examples of how you might document skin signs:

- Pink, warm, dry
- Pale, cool, moist
- Flushed, hot, moist
- Flushed, hot, dry

diaphoretic ▶ excessively sweaty. Commonly caused by exertion or a medical problem such as heart attack or shock.

TABLE 12.5	Skin Signs
SKIN COLOR	**SIGNIFICANCE/POSSIBLE CAUSES**
Pink	Normal in light-skinned patients; normal in inner eyelids, lips, and nail beds of dark-skinned patients
Pale	Constricted blood vessels possibly resulting from blood loss, shock, decreased blood pressure, emotional distress
Blue (cyanotic)	Lack of oxygen in blood cells and tissues resulting from inadequate breathing or heart function
Red (flushed)	Heat exposure, high blood pressure, emotional excitement; cherry red indicates late stages of carbon monoxide poisoning
Yellow (jaundiced)	Liver abnormalities
Blotchiness (mottling)	Occasionally in patients in shock
TEMPERATURE AND CONDITION	**SIGNIFICANCE/POSSIBLE CAUSES**
Cool, moist	Shock, heart attack, anxiety
Cold, dry	Exposure to cold, diabetic emergency
Hot, dry	High fever, heat emergency, spine injury
Hot, moist	High fever, heat emergency, diabetic emergency

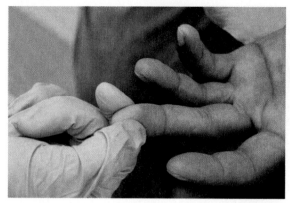

Figure 12.11 Checking capillary refill using the pad of the finger.

To evaluate skin color in dark-skinned patients, use one or more of these methods:

- *Oral mucosa.* Inspect the inside of the lower lip. This area should be pink and moist.
- *Conjunctiva.* This is the tissue on the inside of the skin that surrounds each eye. By simply pulling down gently on the lower eyelid, you will expose this area. It, too, should be pink and moist.
- *Nail beds.* This is the tissue that lies below each fingernail and toenail and can typically be seen through the nail. Of course, if the patient is wearing nail polish, this will not be an option.
- *Palms.* The palms of the hands are generally lighter in color, regardless of skin pigmentation. They are also full of capillaries, and a simple capillary refill test (described in the following section) can provide some indication as to perfusion status in the hand.

Capillary Refill

capillary refill ▶ time it takes for the capillaries to refill after being blanched. Normal capillary refill time is 2 seconds or less.

Another tool used to evaluate circulatory status and perfusion is the capillary refill test. Because the skin is full of very small vessels called capillaries, compressing the skin with a finger or two will temporarily squeeze the blood from the capillaries, causing the normally pink skin to appear blanched or white (Figure 12.11). When the pressure is released, the skin can be observed becoming pink again as blood returns to the capillaries. The time it takes for the blood to return to the capillaries is called the **capillary refill** time and should be 2 seconds or less. Capillary refill time increases as skin perfusion decreases.[3]

This test is commonly used on adults to evaluate the circulatory status in an extremity by evaluating capillary refill time in a finger or a toe. In infants and small children, this test can be applied just about anywhere on the body and is used as a test for general perfusion status.

The capillary refill test for older children and adults is best performed using a nail bed or the pad of a finger or toe. Follow these steps to assess capillary refill:

JEDI

The diversity of human skin tones is vast. If you are unable to determine capillary refill in the extremities, ask the responsive patient to help you determine if changes in skin color are normal for them. For the unresponsive patient, you can look to the mucous membranes in the eyes or mouth to get a sense of perfusion. Remember, a bluish or grayish skin tone is never normal.

1. Select an appropriate finger or toe (the larger the better).
2. Using your thumb and index finger, squeeze the pad of the patient's finger or toe from both sides. Observe the pad as it blanches.
3. Quickly release the pressure, and observe the color return to the pad. Note the time it takes for color to return. Normal color should return in 2 seconds or less.
4. Document your findings.

A delayed capillary refill time may be a sign of impaired circulation due to injury or a sign of poor perfusion due to shock. There are many factors that can affect the reliability of capillary refill time, such as the temperature of the environment, medical conditions, and medications. Capillary refill is just one tool to use in your overall assessment of the patient.

Pupils

Whether you realize it or not, you have probably become quite good at assessing an individual's condition by looking into their eyes. Emotions such as fear, worry, anxiety, and pain can all be seen in the eyes. As an Emergency Medical Responder, you will be assessing the eyes for very specific characteristics: pupil size and shape, equality of pupil size, and reactivity to light (Figure 12.12A–C).

Size and Shape   When you first look at the eyes, note their general condition and identify any obvious injury or deformity. Pay particular attention to the dark circles in the center of each eye known as the pupil. Note the size and shape of each pupil. Many EMS penlights have a pupil gauge printed on the side to aid in the determination of pupil size. Ensure that both pupils are round.

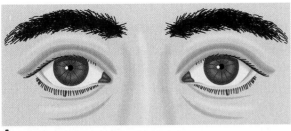

A   Constricted pupils

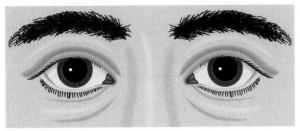

B   Dilated pupils

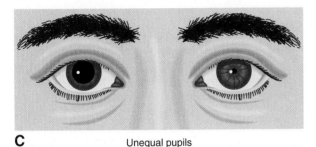

C   Unequal pupils

Figure 12.12 (A) Constricted pupils. (B) Dilated pupils. (C) Unequal pupils.

REMEMBER

Pupils are the EMR's window to a patient's brain perfusion. For the pupils to react normally to light, the brain must receive normal perfusion with oxygenated blood and glucose and not be altered by toxins such as narcotics. Abnormalities in pupil size and reactiveness to light indicate poor perfusion to the brain and should lead you to categorize your patient as a high priority.

Equality   Observe both pupils to ensure that they are the same size. Keep in mind that dark-colored eyes are much more difficult to assess than light-colored eyes. It is also important to note that unequal pupils are a normal finding in some people. When you encounter a patient with unequal pupils, always ask if this is a normal condition for them.

Reactivity to Light   One of the important signs of good perfusion is pupils that respond briskly to the presence or absence of light. Pupils should respond to the sudden introduction of light by constricting and, in contrast, should dilate when light to the pupil is blocked. There are at least two methods that can be used to assess pupil reaction, and each depends on the ambient light in the environment.

In a well-lit area such as a bright room or on a bright, sunny day, it may be of no use attempting to shine a light into someone's eyes. The pupils will likely already be constricted due to the large amount of ambient light. In this situation, you will have better results covering both eyes with your hand for several seconds, then observing the pupils constrict when you take your hand away. You must learn to be patient when using this method because it may take some time for the pupil to dilate after you cover the eye. It is a good practice to ask at least two or three questions pertaining to the patient's medical history while you cover each eye. This will allow enough time for the pupil to dilate while avoiding an awkward silence.

In situations where there is not a lot of ambient light, an artificial light source such as a penlight or flashlight will be necessary. Ask the patient to stare straight ahead as you hold the light just outside their field of vision. With the light turned on, quickly move the light from the side directly toward their pupil. Watch closely for the pupil to constrict as the light hits it. Then move the light away and watch the pupil dilate slightly and return to its original size.

Both pupils should react to the change in light with the same speed. Pupils that respond slowly to the change in light are documented as sluggish. Pupils that do not respond at all are referred to as fixed. This can be seen in some patients with severe head injury or in cardiac arrest; the pupils gradually become fixed and dilated.

An acronym widely used in EMS to help providers remember the characteristics of pupils is PERRL, which stands for:

Pupils
Equal
Round
Reactive
Light

Table 12.6 lists observations you may make when assessing a patient's pupils and lists possible causes.

TABLE 12.6	**Pupils**
OBSERVATION	**POSSIBLE PROBLEM**
Dilated, nonreactive pupils	Shock, cardiac arrest, bleeding, certain medications, head injury
Constricted, nonreactive pupils	Central nervous system damage, certain medications
Unequal pupils	Stroke, head injury

"I don't understand," Morgan says, looking over the shoulders of the ambulance personnel as they are loading Luis onto a stretcher and hooking him up to a heart monitor and oxygen. "Look at his vitals. He was doing better after 10 minutes, and then suddenly his skin turned white as a ghost, his pulse was soaring, and he was practically gasping like a fish."

"You did everything just fine," a paramedic says, taking the list of vitals and paper bag of medications from Morgan's shaking grip. "Sitting him up, keeping him comfortable, and keeping track of his vitals as you did probably kept him from getting worse sooner. We have a better chance of getting him to a doctor because of you."

The loud clatter of the stretcher and the medical chatter of the ambulance crew drowns out Morgan's goodbye to Luis as he is wheeled out to the ambulance without a second look back.

Eduardo puts his hand on Morgan's shoulder and sighs. "To think I almost called in sick today."

Summary

- Gathering information (history) about your patient and their chief complaint and obtaining complete and accurate vital signs are two important aspects of a good patient assessment.
- Properly introduce yourself and get the patient's name right away. Establishing a rapport from the beginning will make the patient comfortable and more cooperative.
- Whenever possible, direct your questions to the patient.
- Speak clearly and confirm that the patient hears, understands, and answers each question before you ask another.
- Use the SAMPLE tool to help guide your questions, and always document the patient's answers.
- Obtain a set of vital signs as soon as practical to establish a good baseline for comparison of subsequent vital signs.
- When practical, repeat vital signs and compare them to previous readings to establish trends in the patient's condition.

- Remember that most vital signs have multiple characteristics; document all characteristics for each vital sign.
- You will assess respirations for rate, depth, and ease. The normal range for respirations is 10 to 30 breaths per minute.
- You will assess pulses for rate, strength, and rhythm. The normal range for pulse rate is 60 to 100 beats per minute.
- Blood pressure is measured in millimeters of mercury (mm Hg) and includes a systolic (contraction) and diastolic (resting) reading.
- You will assess skin for color, temperature, and moisture. The normal findings for skin are pink, warm, and dry.
- You will assess pupils for equality, shape, reactivity to light. Normal pupils are equal, round, and react briskly to changes in light.

Take Action

Making History

You can practice performing a SAMPLE history with the help of friends and family. Make up a set of flashcards, one for each letter of the SAMPLE acronym. On one side, put the letter and the word it represents. On the opposite side, write several questions that pertain to the letter. Now use the flashcards to help you practice performing a SAMPLE history on friends and family members.

Practice Makes Proficient

Developing proficiency with taking vital signs takes considerable practice. Fortunately, there is rarely a shortage of people to practice on. There are no special tools necessary to practice most vital signs (excluding blood pressure), so there is no reason you cannot practice taking vital signs every day.

First on Scene Patient Handoff

Luis is a 53-year-old male whose chief complaint is difficulty breathing. Upon arrival we found Luis in a reclined position. His breathing was rapid and shallow and his skin was pale. He was A&O × 4. Luis is a Spanish speaker so it has been a little challenging getting a good history. He denied any mechanism of injury for trauma. During our assessment, Luis was able to sit up and indicated that this intervention made his breathing easier. Baseline vitals were respirations of 36, shallow with a gurgling sound, pulse was 104, weak, and regular.

First on Scene Run Review

Recall the events of the First on Scene scenario in this chapter, and answer the following questions related to the call. Rationales are offered in the Answer Key at the back of the book.

1. What signs and symptoms did Morgan find, and what might they indicate?
2. What would your treatment be for this patient?
3. Why would sitting Luis up help him?

Quick Quiz

To check your understanding of the chapter, answer the following questions. Then compare your answers to those in the Answer Key at the back of the book.

1. You are caring for an adult patient who appears to be unconscious. When you tap on his shoulder and call out his name, he opens his eyes and attempts to respond. This patient would be classified as ____ on the AVPU scale.
   a. alert
   b. verbal
   c. painful
   d. unresponsive

2. In a SAMPLE history, the *E* represents:
   a. EKG results.
   b. evaluation of the neck and spine.
   c. events leading to the illness or injury.
   d. evidence of airway obstruction.

3. When assessing circulation for a responsive adult patient, you should assess the:
   a. carotid pulse.
   b. brachial pulse.
   c. radial pulse.
   d. pedal pulse.

4. When assessing the pulse, you should assess:
   a. rate, strength, and rhythm.
   b. strength and regularity.
   c. rate and volume.
   d. rate and quality.

5. When assessing a patient's respirations, you must determine rate, depth, and:
   a. regularity.
   b. count of expirations.
   c. ease.
   d. count of inspirations.

6. Five common vital signs are pulse, respirations, blood pressure, pupils, and:
   a. oxygen saturation.
   b. skin signs.
   c. pain level.
   d. capillary refill.

7. Which of the following would be described as a sign?
   a. Chest pain
   b. Headache
   c. Pale skin
   d. Abdominal cramping

8. What can be assessed by watching and feeling the chest and abdomen move during breathing?
   a. Pulse rate
   b. Blood pressure
   c. Skin signs
   d. Respiratory rate

9. Which of the following best describes the reason for obtaining an accurate medical history?
   a. It allows insurance to properly bill the patient.
   b. It allows you to better understand what is happening with the patient.
   c. It helps paramedics complete accurate documentation.
   d. It tells you if the patient is not being truthful in their complaints.

10. The "R" in the OPQRST mnemonic refers to:
    a. respirations.
    b. radial.
    c. remote.
    d. radiate.

11. What are the two pulse points that are referred to as central pulses?
    a. Radial and tibial
    b. Carotid and femoral
    c. Femoral and brachial
    d. Brachial and carotid

12. As blood pressure drops, perfusion is most likely to:
    a. increase.
    b. decrease.
    c. fluctuate.
    d. remain the same.

13. Skin that is bluish in color is called:
    a. pale.
    b. flushed.
    c. cyanotic.
    d. jaundiced.

14. The term *diaphoretic* refers to:
    a. pupil reaction.
    b. skin temperature.
    c. heart rhythm.
    d. skin moisture.

15. When going from a well-lit room to a dark one, you would expect the normal pupil to:
    a. not react.
    b. dilate.
    c. constrict.
    d. fluctuate.

16. Which of the following is most accurate when describing a palpated blood pressure?
    a. It provides only the diastolic pressure.
    b. It must be taken on a responsive patient.
    c. It can be obtained without a stethoscope.
    d. It can be obtained without a BP cuff.

17. A respiratory rate that is lower than ____ breaths per minute for an adult should be considered inadequate.
    a. 4
    b. 6
    c. 8
    d. 10

18. The pressure inside the arteries each time the heart contracts is referred to as the _____ pressure.

    a. diastolic
    b. pulse
    c. systolic
    d. mean

19. Which of the following would best be described as a symptom?

    a. Bruising to the arm
    b. A laceration on the lip
    c. Headache
    d. Diaphoretic skin

20. The term *trending* is best defined as the:

    a. ability to record changes in a patient's condition over time.
    b. name given to the last set of vital signs taken on a patient.
    c. transfer of care from one level of care to another.
    d. ability to improve a patient's condition over time.

Endnotes

1. InformedHealth.org [Internet]. Cologne, Germany: Institute for Quality and Efficiency in Health Care (IQWiG); 2006–. What is blood pressure and how is it measured? 2010 Jun 24 [Updated 2019 May 23]. Available from: https://www.ncbi.nlm.nih.gov/books/NBK279251/
2. "New ACC/AHA High Blood Pressure Guidelines Lower Definition of Hypertension." American College of Cardiology website, updated November 13, 2017. Accessed February 12, 2018, at http://www.acc.org/latest-in-cardiology/articles/2017/11/08/11/47/mon-5pm-bp-guideline-aha-2017
3. McGuire, D., Gotlib, A., King, J. Capillary Refill Time. 2022 Apr 21. In: StatPearls [Internet]. Treasure Island (FL): StatPearls Publishing; 2022 Jan–. PMID: 32491685.

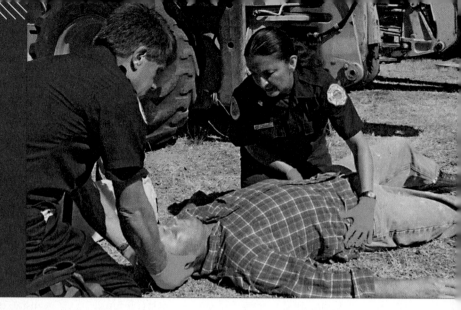

13

Principles of Patient Assessment

Education Standards

Assessment—Scene Assessment, Primary Assessment, History Taking, Secondary Assessment, Monitoring Devices, Reassessment

Competencies

Use scene information and patient assessment findings to identify and manage immediate life threats and injuries.

LEARNING OBJECTIVES

Upon successful completion of this chapter, the student should be able to:

Cognitive

1. Define the chapter key terms.

2. Explain the importance that safety plays at the scene of an emergency.

3. Describe the components of an appropriate scene size-up and the importance of each component.

4. Describe hazards commonly found at emergency scenes (medical and trauma).

5. Explain the role the Emergency Medical Responder plays in ensuring the safety of all people at the scene of an emergency.

6. Differentiate between mechanism of injury and nature of illness.

7. Explain the purpose of the primary assessment.

8. Describe the components of a primary assessment.

9. Differentiate between stable (low priority) and unstable (high priority) patients.

10. Describe the assessment methods used for pediatric and geriatric patients.

11. Explain the purpose of the secondary assessment.

12. Describe the components of a secondary assessment.

13. Differentiate between significant and nonsignificant mechanisms of injury.

14. Describe the components of the BP-DOC assessment tool.

15. Explain the purpose of the reassessment.

Psychomotor

16. Demonstrate the ability to identify immediate and potential hazards to safety.

17. Demonstrate the ability to properly perform a scene size-up.

18. Demonstrate the ability to properly perform a primary assessment.

19. Demonstrate the ability to properly perform a secondary assessment.

20. Demonstrate the ability to properly perform a reassessment.

21. Demonstrate the ability to properly identify and perform appropriate interventions during a patient assessment.

Affective

22. Value the priority that safety plays in the overall assessment and care of the patient.

23. Model a caring and compassionate attitude with classmates and simulated patients.

24. Support the role of the Emergency Medical Responder with respect to patient advocacy.

25. Model an appropriate level of concern for a patient's modesty when exposing the body during an assessment.

KEY TERMS

ABCs (*p. 261*)
accessory muscle use (*p. 276*)
AVPU scale (*p. 262*)
brachial pulse (*p. 264*)
BP-DOC (*p. 272*)
carotid pulse (*p. 263*)
crepitus (*p. 267*)
dorsalis pedis pulse (*p. 276*)
focused secondary assessment (*p. 267*)
general impression (*p. 261*)
guarding (*p. 276*)
immediate life threats (*p. 252*)
interventions (*p. 250*)
jugular vein distention (JVD) (*p. 276*)
manual stabilization (*p. 261*)

mechanism of injury (MOI) (*p. 251*)
medical patient (*p. 251*)
nature of illness (NOI) (*p. 252*)
paradoxical movement (*p. 276*)
patient assessment (*p. 250*)
primary assessment (*p. 251*)
radial pulse (*p. 263*)
rapid secondary assessment (*p. 267*)
reassessment (*p. 252*)
scene size-up (*p. 250*)
secondary assessment (*p. 252*)
track marks (*p. 276*)
trauma patient (*p. 251*)
tracheal deviation (*p. 276*)

One of the most fundamental skills you will learn and develop is patient assessment. The foundation of all emergency care lies in a good physical assessment and patient history. You must assess each patient to detect possible illness or injury and determine the most appropriate emergency care. This assessment must be done in a structured and orderly fashion to minimize the chance of overlooking an important sign or symptom. A good patient assessment almost always leads to good patient care. Likewise, a poor assessment almost always results in poor care. This chapter will help you learn to perform a methodical and thorough patient assessment.

FIRST ON SCENE

"Attention all employees!" The voice from the paging system in the Booker Manufacturing warehouse halts the bustle of the shipping staff. They all turn to look up at the loudspeaker. "All third-shift Medical Emergency Response Team members please report to the number 7 loading dock for a medical emergency."

Two warehouse employees remove their leather gloves and face shields and quickly walk to a white locker with *MERT* stenciled in wide red letters. They open the cabinet, remove two nylon bags, and hurry toward the loading docks at the south end of the building.

"I'll be the patient-care person if you'll do scene control," Joanie says.

"Okay," Lorena replies, fishing a pair of gloves from her bag and putting them on. Lorena is relieved to be with an experienced MERT member. She is new to the company's MERT, and the patient-assessment process is still a little confusing to her.

As the two pass the dock manager's small office and turn left, they are met by a forklift operator. The name embroidered on his shirt is Tariq. "I'm glad you're here," he says quickly. "It's one of the truck drivers. I think he's having a heart attack."

Patient Assessment

LO2 Explain the importance that safety plays at the scene of an emergency.

Performing a good patient assessment is a skill that can continually be improved—the more you practice, the better you get. As you learn to perform a patient assessment, you must learn to differentiate between what is normal and what might be abnormal for any given patient. As you examine the patient and ask questions, you will quickly identify those things that may be abnormal and need attention (Figure 13.1). Emergency Medical Responders and other EMS personnel are trained to identify, prioritize, and care for life-threatening issues first. Once all life threats have been cared for, you will complete a more thorough assessment of the patient, identify less obvious signs and symptoms, and gather a pertinent medical history.

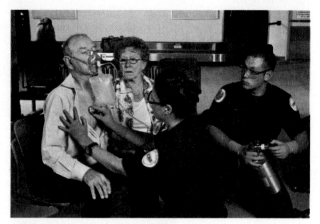

Figure 13.1 A thorough patient assessment is the foundation for the care of all patients.

scene size-up ▶ overview of the scene to identify any obvious or potential hazards; consists of taking BSI precautions, determining the scene safety, identifying the mechanism of injury or nature of illness, determining the number of patients, and identifying the need for additional resources.

interventions ▶ actions taken to correct or stabilize a patient's illness or injury.

A typical patient assessment contains four major components (Figure 13.2):

- *Scene size-up.* The **scene size-up** is a visual overview of the entire scene to identify any obvious or potential hazards prior to entering.
- *Primary assessment.* This is a quick assessment of the patient's airway, breathing, and circulation status, as well as a scan for obvious bleeding. It is designed to detect any immediate life-threatening problems that you can quickly correct.
- *Secondary assessment.* The secondary assessment is a more thorough assessment and has two subcomponents:
  - **History.** This includes all the information you can gather regarding the patient's condition as well as any previous medical history.
  - **Physical exam.** This includes using your hands and eyes to inspect the patient for any signs of illness and/or injury.
- *Reassessment.* This step follows the primary and secondary assessments and is an ongoing process that involves constant monitoring of the patient to detect any changes in condition. The reassessment involves repeating the primary assessment and vital signs and evaluating and adjusting any **interventions** as needed.

While the responsibilities of the Emergency Medical Responder may differ from one EMS system to another, most use an assessment-based approach to patient care. After ensuring one's own personal safety, your first concern is to detect and begin to correct life-threatening problems. The second concern is to identify and provide care for problems that are less serious or may become serious. The third concern is to constantly monitor the patient's condition to quickly detect any changes that may need attention.

CREW RESOURCE MANAGEMENT

Utilizing efficient crew resource management principles is especially important when arriving at the scene and throughout the call. ALL crew members must be always keeping an eye on the safety of the scene and must speak up when they see anything of concern. This will keep everyone aware of the changing environment and ensure the safety of crew members and patients.

SCENE SAFETY

Your patient assessment can put you in contact with a patient's blood and body fluids. Always take appropriate body substance isolation (BSI) precautions. Disposable gloves should always be worn during assessment and emergency care. Eye protection may also be required, depending on the type of emergency and patient condition. Wear any other items of personal protection required for your safety and that of your patients. Follow OSHA, CDC, and local guidelines to help prevent the spread of infectious diseases (see Chapter 3).

patient assessment ▶ standardized approach for performing a physical exam and obtaining a medical history on a patient.

Scene Safety

The components of the **patient assessment** and the order in which they are performed may vary from patient to patient based on their chief complaint. However, ensuring the safety of the scene before you enter is always the first step.

The conditions at a safe scene allow rescuers to access and provide care to patients without danger to themselves. An unsafe scene is one that contains immediate or potential hazards. An example is a motor vehicle crash site, at which it is common to find vehicles or objects that can move or shift position. Immediate hazards include an unstable vehicle

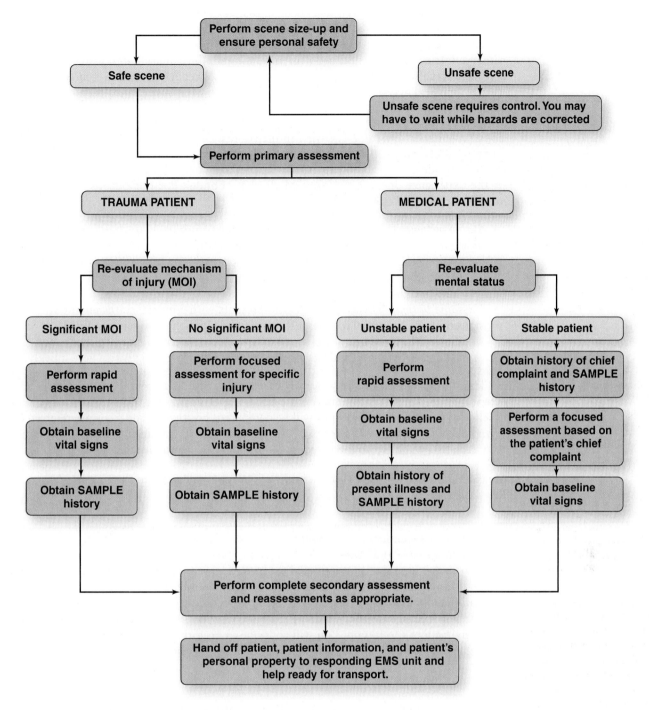

Figure 13.2 Patient assessment algorithm.

and broken glass. In addition, fire could break out or fuel and other fluids could leak and increase the danger, causing the scene to become even more unsafe.

Immediate Life Threats

The **primary assessment** is a set of steps performed to detect life-threatening problems that require immediate attention. The remaining components of the patient assessment change slightly based on each of the four types of patient:

- Unstable **medical patient**
- Stable medical patient
- Unstable **trauma patient** who has sustained a significant **mechanism of injury (MOI)**
- Stable trauma patient who has likely not sustained a significant MOI

primary assessment ▸ quick assessment of the patient's airway, breathing, circulation, and bleeding to detect and correct any immediate life-threatening problems.

medical patient ▸ one who has or describes symptoms of an illness.

trauma patient ▸ one who has a physical injury caused by an external force.

mechanism of injury ▸ force or forces that may have caused injury. Abbrev: MOI.

SCENE SAFETY

If at any point the scene becomes hazardous and your safety and/or the patient's safety is threatened, you must do whatever is necessary to address the hazard and ensure your safety.

The presence of immediate life threats, such as airway problems or uncontrolled bleeding that will be discovered in the primary assessment, also determine the stability of the patient.

At times, the type of patient you are caring for is not so clearly defined. For example, a patient experiencing a medical problem may fall and injure himself, or a medical problem may have actually caused a car crash. Your patient assessment will need to include elements for both medical and trauma patients. The most serious of the patient's problems should guide your assessment.

The Stable versus Unstable Patient In the context of patient care, the terms *stable* and *unstable* can be very subjective and mean different things to different people. The ability to make this determination confidently is based partly on patient presentation and partly on the experience of the Emergency Medical Responder. For our purposes, *stable* and *unstable* are defined as follows:

- *Stable patient.* This is a patient whose condition is not likely to change for the worse in the next few minutes. This could be a patient whose mental status and vital signs are mostly within normal limits and appear to be getting better rather than worse. For the trauma patient, this is a patient who has NOT sustained a significant mechanism of injury (MOI).
- *Unstable patient.* This is a patient who presents with a mental status and/or vital signs that are abnormal for them. It can also be a patient who has sustained a significant MOI and as a result may be experiencing internal bleeding that is not immediately obvious. The unstable patient is at risk for getting worse very quickly.

REMEMBER

A patient who appears to be stable can become unstable without warning.

It is important to obtain a set of vital signs, including mental status, to make a determination if signs and symptoms are changing. This first set of vital signs serve as a baseline to which future vital signs will be compared. For that reason, they are referred to as *baseline vital signs* (see Chapter 12). Any patient whose vital signs and/or mental status are trending toward the abnormal range should be considered unstable.

Medical Patients For a stable medical patient, you will perform the steps described in Key Skill 13.1:

- Perform a scene size-up and a primary assessment.
- Perform a **secondary assessment** based on the patient's chief complaint.
- Obtain baseline vital signs.
- Attempt to obtain a thorough medical history. Interview the patient's family and/or bystanders, if necessary, to determine the patient's chief complaint and **nature of illness (NOI)**.
- Perform a **reassessment**, including the patient's vital signs, to identify any changes in the patient's condition. You will continue to perform the reassessment until higher-trained EMS personnel assume care of the patient.

For an unstable medical patient, you will perform the steps described in Key Skill 13.2:

- Perform a scene size-up and a primary assessment. Care for all **immediate life threats** first.
- Obtain baseline vital signs.
- Attempt to obtain a medical history, if possible. Interview the patient's family and/or bystanders, if necessary, to determine the patient's chief complaint and nature of illness.

Trauma Patients For a stable trauma patient with no significant mechanism of injury, you will perform the steps described in Key Skill 13.3:

- Perform a scene size-up and a primary assessment. Determine the mechanism of injury.
- Conduct a secondary assessment based on the patient's chief complaint.
- Obtain baseline vital signs.
- Perform a reassessment, including vital signs, to identify any changes in the patient's condition.

secondary assessment ▶ complete head-to-toe physical exam, including medical history.

nature of illness ▶ what is medically wrong with the patient; a complaint not related to an injury. Abbrev: NOI.

reassessment ▶ last step in patient assessment, used to detect changes in a patient's condition; includes repeating the primary assessment, reassessing and recording vital signs, and checking interventions. To be repeated as time allows until higher-trained EMS personnel assume care of the patient.

immediate life threats ▶ any condition that may pose an immediate threat to the patient's life, such as problems with the airway, breathing, circulation, or safety.

Focused Secondary Assessment—Responsive/Stable Medical Patient

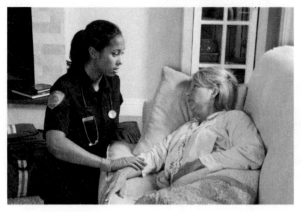

1. Perform a scene size-up and establish the chief complaint.

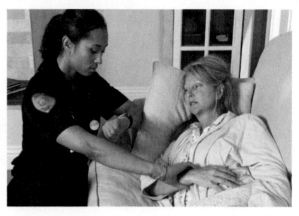

2. Perform a primary assessment. Care for immediate life threats first.

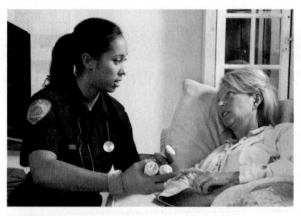

3. Obtain a medical history.

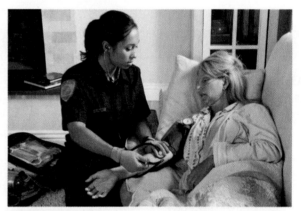

4. Perform a secondary assessment, including vital signs.

Rapid Secondary Assessment—Unresponsive/Unstable Medical Patient

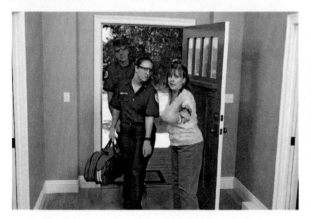

1. Perform a scene size-up as you approach the scene.

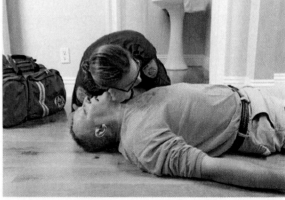

2. Perform a primary assessment. Care for immediate life threats first.

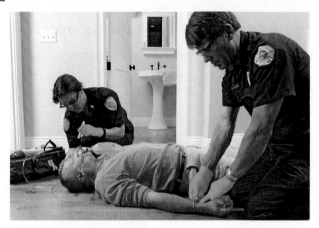

3. Perform a rapid secondary assessment to identify signs of illness. Obtain baseline vital signs. Perform reassessments as often as necessary depending on the patient's condition.

KEY SKILL 13.3

Focused Secondary Assessment—Trauma Patient With No Significant Mechanism of Injury

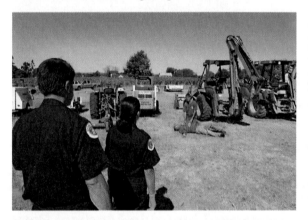

1. Perform a scene size-up as you approach the scene.

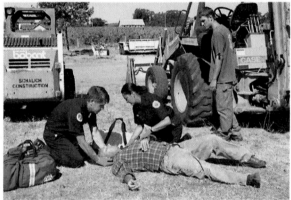

2. Perform a primary assessment. Care for immediate life threats first.

3. Perform a focused secondary assessment based on the patient's injuries. Perform reassessments as often as necessary.

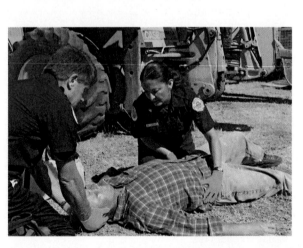

Rapid Secondary Assessment—Trauma Patient With a Significant Mechanism of Injury

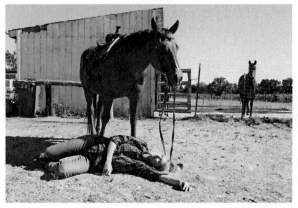

1. Perform a scene size-up as you approach the scene.

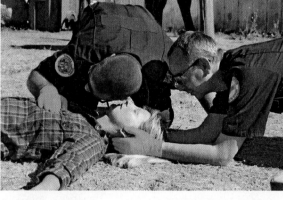

2. Perform a primary assessment. Care for immediate life threats first.

3. Perform a rapid secondary assessment and obtain baseline vital signs. Perform reassessments as often as necessary.

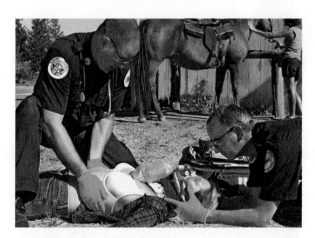

For an unstable trauma patient with a significant MOI, you will perform the steps described in Key Skill 13.4:

- Perform a scene size-up. Determine the mechanism of injury.
- Perform a primary assessment. Manually stabilize the patient's head and neck. Care for any life threats as you detect them.
- Perform a rapid secondary assessment to look for obvious serious injuries.
- Obtain baseline vital signs.
- Perform a reassessment, including vital signs, to identify any changes in the patient's condition.

Scene Size-Up

LO3 Describe the components of an appropriate scene size-up and the importance of each component.

Safety is a primary goal of the scene size-up. The scene size-up actually begins with the information you receive from dispatch before you arrive at the emergency scene. While en route, recall the dispatcher's description of the emergency. Think about the types of injuries or hazards you may find at that particular scene. The factors you will encounter when responding to a vehicle collision will be very different from those you will encounter at the residence of an individual experiencing abdominal pain.

When you arrive on the scene, take appropriate body substance isolation (BSI) precautions and make sure the scene is safe to enter. When the scene is safe to enter, remain cautious and continue to evaluate scene safety throughout the call.

Next, when the call involves a trauma patient, look for the mechanism of injury (MOI). Identify the nature of illness (NOI) for patients who are sick. The nature of illness is usually tied to the patient's chief complaint, but not always (Figure 13.3). Note the number of patients and anticipate any additional resources that may be needed. It is best to call for any needed resources as soon as practical. For all patients, consider the need for spinal precautions as you approach the scene.

To recap, every patient assessment begins with scene size-up (Key Skill 13.5), which includes:

- taking universal precautions.
- determining if the scene is safe for you, other responders, the patient, and bystanders.
- identifying the MOI or NOI.
- determining the number of patients.
- identifying any additional resources needed.
- considering the need for spinal precautions when caring for a trauma patient.

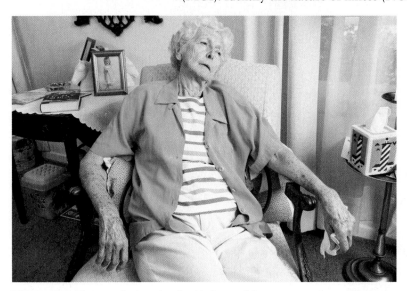

Figure 13.3 The medical patient's chief complaint may not always be obvious as you approach.

KEY SKILL 13.5

Scene Size-Up

TRAUMA PATIENT

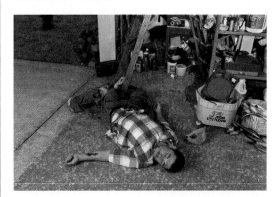

As you approach the trauma patient:

- Take appropriate BSI precautions.
- Determine if the scene is safe for you, the patient, and bystanders.
- Identify and evaluate the mechanism of injury.
- Determine the number of patients.
- Decide if additional resources, such as an ambulance, fire department, law enforcement, helicopter, or utility company, are needed.
- Consider the need for spinal immobilization.

MEDICAL PATIENT

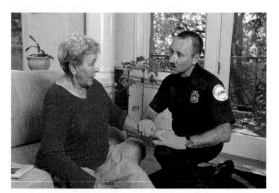

As you approach the medical patient:

- Take appropriate BSI precautions.
- Determine if the scene is safe for you, the patient, and bystanders.
- Identify and evaluate the chief complaint.
- Determine the number of patients.
- Decide if additional resources, such as an ambulance, fire department, law enforcement, or helicopter, are needed.

BSI Precautions

Always take appropriate universal precautions prior to assessing and caring for patients. At the very least, this includes wearing disposable gloves. Wear eye protection and use additional personal protective equipment as needed, depending on the patient's problem. Remember, BSI precautions are meant to protect both you and your patient, so take precautions before you make contact.

Ensuring Safety at the Scene

| LO4 | Describe hazards commonly found at emergency scenes (medical and trauma). |

| LO5 | Explain the role the Emergency Medical Responder plays in ensuring the safety of all people at the scene of an emergency. |

A dangerous and sometimes fatal mistake that responders may make is entering an unsafe or hazardous scene. Never assume that any scene is safe without a careful assessment. Take the time to stop and carefully assess the scene for yourself. If the scene is unsafe, do not enter it. For example, if a scene has the potential for violence and you are not a law enforcement officer, do not enter it until law enforcement indicates it is safe for you to do so. If there is a potential for a hazardous materials release, remain a safe distance away. In fact, you may never actually enter such scenes. Often, appropriately trained and equipped hazardous materials team members will bring properly decontaminated patients to you.

Examples of unsafe scenes include those involving vehicle collisions and traffic, the release of toxic substances, the potential for violence, or the presence of weapons. Also look for signs of domestic disturbances, electrical hazards, potential for fire or explosions, and aggressive animals. Use all your senses to detect unsafe scenes. Remain at a safe distance to keep yourself and others away from harm.

An important rule to remember is: *Do not become a victim yourself.* Every year, many rescuers are injured and some are killed while attempting to care for others at an emergency scene.

Mechanism of Injury or Nature of Illness

| LO6 | Differentiate between mechanism of injury and nature of illness. |

During the scene size-up, you must do your best to identify the mechanism of injury (MOI) for a trauma patient and the nature of illness (NOI) for a medical patient. Information may be obtained from the patient, family members, and/or bystanders, and by carefully looking at the scene for clues.

The MOI is made up of the combined forces that caused the injury. Did the patient fall? Is there a penetrating wound? Were they involved in a motor vehicle crash? For example, a damaged steering wheel in a vehicle should lead you to consider the possibility of a chest injury. A cracked windshield could indicate a head injury. It is wise to suspect spinal injuries in any patient who experienced a fall or blunt trauma (also called blunt force trauma) to the head.

Identifying the NOI is similar to identifying the MOI. In most instances, the NOI will be directly related to the patient's chief complaint. While diagnosing why the patient is having a particular medical problem is not necessary, the NOI will guide you in the appropriate direction for care. Common NOIs include chest pain, difficulty breathing, and abdominal pain. Look at the patient and the area in which they were found for clues:

- Does the patient look like they are having trouble breathing?
- Are they holding their chest or abdomen as if they are in pain?
- Does their position suggest where there might be pain or discomfort?
- Are medications or home oxygen equipment in view?
- Do you detect any odors, such as vomit or urine?

Both the mechanism of injury and the nature of illness allow you to consider what complications could potentially develop. For example, if the patient is complaining of chest pain, consider the possibility of a heart problem and the potential for cardiac arrest. If the patient experienced a fall, consider the forces involved and the potential for injury. Always keep in mind the possibility of a medical condition as the cause of a fall. For example, consider the patient who had a seizure while standing and fell to the ground, injuring their head when it struck the pavement.

Number of Patients and Need for Additional Resources

The next steps in the scene size-up are to determine the number of patients and whether you have sufficient resources to handle the emergency. Once you are certain of the number of patients involved, you must determine if additional resources are needed. More than one ambulance may be required to handle several patients. In fact, you may require additional resources even on calls with only one patient. You may need additional help if a heavy patient must be carried down stairs. You may require the fire department to respond to help with extrication or to make a crash scene safe. Or the patient may require air transport to a specialty medical facility such as a regional trauma center. An important part of the scene size-up is recognizing the need for additional resources and calling for them early.

Arrival at the Patient's Side

Upon arrival at the patient's side, begin by identifying yourself, even if it appears that the patient may be unresponsive. Simply state your name and your role: "I am an Emergency Medical Responder." While many people may not know exactly what an EMR does, the statement should allow you access to the patient and the cooperation of bystanders.

Your next statement to the patient should be: "May I help you?" By answering "yes" to this question, the patient is giving you expressed consent to begin care. The patient may not answer "yes" to your question but instead may simply remain still and allow you to provide care. A patient who is alert and does not refuse your care is said to be providing consent for your care.

Sometimes a patient's fear may be so great that they are confused and will answer "no" or say something like "Just leave me alone." Gaining the patient's confidence by talking with them is usually easy. If the patient is unresponsive or unable to give expressed consent, a legal form of consent called implied consent allows you to care for the patient. This means that if the patient were able to do so, it is implied that they would consent to care. (Review Chapter 2 for a more detailed discussion of consent.)

Remember, upon arrival and after conducting a scene size-up, you must:

1. State your name and identify yourself as a trained Emergency Medical Responder. Let the patient and bystanders know that you are with the EMS system.
2. Gain consent from the patient to provide care.

If someone is already providing care to the patient when you arrive, identify yourself as an Emergency Medical Responder. If the individual's training is equal to or at a higher level than your own, ask if you may assist. When appropriate, you should still introduce yourself to the patient and let them know you are there to assist.

If you have more training than the individual who has begun care, respectfully ask to take over care of the patient and ask the original responder to assist you. You might start by simply offering to take over care. You can say something like, "Would you like me to take the lead, or are you okay with continuing?" Thank the individual for their assistance. Never criticize or argue with anyone who may have initiated care.

JEDI

Your introduction sets the tone for your entire patient assessment. Be mindful of positioning yourself at the patient's eye level and asking the patient their name and pronouns when possible. Be careful to not make assumptions about the patient's gender, as it may not always be obvious.

"Darn it, Tariq!" the driver says loudly. "I told you it's not a heart attack! I think I pulled a muscle in my chest." The older man is sitting on a pallet of boxes with his hand pressed to the center of his chest.

"Hello, sir," Joanie says as she kneels beside the patient. "I'm Joanie. This is Lorena. We're Emergency Medical Responders with the company's medical emergency response team. Do I have permission to make sure that you're okay?"

The driver sighs, rolls his eyes, and says, "Yes, but I'm fine."

"Great." Joanie smiles. "That makes it a good day for both of us, doesn't it? What's your name?" She then touches the driver's wrist with her gloved hand and pauses to feel for a pulse.

"Brad," the driver says between rapid breaths. At first, Brad's pulse is weak and somewhat irregular, and Joanie notices that he is growing pale and anxious. After a few moments, his pulse takes on a more regular rhythm and his color returns.

Primary Assessment

LO7 Explain the purpose of the primary assessment.

LO8 Describe the components of a primary assessment.

The primary assessment is designed to help the Emergency Medical Responder detect and correct all immediate threats to life. Immediate life threats typically involve the patient's airway, breathing, circulation, or bleeding, and each is corrected as it is found. The primary assessment begins as soon as you reach the patient and gain the patient's consent to treat.

The primary assessment has seven components (Key Skills 13.6, 13.7, and 13.8):

- Form a general impression of the patient.
- Assess the patient's mental status. Initially, this may mean determining if the patient is responsive or unresponsive.
- Assess the patient's airway.
- Assess the patient's breathing.
- Assess the patient's circulation.
- Assess for uncontrolled bleeding.
- Make an initial decision on the priority or urgency of the patient for transport.

KEY SKILL 13.6

Primary Assessment—Trauma Patient With No Significant MOI

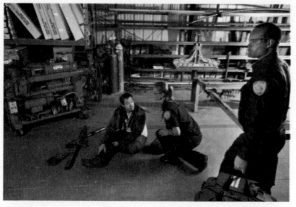

1. Size up the scene and form a general impression of the patient.

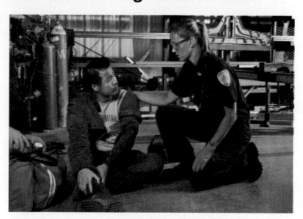

2. Evaluate the mental status of the patient.

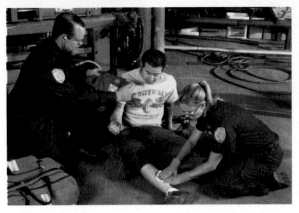

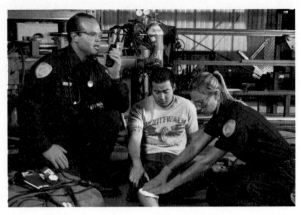

3. Address any issues relating to the airway, breathing, and circulation.

4. Determine patient priority for transport.

KEY SKILL 13.7

Primary Assessment—Medical Patient

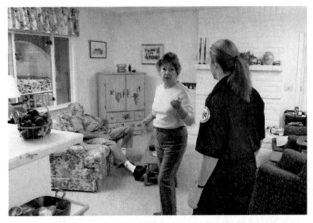

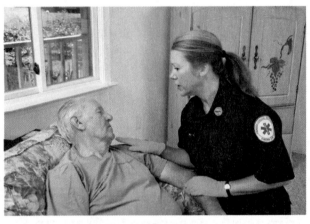

1. Size up the scene and form a general impression of the patient.

2. Assess the patient's mental status.

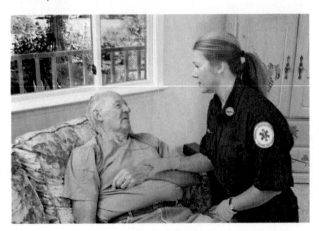

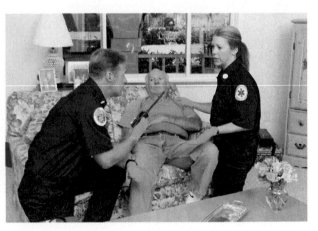

3. Assess the patient's airway, breathing, and circulation.

4. Determine patient priority for transport.

Primary Assessment—Unresponsive Patient (Medical or Trauma)

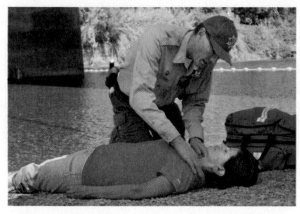

1. Determine level of responsiveness (stable/unstable).

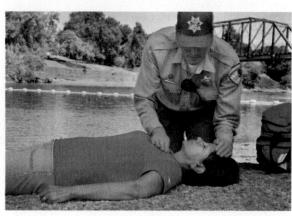

2. Ensure an open airway and adequate breathing.

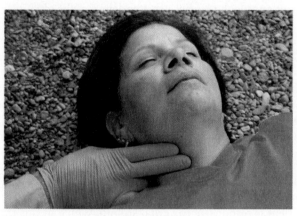

3. Check for the presence of a pulse.

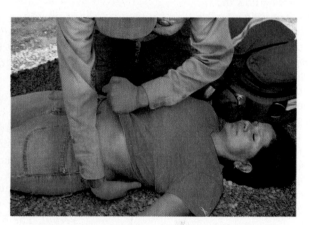

4. Look for and control all major bleeding. Determine patient priority for transport.

While conducting the primary assessment, you will look for life-threatening problems in three major areas, known as the **ABCs** of emergency care:

- *Airway.* Is the patient's airway open and clear?
- *Breathing.* Is the patient breathing adequately?
- *Circulation.* Does the patient have an adequate pulse? Is there serious bleeding? Are there signs of obvious blood loss?

ABCs ▶ patient's airway, breathing, and circulation as they relate to the primary assessment.

During the primary assessment, if a life-threatening problem is detected, it may be necessary to start simultaneous actions focused on caring for these problems. For example, a trauma patient may require **manual stabilization** of their head and neck at the same time you are opening the patient's airway, providing ventilations, and controlling bleeding. A medical patient may require you to assess their mental status at the same time you are taking a pulse and assessing their breathing. Simultaneous actions can prove to be very challenging. The more you practice your assessment, the better you will become at completing it efficiently.

manual stabilization ▶ using your hands to physically hold the body part and keep it from moving.

General Impression

As you approach your patient, you will be forming a **general impression** of the patient and the patient's environment. Your general impression is your first assessment of the patient's overall condition. The general impression will help you decide the seriousness of

general impression ▶ first informal impression of the patient's overall condition.

AVPU scale ▶ memory aid for the classifications of levels of responsiveness; the letters stand for *alert, verbal, painful,* and *unresponsive.*

the patient's condition based on their level of distress and mental status. You also might be given information by the patient or bystanders at this time, such as the reason EMS was called. In most cases, the reason EMS was called can be determined by identifying the patient's chief complaint.

The general impression consists of the following elements: approximate age, sex, and level of distress or responsiveness. For example: *I see an approximately 30-year-old man in moderate distress* or *I see an approximately 60-year-old woman who appears to be unresponsive.*

Emergency Medical Responders always form a general impression when they first see a patient, even if they are not immediately aware of doing so. With experience, you will learn to form one based on intuition and observation. You may notice if the patient looks very ill, pale, or cyanotic. You may immediately see serious injuries or that the patient looks alert. This impression forms an early opinion of how seriously ill or injured the patient is. Your decision to request immediate transport or to continue assessing the patient may be based solely on your general impression.

Mental Status

Your general impression of a patient begins by determining the patient's level of responsiveness. You must quickly determine if they are responsive or unresponsive. Sometimes this is obvious as you approach. A responsive patient may be obviously awake and interacting with those around them. An unresponsive individual may not be so obvious. You must kneel beside the patient, tap their shoulder, and state loudly something like, "Are you okay?" or "Can you hear me?" If they respond, you know they are not totally unresponsive.

If it is a trauma patient or you have reason to suspect a spinal injury, place your hands on both sides of their head before attempting to elicit a response. This will help stabilize the head and prevent the patient from moving too much in response to your questioning.

Classify the patient's mental status using the **AVPU scale**, which describes the patient's ability to respond to various stimuli (see Chapter 12):

A — *Alert.* The patient is alert and spontaneously interacting with the environment around them.

V — *Verbal.* The patient is responsive to verbal stimuli, which means they respond when you speak to them or ask a question. They may or may not provide any meaningful information.

P — *Pain.* The patient is responsive only to painful stimuli. This patient appears to be unconscious and does not respond to your verbal commands or questions. However, they respond by groaning or pulling away when you provide some type of painful stimulus, such as rubbing the sternum with your knuckles or pinching the muscle above the shoulder near the neck.

U — *Unresponsive.* The patient is unconscious or completely unresponsive. This patient does not offer any type of response to verbal or painful stimulus.

The designation "alert" has various levels. A patient who is able to tell you only their name and where they are can be described as "alert and oriented ×2," or simply A&O × 2. The individual who knows who they are, where they are, the time of day, and what has happened to them would be described as A&O × 4.

The designation "verbal" does not necessarily mean that the patient is answering your questions or initiating a conversation. Instead, the patient may speak, grunt, groan, or say, "huh." It is possible that the patient may have a medical condition such as a stroke or a problem associated with trauma such as a head injury. Either of those conditions may cause the patient to lose the ability to speak.

Try to assess mental status without moving the patient. But if the patient is unresponsive, you may need to reposition them to open their airway, check for breathing and pulse, or look for serious bleeding.

Always suspect the presence of neck or spinal injuries in the unresponsive trauma patient. Despite the possibility of a spinal injury, it may be necessary to carefully move the patient so you can check for and address life-threatening problems. (Review Chapter 6 for information on moving a patient safely.)

Airway and Breathing

If the patient is unresponsive, check for adequate breathing by observing the chest rise and fall. Shallow or absent respirations require immediate attention. Gasping respirations in the unresponsive patient are called *agonal respirations*. They should not be considered normal respirations. If your patient is unresponsive and there are no signs of breathing, check for a carotid pulse and begin CPR if there is no pulse. You must also visually inspect the mouth and airway for evidence of a foreign body obstruction.

If the patient is breathing, there will always be circulation, even if you cannot palpate a pulse. At this point, you can move on to checking for obvious bleeding. Now is the time to consider the need for supplemental oxygen. Delegate this task to another rescuer so you may continue with your assessment.

Circulation

Circulation refers to the flow of blood as it is circulated with each beat of the heart. It can be implied that a responsive patient who is breathing also has a pulse. For the unresponsive patient, you must locate and assess a pulse to confirm adequate circulation. The assessment of circulation also includes observing for and controlling any obvious serious bleeding.

Check for a Pulse If the patient is not breathing, check for a **carotid pulse** at the neck (Figure 13.4A). The carotid pulse at the neck is considered more reliable than the **radial pulse** at the wrist (Figure 13.4B). The radial pulse may not be present if the patient has a very low blood pressure.

To assess the carotid pulse, first locate the patient's larynx (Adam's apple). Place the tips of your index and middle fingers directly over the midline of this structure. Now, slide your fingertips to the side of the neck closest to you. Do not slide your fingertips to the opposite side of the patient's neck because this may apply improper pressure on the airway. You should detect a pulse in the groove between the trachea and the large muscle on the side of the neck. It is important to check only one carotid pulse point at a time to avoid reducing blood flow to the brain. Only moderate pressure is needed to feel it. Check for a carotid pulse for 5 to 10 seconds. Frequent practice will make this skill easy to master.

It is not important during the primary assessment to count the exact rate of the pulse. You only want to confirm the presence of a pulse. If there is no pulse, begin CPR.

carotid pulse ▶ pulse that can be felt on either side of the neck. Palpate only one side at a time.

radial pulse ▶ pulse that can be felt on the anterior aspect of the wrist on the same side as the thumb.

REMEMBER

If you cannot feel a radial pulse, check for a carotid pulse. When there is no radial pulse, the patient may still have a carotid pulse. Never begin CPR without first checking the carotid pulse.

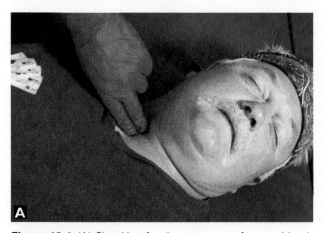 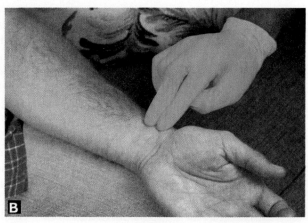

Figure 13.4 (A) Checking for the presence of a carotid pulse on an unresponsive patient. (B) Checking for the presence of a radial pulse on a responsive patient.

If the patient is not breathing but does have a pulse, the patient may have an airway obstruction or they may be in respiratory arrest. You must take immediate action to ventilate the patient before the heart stops. (See Chapter 9.)

Check for Serious Bleeding   The next step is checking for serious uncontrolled bleeding. While any uncontrolled bleeding may eventually become life threatening, during the primary assessment you will only be concerned with profuse bleeding. Quickly scan the patient from head to toe and look for evidence of bleeding. Be sure to observe under the patient as best as you can. Blood that is bright red and spurting may be coming from an artery. Because blood in arteries is under a great deal of pressure, large amounts of blood may be lost through arterial bleeding in a short period of time. Flowing blood that is darker in color is most likely coming from a vein. Even if the bleeding is slow, it may be life threatening if the patient has been bleeding for a long period of time. Look at the amount of blood that has been lost on the ground, clothing, and in the hair.

Assessment of circulation may be altered slightly when you immediately see profuse bleeding. In this case, attempt to control the bleeding as soon as it is discovered. (Methods of controlling serious bleeding are covered in Chapter 18.) Do what you can to control it, but never neglect the patient's airway and breathing status.

Patient Priority

LO9   Differentiate between stable (low priority) and unstable (high priority) patients.

The Emergency Medical Responder understands the local EMS system and is usually the first medically trained individual on the scene. You will know whether Basic Life Support or Advanced Life Support is available as well as the capability of the hospitals near you. You will be expected to provide notification to responding agencies with the number of patients and the severity of their conditions. This information determines the urgency of the response and alerts them to the type of care that may be required. In some areas, this may result in the launching of medical helicopters or the dispatching of additional resources. As the first qualified eyes on the scene, you play a vital role.

As soon as you have enough information about your patient, you will want to establish a priority for transport. A high-priority patient should be transported immediately, with as little time spent on the scene as is practical. High-priority conditions include unresponsiveness, breathing difficulties, severe bleeding or shock, complicated childbirth, chest pain, and any severe pain. Consider calling for an ALS ambulance for all high-priority patients.

Special Considerations for Infants and Children

LO10   Describe the assessment methods used for pediatric and geriatric patients.

Assessment of an infant or child differs from that of an adult in a few ways. It is important to realize that children are not merely little adults. They react to illness and injury in different ways.

Infants and children are often shy and distrustful of strangers. A responsive infant or a child who pays no attention to you or what you are doing may be seriously ill. When checking the mental status of an unresponsive infant, talk directly to them and gently flick the bottoms of the infant's feet.

Opening the airway of an infant involves moving the head into a neutral position, not tilting it back, as with an adult.[1] Opening the airway of a child requires only a slight extension of the neck by tilting the head back only slightly.

Respiratory and pulse rates are faster in infants and children than in adults. The easiest pulse to locate in an infant or a small child is the **brachial pulse** (Figure 13.5). The pulse points in the neck and wrist are difficult to locate in small patients due to the amount of body fat in these areas.

brachial pulse ▶ pulse that can be felt in the medial side of the upper arm between the elbow and shoulder.

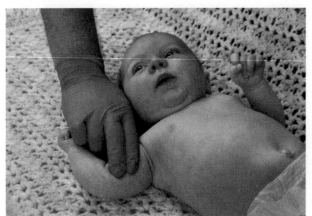

Figure 13.5 Checking for the presence of a brachial pulse in an infant.

An additional technique used for checking an infant's or a child's circulation is capillary refill. When the end of a finger is gently pressed, it turns white because the pressure forces out the blood. When the pressure is released, the skin or nail bed turns pink again, usually in less than 2 seconds. This is a good way to evaluate the circulation status of an infant or a child. If it takes longer than 2 seconds for the nail bed to become pink again or if it does not return to pink at all, there may be a problem with circulation, as in the case of shock.

For infants less than 1 year of age, you may perform the same test on the top of their foot or back of their hand. For patients with darker skin, you may use the palm of the hand or the bottom of the foot. To judge the amount of time it takes for the blood to flow back, count "one-one thousand, two-one thousand," or simply say "capillary refill."

Usually, when adult patients have a serious problem, they become worse gradually. The downward trend often can be spotted in time to take appropriate action. However, an infant's or a child's body can compensate so well for a problem such as blood loss that he or she may appear stable for some time and then suddenly become much worse.[2] Children can actually maintain a near-normal blood pressure up to the time when almost half of their total blood volume is gone. That is why blood pressure is not a reliable assessment of a child's circulation. Checking capillary refill time is more reliable.

A child's condition can change very quickly. It is vital for the Emergency Medical Responder to recognize the seriousness of a child's illness or injury early, before it is too late. You will learn about other considerations in approaching and assessing infants and children in Chapter 24.

Alerting Dispatch

If you have called for additional resources, such as an ambulance or helicopter, it may be helpful to give them an update of the patient's condition. Your update should include information about the patient such as mental status, age, sex, chief complaint, airway and breathing status, and circulation status along with whatever interventions you have performed.

Secondary Assessment

LO11 Explain the purpose of the secondary assessment.

LO12 Describe the components of a secondary assessment.

A secondary assessment should be performed only after the primary assessment is complete and all immediate life threats have been found and corrected. If you have a patient with a life-threatening problem that you must continually care for (performing CPR on a cardiac-arrest patient, for example), you may not be able to start or complete a secondary assessment.

The main purpose of the secondary assessment is to discover and care for the patient's specific injuries or medical problems. It is a very systematic approach.

The secondary assessment includes a physical examination that focuses on the patient's chief complaint, typically a specific injury or medical complaint. It includes obtaining a patient history and taking vital signs. The order in which the steps are accomplished is based on the type of emergency the patient is experiencing (Table 13.1).

Recall that the list of signs may differ slightly from system to system, but most EMS systems include the following in their list of vital signs: respirations, pulse, blood pressure (BP), skin signs, pupils, and mental status. In some areas, Emergency Medical Responders also include assessment of blood pressure and oxygen saturation. The first set of vital signs taken on any patient are the *baseline vital signs*. All subsequent vital signs should be compared to the baseline set to identify developing trends.

Objective findings (signs) can be seen, felt, heard, smelled, or in some way measured scientifically. *Subjective findings* (symptoms) are information reported by the patient based on what they are feeling and experiencing. Many signs and symptoms you find during the physical exam are the result of the body's compensatory mechanisms. For example, to compensate for blood loss, the body will increase pulse and breathing rates and close

TABLE 13.1	Secondary Assessment	
Trauma Patient	**Medical Patient**
Unstable: Significant MOI	**Unstable**
1. Perform a rapid secondary assessment.	1. Perform a rapid secondary assessment.
2. Take vital signs.	2. Gather a patient history.
3. Gather patient history.	3. Take vital signs.
Stable: No significant MOI	**Stable**
1. Perform a focused secondary assessment.	1. Perform a focused secondary assessment.
2. Take vital signs.	2. Gather a patient history.
3. Gather patient history.	3. Take vital signs.

down, or constrict, blood vessels in the extremities, all of which results in pale, cool skin. These actions are attempts by the body to circulate an adequate amount of oxygenated blood to the cells and vital organs (perfusion). Inadequate blood flow can lead to shock.

Abnormal findings during your exam indicate a problem that should not be ignored. However, unless the problem is likely to get worse, do not interrupt your assessment. You can stop bleeding from getting worse, but there is little you can do to stop a broken leg from getting worse. It is important to complete your examination once all immediate life threats have been addressed.

Trauma Patient

LO13 Differentiate between significant and nonsignificant mechanisms of injury.

Your approach and assessment of the trauma patient will differ slightly from that of the medical patient. Your evaluation of the mechanism of injury (MOI) is especially important when determining the priority of the trauma patient.

The MOI describes how the patient was injured. What were the forces involved that contributed to the patient's injuries? Common mechanisms of injury include:

- Blunt trauma (also called blunt force trauma) from a fall or being struck by a blunt object
- Penetrating injury, such as a wound caused by a bullet or knife
- Crush injury, as when the torso, limb(s), or other body part is squeezed or compressed, as might occur in a vehicle accident

In addition to the specific forces involved, the location on the body where the forces were applied requires your close attention. Some areas of the body contain vital organs and/or major blood vessels. The head, chest, abdomen, pelvis, and thighs are very vulnerable areas; there is an increased risk of death if one or more of these areas is damaged. You will want to pay close attention as you determine the MOI and if these areas are affected.

Multi-system trauma refers to injuries that may have affected multiple body systems. As you know, the chest and abdomen contain many vital and nonvital organs. When someone experiences trauma to these areas and there is a high likelihood that multiple body systems may be affected, the patient is said to have experienced multi-system trauma. These patients should always be considered unstable and cared for accordingly.

In contrast, a patient may sustain a significant injury that does not involve multi-system trauma, as with a patient who has a lower leg and foot crushed by a heavy piece of machinery. While the isolated injury to the lower leg is painful, it does not involve multiple body systems and, therefore, the patient may be categorized as stable.

The approach to the trauma patient will differ slightly for the patient with an isolated injury (stable) versus the patient with a high likelihood of multi-system trauma (unstable).

REMEMBER

One of the most difficult lessons to learn when assessing the trauma patient is to not be distracted by bloody and sometimes graphic injuries. Do not let them distract you from performing your assessment. Less obvious injuries can still be life threatening.

For the isolated injury, we might begin the secondary assessment focusing on the injured leg. On the other hand, for the patient who has sustained multi-system trauma, we begin the secondary assessment with a *rapid trauma assessment*, which is a very quick, hands-on assessment of the most vulnerable areas (head to thighs) looking for any evidence of obvious trauma such as bleeding, pain, deformities, open wounds, or **crepitus**. The rapid trauma assessment should only take 60 to 90 seconds to complete.

crepitus ▶ grating noise or the sensation felt when broken bone ends rub together.

The trauma patient is classified as either stable or unstable depending on the presence of immediate life threats discovered during the primary assessment and the evaluation of the MOI. Your assessment will differ slightly for each type of patient depending on your findings.

To assess a trauma patient with no significant MOI, begin by performing a **focused secondary assessment** on the area the patient tells you is injured (Key Skill 13.9). Next you will obtain vital signs and gather a patient history. Provide continued care during reassessments.

focused secondary assessment ▶ examination conducted on stable patients, focusing on a specific injury or medical complaint.

To detect and care for serious injuries in a patient with a significant MOI, you will begin by performing a **rapid secondary assessment** from the head to the thighs, looking for obvious injuries (Key Skill 13.10). Next you will obtain vital signs and gather a patient history. If time and the patient's condition allow, perform a complete secondary assessment.

rapid secondary assessment ▶ quick head-to-toe assessment of the most critical patients.

KEY SKILL 13.9

Focused Secondary Assessment—Trauma With No Significant MOI

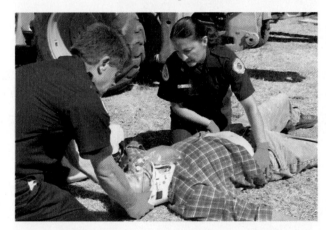

1. Examine the area the patient tells you is injured.

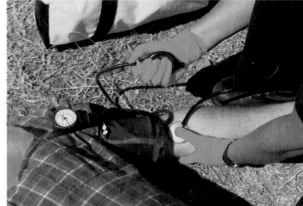

2. Obtain baseline vital signs.

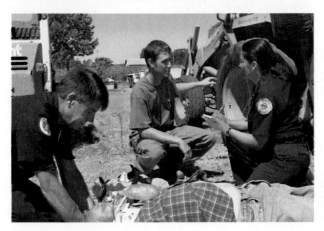

3. Gather a patient history.

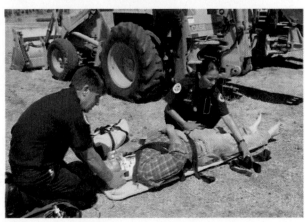

4. Provide appropriate care for the injury.

Rapid Secondary Assessment—Significant MOI or Unstable Medical Patient

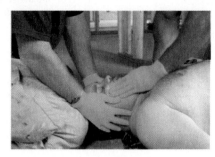

1. If appropriate, stabilize the patient's head and neck. Then palpate the head and face.

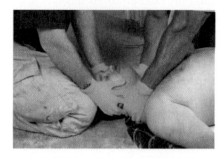

2. Palpate the patient's neck. Apply a cervical collar if appropriate.

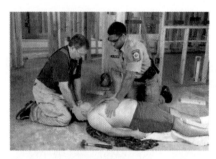

3. Palpate the chest.

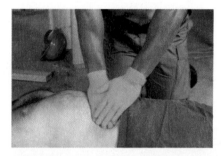

4. Palpate each quadrant of the abdomen.

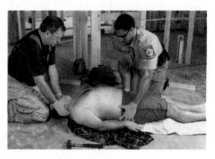

5. Palpate the pelvis.

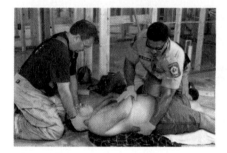

6. Palpate the back by sliding your hands under the patient.

7. Palpate all four extremities.

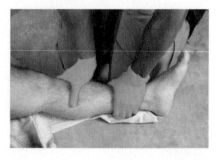

Significant mechanisms of injury for an adult include:

- Ejection from a vehicle
- Rollover vehicle crash
- High-speed vehicle crash
- Vehicle colliding with pedestrian
- Motorcycle crash
- Falls greater than 10 feet
- Penetrations of the head, neck, chest, or abdomen

Significant mechanisms of injury for a child include:

- Falls greater than 10 feet
- Bicycle collision
- Medium-speed vehicle crashes

Medical Patient

The secondary assessment for a medical patient and a trauma patient are similar, but the order and emphasis are different. For a medical patient, you are more concerned with their medical history. For the unstable medical patient, perform a rapid secondary assessment to determine if there are any obvious signs of illness. Obtain baseline vital signs. Gather a patient history, if possible. Provide care as needed.

For the stable medical patient (Key Skill 13.11), gather a patient history, observing signs and symptoms while asking about the history of the illness. The patient's chief

---

KEY SKILL 13.11

Focused Secondary Assessment—Stable Medical Patient

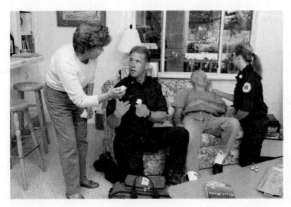

1. Gather a patient history.

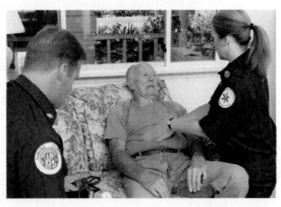

2. Perform a focused secondary assessment based on the patient's chief complaint.

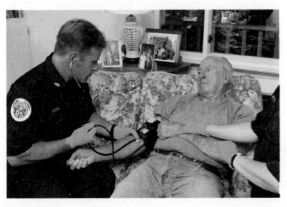

3. Obtain baseline vital signs.

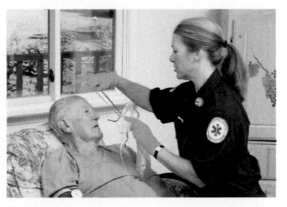

4. Provide the appropriate care as indicated.

complaint helps direct the questioning. Perform a focused secondary assessment based on the patient's problem areas. Obtain baseline vital signs. Provide care as needed. Provide continued care during reassessments.

Patient History

Much of the information you gather will come from the patient directly. You must become proficient at asking all the appropriate questions depending on the chief complaint.

Interview the Patient   An alert patient is your best source of information. Ask questions clearly at a normal rate and in a normal tone of voice. Avoid leading questions such as, "Does your pain feel like heartburn?" Statements such as "I'm here to help you" or "I'm doing everything I can to help you" are more appropriate.

When interviewing a patient who is alert, ask the following questions:

- *What is your name?* Remember their name and use it often. If your patient's mental status decreases, you can call the patient by name to elicit a response.
- *How old are you?* You need to know the general age of your adult patient. But the exact age of a child is important because it may determine what type of care is provided. Ask all children their ages. It may be appropriate to ask an adolescent their age to be certain that they are a minor. If a parent or guardian isn't present, ask, "How can I contact your parents?" Children may be upset at being hurt or ill without a parent there to help them. Always reassure them that someone will contact their parents.
- *What is going on today?* The response is usually is the patient's chief complaint. No matter what is wrong, ask if there is any pain. As you learn more about various illnesses and injuries, you will learn additional questions to ask.
- *How did this happen?* Knowing how a trauma patient was injured will help direct you to problems that may not be noticeable or obvious to you or the patient. If your patient is lying down, determine if they got into that position on their own or if they fell, were knocked down, or were thrown. Do this for patients with medical problems as well. Remember, the injury may be the result of a medical problem. For example, the patient may have fainted or had a seizure which caused them to fall and injure themselves. This information may indicate the possibility of a spinal injury or internal bleeding.
- *How long have you felt this way?* You want to know if the patient's problem occurred suddenly or if it has been developing for a few days or over a longer period of time.
- *Has this happened before?* This question is especially important for medical patients. You want to know if this is the first time or if it is a chronic (recurring) problem.
- *Do you have any current medical problems?* Has the patient been feeling ill lately? Have they seen or are they being treated by a doctor for any problems?
- *Do you take any medications?* Your patient may not be able to tell you the exact name of a medication they are taking, especially if there are several. They may be able to tell you general medication categories, such as "heart pills" or "blood pressure pills." Be sure to ask about over-the-counter medications as well. Routine use of simple medications such as aspirin may alter the treatment the patient receives at the hospital.

  Depending on the situation, it may be appropriate to ask if they have taken any recreational drugs. This is a question that requires some trust by your patient. You may want to wait until you have established a rapport with your patient before asking this one. You are more likely to get an honest answer if they trust you.
- *Do you have any allergies that you know of?* Allergic reactions can vary from simple hives or itching to life-threatening airway problems and shock. Also ask what happens when they are exposed to the source of the allergy. For instance, does the patient simply develop a rash, get itchy, or do they develop difficulty breathing?
- *When did you last eat?* This is an important question if your patient is a candidate for surgery. It is also important information when dealing with a patient experiencing a diabetic emergency.

Recall from Chapter 12 that the SAMPLE history tool is commonly used in obtaining a patient history. The letters serve as a memory aid for questions that should be asked:

S — Signs/symptoms
A — Allergies
M — Medications
P — Pertinent past medical history
L — Last oral intake
E — Events leading to the illness or injury

When taking a history, do your best to get down at eye level with the patient and establish eye contact. This will improve personal communication and build the patient's confidence in you. If you look away while asking questions or while listening to answers, it may indicate to your patient that you are not as concerned as you should be or are not giving them your full attention. A simple appropriate touch can also improve communication. You touch the patient's forehead to note relative skin temperature and moisture and, by touching the patient, you are also showing care and concern. However, respect a patient's wish not to be touched. Your calm, caring, and professional attitude can often do as much for the patient as any medical care you provide.

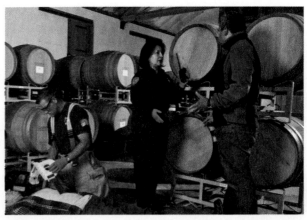

Figure 13.6 When caring for an unresponsive patient, look to family members, friends, or bystanders for additional information.

Interview Bystanders   You may encounter a patient who is unresponsive or unable to answer your questions regarding their history. If this is the case, you must depend on family, friends, or bystanders for information (Figure 13.6). Ask specific, directed questions to shorten the time required to obtain the information. Questions to bystanders may include:

- *What is the patient's name?* If the patient is a minor, ask if the parents are there or if they have been contacted.
- *What happened? or Did you see what happened?* If the patient fell from a ladder, did they appear to faint or pass out first? Were they hit on the head by something?
- *Did you see anything else?* For example, was the patient holding their chest before the fall? This gives the bystander a chance to think again and add anything they remember.
- *Did the patient complain of anything before this happened?* You may learn of chest pain, nausea, or shortness of breath.
- *Do you know if the patient has any known medical problems?* Family or friends who know the patient may know their medical history such as heart problems, diabetes, allergies, or other problems that may be related to the patient's current condition.
- *Does the patient take any medications?* Again, family or friends who know the patient may be aware of the medications they take.

Locate Medical Identification Jewelry   Medical identification jewelry can provide important information if the patient is unresponsive and a history cannot be obtained from family, friends, or bystanders. A common form of medical identification jewelry is the MedicAlert medallion, worn as a bracelet or necklace. One side of the device has a Star of Life emblem. Information pertaining to the patient's medical history, including any allergies, is engraved on the reverse side along with a phone number for additional information.

Vital Signs

Vital signs can alert you to problems that require immediate attention (see Chapter 12). Taken at regular intervals, they can help you determine if the patient's condition is getting better, worse, or staying the same (Figure 13.7). For most Emergency Medical Responders, vital signs include respirations, pulse, blood pressure (BP), skin signs, pupils, and mental status. In some areas, Emergency Medical Responders also include assessment of blood pressure and oxygen saturation.

REMEMBER

Once you learn that a patient has been prescribed medications by their doctor, you must always ask the next question: "Are you taking all your medications as prescribed?" Many patients are not compliant with taking their medications, sometimes due to forgetfulness or financial constraints, and this can make a simple medical problem much worse.

JEDI

Always ask permission before touching a responsive patient. Much of the patient assessment requires physical touch, so be sure that your touch is appropriate and deliberate. This means using cupped hands and telling the patient what you are doing. This can help involve the patient in their own care and also ease any anxiety they may have about being touched.

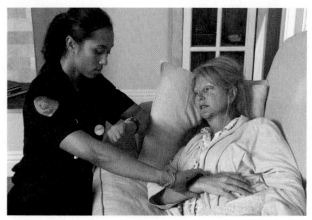

Figure 13.7 Establishing a baseline set of vital signs is an important aspect of your patient assessment.

Compare all other vital sign readings to the baseline vital signs. This comparison helps determine if the patient is stable or unstable, improving or growing worse, and benefiting or not benefiting from the care you are providing. For example, comparing baseline vital signs before and after administering oxygen can tell the EMTs who take over patient care objective information about how that intervention may be affecting the patient.

Certain abnormal vital signs point to possible serious medical or traumatic conditions. For example, cool, moist skin; a rapid, weak pulse; and increased breathing rate can indicate possible shock in the presence of a significant MOI. Hot, dry skin with a rapid pulse could indicate a serious heat-related emergency. Abnormal vital signs are one of the indicators that the patient is a high priority for immediate transport.

For an adult, a continuous pulse rate of less than 60 beats per minute or more than 100 beats per minute is considered abnormal. Likewise, a respiratory rate of more than 30 breaths per minute or less than 10 breaths per minute may be a sign of a serious condition. You should be concerned about these vital signs because they may indicate a patient who is unstable. Stay alert and monitor the patient closely. Keeping the patient quiet or at rest, caring for shock, and reassuring the responsive patient can make a difference in the outcome.

FIRST ON SCENE (*continued*)

"Are you having trouble breathing, Brad?" Joanie watches the driver's chest and counts his shallow, rapid breaths at 28 per minute.

"A little," the man says. "That's not a big deal, though, right? I mean, I was just unloading boxes."

"Honestly, Brad, it could be a big deal. I'm not really trained to make that determination." Joanie turns to Lorena and says, "Why don't you go ahead and call 911?"

"Oh! Hold on a minute," the driver protests as he stands up. "I'm . . . I'm . . . I think . . ." He grows pale again, and Joanie helps him sit back on the pallet of boxes.

"Just relax, Brad," Joanie says and places a nonrebreather mask on his face. She can hear Lorena talking to the 911 operator through the thin walls of the dock manager's office.

BP-DOC ▶ memory aid used to recall what to look for in a physical exam of a trauma patient; the letters stand for *bleeding, pain, deformities, open wounds,* and *crepitus.*

Physical Exam

LO14 Describe the components of the BP-DOC assessment tool.

If your trauma patient has no significant MOI and appears to have an isolated minor injury, perform a focused assessment on the injury site and the area close to it. If the patient has a significant MOI or is unresponsive, perform a rapid secondary assessment. You must use as many of your senses as possible when performing the physical exam. Use your eyes, ears, hands, and nose to detect any abnormal findings in your patient.

The physical exam of a medical patient may be brief. If the patient is responsive, perform a focused secondary assessment based on the patient's chief complaint. If the patient is unstable or unresponsive, conduct a rapid secondary assessment of the entire body.

When assessing a trauma patient, the **BP-DOC** memory aid may be useful to help you remember what to look for during the physical exam:

B — Bleeding
P — Pain
D — Deformities
O — Open wounds
C — Crepitus (a grating noise or sensation often felt with broken bones)

Rapid Secondary Assessment—Trauma Patient with Significant MOI The rapid secondary assessment is a head-to-thighs physical exam of the patient that should take no more than 90 seconds to complete. It is performed on patients who have a high likelihood of multi-system trauma. These patients will most likely have a high priority for transport. Do not move the patient unless absolutely necessary. Keep in mind that neck and spinal injuries may be present. To save time, another Emergency Medical Responder may take vital signs while you perform the exam.

It is not usually necessary to remove the patient's clothing during a physical exam. Of course, you may remove or readjust clothing that interferes with your ability to examine the patient. Cut away, lift, slide, or unbutton clothing covering a suspected injury site, especially the chest, back, and abdomen, so you can fully inspect the area. Also check the patient's clothing for evidence of bleeding. If you have any reason to suspect serious injury to or uncontrolled bleeding from the back, you may need to carefully roll the patient to inspect the back. Use care to keep the head and spine in alignment as you do it.

Suspect internal injuries if your patient indicates pain in the area or tenderness when you touch the area during your exam. If the patient is unresponsive, you may wish to remove or rearrange clothing covering the chest, abdomen, and back to examine those areas of the body completely. If you must remove or rearrange the clothing of a responsive patient, tell them what you are doing and why. Take great care to respect the modesty of the patient and to protect them from harsh weather conditions and temperatures.

To perform a secondary assessment (Key Skill 13.12):

1. Check the head for bleeding and deformities. Deformities can be any abnormal bulge, bump, or swelling that you see or feel. Take care not to move the patient's head. Run your fingers through the patient's hair, looking for blood. Check your gloves for blood. Check the face for pain, deformities, or discoloration. Check for symmetry of facial muscles by asking the patient to smile or show their teeth. If, when they smile or show you their teeth, only one side of the face or mouth is able to move, this is a sign of abnormal symmetry. Look for any fluids that may be leaking from the ears, nose, or mouth.
2. Examine the patient's eyes for signs of injury. Check the pupils for size, equality, and reaction to light. A penlight would be helpful for this. If you are outside in bright sunlight, cover the patient's eye with your hand. Remove your hand quickly and watch for reaction of the pupil to the light. Observe the conjunctiva (inner surface of the eyelids). The tissue should be pink and moist. A pale color may indicate poor perfusion.

KEY SKILL 13.12

Secondary Assessment

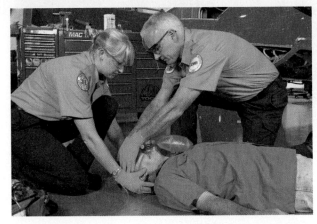

1. Use both hands to palpate the scalp as you inspect the head.

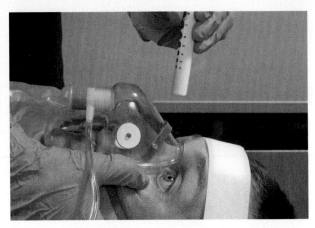

2. Check the pupils for equality and reaction to light.

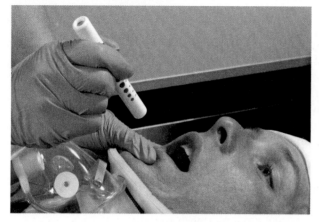

3 Inspect the mouth for anything that may cause an airway obstruction.

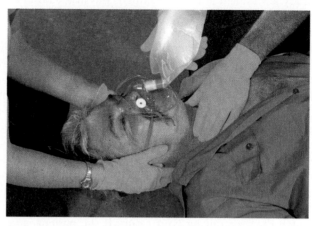

4. Inspect the neck for pain and deformities.

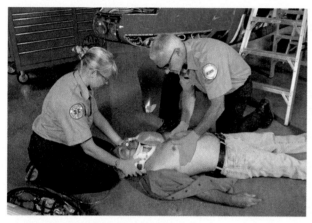

5. Use both hands to palpate the chest.

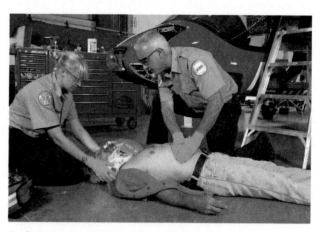

6. Palpate the abdomen for pain and deformities.

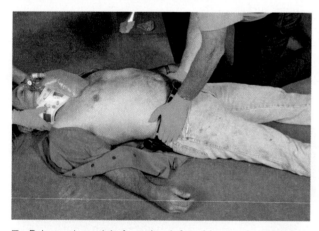

7. Palpate the pelvis for pain, deformities, and wetness.

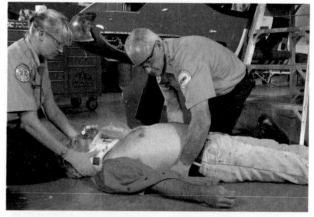

8. Palpate the lower back for pain and deformities.

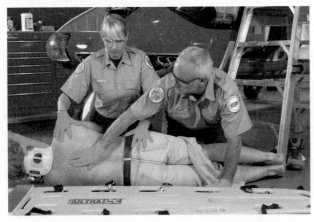

9. When appropriate, roll the patient to inspect the entire back.

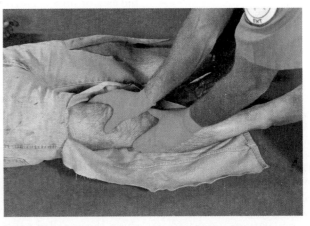

10. Palpate the legs and feet for pain and deformities.

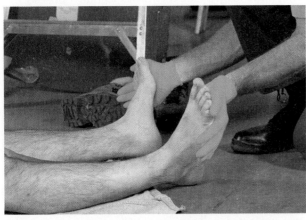

11. Assess distal circulation, sensation, and motor function in each foot.

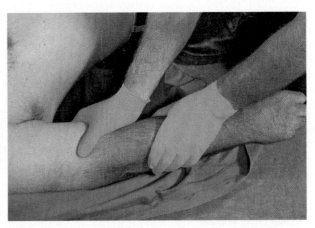

12. Palpate the arms and hands for pain and deformities.

13. Assess distal circulation, sensation, and motor function in each hand.

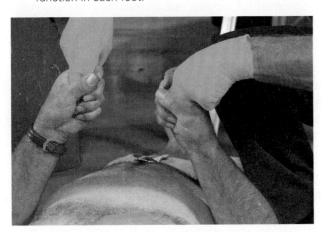

tracheal deviation ▶ shifting of the trachea to either side of the midline of the neck caused by the buildup of pressure inside the chest (tension pneumothorax).

jugular vein distention ▶ abnormal bulging of the veins of the neck indicating cardiac compromise or possible injury to the chest. Abbrev: JVD.

accessory muscle use ▶ use of the muscles of the neck, chest, and abdomen to assist with breathing effort.

paradoxical movement ▶ movement of an area of the chest wall in the opposite direction to the rest of the chest during respiration; an indication of chest wall trauma.

guarding ▶ protection of an area of pain by the patient; spasms of muscles to minimize movement that might cause pain.

dorsalis pedis pulse ▶ pulse located on the top of the foot.

track marks ▶ small dots of infection, scarring, or bruising that form a track along a vein; may be an indication of IV drug abuse.

REMEMBER

In a secondary assessment of a trauma patient, each area of the body is checked for BP-DOC plus other problems specific to the area.

---

3. Inspect the ears and nose for drainage, clear or bloody. Clear or bloody fluids in the ears or nose are strong indications of a skull fracture. Also inspect the nose for singed nostrils, which may indicate the inhalation of toxic smoke. Flaring nostrils may be a sign of respiratory distress.

4. Inspect the mouth for foreign material, bleeding, and tissue damage. Look for broken teeth, loose bridges, or dentures. Check for chewing gum, food, vomit, and foreign objects that may cause an airway obstruction.

5. Check the neck—front and back—for pain and deformities. Look for any medical identification jewelry. Also notice if the patient has a stoma or evidence of **tracheal deviation** (any shift of the trachea to one side). Observe for **jugular vein distention (JVD)** and **accessory muscle use.**

6. Use both hands to inspect the chest—front and sides—for pain and deformities. If necessary, bare the chest. Gently apply pressure to all sides of the chest with your hands. Observe for equal expansion of both sides of the chest. Note any portion that appears to be floating or moving in opposite directions to the rest of the chest; this is called **paradoxical movement**. It could indicate an injury called a *flail chest,* in which two or more ribs are fractured in two or more places. When baring the chest of feminine-presenting patients, provide them with as much privacy as possible.

7. Inspect the abdomen for any signs or symptoms of trauma such as pain, deformities, distention, rigidity, or **guarding**. Gently press on each quadrant of the abdomen with your fingers, noting any areas that are rigid, swollen, or painful. As you press on the area, ask the patient if it hurts more when you press down or when you let go.

8. Inspect the pelvis for pain and deformity. Note any obvious injury to the genital region. Look for wetness caused by incontinence (loss of bladder control) or bleeding. Do not expose the area unless you suspect there is an injury. In male patients, priapism (persistent erection of the penis) may be a sign of serious spinal cord injury.

9. Feel the lower back for pain and deformity. Gently slide your gloved hands into the area of the lower back that is formed by the curve of the spine. Check your gloves for blood. If spinal injury is not suspected, roll the patient to inspect the entire back for pain and deformity.

10. Examine each leg and foot individually. Compare one limb to the other in terms of length, shape, and deformity.

11. Check for distal circulation, sensation, and motor function. Check the **dorsalis pedis pulse**, which is located on top of the foot just lateral to the large tendon of the big toe.

12. Examine the upper extremities from the shoulders to the fingertips. Examine each limb separately for pain and deformities.

13. Check for distal circulation, sensation, and motor function in each hand. Note any weakness, numbness, or tingling. Observe for evidence of **track marks** or medical identification jewelry.

Secondary Assessment—Trauma Patient with No Significant MOI When your trauma patient has no significant MOI, the steps of the secondary assessment are appropriately simplified. Instead of examining the patient from head to toe, focus your assessment on just the areas the patient says are painful or that you suspect may be injured because of the MOI. The assessment includes a physical exam, vital signs, and a patient history.

Deciding which areas of the patient's body to assess depends partly on what you see and partly on the patient's chief complaint. Be sure to consider potential injuries based on the MOI. For example, if the patient's chief complaint is pain in their leg after falling down stairs, consider possible back or neck injuries and care for the patient accordingly. Use the memory aid BP-DOC to help you remember what signs you are looking for as you perform your assessment.

Rapid Secondary Assessment—Unresponsive Medical Patient The rapid secondary assessment of an unstable medical patient is almost the same as the rapid assessment of a trauma patient with a significant MOI. You will rapidly assess the patient's head, neck, chest, abdomen, pelvis, and extremities. As you assess each area of the body, look for signs of illness:

- *Neck:* Look for accessory muscle use, neck vein distention, and medical identification jewelry.
- *Chest:* Check for equal chest rise and fall and signs of rash.
- *Abdomen:* Assess for tenderness, distention, or rigidity.
- *Pelvis:* Check for incontinence of urine or feces.
- *Extremities:* Check circulation, sensation, motor function, and for medical identification jewelry.

Secondary Assessment—Stable Medical Patient The secondary assessment of a stable medical patient is usually brief. The most important assessment information is obtained through the patient history and vital signs. Note the patient's chief complaint and focus the exam on that body part or area. For example, if the patient complains of abdominal pain, focus your exam on the entire abdomen.

Recall the OPQRST assessment tool described in Chapter 12. Each letter represents a word or words meant to trigger specific questions that you should ask. OPQRST is especially helpful when the chief complaint is related to pain or shortness of breath.

O — *Onset.* Questions focus on when the pain or symptoms began. For example, "What were you doing when the pain began?" or "When did you first began to feel short of breath?"

P — *Provocation.* Questions focus on what provokes pain or makes the pain lessen. For example, "Does anything you do make the pain better or worse?" or "Does it hurt when I push here?"

Q — *Quality.* Questions focus on what the pain or symptom feels like. For example, "Can you describe how your pain feels?" or "Is the pain sharp or dull?" or "Is it steady, or does it come and go?"

R — *Region/radiate.* Ask where the pain is originating (region) and to where it may be moving or radiating. For example, "Can you point to where the pain is the worst?" "Does your pain move to any other part of your body?"

S — *Severity.* A standard pain scale is typically presented like this: "On a scale of 0 to 10, with 10 being the worst pain you have ever felt, how would you rate your pain right now?" Also ask the patient to rate the severity of the pain when it first began. Once you have been with the patient a while, you will want to ask the severity question again to see if their pain has gotten better or worse.

T — *Time.* Ask the patient how long they have been experiencing the pain or discomfort. For example, "When did you first begin having pain today?" or "How long have you had this pain?".

Avoid leading questions such as "Is the pain very sharp and radiating?" Instead, provide the patient with choices and then allow them to choose. It is also important to use the patient's own words when documenting the call or transferring care to higher-trained personnel. For example, if the patient tells you they feel as though an anvil is sitting on their chest, quote their words to describe the pain. Do not paraphrase or attempt to translate what was said into medical terminology.

REMEMBER

It is not necessary to learn each and every memory tool for assessment. The important thing is to find one you understand and are comfortable with and use it consistently.

Completing the Exam Upon completing the physical exam of the patient, you must consider all the signs and symptoms found that could indicate an illness or injury. Certain combinations of signs and symptoms can point to one specific problem. A finding as simple as pain in a certain region of the body may be significant.

During your assessment and throughout the time you are providing care, remember the first rule of emergency care: *Do no further harm.* Be sure to do only what you have been trained to do and avoid aggravating existing injuries.

Remember these key principles of patient assessment:

- Do no further harm.
- An altered mental status is almost always a sign of a serious problem.
- Patients who appear stable may worsen rapidly. You must be alert to all changes in a patient's condition.
- Unless you are certain that the patient is free of spinal injury, assume every trauma patient has a spinal injury.
- Keep patients engaged in your exam by telling them what you are doing.
- Monitor vital signs as frequently as every 5 minutes for unstable patients.
- If it hurts, look at it. Expose the area if necessary.

FIRST ON SCENE (continued)

"Okay, Brad," Joanie says as she kneels, facing him. "While we wait for the ambulance, let's talk about your chest pain." The driver, now wide-eyed and frightened by his symptoms, nods. "I already know that you were unloading the truck when the pain started, right?"

"Yes," Brad says, his voice somewhat muffled by the oxygen mask.

"Does anything make it better or worse? You know, like if you move a certain way or push on it?"

Brad moves his upper body back and forth and presses harder on his chest. "No," he answers.

The sound of sirens can be heard from the parking lot next to the loading dock. "Okay." Joanie is now writing in a small notebook. "What does the pain feel like?"

The driver thinks for a moment and pulls the mask up to speak. "Like a pressure. Like a heavy weight sitting on my chest."

Reassessment

LO15 Explain the purpose of the reassessment.

When performing the reassessment, repeat the primary assessment, reassess vital signs, and check any interventions to ensure that they are still effective. Reassess the patient, watching closely for any changes in their condition. Elements of the reassessment are:

- Ensure that ABCs are all appropriate.
- Reassess vital signs and compare with baseline vital signs.
- Check and adjust interventions as appropriate.

Repeating assessments and noting any changes in the patient's condition are ways of trending their condition. Patients will get better, worse, or stay the same. Seriously ill or injured patients should be reassessed every 5 minutes. A good rule to follow is that by the time you finish a reassessment from start to finish, it is time to start over with the beginning of the next reassessment. Patients who are not seriously ill or injured should be reassessed no less than every 15 minutes.

When additional EMS providers arrive at the scene, it is important to communicate with them clearly and effectively. Give the responding EMTs a verbal report that includes:

- Name and age of patient
- Chief complaint
- Mental status
- ABCs: airway, breathing, and circulatory status
- Physical findings
- Patient history
- Interventions applied and the patient's responses to them

Some EMS systems also require the Emergency Medical Responder to provide a written report to the transport crew. It usually includes the same information as the verbal report.

The written report and the information in it will become part of the transport crew's patient care report. Accuracy is important in any verbal or written report because care given by the responding EMTs and the hospital emergency department staff may be based, in part, on your evaluation of the patient.

FIRST ON SCENE WRAP-UP

Before Joanie can ask the next question, Lorena leads a group of firefighters to the loading dock. They are carrying several bags and a bright green AED. "Okay," the firefighter in the lead says, pulling on a pair of purple exam gloves. "Who do we have here?"

Joanie introduces Brad and explains the situation. Just as she finishes, an ambulance crew arrives, rolling a wheeled stretcher across the loading dock floor. In a short time, the ambulance crew has obtained a set of vitals, loaded the patient onto the stretcher, switched the nonrebreather mask onto their

oxygen tank, and rolled Brad out to the waiting ambulance. Joanie and Lorena watch the firefighters and ambulance crew load up into their vehicles and drive out of the parking lot.

"Wow," Lorena says as they return to the building. "That went just like clockwork."

"Yes, it did." Joanie pats Lorena on the shoulder as they walk back into the darkness of the loading dock. "And next time, you get to do patient care."

Summary

- Patient assessment is one of the most important skills you will learn as an Emergency Medical Responder. A good assessment will result in good care.
- You must detect life-threatening problems and correct them as quickly as possible. Then you must detect problems that may become life threatening if left without care.
- Always perform a scene size-up first. Always make sure the scene is safe to enter before you enter it. Then gain information quickly from the scene, the patient, and bystanders. If possible, determine the patient's nature of illness or mechanism of injury.
- During the primary assessment, determine if the patient is responsive. If you suspect a spinal injury, maintain manual stabilization of the head and neck. Make certain that the patient has an open airway, adequate breathing, and a pulse. Control all serious bleeding.
- During the secondary assessment, look over the patient. Check for medical identification jewelry. Begin gathering information by asking questions and listening. The more organized your interview and physical exam are, the better your chances of gaining the needed information. Use the SAMPLE, BP-DOC, and OPQRST assessment tools as appropriate.
- Take the patient's vital signs. Remember that baseline vital signs—plus repeated vital signs over time—are valuable to the personnel who take over patient care.
- The physical exam of a patient varies somewhat depending on whether the patient is a medical or trauma patient. A physical exam consists of the following:
  - *Head.* Check the scalp for cuts, bruises, and swelling, and the skull and facial bones for deformities, depressions, and other signs of injury. Inspect the eyes for injury, and check pupil size, equality, and reaction to light. Look for blood, clear fluids, or bloody fluids in the nose and ears. Examine the mouth for airway obstructions and blood.
  - *Neck.* Examine the cervical spine for tenderness and deformities. Note any accessory muscle use. Note obvious injuries and look for medical alert jewelry.
  - *Chest.* Examine the chest for tenderness, open wounds, crepitus, bruises, and rashes. Look for equal rise and fall of the chest.
  - *Abdomen.* Examine the abdomen for tenderness, open wounds, bruises, and rashes.
  - *Lower back.* Examine for tenderness, open wounds, bruises, and rashes. Check the rest of the back last and only if it is safe to roll the patient (no suspected spinal injuries).
  - *Pelvis.* Press in and down to check for stability and pain and note any signs of injuries.
  - *Genital region.* Note any obvious injuries. Look for wetness. Note the presence of priapism when examining male patients.
  - *Extremities.* Examine for tenderness, open wounds, and deformities. Check for distal circulation, sensation, and motor function. In pediatric patients, check for capillary refill. Look for medical identification jewelry.
- While EMTs usually complete a more detailed secondary assessment en route to the hospital, in some systems, Emergency Medical Responders may assist by repeating the primary assessment and vital signs. If you also assist with the reassessment, note any changes in patient condition and/or the need for additional interventions.

Take Action

Hide and Seek

Becoming adept at thorough and efficient patient assessment can take years and hundreds of patients. For that reason, it is important to practice this skill often, especially if you are not in a job where you are assessing patients regularly.

For this exercise, gather several small- to medium-sized items such as an oral airway (OPA), nasal airway (NPA), large coin, pencil or pen, eraser, and so on. Use some tape and secure several items in random places on your body beneath your clothing. You might hide them at the lower back, behind the knee, under the arm, and inside the ankle. Once you have several items secured beneath your clothing, find a classmate who is willing to practice patient assessment. Do not let them know that you have items hidden on your body.

Now lie down and think of a simple scenario that you can use to set the stage for your practice session. Let your partner perform a complete assessment and see how many of the objects they can find. If they find an item, just tell them that it represents a deformity and to continue with the exam. When they are finished with the exam, reveal all the items. Was your classmate able to locate all of them? Why do you suppose they may have missed some? This is a great way to reinforce the importance of a thorough physical exam.

First on Scene Patient Handoff

Brad is a 45-year-old male who started to experience a sudden onset of chest pain while unloading pallets. He is A&O × 4 and describes the pain as a heavy weight on his chest. Brad denies any trauma as well as any previous history of heart problems. Baseline vitals were RR 28 and labored, HR 140 strong and regular. Skin was pale, warm, and dry. We have him on 12 liters of oxygen by NRB, and he states the oxygen may be helping his pain.

First on Scene Run Review

Recall the events of the First on Scene scenario in this chapter, and answer the following questions related to the call. Rationales are offered in the Answer Key at the back of the book.

1. Why should you ask permission to help an individual?
2. For this call, why would scene control be important?
3. As an Emergency Medical Responder, how could you help this patient with these signs and symptoms?
4. Why might this patient not want the ambulance called?

Quick Quiz

To check your understanding of the chapter, answer the following questions. Then compare your answers to those in the Answer Key at the back of the book.

1. Which of the following is NOT a component of an appropriate scene size up?
   a. Determining the number of patients
   b. Assessing the airway
   c. Manually stabilizing the cervical spine
   d. Donning gloves and safety goggles

2. After arriving on scene but before making patient contact, you should:
   a. perform a primary assessment.
   b. contact medical direction.
   c. perform a secondary assessment.
   d. take BSI precautions.

3. A patient has been involved in a rollover vehicle collision. In this scenario, the rollover is an example of the:
   a. mechanism of injury.
   b. nature of illness.
   c. chief complaint.
   d. causative factor.

4. Which of the following BEST describes the purpose of the primary assessment?
   a. Identify scene hazards.
   b. Obtain a complete history.
   c. Identify and treat life-threatening conditions.
   d. Perform a full body exam.

5. In a SAMPLE history, the *E* represents:
   a. EKG results.
   b. evaluation of the neck and spine.
   c. events leading to the illness or injury.
   d. evidence of airway obstruction.

6. A patient presents with their eyes closed, but moans when you pinch their trapezius muscle. This patient would fall into which category of the AVPU scale?
   a. Alert
   b. Painful
   c. Verbal
   d. Unresponsive

7. Which of the following would NOT typically happen during the primary assessment?
   a. Inserting an airway adjunct
   b. SAMPLE history
   c. Controlling bleeding
   d. Evaluating mental status

8. An older adult patient is having trouble breathing. In this case, "trouble breathing" is an example of the:
   a. nature of illness.
   b. mechanism of injury.
   c. medical history.
   d. respiratory rate.

9. The steps of a primary assessment include forming a general impression, assessing mental status, assessing ABCs, and:
   a. collecting a history.
   b. determining priority for transport.
   c. performing a secondary assessment.
   d. obtaining vital signs.

10. When performing a patient assessment on an infant or child, it is important to remember that:
    a. you should only speak to the parent or caregiver.
    b. a child's condition can change very quickly.
    c. children are rarely truthful about what happened to them.
    d. children will not be able to understand what you are doing.

11. A patient who presents with normal vital signs and shows no indications of a life-threatening problem may be described as:

    a. routine.
    b. normal.
    c. unstable.
    d. stable.

12. When assessing a trauma patient who has a significant mechanism of injury, the BP-DOC assessment tool is designed to look for:

    a. evidence of a crime.
    b. signs of traumatic injury.
    c. abnormal vital signs.
    d. signs of shock.

13. You have arrived to find a conscious and alert older adult man complaining of moderate abdominal pain. When assessing an older adult patient, you should:

    a. speak only to the patient's caregiver as the patient might have dementia.
    b. address older adults by using their last names with *Mr.*, *Ms.*, or *Mrs.*
    c. assume they will need you to speak very loudly in order to hear you.
    d. repeat your questions several times to make sure they understand.

14. You have arrived to find a conscious and alert child with obvious deformity to his right forearm. You should:

    a. perform a primary assessment.
    b. obtain a SAMPLE history.
    c. perform a focused secondary assessment.
    d. obtain a set of vital signs.

15. The secondary assessment is designed to:

    a. identify life-threatening conditions.
    b. collect a detailed medical history.
    c. identify any allergies.
    d. find and treat non-life-threatening injuries or conditions.

Endnotes

1. Jeff Harless, Ramesh Ramaiah, and Sanjay M. Bhananker, "Pediatric Airway Management," *International Journal of Critical Illness and Injury Science,* Vol. 4 (2014): 65–70.
2. Bettencourt, A.P., Gorman, M., Mullen, J.E, "Pediatric Resuscitation," *Critical Care Nursing Clinics of North America*, Vol. 33, No. 3 (September 2021): 287–302. doi: 10.1016/j.cnc.2021.05.005. Epub 2021 Jul 7. PMID: 34340791; PMCID: PMC8445069.

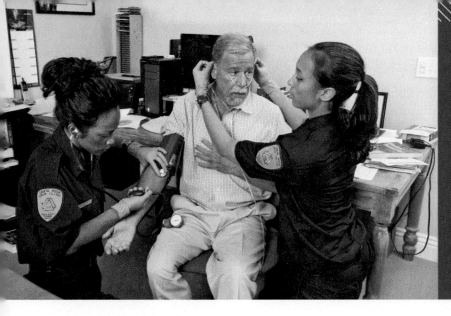

14

Caring for Cardiac Emergencies

Education Standards

Medicine—
Cardiovascular

Competencies

Recognizes and manages life threats based on assessment findings of a patient with a medical emergency while awaiting additional emergency response.

LEARNING OBJECTIVES

Upon successful completion of this chapter, the student should be able to:

Cognitive

1. Define the chapter key terms.
2. Review cardiovascular anatomy and physiology (see Chapter 4).
3. Describe the normal flow of blood through the heart.
4. Explain the common causes of cardiac compromise.
5. Describe the signs and symptoms of a patient experiencing cardiac compromise.
6. Differentiate and explain the pathophysiology of angina, myocardial infarction, and heart failure.
7. Explain the appropriate assessment and care for a patient experiencing cardiac compromise.

Psychomotor

8. Demonstrate the ability to appropriately assess and care for a patient experiencing cardiac compromise.

Affective

9. Value the importance of caring for all patients with chest pain as though it were cardiac compromise.

KEY TERMS

angina (*p. 286*)
cardiac compromise (*p. 286*)

conduction pathway (*p. 284*)
heart failure (*p. 288*)

According to the most recent statistics from the Centers for Disease Control and Prevention (CDC), heart disease is the number one killer among adults in the United States.[1] As discussed in previous chapters, the heart is at the center of the cardiovascular system, which also includes the blood vessels and blood. The cells of the body require a constant supply of well-oxygenated blood to function properly. This is known as perfusion. Good perfusion depends on the heart's ability to circulate blood throughout the body at a constant and steady pressure (blood pressure). When illness or injury affects the heart's function, it is unable to maintain a pressure necessary to support adequate perfusion. This chapter discusses some of the more common conditions that affect the heart's ability to pump adequately, the consequences that often result, and the care you will need to provide to support these patients.

FIRST ON SCENE

Police officer Taylor forgot his lunch on the kitchen table when he left for work this morning. It is a move he regrets the moment one of the dispatchers advises him, while stifling a giggle, that his wife has dropped it off at the front desk. The giant smiley face drawn on the brown paper bag and the block letters spelling out his name make his face flush and sends quiet laughter through the department's administrative staff. This is Alexandra's way of ensuring that he never forgets his lunch again.

He is walking out the lobby doors toward his patrol car, lunch bag in hand, when the squeal of tires catches his attention.

A blue compact car skitters across the lanes in front of the police station and slides to a halt about 10 feet from where Taylor is standing. A panicked woman stumbles from the driver's side, yelling for help.

"My dad!" she shouts, pointing back at the car. "There is something wrong with my dad. I think it's his heart!"

Taylor drops the paper bag onto the pavement and rushes to the passenger door. An older man is slumped against the window, eyes closed tightly, seemingly in pain.

Normal Heart Function

LO3   Describe the normal flow of blood through the heart.

When functioning properly, the heart is an amazingly efficient pump that beats an average of 100,000 times per day. It also circulates 6,000 to 7,500 liters of blood each day. Blood flows through the heart beginning with the right atrium (Figure 14.1). It then flows down into the right ventricle. From there, it flows into the lungs, where it drops off carbon dioxide and picks up oxygen. It returns from the lungs, enters the left atrium, and then flows down into the left ventricle. The left ventricle is the largest and strongest chamber of the heart and must force blood out to the entire body. The heart muscle itself receives its blood supply from tiny vessels called *coronary arteries*. Many of the problems related to the heart are the result of the coronary arteries becoming narrowed or blocked, causing a decrease in the normal blood flow to the heart.

The heart contains a sophisticated electrical system that keeps it beating every minute of every day. The heart's conduction system consists of a network of nodes (groups of cells), specialized cells and fibers, and electrical signals. The **conduction pathway** is the route that electrical signals travel within the heart (Figure 14.2). The electrical signal originates in the sinoatrial (SA) node at the top of the heart in the right atrium. It continues down through the center of the heart, eventually reaching the right and left ventricles. These electrical signals produce coordinated contractions of the heart.

conduction pathway ▶ route of electrical impulses within the heart.

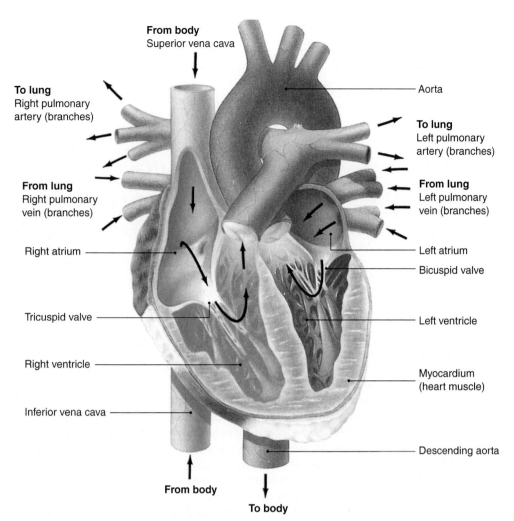

Figure 14.1 Major anatomy of the heart, including blood flow through the chambers.

From body
Superior vena cava

To lung
Right pulmonary artery (branches)

Aorta

To lung
Left pulmonary artery (branches)

From lung
Right pulmonary vein (branches)

From lung
Left pulmonary vein (branches)

Right atrium

Left atrium

Bicuspid valve

Tricuspid valve

Left ventricle

Right ventricle

Myocardium (heart muscle)

Inferior vena cava

Descending aorta

From body

To body

Damage to the conduction pathway can lead to an abnormal heart rhythm that impairs the ability of the heart to pump blood. If the amount of blood pumped is significantly reduced, the patient will develop signs and symptoms of poor perfusion.

Cardiac Compromise

LO4 Explain the common causes of cardiac compromise.

LO5 Describe the signs and symptoms of a patient experiencing cardiac compromise.

LO6 Differentiate and explain the pathophysiology of angina, myocardial infarction, and heart failure.

The term **cardiac compromise** describes specific signs and symptoms that indicate some type of emergency relating to the heart. Medical conditions such as myocardial infarction (also called a heart attack), angina pectoris, and heart failure are some of the most common causes of cardiac compromise. Common signs and symptoms of cardiac compromise are:

- Chest discomfort, typically described by patients as pain or a dull pressure, tightness, or a squeezing sensation in the chest. The discomfort may also radiate to the arms, shoulders, back, neck, or jaw.

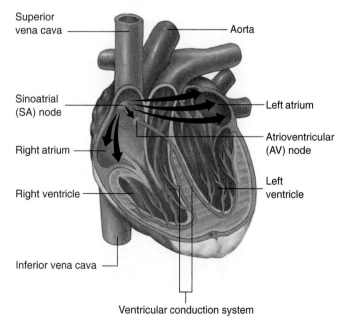

Superior vena cava

Aorta

Sinoatrial (SA) node

Left atrium

Atrioventricular (AV) node

Right atrium

Left ventricle

Right ventricle

Inferior vena cava

Ventricular conduction system

Figure 14.2 The heart's conduction pathway, highlighted in green.

- Diaphoresis (sudden onset of sweating)
- Dyspnea (shortness of breath)
- Nausea/vomiting
- Anxiety, irritability
- Feeling of impending doom
- Abnormal pulse (may be rapid, slow, and/or irregular)
- Abnormal blood pressure (may be high or low)

Cardiac compromise has many causes and can present with one or all of the above signs and symptoms. As an Emergency Medical Responder, you must use your assessment skills to quickly gather a patient history and perform a physical exam to identify the potential for cardiac involvement. When in doubt, provide care for the worst possible scenario and call for an advanced life support (ALS) ambulance.

Cardiac arrest is the ultimate form of cardiac compromise and results in stoppage of the heart. Cardiac arrest can occur for many reasons, including heart attack, trauma, allergic reaction, or overdose. Sudden cardiac arrest is most common in adults and is most often caused by a heart attack. Care for patients in cardiac arrest is covered in detail in Chapter 11.

Angina Pectoris

Angina pectoris, commonly called, **angina**, is a common cause of cardiac compromise. *Angina pectoris* literally means "pain in the chest." Angina occurs when one or more coronary arteries are unable to provide an adequate supply of oxygenated blood to the myocardium (heart muscle). While it is similar to a heart attack, with angina, the coronary blood flow is not completely cut off. There is also no actual damage to the heart muscle. Although the supply of oxygenated blood is never cut off entirely, the pain is caused by the muscles starving for more blood and oxygen. Angina can be caused by a partial blockage or spasm of a coronary artery[2] or when the supply of blood from the coronary arteries is not sufficient to meet the demands of the heart muscle.

Chest pain caused by angina is often triggered by exertion such as physical activity, which creates a demand on the heart muscle that the coronary arteries are unable to meet. The pain increases until the patient stops the activity and rests. In the case of angina, when the demand on the heart returns to normal, the pain begins to subside and eventually goes away. In the case of a heart attack, the chest pain does not improve with rest because there is a complete blockage of the coronary artery. Some patients are prone to angina attacks and must take medication such as nitroglycerin to help reduce the workload of the heart. (Nitroglycerin is discussed in more detail later in this chapter.) Angina alone is not life threatening, but it can be a sign of an impending heart attack.

The signs and symptoms of angina are nearly identical to those of a heart attack. For that reason, it is important to care for all suspected cardiac-related pain as though the patient is having a heart attack and to seek immediate advanced medical care.[3]

Myocardial Infarction

Recall from Chapter 11 that *myocardial infarction (MI)* is the medical term for what is commonly known as a heart attack. *Myo-* means muscle, *cardial* means heart, and *infarction* means a deadening of tissue due to a loss of adequate blood supply. The myocardium (heart muscle) must have an adequate supply of well-oxygenated blood to continue to function properly. The heart receives its blood supply through the coronary arteries (Figure 14.3). When these arteries become excessively narrow or blocked from disease (atherosclerosis), spasm, or a clot and can no longer supply the myocardium with enough oxygenated blood, the tissue of the heart begins to die.[4]

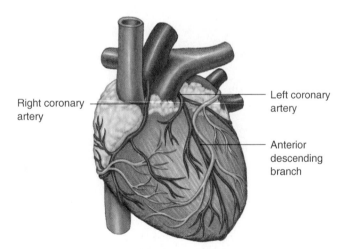

Right coronary artery
Left coronary artery
Anterior descending branch

Figure 14.3 The coronary arteries supply blood to the heart muscle (myocardium).

It is important to understand that myocardial infarction and cardiac arrest are not the same thing. Patients in cardiac arrest are unresponsive, apneic (not breathing), and have no pulse. Those patients should receive immediate CPR and the application of an automated external defibrillator (AED). While it is true that most cardiac arrests are the result of an MI, most MIs do not result in cardiac arrest.

Many factors will ultimately determine whether a heart attack will result in a cardiac arrest. The most common are the location of the damage in the heart and how much heart muscle actually dies. Damage that occurs over an important electrical pathway or to a large area of the heart muscle is more likely to cause cardiac arrest.

The following are common signs and symptoms of a heart attack (Figure 14.4):

- Chest or upper abdominal sensations of pain, pressure, tightness, or heaviness. Some patients describe a burning sensation that can easily be mistaken for indigestion.
- The pain or discomfort may be described as behind or below the sternum (substernal) and radiate to either one of the arms or shoulders. In some cases, the pain may extend to the back, neck, jaw, or upper abdomen.

These are the classic signs and symptoms of a cardiac-related event. However, cardiac compromise can present in other ways. Patients most likely to display signs and symptoms other than those noted above are women, people with diabetes, and older adults. While these individuals may present with common signs and symptoms, it is important to remain suspicious even if the more classic signs and symptoms are absent. Indications of cardiac compromise in these patients may appear as flu-like signs and symptoms, such as nausea and vomiting, indigestion, or a feeling of general weakness. The patient may simply tell you, "I don't feel right," or "Something is wrong with me, but I don't know what it is."

As an Emergency Medical Responder, you must be very aware of all possible presentations of cardiac compromise and not just the stereotypical image of a man suddenly grasping his chest and falling to the ground. You must be very suspicious when older adults, female patients, and patients with a history of diabetes insist that they have the flu or just don't feel well. Provide care as if they are experiencing cardiac compromise.

> **REMEMBER**
>
> Not everyone who is having a heart attack will have chest discomfort or chest pain. Sometimes patients present with shortness of breath, weakness, nausea, vomiting, and pale skin. Any combination of these should be cause for concern, and a more advanced provider should evaluate the patient.

DISTINGUISHING ANGINA PECTORIS FROM MYOCARDIAL INFARCTION

	Angina Pectoris	Myocardial Infarction
Location of Discomfort	Substernal or across chest	Same
Radiation of Discomfort	Neck, jaw, arms, back, shoulders	Same
Nature of Discomfort	Dull or heavy discomfort with a pressure or squeezing sensation	Same, but maybe more intense
Duration	Usually 2 to 15 minutes, subsides after activity stops	Lasts longer than 10 minutes
Other Symptoms	Usually none	Perspiration, pale gray color, nausea, weakness, dizziness, lightheadedness
Precipitating Factors	Extremes in weather, exertion, stress, meals	Often none
Factors Giving Relief	Stopping physical activity, reducing stress, nitroglycerin	Nitroglycerin may give incomplete or no relief

Figure 14.4 Both myocardial infarction and angina can present with symptoms of chest pain. Treat all cases of chest pain as a true cardiac emergency.

After requesting an ambulance using his shoulder microphone, Taylor carefully opens the car door and kneels in front of the man.

"He wasn't feeling well, and I was taking him to the doctor." The woman stands above Taylor, tears streaming down her cheeks.

"Where do you hurt?" Taylor asks the man.

"My chest," the man replies. "It's my chest. It feels tight and I'm having trouble breathing." He grimaces with pain.

"Go into the lobby, tell them that I've called an ambulance and that we need the AED," Taylor says to the woman, accentuating each letter.

Heart Failure

heart failure ▶ condition that develops when the heart is unable to pump blood efficiently, causing a backup of blood and other fluids within the circulatory system; also called *congestive heart failure*.

Sometimes called *congestive heart failure (CHF)*, **heart failure** describes a condition that develops when the heart is unable to pump blood efficiently. Heart failure can occur slowly over time; this is known as chronic heart failure. It also can occur suddenly following a heart attack (acute heart failure). Because the heart muscle is weakened, it is unable to pump blood efficiently. When this happens, pressure rises in the blood vessels. Left untreated, heart failure can cause fluid to be pushed out of the circulation and into the alveoli within the lungs, resulting in difficulty breathing (left-sided heart failure). It can also result in swelling in the lower extremities, which is often evidence of right-sided heart failure.[5] Although some patients with heart failure have a chief complaint of chest pain, most have a chief complaint of difficulty breathing.

A patient with heart failure will complain of trouble breathing because the fluid backing up in the vessels of the lungs moves out of the circulatory system into the tissue and into the alveoli (small air sacs) of the lung. When the patient lies flat, it is easier for the fluid to move into the lungs, resulting in a sense of suffocation. When the patient sits up, the fluid drains to the lower areas of the lung, and breathing gets easier.

Heart failure can be both chronic (ongoing) and acute (sudden). Causes of chronic heart failure include diseased heart valves, hypertension (high blood pressure), and various lung diseases. A patient can also experience an acute episode of heart failure following a heart attack.

Much like angina and heart attack, the patient with acute heart failure may complain of chest pain, difficulty breathing, or both. These patients typically have a history of cardiac problems and, for that reason, will likely be taking a number of prescribed medications. Many patients with heart failure have difficulty breathing while lying down. The patient may tell you that they cannot lie down and need to sit upright or that they must sleep in a recliner to enable breathing during the night.

Patients with chronic heart failure will often have swelling in their feet and ankles that sometimes extends up the legs. This is a result of the inability of the heart to move blood effectively. The jugular vein is the large vein on the side of the neck. It returns blood from the head directly into the superior vena cava. Heart failure causes the large veins to bulge and, therefore, you may see jugular vein distention (JVD) as a result of the increased pressure inside the circulatory system.

The signs and symptoms of heart failure include the following (Figure 14.5A and B):

- Shortness of breath
- Chest pain/discomfort
- Rapid pulse rate
- Edema of the lower extremities
- Jugular vein distention (JVD)
- Pale, moist skin
- Altered mental status due to a decrease in perfusion to the brain
- Increased difficulty breathing while lying flat

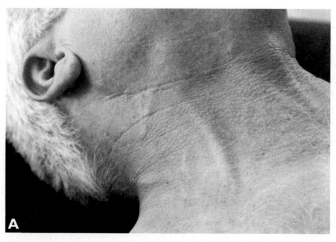
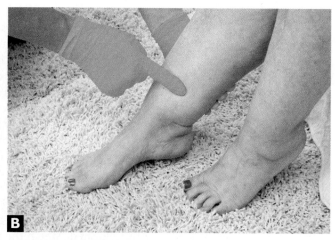

Figure 14.5 Signs of heart failure include (A) bulging neck veins and (B) edema of the lower extremities.

Taylor is thrilled to hear ambulance sirens approaching as he finishes getting a medical history from the patient. His calm demeanor and quick action seem to have somewhat calmed the older man.

"Here!" the patient's daughter shouts as she returns from the police station, carrying a first-aid bag. Several records clerks follow her, with worried looks on their faces.

"Put it down right there," says Taylor as he points to the ground next to him. Taylor digs through the first-aid bag, pulling out an oxygen mask and placing it on the patient. "This is going to help your pain," he tells the patient as he places the clear mask over the man's face. "Just breathe normally. This is oxygen and it should help with your breathing," he says in a reassuring voice.

Emergency Care for Cardiac Compromise

LO7 Explain the appropriate assessment and care for a patient experiencing cardiac compromise.

The care you provide for patients with suspected cardiac compromise depends on a thorough medical history and physical exam. The OPQRST assessment tool introduced in Chapter 12 is useful for gathering a history of the chief complaint.

Assessment

When your patient's chief complaint is chest pain, gather a patient history first, focusing your questions on the chief complaint. The OPQRST tool is commonly used to assess pain. Be sure to look the patient in the eyes as you ask questions to be certain that they understand the questions and are not distracted by what is happening to them. Remember that the patient is likely to be frightened. Speak clearly and allow plenty of time for the patient to respond to each question. Although it may not change how you treat the patient, this information will be valuable to the health care provider who will be treating the patient at the hospital.

Following is a review of OPQRST and some sample questions for each component:

O—*Onset.* "What were you doing when the pain/discomfort began?" With this question, you are trying to determine if the patient was at rest or may have been involved in some physical activity when the pain began.

P—*Provocation.* "Does anything you do make the pain or discomfort better or worse?" This question helps determine if any movement or change in position makes the pain better or worse. Cardiac-related chest pain is typically a constant pain that will not change with palpation or position. Although the patient may feel as though they can breathe easier in one position or another, the pain or discomfort will not usually change.

Q—*Quality.* "Can you describe how your pain/discomfort feels?" Allow the patient to describe the pain/discomfort in their own words, without leading them. It is helpful to offer contrasting choices and allow the patient to select the most appropriate word. For example, you might ask, "Is your pain sharp or dull?" or "Is your discomfort steady, or does it come and go?"

R—*Region/radiate.* "Can you point with one finger to where the pain or discomfort is the most intense?" "Does your pain move to any other part of your body?" The focus of these questions is to determine where the pain/discomfort is located. Watch the patient carefully to see if they are able to pinpoint the pain or if they make any gestures to suggest that the pain is spread out and perhaps radiating.

S—*Severity.* "On a scale of 1 to 10, with 10 being the worst pain you have ever felt, how would you rate your pain?" It is important to ask this question three different times. The first time you ask, you are trying to determine the level of pain/discomfort at that moment. You must then ask, "What level was the pain when it first began?" This will provide insight into whether the pain has gotten better, worse, or stayed the same. You will then ask the question again after you have provided some care to the patient.

T—*Time.* "When did you first begin feeling this pain or discomfort?" In many cases of cardiac compromise, time plays an important factor. Although it should not affect how you care for your patient, it will be an important part of the history you obtain. Ask when the pain/discomfort first began. Also find out if the patient felt ill or had any other symptoms prior to its onset. Many patients experience nausea, lightheadedness, shortness of breath, and fatigue long before the pain or discomfort begins.

Emergency care for a patient with signs and symptoms of cardiac compromise is similar to care provided for other medical complaints:

1. Maintain an open airway.
2. Make certain someone activates the EMS system and requests ALS services if available.
3. Allow the patient to maintain a position of comfort. This will usually provide the greatest ease when breathing.
4. If the patient is alert, they should be assisted to a sitting position. Administer oxygen if trained to do so.
5. Reassure the patient and calm them, if possible.

If the patient is in cardiac arrest (no pulse and not breathing), have someone activate EMS while you begin CPR. Otherwise, complete the assessment as required, carefully noting the patient's signs and symptoms. If the patient is unresponsive when you arrive, gain what information you can from family, friends, or bystanders.

Oxygen Saturation

For patients with signs and symptoms of cardiac compromise, the American Heart Association recommends using a pulse oximeter to monitor peripheral oxygen saturation. (See Appendix 1.) Any patient with an oxygen saturation (SpO_2) of less than 94 percent

> **REMEMBER**
>
> Continue to monitor the cardiac patient and provide care, even if the pain stops. Do not cancel your request for an EMT or more advanced EMS response just because the patient states that they are feeling better.

should receive supplemental oxygen. In most instances, a nasal cannula can be used to administer the oxygen and bring the SpO$_2$ up to between 94 and 99 percent. The use of a pulse oximeter should be considered a part of obtaining vital signs.

Emergency Care

When caring for a patient with signs and symptoms indicating cardiac compromise, you should perform the following steps as part of the assessment:

1. Take appropriate BSI precautions.
2. Perform a primary assessment and support the ABCs (airway, breathing, and circulation) as necessary.
3. Obtain a medical history.
4. Obtain vital signs.
5. If trained to do so, provide oxygen per local protocols.
6. Keep the patient at rest. Provide emotional support and reassure the patient.
7. Allow the patient to maintain a position of comfort, which is usually sitting upright.
8. Assist the patient with their prescribed dose of nitroglycerin or aspirin if your protocols permit. Consult medical direction.
9. Continue to monitor vital signs.

Remember to conduct yourself in a calm, professional manner when caring for your patient. This is particularly important when caring for patients with chest pain. These patients can be anxious, restless, or in denial. Their chances for survival may be increased if they can be kept calm and at rest.

A patient may ask if they are having a heart attack. It is best to respond by saying, "Your pain could be a lot of things, but let's not take chances." Do all you can to keep the patient calm and still. Remain calm yourself and talk to your patient. Let the patient know that resting is an important part of their care.

Medications

Some patients with a history of heart problems have been prescribed medications to take when having chest pain. Always ask if a health care provider has given the patient any medications for the current problem. If medications such as nitroglycerin or aspirin have been prescribed, then assist the patient in taking them only if your local protocols allow.

Patients who have a history of angina usually have nitroglycerin tablets or spray to take when having chest pain (Key Skill 14.1). Chest pain could indicate that the heart muscle needs more oxygen. Placing a nitroglycerin tablet or giving one spray under the patient's tongue will allow the drug to rapidly enter the bloodstream. Nitroglycerin dilates (enlarges) blood vessels, causing a decrease in blood pressure and reducing the workload on the heart. This can cause the patient to become dizzy or lightheaded. Patients receiving nitroglycerin should be sitting or lying down to avoid fainting. (Nitroglycerin in the form of transdermal patches can pass through the skin and be picked up by the circulatory system. However, the patches are too slow to be of use in a cardiac emergency.)

In recent years, the use of aspirin for the treatment of suspected heart attack has become commonplace in hospitals and EMS systems (Key Skill 14.2). In fact, pharmaceutical companies promote the use of aspirin for this purpose. As an Emergency Medical Responder, you may encounter patients who have recently taken aspirin or who may want to take some while in your care. Follow your local protocols when assisting any patient with the administration of medication.

REMEMBER

Recent studies indicate that high-concentration oxygen may be harmful to the heart, even in the case of myocardial infarction. The American Heart Association recommends oxygen only if the patient has an oxygen saturation of less than 94 percent or is in respiratory distress. Follow your medical director's recommendations.

JEDI

Be aware of the atypical signs and symptoms of a cardiac event. Many women report having pain in areas such as the upper or lower back, abdomen, neck, or jaw as opposed to the chest. Some people report nausea, lightheadedness, or shortness of breath at rest, with no chest pain. Know all the ways an MI can present and treat the case as urgent until further evaluation at a medical facility can be completed.

SCENE SAFETY

It is important to always wear protective gloves when handling medications. Some medications, such as transdermal patches, gels, and pastes, can be absorbed directly through the skin. If these medications come in contact with your skin, you may experience the effects intended for the patient.

Administering Nitroglycerin

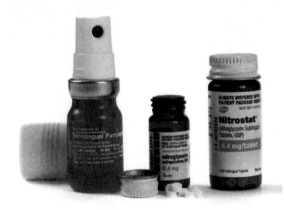

Medication Name
- Generic: nitroglycerin
- Trade: Nitrostat, NitroTab, Nitrolingual

Indications
All of the following conditions must be met:
- Patient complains of chest pain.
- Patient has a history of cardiac problems.
- Patient's health care provider has prescribed nitroglycerin.
- Systolic blood pressure is greater than 100 mm Hg. (Local protocols may vary.)
- Medical direction authorizes administration of the medication.

Contraindications
- Patient has a systolic blood pressure below 100 mm Hg. (Local protocols may vary.)
- Patient has a head injury.
- Patient has already taken the maximum prescribed dose.
- Patient has taken an erectile dysfunction (ED) medication in the past 24 hours (e.g., Viagra, Cialis). These medications also cause dilation of the blood vessels.
- Altered mental status.

Medication Form
Tablet or sublingual spray

Dosage
One dose is equal to 0.4 mg. Repeat it in 3 to 5 minutes. If no relief, systolic blood pressure remains above 100 (local protocols may vary), and authorized by medical direction, administer up to a maximum of three doses. Spray is typically prescribed for one metered spray, followed by a second in 15 minutes.

Steps for Assisting the Patient
1. Perform a focused secondary assessment for the cardiac patient.
2. Obtain vital signs including blood pressure. (Systolic pressure must be above 100. Local protocols may vary.)
3. Contact medical direction if there are no standing orders.
4. Ensure right medication, right patient, right dose, right route, and right time. Check the expiration date.
5. Ensure that the patient is alert.
6. Question the patient regarding any improvement following the last dose.
7. Ask the patient to lift their tongue, and place a tablet or spray dose under the tongue. If you are assisting, be sure you are wearing gloves.
8. Have the patient keep their mouth closed with the tablet under their tongue (without swallowing) until the medication is dissolved and absorbed.
9. Recheck blood pressure within 2 minutes.
10. Record administration, route, and time.
11. Perform a reassessment.

Actions
- Dilates blood vessels.
- Decreases workload of heart.

Side Effects
- Hypotension (lowers blood pressure)
- Headache
- Pulse rate changes
- Dizziness, lightheadedness

Reassessment Strategies
- Monitor vital signs.
- Ask patient about the effect on pain relief.
- Seek medical direction before readministering.
- Document changes in the patient's condition.
- Provide oxygen as appropriate.

Administering Aspirin

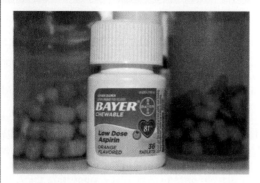

Medication Name
- Generic: aspirin or acetylsalicylic acid (ASA)
- Trade: Aspirin, Bufferin, Ecotrin

Indications
- Mild to moderate pain
- Fever
- Inflammation
- Cardiac chest pain

Contraindications
- Known allergy to aspirin
- History of bleeding disorders
- History of ulcers

Medication Form
Tablet

Dosage
One standard dose (adult tablet) is 325 mg or four low-dose (81 mg) tablets.

Steps for Assisting the Patient
1. Perform a focused secondary assessment for the cardiac patient.
2. Obtain vital signs.
3. Contact medical direction if there are no standing orders.
4. Ensure right medication, right patient, right dose, right route, and right time. Check the expiration date.
5. Ensure that the patient is alert.
6. Assist the patient as they chew and swallow the tablet(s).
7. Record administration, route, and time.
8. Perform a reassessment.

Actions
- Reduces the likelihood of clot formation

Side Effects
- Heartburn
- Nausea

Reassessment Strategies
- Monitor vital signs.
- Document changes in the patient's condition.
- Provide oxygen as appropriate.

FIRST ON SCENE WRAP-UP

Taylor is still writing down details of the patient's medical history when the paramedic from the ambulance touches his shoulder. "You've done a great job, Officer," she says. "I can take it from here."

Taylor stands and watches as the EMS personnel apply a heart monitor to the man's exposed chest. "His skin certainly looks better than it did just a few minutes ago," Taylor states as he moves back and makes way for the ambulance crew.

"Thank you, thank you!" the patient's daughter shouts, wrapping her arms around Taylor's midsection. She then rushes over to where her father is being loaded into the ambulance.

Taylor sighs, wipes the sweat from his face, and picks up his discarded lunch, smiling now at the cartoon face scrawled on the side. Regardless of what is in the bag, he knows that it will be the best lunch ever.

Summary

- A properly functioning heart is at the core of a healthy cardiovascular system.
- Blood flows through the heart beginning at the right atrium, then to the right ventricle, then to the lungs. It returns to the left atrium and down to the left ventricle. From there, it is pumped to the rest of the body.
- Each heartbeat is generated by an electrical impulse that travels along the conduction pathway.
- When normal heart function is disrupted, the patient will display signs and symptoms of cardiac compromise.
- Signs and symptoms of cardiac compromise include chest pain or discomfort that begins in the chest and may radiate to the shoulders, arms, neck, or jaw; shortness of breath; pale, moist skin; nausea; and weakness.
- Angina is caused by an insufficient supply of oxygenated blood to the myocardium.
- A myocardial infarction occurs when a portion of the myocardium dies due to inadequate blood supply.
- Heart failure, also known as congestive heart failure (CHF), occurs when the heart is weakened and can no longer pump blood efficiently. Blood and other fluids then back up in the system, causing edema of the lower extremities and fluid in the lungs.
- Care for cardiac compromise involves supporting the ABCs, applying supplemental oxygen, obtaining a thorough medical history, and monitoring vital signs.
- Patients with signs and symptoms of cardiac compromise should be considered unstable and in need of immediate transport. Initiate ALS transport if available.

Take Action

There are many causes of cardiac compromise. Most of them share at least one common symptom: pain. While you will likely care for anyone with chest pain as though they are having a heart attack, there are subtle and not-so-subtle differences in the three most common causes of cardiac compromise: angina, myocardial infarction, and heart failure.

This activity will help you learn the specific signs and symptoms for each of the three conditions. Using index cards, write the name of each condition on one side of a card—one card per condition, for a total of three cards. Now, using your text and the internet, research the specific signs and symptoms of each condition. Write as many signs and symptoms as you can find on the reverse of each respective card.

You will now have a very effective study tool for learning the different presentations for the three conditions. It is important to remember that as an Emergency Medical Responder you will always provide care for the worst possible cause of chest pain and not waste time trying to figure out the exact cause.

First on Scene Patient Handoff

Mr. Pannell is a 70-year-old male with a chief complaint of gradual onset of substernal chest pain that he states radiates to both shoulders and his jaw. His daughter states that he began feeling unwell earlier this morning, and she was taking him to see his doctor when his chest pain got worse. The patient states that he is short of breath and denies any previous medical history. He was pale and diaphoretic when he arrived here, and we put him on 12 L by nonrebreather mask just prior to your arrival.

First on Scene Run Review

Recall the events of the First on Scene scenario in this chapter, and answer the following questions related to the call. Rationales are offered in the Answer Key at the back of the book.

1. Should Taylor have checked the scene for safety first? Why or why not?
2. What signs observed in the patient were suggestive of heart problems?
3. What information would you give the paramedics when they arrive?

Quick Quiz

To check your understanding of the chapter, answer the following questions. Then compare your answers to those in the Answer Key at the back of the book.

1. Blood returning to the heart from the lungs enters the heart at the:
   a. right atrium.
   b. left atrium.
   c. right ventricle.
   d. left ventricle.

2. You are caring for a 44-year-old man who began experiencing chest pain and shortness of breath while jogging. His pain went away completely about 20 minutes after he stopped to rest. The most likely cause of his chest pain is:
   a. myocardial infarction.
   b. heart failure.
   c. angina.
   d. muscle strain.

3. You have completed your secondary assessment for a 65-year-old woman who has a long history of cardiac problems. She is complaining of chest pain and difficulty breathing. You should:
   a. place her in a supine position.
   b. administer high-flow oxygen.
   c. obtain a medical history.
   d. obtain her vital signs.

4. The myocardium receives its blood supply from:
   a. coronary arteries.
   b. myocardial arteries.
   c. the conduction pathway.
   d. the aorta.

5. Which of the following is NOT a common cause of cardiac compromise?
   a. Angina pectoris
   b. Myocardial infarction
   c. Cardiac arrest
   d. Heart failure

6. Which of the following statements best describes the relationship between a heart attack and sudden cardiac arrest?
   a. A heart attack and sudden cardiac arrest are the same thing.
   b. Sudden cardiac arrest is a leading cause of heart attack.
   c. Heart attack results in tissue damage; sudden cardiac arrest does not.
   d. Heart attack is a leading cause of sudden cardiac arrest.

7. You have arrived on the scene of an unresponsive female whom you find to be without a pulse and apneic. You should:
   a. begin chest compressions.
   b. administer oxygen.
   c. provide two breaths.
   d. place her in the recovery position.

8. You have completed your secondary assessment for a 52-year-old woman who has a chief complaint of nausea and general fatigue. She is pale and sweaty and has a history of diabetes, and you suspect she is experiencing cardiac compromise. You should:
   a. consider administering oxygen.
   b. administer oral glucose.
   c. obtain vital signs.
   d. perform a primary assessment.

9. Which of the following BEST describes the pathophysiology of angina pectoris?
   a. A lack of blood flow caused by narrowing of the coronary arteries causes temporary chest pain.
   b. A blood clot completely obstructs blood flow through a coronary artery causing death of heart tissue.
   c. Poor heart function causes a backup of blood and other fluids within the circulatory system.
   d. A complete cessation of heart function causes sudden death.

10. You are caring for a 72-year-old woman with a chief complaint of shortness of breath. You observe edema of the lower extremities and distended neck veins. She states that it is more difficult to breathe while lying down. Her signs and symptoms are most likely caused by:
    a. myocardial infarction.
    b. angina pectoris.
    c. heart failure.
    d. congestive infarction.

Endnotes

1. Centers for Disease Control and Prevention, National Center for Health Statistics. Multiple Cause of Death 1999-2020 on CDC WONDER Online Database, released December 2016. Data are from the Multiple Cause of Death Files, 1999-2015, as compiled from data provided by the 57 vital statistics jurisdictions through the Vital Statistics Cooperative Program. Accessed September 22, 2022, at http://wonder.cdc.gov/mcd-icd10.html

2. Jamshid Alaeddini and Jamshid Shirani, "Angina Pectoris," Medscape web site, updated July 19, 2018. Accessed September 22, 2022, at http://emedicine.medscape.com/article/150215-overview

3. Singletary, E.M., Zideman, D.A., Bendall, J.C., Berry, D.C., Borra, V., Carlson, J.N., Cassan, P., Chang, W.T., Charlton, N.P., Djärv, T., Douma, M.J., Epstein, J.L., Hood, N.A., Markenson, D.S., Meyran, D., Orkin, A.M., Sakamoto, T., Swain, J.M., Woodin, J.A. "First Aid Science Collaborators. 2020 International Consensus on First Aid Science with Treatment Recommendations," *Circulation* Vol. 142, No. 16, Suppl. 1 (October 20, 2020):S284–S334. doi: 10.1161/CIR.0000000000000897. Epub 2020 Oct 21. PMID: 33084394.

4. A. Maziar Zafari, S.V. Reddy, A.M. Jeroudi, and S.M. Garas, "Myocardial Infarction," Medscape web site, updated September 15, 2015. Accessed September 22, 2022, at http://emedicine.medscape.com/article/155919-overview

5. Ioana Dumitru and Mathue M. Baker, "Heart Failure," Medscape web site, updated July 2, 2022. Accessed September 22, 2022, at http://emedicine.medscape.com/article/163062-overview#aw2aab6b2b2

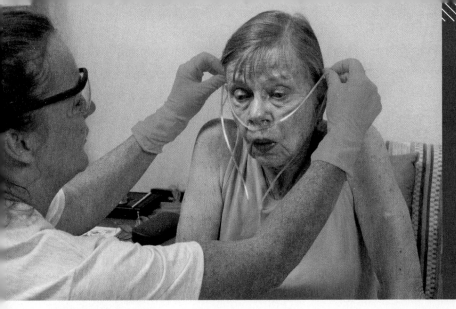

15

Caring for Respiratory Emergencies

LEARNING OBJECTIVES

Upon successful completion of this chapter, the student should be able to:

Cognitive

1 Define the chapter key terms.

2 Review respiratory anatomy and physiology (see Chapter **4**).

3 Explain the common causes of respiratory compromise.

4 Describe the signs and symptoms of a patient experiencing respiratory compromise.

5 Explain the pathophysiology of respiratory compromise.

6 Describe the appropriate assessment of and care for a patient experiencing respiratory compromise.

Psychomotor

7 Demonstrate the ability to appropriately assess and care for a patient experiencing respiratory compromise.

Affective

8 Recognize the fear that a respiratory emergency can cause.

9 Value the importance of reassurance when caring for a patient with a respiratory emergency.

Education Standards

Medicine—Respiratory

Competencies

Recognizes and manages life threats based on assessment findings of a patient with a medical emergency while awaiting additional emergency response.

KEY TERMS

asthma (*p. 304*)
bronchitis (*p. 303*)
chronic obstructive pulmonary disease (COPD) (*p. 302*)
cyanosis (*p. 299*)
emphysema (*p. 304*)

hypercarbia (*p. 299*)
hyperventilation (*p. 306*)
stridor (*p. 301*)
tripod position (*p. 301*)
wheezing (*p. 301*)

There are few things more important than the ability to breathe properly. Calls for "difficulty breathing" and "respiratory distress" are all too common in the world of EMS. A number of conditions can affect an individual's ability to breathe. Without adequate oxygen, body systems begin to struggle and will eventually shut down altogether. This chapter will discuss the signs and symptoms of inadequate breathing, the common causes of inadequate breathing, and how you can provide optimal care for these patients until more advanced help arrives.

FIRST ON SCENE

The ground rumbles beneath Scott's feet as screams pierce the air high above him. Scott looks up, unconcerned. It's just another day at the theme park. Scott has just dropped off a young girl who scraped her knee at the clinic and is walking toward the emergency services golf cart he parked in the shade.

Scott looks longingly at the ice cream cart beside the carousel. *Wow, no lines,* he thinks. *A 45-degree turn is all it would take to get a double scoop of my favorite ice cream.* Suddenly, his radio sounds off. "Dispatch to Medical One. What is your location?"

"Medical One at the carousel," Scott responds, a bit disappointed that he will now not be able to enjoy a large scoop of mint chocolate chip ice cream.

"Medical One, Park Services is requesting a response at the Crusher roller coaster. Sounds like a young female with difficulty breathing. You will be meeting Cal from security."

Scott leaps into the front seat of the golf cart and speeds off in the direction of the Crusher.

Overview of Respiratory Anatomy

As you learned in Chapter 4, the respiratory system (Figure 15.1) is responsible for the intake of oxygen and the removal of carbon dioxide. The primary structures associated with the respiratory system include the nasopharynx (nose), oropharynx (mouth), trachea, lungs, bronchi, bronchioles, alveoli, and associated muscles related to breathing.

Figure 15.1 Overview of the respiratory system.

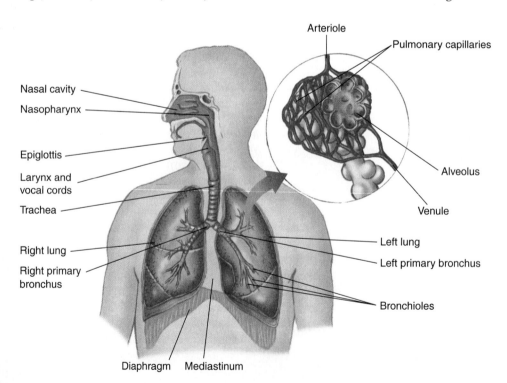

The respiratory system is divided into two sections: the upper and lower respiratory tracts. The upper tract consists of the nose, mouth, pharynx, and larynx. All structures of the upper tract are located outside of the chest cavity.

The lower respiratory tract consists of the trachea and the bronchi, bronchioles, alveoli (air sacs), and connective tissues of the lungs. The diaphragm is the primary muscle of respiration and contracts and relaxes to move air in and out of the lungs.

After air enters the body through the nose and mouth, it passes down the trachea and enters the lungs through the right and left bronchi. From there, the air passes through smaller passages called bronchioles and eventually ends up at the alveoli. The alveoli are surrounded by tiny blood vessels that drop off carbon dioxide while picking up fresh oxygen.

Respirations are normally controlled by the autonomic nervous system. The control center for the respiratory drive is located in an area called the *medulla*, which is the lower portion of the brain stem.

Respiratory Compromise

LO3 Explain the common causes of respiratory compromise.

Any time an individual experiences a condition that affects their ability to breathe adequately, it is referred to as respiratory compromise. Respiratory compromise can result from trauma or a medical condition. It can come on suddenly or develop slowly over time (Key Skill 15.1).

When breathing becomes compromised, the body does not receive an adequate supply of oxygen. If left untreated, this could lead to a condition known as *hypoxia*, which is an abnormally low level of oxygen in body tissues and cells. Signs of hypoxia include altered mental status, pale skin, and **cyanosis** of the lips and nail beds.

Breathing can also become compromised due to inadequate ventilations. Ventilations become inadequate when they become too shallow or too weak or when air becomes trapped in the lower airways, as occurs in emphysema and asthma. As the ventilatory rate drops, **hypercarbia** can develop, which is the condition of having too much carbon dioxide in the blood.

cyanosis ▶ bluish appearance of tissues caused by a lack of sufficient oxygen in the blood.

hypercarbia ▶ abnormally high level of carbon dioxide in the blood.

Respiratory Distress

Respiratory distress, also known as dyspnea, is the body's normal response to an inadequate supply of oxygen and an increase in the level of carbon dioxide in the blood. It is characterized by an increased work of breathing (the amount of energy required to breathe in and out). An increased work of breathing is characterized by an elevated respiratory rate, the use of accessory muscles to expand and contract the chest, an upright (often tripod) posture, and the inability to speak in complete sentences. In most cases, it is easy to spot a patient in respiratory distress because you can see that they have an increased work of breathing.

If the cause of the respiratory compromise is not corrected, it can lead to respiratory failure. Respiratory failure occurs when the body's normal compensatory mechanisms fail, the breathing rate slows, and tidal volume gets shallower. The patient in respiratory failure will almost always have an altered mental status. If not corrected, respiratory failure will quickly lead to respiratory arrest (complete cessation of breathing) and death.

There are many reasons a patient may experience respiratory compromise. Common causes encountered by Emergency Medical Responders include:

- Hyperventilation
- Asthma
- Chronic bronchitis
- Emphysema
- Traumatic injury
- Pneumonia
- Pulmonary edema

Respiratory compromise can also be caused by exposure to a poison, inhaling toxic fumes or a toxic substance, or a severe allergic reaction.

> **REMEMBER**
>
> One of the first things the body does when it recognizes an increase in carbon dioxide in the blood is to increase the breathing rate. This serves to blow off excess carbon dioxide in an attempt to stabilize the balance between oxygen and carbon dioxide.

Caring for Patients with Respiratory Compromise

Signs and Symptoms of Respiratory Compromise

- Shortness of breath
- Increased work of breathing
- Noisy breathing
- Altered mental status
- Restlessness, anxiety, and/or confusion
- Use of accessory muscles: neck, chest, abdomen
- Pursed-lip breathing
- Pale or bluish (cyanotic) skin color
- Numbness or tingling in the hands or feet
- Spasms of the fingers and toes (possible hyperventilation)

Emergency Care

1. Perform a primary assessment and support the ABCs as necessary.
2. Ensure an open airway. Check for an airway obstruction.
3. Obtain a patient history.
4. Administer oxygen per local protocols.
5. Check to see if the patient is allergic to anything at the scene.
6. Keep the patient at rest and try to calm them.
7. Monitor the ABCs and vital signs.
8. Assist with metered-dose inhaler per local protocols and medical direction.

Chronic Obstructive Pulmonary Disease (COPD)

Signs and Symptoms

- History of respiratory problems
- Persistent cough
- Shortness of breath
- Tightness in chest
- Swelling (edema) in lower extremities
- Rapid pulse
- Barrel (enlarged) chest
- Dizziness
- Pale or bluish (cyanotic) skin color

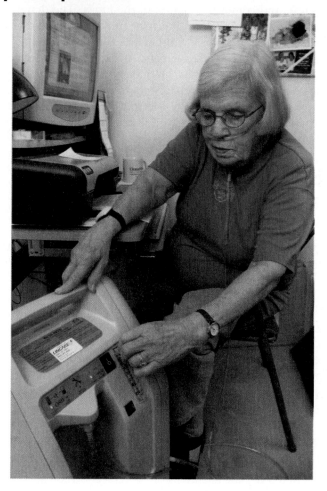

Emergency Care

Provide the same care as you would for respiratory distress. Do what you can to reduce stress. If you are allowed to provide oxygen, follow local guidelines for the COPD patient.

The first step in the management of a patient with respiratory compromise is to be able to differentiate adequate breathing from inadequate breathing.

Adequate Breathing

Adequate breathing is breathing that is sufficient to support life. It is easy and effortless. The diaphragm, the primary muscle of respiration, smoothly moves downward as we breathe in (inhale) and upward as we breathe out (exhale). Adequate breathing is characterized by a normal respiratory rate, depth, and very little effort to breathe. Breathing should not be hard work. One should be able to speak in full sentences without having to catch a breath.

To get a better understanding of what adequate breathing looks like, take a moment to notice the character of your own breathing. Close your eyes for a few moments and notice the movement of air as it enters your nose and mouth. Notice the movement of your chest and abdomen as the air fills your lungs. Pay attention as air rises up through the airways and exits your nose and mouth. Notice how quiet and calm this process is.

If you are near other people, try to observe their breathing. Are they breathing through their nose or mouth? Perhaps both? Can you see the movement of their chest and abdomen? Which area seems to be moving more—their chest or abdomen? This may differ from individual to individual, depending on the position they are in. As you will see, normal breathing by a healthy individual seems very subtle.

Characteristics of normal breathing include:

- Normal limits, 10 to 30 breaths per minute for an adult.
- Average respiratory rate is 12 to 20 for an adult. Respiratory rates can be as high as 60 for a newborn and steadily decrease with age.
- Normal depth (tidal volume). Normal breaths are not too shallow and not too deep. Your best indicator is an obvious rise and fall of the chest and/or abdomen with each breath.
- Work of breathing. This describes how much effort it takes for the patient to move each breath in and out. Normal respirations are effortless and unlabored as the diaphragm moves up and down with each breath.

Normal ranges for infants and children will vary significantly by age, with pulse and breathing rates being fastest at birth and gradually slowing down as age increases until they stabilize in the early teens. (See Chapter 24 for typical vital sign ranges for infants and children.)

Along with assessing rate, depth, and work of breathing, you must assess the rhythm of a patient's breathing. Respiratory rhythm should be regular. Breaths should occur at regular intervals and last the same amount of time. Exhaling should take about twice as long as inhaling.

Inadequate (Abnormal) Breathing

Inadequate breathing, also known as abnormal breathing, is breathing that is not sufficient to support life. Left untreated, this condition will eventually result in death. For most patients, the most obvious early sign of inadequate breathing is an increase in the work of breathing—breathing will appear labored and difficult. This is often called respiratory distress. If the patient does not receive prompt treatment, their condition can worsen quickly, advancing to respiratory failure, which is characterized by decreased respiratory effort and altered mental status.

Common signs of inadequate breathing include:

- Increased work of breathing
- Increased respiratory rate (early sign)
- Decreased respiratory rate (late sign)
- Respirations that are too deep or too shallow
- Irregular breathing rhythm
- Audible breath sounds, such as gurgling, snoring, stridor, or wheezing

Stridor is an abnormal, high-pitched breathing sound caused by disrupted airflow. **Wheezing** is a high-pitched whistling sound created when air passes through narrowed airways. It is most often heard when the lungs are auscultated with a stethoscope. In extreme cases, wheezing can be heard without a stethoscope.

When breathing becomes difficult, the patient has to work extra hard to move air in and out of the lungs. Labored breathing is usually obvious because the patient will be sitting upright, mouth open, and struggling to breathe. A person experiencing dyspnea often maintains what is known as a **tripod position**, in which they are seated or standing with their hands on their knees, shoulders arched upward, and head forward. This position allows for unrestricted movement of the muscles used for respiration. Other muscles, such as those between the ribs (intercostal) and in the neck and abdomen, begin to assist the diaphragm. They are called accessory muscles because they assist only when the diaphragm alone is not able to move enough air. During cardiac arrest, a patient may exhibit reflexive gasping breaths called agonal breaths or agonal respirations. These gasping breaths should not be considered normal respirations.

stridor ▶ abnormal, high-pitched breathing sound caused by disrupted airflow.

wheezing ▶ coarse whistling sound often heard in the lungs when a patient with respiratory compromise exhales. May also be heard on inspiration.

tripod position ▶ body position characterized by sitting forward with hands on knees or standing, leaning forward, with hands on knees, in an attempt to ease breathing.

Respiratory compromise may be caused by a variety of conditions, including chronic medical problems such as asthma, a sudden medical crisis such as a blood clot in the lung (pulmonary embolism), or an injury such as blunt trauma to the chest. Always listen to what a patient tells you about how they perceive the problem before attempting to make a determination of their condition.

Patients with certain respiratory conditions may have medications that need to be inhaled. They will want to take the medication but may be too upset or frightened to use the inhaler properly. Some jurisdictions allow Emergency Medical Responders to help patients use an inhaler. Check your local protocols and always call for medical direction before assisting a patient with medications.

Chest Trauma   Injuries to the chest such as blunt trauma or a penetrating injury can damage the muscles and bones of the chest wall, making it difficult and painful for the patient to breathe, leading to inadequate breathing. Damage can also occur to the lungs and trachea that may disrupt the normal exchange of gases and lead to inadequate breathing. Bleeding can also occur inside the chest cavity, reducing the effectiveness of respirations.

Pulmonary Edema   The accumulation of fluid inside the lungs is known as pulmonary edema; this is a common complication for many patients with a history of cardiac compromise. The presence of fluid in the lungs can be heard with a stethoscope and, in extreme cases, can be heard without a stethoscope. It presents as a "crackling" sound each time the individual breathes in or out.

Pneumonia   Pneumonia is caused by an infection of one or both lungs and results in the accumulation of thick mucus called pus. The pus fills the alveoli and prevents the exchange of oxygen and carbon dioxide, resulting in respiratory compromise.

Signs and Symptoms of Respiratory Compromise

LO4 | Describe the signs and symptoms of a patient experiencing respiratory compromise.

LO5 | Explain the pathophysiology of respiratory compromise.

For most cases of respiratory compromise, any or all of the following signs and symptoms may be noticed (Figure 15.2):

- Labored or difficulty breathing; a feeling of suffocation
- Audible breathing sounds
- Rapid or slow rate of breathing
- Abnormal pulse rate (too fast or too slow)
- Pale or bluish skin color, particularly of the lips and nail beds
- Maintaining a tripod position
- Altered mental status

Chronic Obstructive Pulmonary Disease   A group of respiratory conditions are classified as **chronic obstructive pulmonary disease (COPD)**. These include chronic bronchitis and emphysema.

The signs and symptoms of COPD include:

- History of cigarette smoking
- Persistent cough
- Chronic shortness of breath
- Pursed-lip breathing
- Maintaining a tripod position
- Fatigue
- Tightness in the chest
- Wheezing
- Barrel (enlarged) chest

chronic obstructive pulmonary disease ▶ general term used to describe a group of lung diseases that cause respiratory distress and shortness of breath. Abbrev: COPD.

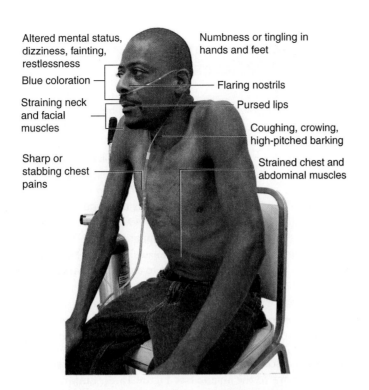

Altered mental status, dizziness, fainting, restlessness

Blue coloration

Straining neck and facial muscles

Sharp or stabbing chest pains

Numbness or tingling in hands and feet

Flaring nostrils

Pursed lips

Coughing, crowing, high-pitched barking

Strained chest and abdominal muscles

Figure 15.2 Signs and symptoms of respiratory compromise.
(Ray Kemp/911 Imaging)

In advanced cases, there may be altered mental status, a strong desire to remain sitting (even when asleep), and pale or blue appearance of the skin, lips, and nail beds.

COPD can be difficult to distinguish from heart failure, but you do not have to make that distinction. For Emergency Medical Responders, emergency care is the same for both conditions.

Bronchitis **Bronchitis** is a disease process that causes swelling and thickening of the walls of the bronchi and bronchioles. In addition to swelling of the tissues, bronchitis causes an overproduction of mucus in the air passages (Figure 15.3). Both of these conditions cause the airways to become restricted, resulting in difficulty breathing. Chronic bronchitis is defined as a productive cough that continues for three consecutive months and occurs for at least two consecutive years.

bronchitis ▸ lung condition characterized by inflammation of the bronchial airways and mucus formation; a form of COPD.

Classic signs and symptoms of chronic bronchitis include:

- Overweight
- Mild to moderate shortness of breath
- Pale complexion
- Productive cough
- Wheezing

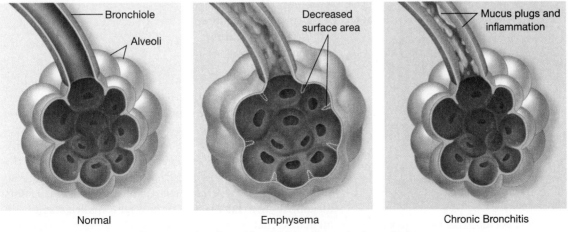

Bronchiole

Alveoli

Decreased surface area

Mucus plugs and inflammation

Normal

Emphysema

Chronic Bronchitis

Figure 15.3 Emphysema affects the alveoli, and bronchitis affects the bronchioles.

Scott pulls up to the roller coaster and finds a group of park guests surrounding a teenage girl sitting on the grass. He grabs his response bag and runs up to the young woman, who is gasping loudly with each breath. Two other girls are on either side, holding her forward.

"Can anyone tell me what happened here?" Scott says, as he opens his jump bag.

"Her name is Natalie," one of the girls says. "I told her not to go on this stupid ride but, of course, since Cor was going on it—"

"She's hyperventilating," the other girl shouts. "I've seen this before. I'm a babysitter and am first-aid certified!"

"Okay, okay, thank you," Scott says, trying to concentrate on Natalie, who is turning white as a sheet, her eyes closing slowly. "Natalie, I'm going to help you but, before I can, can you tell me what you were doing when you started having trouble breathing?"

"I was just . . . standing in line . . . for the ride," Natalie says in short bursts of words between breaths.

"Do you have any breathing problems, such as asthma?" Scott asks as he prepares an oxygen cylinder.

Natalie shakes her head no.

"Has this ever happened before?"

Once again, Natalie shakes her head no.

"Are you allergic to anything? Maybe a bee sting or food?" Scott asks.

Natalie shakes her head again.

---

emphysema ▶ progressive lung condition characterized by destruction of the alveoli; a form of COPD.

Emphysema   Most often associated with cigarette smoking, **emphysema** is a lung disease that causes permanent damage to the alveoli (see Figure 15.3). Emphysema is also common in individuals who have been exposed to environmental toxins over a long period of time, such as coal miners. The majority of patients with emphysema are middle aged or older and spend most of their energy just trying to breathe.

Emphysema causes destruction of the alveoli, making them useless for the exchange of oxygen and carbon dioxide. In addition, it causes the lungs to become less elastic, causing carbon dioxide to become trapped.[1] The loss of lung elasticity and the resulting accumulation of air cause the chest wall to expand over time. This is often described as a "barrel chest" appearance.

Another classic sign of the patient with emphysema is what is called "pursed-lip" breathing. The patient will purse or pucker their lips while forcing exhaled air out. This increases the exhalation phase and causes a back pressure deep within the lungs, which is believed to assist with keeping the alveoli open, promoting gas exchange. Wheezes are another common sign and can sometimes be heard without a stethoscope (audible wheezes).

Common signs and symptoms of emphysema include:

- Moderate to severe shortness of breath
- Thin or underweight appearance
- Large (barrel) chest
- Nonproductive cough
- Extended exhalations
- Pursed-lip breathing
- Wheezing

asthma ▶ condition affecting the lungs, characterized by narrowing of the air passages and wheezing.

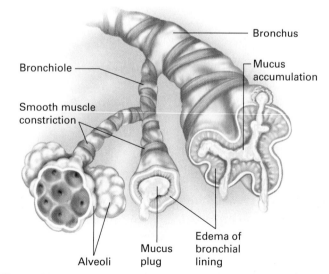

Figure 15.4 Asthma causes the bronchioles to narrow and fill with mucus.

Asthma   **Asthma** is a reactive airway disease that affects millions of people in the United States.[2] Asthma is a disease of the lower airway caused by an increased sensitivity (reaction) to a variety of irritants such as pollen, pollutants, and even exercise. When exposed to these irritants, the bronchioles spasm and constrict. Once irritated, they also swell and produce excess mucus (Figure 15.4). These factors all contribute to making the air passages smaller, resulting in an acute onset of respiratory distress. The narrowing of the air passages will often lead to wheezing.

Most individuals with asthma have few or no symptoms between acute attacks. Asthma patients often carry a metered-dose inhaler containing medication that they inhale into their lungs when they feel an asthma attack coming on (Key Skill 15.2). The medications are called *bronchodilators* because they dilate the bronchiole passages to help make breathing easier. If left untreated, an asthma attack can be severe enough to cause respiratory arrest and even death.

KEY SKILL 15.2

Administering Medication Using a Metered-Dose Inhaler

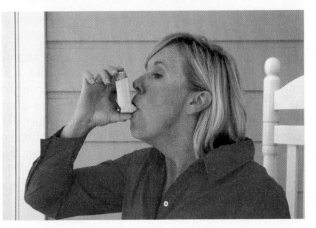
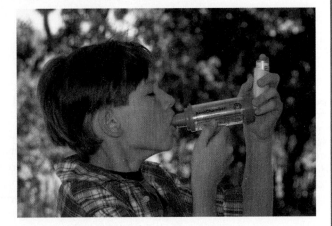

Medication Name

Generic: albuterol, ipratropium, metaproterenol
Trade: Proventil, Ventolin, Atrovent, Alupent, Metaprel

Indications

Meets all of the following criteria:

- Patient exhibits signs and symptoms of respiratory difficulty.
- Patient has their own prescribed inhaler.
- Medical direction gives the Emergency Medical Responder specific authorization to use.

Contraindications

- Altered mental status (such that the patient is unable to use the device properly).
- No permission has been given by medical direction.
- Patient has already taken the maximum prescribed dose prior to the rescuer's arrival.

Medication Form

Handheld metered-dose inhaler

Dosage

Number of inhalations based on medical direction's order or health care provider's order

Steps for Administration

1. Obtain an order from medical direction.
2. Confirm the patient is alert enough to use the inhaler.
3. Ensure it is the patient's own prescription.
4. Check the expiration date of the inhaler.

5. Check if the patient has already taken any doses.
6. Shake the inhaler vigorously several times.
7. Have the patient exhale deeply.
8. Have the patient put their lips around the mouthpiece of the inhaler.
9. Have the patient depress the inhaler to release the medication and begin to inhale slowly and deeply.
10. Instruct the patient to hold their breath for as long as is comfortable so the medication can be absorbed.
11. Allow the patient to breathe a few times and repeat with a second dose if so ordered by medical direction.
12. If the patient has a spacer device for use with the inhaler (a chamber that attaches between the inhaler and the patient's mouth to allow for more effective use of the medication), it should be used.
13. Provide oxygen as appropriate.

Actions

Dilates bronchioles, reducing airway resistance

Side Effects

Increased pulse rate
Anxiety
Nervousness

Reassessment Strategies

1. Monitor vital signs.
2. Adjust oxygen as appropriate.
3. Reassess level of respiratory distress.
4. Observe for deterioration of the patient. If breathing becomes inadequate, provide artificial ventilations.

Using your crew resources wisely is especially important on calls involving respiratory emergencies. While one person is getting a history from the patient, the other can get a history from friends, family, or bystanders. It's crucial to work together to get a full picture of the situation.

The signs and symptoms of asthma include:

- Moderate to severe shortness of breath
- Wheezing
- Nonproductive cough
- Anxiety

Hyperventilation Syndrome   Normal breathing can be affected by an emotional response or a sudden onset of anxiety. When this happens, breathing often becomes rapid, deep, and difficult to control. The body needs a proper balance of oxygen and carbon dioxide. **Hyperventilation** occurs when the individual breathes out and eliminates an excess amount of carbon dioxide. Most cases of hyperventilation are caused by anxiety and do not represent a true medical emergency. However, conditions such as a pulmonary embolism (blockage of an artery in the lung) or overdosing on certain drugs can also cause hyperventilation. These are true emergencies.

In some instances, hyperventilation can be a sign of something more serious, such as an impending heart attack or other serious medical condition. Activate the EMS system and provide care for respiratory distress. Be alert for cyanosis or other signs and symptoms of inadequate breathing. Monitor the patient for changes in vital signs, which may indicate serious medical problems.

Regardless of the underlying cause, your priority in the care of these patients is to reduce anxiety by reassuring and comforting them. Though hyperventilation is rarely life threatening, it can be very frightening. They feel as if they are not able to breathe, and this often makes the situation worse. Signs and symptoms of anxiety-driven hyperventilation include:

- Moderate to severe shortness of breath
- Anxiety
- Numbness or tingling of the fingers, lips, and/or toes
- Dizziness
- Spasms of the fingers and/or toes
- Chest discomfort

hyperventilation ▶ temporary condition characterized by uncontrolled, rapid, deep breathing that is usually self-correcting; often caused by anxiety but may have more serious causes.

FIRST ON SCENE (*continued*)

"Okay," Scott says, unraveling his oxygen tubing. "I just want to rule out an allergic reaction. I'm going to get this oxygen ready. Can you work on slowing your breathing for me?"

Natalie opens her eyes and nods, though her breathing is almost uncontrollable.

"Natalie, you're doing great," Scott says, holding the oxygen mask close to her mouth and nose. She forcefully pushes the mask away when he tries to attach it, so he holds it as close to her face as she will allow. Her face is dripping with sweat, her hands are shaking, and she is crying.

"She needs a paper bag!" one of her friend's shouts. "I told you, she's hyperventilating."

"Thanks again," Scott says automatically, as he counts Natalie's breaths again. Her respiratory rate is 32. "Natalie, I know this coaster was scary, but it's okay. You're safe now. Can you breathe with me?"

She nods and watches Scott carefully. He breathes in slowly and breathes out even more slowly. Natalie tries copying his breathing but keeps cutting each breath with a sharp intake. "You're doing fine," Scott encourages her. "Just keep breathing with me."

The care of the patient with hyperventilation should focus on calming the patient. You may need to remove them from an environment that could be contributing to their anxiety and assist them with slowing their breathing. It is not recommended to have the patient breathe into a paper bag or similar device because this could make the situation worse if there is an underlying medical problem. If your local protocols allow, you may use low-flow oxygen while helping to calm the patient and slow their breathing.

Emergency Care for Respiratory Compromise

LO6 Describe the appropriate assessment of and care for a patient experiencing respiratory compromise.

Your assessment of the patient with respiratory compromise will begin as you enter the scene and first see the patient. You must begin by observing their body position and body language. Are they sitting, standing, or lying down? Do they appear to be conscious or unresponsive? Your assessment of an unresponsive patient will need to be much more aggressive than that for a responsive patient. You must kneel beside the patient and place your ear next to their nose and mouth to confirm they have a patent airway. You must also determine the characteristics of their breathing (rate, depth, and work of breathing). You must provide positive pressure ventilations if you determine breathing is inadequate.

When assessing a responsive patient, pay attention to the level of distress and facial expression. Do they appear to be anxious and frightened? If so, the situation is likely getting worse. Introduce yourself and immediately begin to reassure the patient. Tell them that you are going to help them breathe easier. As you begin to gather a history, pay attention to the patient's ability to speak clearly and in full sentences. One of the classic signs of moderate to severe distress is the inability to speak in full sentences. A patient in moderate to severe distress will be able to speak only a few words before having to stop for a breath.

Listen for sounds as they breathe. Noisy breathing is always a sign of some form of airway obstruction. It may sound like gurgling, which usually indicates fluid in the airway. If the sound is more like snoring, either swelling of the upper airway or partial blockage caused by the tongue may be the issue. The problem usually can be corrected with proper positioning of the head. Wheezing may be heard, usually with a stethoscope, but severe cases can be heard without one.

Pulse Oximetry   The pulse oximeter is a simple tool that can be used to assess how much oxygen is getting to the patient's blood (Figure 15.5). It is most commonly placed on a finger and measures the level of oxygen saturation in the blood. A normal range for oxygen saturation is 94 to 99 percent. (See Appendix 1 for more about pulse oximetry.)

General Care   The care for any patient with respiratory compromise is the same, regardless of the cause (Table 15.1). Perform the following steps:

1. Take appropriate BSI precautions.
2. Perform a primary assessment and support the ABCs as necessary.
3. Ensure a patent airway. Administer oxygen per local protocols.
4. Allow the patient to maintain a position of comfort.
5. Arrange for ALS response if available.
6. Assist with prescribed medication per local protocols and medical direction (see Appendix 2).
7. Obtain vital signs.
8. Continue to monitor the patient and provide reassurance.

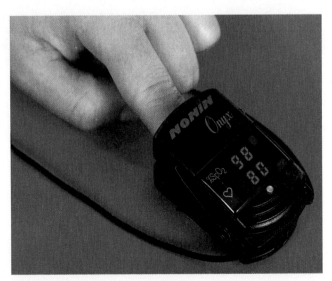

Figure 15.5 A pulse oximeter will measure and display both oxygen saturation and pulse rate.

TABLE 15.1   **Indications and Care for a Compromised Airway**

PRIMARY EXAM FINDING	PROBABLE CAUSE	IMMEDIATE ACTION	SUBSEQUENT ACTIONS
Gurgling	Fluid in airway (blood, secretions, vomit)	Roll patient on side and/or suction.	Monitor airway and breathing continuously.
Snoring	Tongue acting as partial airway obstruction	Manual airway maneuver (head-tilt/chin-lift or jaw-thrust).	OPA, NPA. Monitor airway and breathing continuously.
Stridor	Swelling of the soft tissues of the throat; partial foreign-body obstructions	Consider supplemental oxygen. If partial foreign-body obstruction, follow American Heart Association guidelines for removal of obstruction.	Monitor airway and breathing continuously.
Signs of hypoxia	Inadequate ventilations	Assist ventilations with bag-mask device. Consider supplemental oxygen.	Monitor airway and breathing continuously.
Inadequate or absent breathing	Respiratory failure or arrest	Assist ventilations with bag-mask device. Consider supplemental oxygen.	Monitor chest rise with each ventilation.
Inadequate or absent breathing	Foreign-body airway obstruction	Follow American Heart Association guidelines for removal of obstruction.	Provide care for air obstruction or assist breathing as necessary.

Positive Pressure Ventilations   When the normal breathing rate for a patient becomes too slow or too shallow, as in respiratory failure, it may be necessary to provide positive pressure ventilations.[3] Simply applying supplemental oxygen by a mask or cannula will not be enough. Use an appropriate bag-mask device to provide manual ventilations when breathing is determined to be inadequate and the patient is no longer alert (Figure 15.6). Place the mask firmly over the patient's face and provide ventilations at a rate appropriate for the patient's age. If the patient is still attempting to breathe, try to time your manual ventilations with the patient's inhalations. Provide just enough squeeze of the bag to see slight chest rise.

Figure 15.6 When breathing is inadequate and the patient is no longer alert, provide positive pressure ventilations with a bag-mask device.

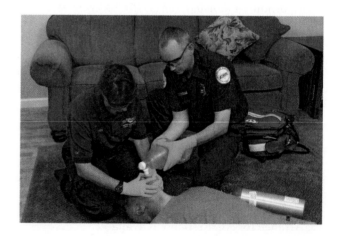

Metered-Dose Inhalers   Patients with a history of respiratory problems usually have been prescribed medication in the form of a metered-dose inhaler (MDI). An MDI is a small device that stores and delivers medication that the patient inhales into the lungs. The patient places their lips around the mouthpiece and squeezes the device to deliver one carefully measured "puff" (dose) of medication. Whenever possible, encourage the patient to take their medication exactly as prescribed by their doctor. Like all medications, MDIs have an expiration date. Prior to allowing the patient to self-administer the medication, check the expiration date to make sure that it has not expired. It is not recommended that you allow the patient to self-administer any medication that has expired. (See Appendix 2 for more information on metered-dose inhalers.)

FIRST ON SCENE WRAP-UP

"She won't need transport," the EMS crew leader says after assessing Natalie. She sits on the grass, holding the mask close to her face, her breathing returning to normal. "Her respiration rate is about 18 now, and her pulse rate and blood pressure have returned to normal. She's been advised to not go on any more roller coasters today."

"That's good. I wasn't sure if I could get her to catch her breath before she passed out altogether," says Scott.

"You did fine," the medic assures. "And her friends said they watched a medical drama last night and were ready to save Natalie if you couldn't."

Scott laughs. "That's reassuring. Now I can breathe easier myself."

Summary

- Respiratory compromise (difficulty breathing) is one of the most common calls you will encounter as an Emergency Medical Responder.
- Respiratory distress is the body's normal response to an inadequate supply of oxygen and is characterized by increased work of breathing, increased breathing rate, and the use of accessory muscles.
- If left untreated, respiratory distress can lead to respiratory failure and, eventually, respiratory arrest and death.
- Common causes of respiratory compromise include asthma, bronchitis, emphysema, and hyperventilation.
- Asthma is a disease of the lower airways characterized by spasms and swelling of the bronchioles, resulting in narrowing of the airways. Asthma can be triggered by environmental factors such as allergens, dust, stress, and exercise.
- Bronchitis is an inflammation of the bronchi and bronchioles that results in an overproduction of mucus within the airways. The disease is characterized by a productive cough. Chronic bronchitis may last for months.
- Emphysema causes a loss of elasticity of the lung tissue and destruction of alveoli. The result is poor gas exchange and a trapping of excess carbon dioxide within the lungs. Emphysema is a slow, progressive disease that results in severe respiratory distress.
- Hyperventilation syndrome is most often associated with situations of high stress or anxiety. It begins when stress or anxiety causes the patient to breathe rapidly. If not controlled, it will result in a loss of too much carbon dioxide, and other signs and symptoms will appear. It can usually be treated by helping the patient calm down and control their breathing.
- Care for respiratory compromise is the same regardless of the cause. It includes support of the ABCs, providing supplemental oxygen, and calming and reassuring the patient.
- Allow the patient to maintain a position of comfort, and do not force them to lie down unless they become unresponsive.
- Respiratory compromise is often a true emergency, and rapid transport by an ALS ambulance is often the most appropriate care.
- When the patient has been prescribed a metered-dose inhaler, allow them to self-administer the medication exactly as the doctor has prescribed.

Take Action

Sneak a Peek

Being able to observe a patient from a distance and quickly make an assessment of their breathing status is an important skill. It can be a bit challenging. For this activity, practice assessing the respiratory status of people around you without their being aware of what you are doing.

You can begin right at home. While you and others are sitting quietly watching television, pick someone and try to count their respirations. Remember, one inspiration plus one expiration equals one respiration. Continue to count the respirations for everyone in the room, getting their minute rate each time. One of the first things you will notice is that "normal" respirations for a person at rest are quite shallow. You can also observe the breathing of people who are asleep.

First on Scene Patient Handoff

Natalie is a 15-year-old female with a chief complaint of sudden onset of difficulty breathing while standing in line for the roller coaster. Natalie was in the tripod position when we arrived and appeared to be in moderate distress. She was able to answer questions with one- and two-word sentences. She denies any history of respiratory problems and states that this has never happened before. She responded well to our coaching to slow her breathing rate and would not tolerate an oxygen mask. Upon our arrival she was pale and diaphoretic, her respirations were 32, shallow and labored, and her pulse was 110, strong and regular.

First on Scene Run Review

Recall the events of the First on Scene scenario in this chapter, and answer the following questions related to the call. Rationales are offered in the Answer Key at the back of the book.

1. Did Scott ask all the proper questions to find out the problem? Why or why not?
2. How would you treat this patient if she were hyperventilating?
3. Should Scott have called an ambulance? Why or why not?

Quick Quiz

To check your understanding of the chapter, answer the following questions. Then compare your answers to those in the Answer Key at the back of the book.

1. You are caring for a patient with difficulty breathing. She states that she has a history of asthma. You understand asthma to be a disease of the:

   a. upper airway.
   b. lower airway.
   c. alveoli.
   d. trachea.

2. The respiratory control center, located deep within the brain, primarily monitors the level of ____ to maintain proper respiratory rate and volume.

   a. carbon dioxide
   b. carbon monoxide
   c. oxygen
   d. glucose

3. Your patient has been in respiratory distress for approximately 30 minutes. Your assessment reveals pale skin and cyanosis of the lips. These are signs of:

   a. heart failure.
   b. asthma.
   c. hypoxia.
   d. respiratory arrest.

4. You are caring for a patient complaining of shortness of breath. Her respiratory rate is 24 with good tidal volume. During the primary assessment, you should:

   a. provide supplemental oxygen.
   b. take a set of vital signs.
   c. perform a rapid secondary assessment.
   d. place her in the recovery position.

5. You are caring for a 17-year-old female who began experiencing difficulty breathing during soccer practice. You find her on her knees in the tripod position with a respiratory rate of 24 and shallow, and you can hear wheezing as she breathes. She has taken two puffs from her inhaler with no relief. Her condition is most likely caused by:

   a. bronchitis.
   b. asthma.
   c. emphysema.
   d. hyperventilation.

6. Emphysema is characterized by which of the following sets of signs and symptoms?

   a. History of smoking, barrel-shaped chest, and chronic hypoxia
   b. Fluid in the lungs and trouble breathing while lying down
   c. Rapid breathing, spasm of the hands, and normal blood oxygen levels
   d. Exercise-induced shortness of breath and wheezing

7. Which medical condition causes inflammation of the bronchioles, excess mucus production within the airways, and a chronic productive cough?

   a. Asthma
   b. Bronchitis
   c. Emphysema
   d. Hyperventilation

8. You have been dispatched to a call for respiratory distress and find a 67-year-old man in severe distress. He has a history of emphysema and is on home oxygen at 2 L per minute by cannula. His respirations are 32 and very shallow, and he is lethargic and unable to speak more than two or three words at a time. His airway appears clear. You should:

   a. increase the home oxygen to 6 LPM.
   b. place him on a nonrebreather mask at 15 LPM.
   c. provide positive pressure ventilations.
   d. remove the home oxygen.

9. You are caring for a 22-year-old woman with difficulty breathing. She has no prior medical history and states that she began having trouble breathing following an argument with her boyfriend. She states that her fingers are numb and tingly. You should:

   a. provide low-flow oxygen and attempt to calm her down.
   b. provide high-flow oxygen and transport.
   c. not provide oxygen.
   d. massage her hands and fingers while calming her down.

10. Which of the following medical conditions is characterized by a narrowing of the lower airways, often associated with exercise or allergies?

    a. Asthma
    b. Bronchitis
    c. Emphysema
    d. Hyperventilation

Endnotes

1. Decramer M., Janssens W., Miravitlles M. "Chronic Obstructive Pulmonary Disease," *Lancet*, Vol. 379, No. 9823 (April 2012): 1341–1351. doi:10.1016/S0140-6736(11)60968-9. PMID 22314182. Accessible online as of September 22, 2022, at https://www.ncbi.nlm.nih.gov/pmc/articles/PMC7172377/

2. David Markenson, J.D. Ferguson, L. Chameides, P. Cassan, K.L. Chung, J. Epstein, L. Gonzales, R.A. Herrington, J.L. Pellegrino, N. Ratcliff, and A. Singer, "2015 American Heart Association and American Red Cross Guidelines for First Aid," *Circulation*, Vol. 132 (2015): S269–S311, originally published October 14, 2015.

3. Bucher J.T., Vashisht R., Ladd M., et al. Bag Mask Ventilation. [Updated 2022 Jun 27]. In: StatPearls [Internet]. Treasure Island (FL): StatPearls Publishing; 2022 Jan–. Available from: https://www.ncbi.nlm.nih.gov/books/NBK441924/

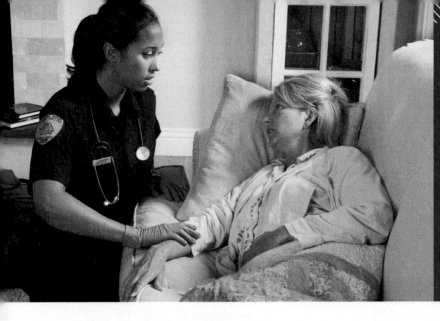

16

Caring for Common Medical Emergencies

LEARNING OBJECTIVES

Upon successful completion of this chapter, the student should be able to:

Cognitive

1. Define the chapter key terms.
2. List common causes of altered mental status.
3. Describe the signs and symptoms of a patient with an altered mental status.
4. Explain the appropriate assessment and care for a patient with an altered mental status.
5. Describe the signs and symptoms of a patient experiencing a generalized seizure.
6. Explain the appropriate assessment and care for a patient experiencing a generalized seizure.
7. Describe the signs and symptoms of a patient experiencing a stroke.
8. Explain the appropriate assessment and care for a patient experiencing a stroke.
9. Describe the signs and symptoms of a patient experiencing a diabetic emergency.
10. Differentiate between the signs and symptoms of hyperglycemia and hypoglycemia.
11. Explain the appropriate assessment and care for a patient experiencing a diabetic emergency.
12. State when it is most appropriate to contact the poison control center.
13. Describe the signs and symptoms of a patient experiencing an overdose or poisoning.
14. Explain the appropriate assessment and care for a patient experiencing an overdose or poisoning.
15. Describe the signs and symptoms of a patient experiencing carbon monoxide poisoning.
16. Describe the signs and symptoms of a patient experiencing sepsis.
17. Explain the appropriate assessment and care for a patient experiencing sepsis.
18. Describe the signs and symptoms of an allergic reaction.
19. Explain the appropriate assessment and care for a patient experiencing anaphylaxis (severe allergic reaction).
20. Describe the signs and symptoms of a patient experiencing an emergency related to renal failure.
21. Explain the special considerations that apply to caring for a patient undergoing hemodialysis.
22. Describe the signs and symptoms of a patient experiencing a suspected behavioral emergency.
23. Explain the appropriate assessment and care for a patient experiencing a suspected behavioral emergency.

Education Standards

Medicine—Neurology, Immunology, Endocrine Disorders, Psychiatric, Toxicology, Genitourinary/Renal

Competencies

Recognizes and manages life threats based on assessment findings of a patient with a medical emergency while awaiting additional emergency response.

Psychomotor

24 Demonstrate the ability to appropriately assess and care for a patient experiencing an altered mental status.

Affective

25 Value the significance of an altered mental status as a sign of an unstable patient.

KEY TERMS

altered mental status (*p. 315*)
anaphylaxis (*p. 333*)
behavioral emergency (*p. 335*)
clonic muscle activity (*p. 318*)
convulsions (*p. 318*)
diabetes (*p. 323*)
epilepsy (*p. 319*)
febrile seizure (*p. 318*)
generalized seizure (*p. 318*)
hemodialysis (*p. 335*)

hyperglycemia (*p. 323*)
hypoglycemia (*p. 324*)
overdose (*p. 325*)
partial seizure (*p. 318*)
postictal (*p. 319*)
sepsis (*p. 333*)
status epilepticus (*p. 320*)
stroke (*p. 320*)
tonic muscle activity (*p. 318*)

All emergencies can be categorized as medical or trauma. Emergencies that result in injury, such as from a fall or vehicle crash, are classified as trauma. Emergencies related to an illness of some kind are medical emergencies. You must be prepared to provide appropriate emergency care to patients with a wide range of medical conditions. This chapter provides an overview of common medical emergencies, including stroke, seizures, poisoning, overdose, and diabetic emergencies, and addresses appropriate emergency care.

 FIRST ON SCENE

"Jordan! Jordan! Wake up!" Jordan shoots up in bed and quickly looks around the dorm room. Nothing seems out of place. His vacationing roommate's movie posters still hang at odd angles on the walls. Clothing and books are still scattered around in piles. Just as he starts to lie back down, someone pounds on the door, rattling it with each impact.

"Jordan! Are you in there?" He slides out of bed and stomps to the door.

"What?" he shouts, as he pulls the door open. The look on the freshman's face tells him immediately that something is really wrong.

"There's this girl down in our room." Kaden is wide-eyed and whispering hoarsely. "And she's like, like, having some sort of . . . I think she's dying or something!"

Jordan has been considered the dorm "doctor" ever since he completed an Emergency Medical Responder course. He quickly grabs a shirt and pulls it on as he runs down the hall.

Medical Emergencies

The reasons a patient may require an EMS response are limitless. However, the majority of calls are related to an illness of some kind. Medical emergencies can result from literally hundreds of causes. Some of the more common medical emergencies seen by EMS are caused by infections, poisons, allergic reactions, and the failure of one or more of the body's organ systems.

You must assess each patient carefully and determine the chief complaint as well as any signs and symptoms that might be present. The patient, a family member, or a friend may be able to tell you if the patient has a medical history, such as an existing disease or condition. However, in most cases, what you observe and what the patient describes will be your main sources of information as to the patient's underlying problem.

Sometimes, a patient's underlying medical emergency may be hidden because of an injury. For example, a patient with diabetes may collapse because of very low blood sugar or may be involved in a vehicle crash and become injured. As an Emergency Medical Responder, your primary job will be to provide care for the patient's most obvious problem—in this example, their injuries. The medical problem, however, should not go unnoticed or untreated. During your assessment of a trauma patient, keep in mind that there may be an underlying medical problem.

Signs and Symptoms of a General Medical Complaint

To detect a medical emergency, you must be aware of common signs and symptoms, such as:

- Altered mental status
- Abnormal vital signs
- Tenderness or rigidity in the abdomen
- Weakness
- Rash

A patient may describe one or more of the following symptoms:

- Pain
- Dizziness/feeling light-headed
- Shortness of breath
- Fever or chills
- Nausea
- Chest or abdominal pain
- Unusual bowel or bladder activity
- Thirst, hunger, or odd tastes in the mouth

Assessment

Emergency care for medical emergencies is based on the patient's signs and symptoms. That is why it is so important to complete an appropriate patient assessment (see Chapters 12 and 13). For general medical complaints, you should:

1. Take appropriate BSI precautions and complete a scene size-up before you begin emergency medical care.
2. Perform a primary assessment.
3. Perform a secondary assessment focusing on the chief complaint, including patient history and physical exam.
4. Complete appropriate reassessments.
5. Comfort and reassure the patient while awaiting additional EMS resources.

When assessing the patient, keep in mind the following:

- If the patient appears or feels unusual in any way, suspect that there is a medical emergency.
- If the patient has abnormal vital signs, conclude that there is a medical emergency.

Altered Mental Status

Altered mental status (AMS) is one of the most common complaints to which you will respond. For this reason, it is important to be familiar with common causes, as well as the assessment of and care for a patient with an altered mental status. Although there are many potential causes of altered mental status, regardless of the cause, your assessment and emergency care will follow the same basic steps.

altered mental status ▶ state characterized by a decrease in the patient's alertness and responsiveness to their surroundings. Abbrev: AMS.

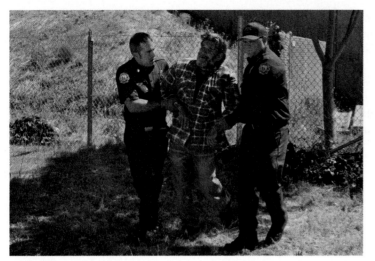

Figure 16.1 A patient with an altered mental status is often confused and not aware of their surroundings.

Evaluating Mental Status

LO2 List common causes of altered mental status.

A normal mental status is characterized by a complete and accurate awareness of one's surroundings. For instance, at any point in time, an individual with a normal mental status would be aware of who they are (person), where they are (place), the current day and time (time), and the events going on around them (event). When alert and oriented to all four elements, an individual is said to be "alert and oriented times four," or simply "A&O × 4." An individual who can tell you who they are and where they are but is unsure of the day/time and events is described as "A&O × 2."

An altered mental status is characterized by a decrease in the patient's alertness and responsiveness to their surroundings. This may appear as confusion and/or slowness to respond (Figure 16.1). Several conditions can cause a patient to experience an altered mental status. Among them are those shown in the following list and in Figure 16.2:

- Seizure
- Stroke
- Diabetic emergency
- Poisoning and overdose
- Hypoxia
- Shock
- Infection
- Head injury
- Psychiatric condition
- Kidney failure

Before you can make any judgment about a patient's mental status, you must first understand their baseline mental status. Baseline mental status is their mental status prior

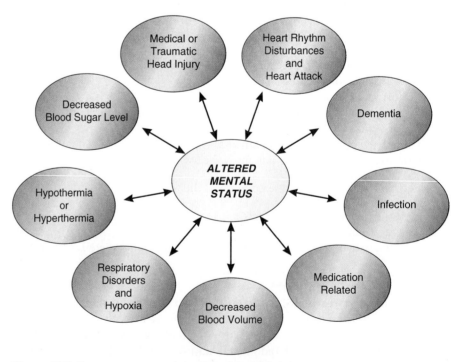

Figure 16.2 Common causes of an altered mental status.

to experiencing a medical emergency. For instance, your mental status at this moment is likely to be alert and oriented to person, place, time, and event. You are completely alert and aware of your surroundings. Some patients you encounter will not have a normal mental status. A patient who has dementia will often be confused and disoriented much of the time, and it may be difficult for you to determine if their confusion is new or their normal state.

In some cases, you must rely on family, friends, and/or caregivers to provide you with a description of the individual's normal mental status. They can usually tell you if the patient appears altered or if their status is normal for them.

Glasgow Coma Scale

The Glasgow Coma Scale is a standardized tool used to describe the level of responsiveness of a patient using specific criteria. This tool is most commonly used at the EMT and paramedic levels of care, but Emergency Medical Responders should be familiar with it. Originally developed as a tool for assessing trauma patients, it is useful for medical patients as well. The highest (best) score is a 15, and the lowest (worst) score is a 3. Scores depend on patient responses to three criteria: eye opening, verbal response, and motor response (Figure 16.3).

Signs and Symptoms of Altered Mental Status

LO3 Describe the signs and symptoms of a patient with an altered mental status.

Common signs and symptoms of altered mental status include:

- Confusion
- Incoherent speech
- Drowsiness
- Abnormal behavior
- Lack of awareness of surroundings
- Combativeness
- Repetitive questions
- Syncope (collapse or fainting)
- Unresponsiveness

Assessing the Patient with an Altered Mental Status

LO4 Explain the appropriate assessment and care for a patient with an altered mental status.

Assessment of a patient with an altered mental status should be focused on observation and obtaining as complete a medical history as possible. Understanding the common causes of altered mental status becomes important here (Figure 16.4). As you examine the patient's surroundings and communicate with the patient and any available family members, friends, or caregivers, you usually will be able to determine whether the patient's condition is being caused by a medical issue such as diabetes, stroke, or poisoning, or by a trauma-related issue such as a head injury.

Glasgow Coma Scale	
Eye Opening	
Spontaneous	4
To verbal command	3
To pain	2
No response	1
Verbal Response	
Oriented and converses	5
Disoriented and converses	4
Inappropriate words	3
Incomprehensible sounds	2
No response	1
Motor Response	
Obeys verbal commands	6
Localizes pain	5
Withdraws from pain (flexion)	4
Abnormal flexion in response to pain (decorticate rigidity)	3
Extension in response to pain (decerebrate rigidity)	2
No response	1

Figure 16.3 Glasgow Coma Scale.

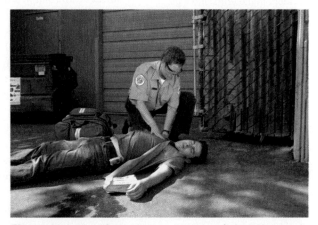

Figure 16.4 Identifying the exact cause of altered mental status can be very difficult.

The AVPU scale (discussed in Chapters 12 and 13) is one tool used to categorize the mental status of patients. It provides four general categories for assessment of a patient's mental status: alert, verbal, painful, and unresponsive.

When the patient is awake and aware of their surroundings, it is stated that the patient is alert and oriented times four (A&O × 4), which means the patient is:

A—Alert	A&O × 1 to person (individual)—They can tell you their name.
	A&O × 2 to place—They can also tell you where they are.
	A&O × 3 to time—They can also tell you exactly or approximately what time it is.
	A&O × 4 to event—They can also tell you about the event.
V—Verbal	Patient responds only to verbal stimuli (yelling or raised voice).
P—Painful	Patient responds only to painful stimuli.
U—Unresponsive	Patient does not respond to any stimuli.

The more altered a patient's mental status appears to be, the more aggressive care may need to be. For instance, if a patient is unresponsive, they may not be able to manage their own airway. In this case, you will need to monitor and manage their airway and be alert for vomiting. If the patient is behaving violently, you must ensure your safety and call for additional resources, such as law enforcement.

General guidelines for the emergency care of the patient with an altered mental status are:

1. Take BSI precautions and perform a primary assessment.
2. Monitor the patient's airway and breathing.
3. Administer oxygen per local protocols.
4. Monitor vital signs.
5. Provide emotional support.
6. Position the patient properly for comfort and protection of the airway.
7. Do not administer anything by mouth.
8. Continue to monitor the patient while awaiting EMS arrival.

Seizures

LO5 Describe the signs and symptoms of a patient experiencing a generalized seizure.

LO6 Explain the appropriate assessment and care for a patient experiencing a generalized seizure.

A sudden, abnormal burst of electrical activity in the brain that causes a sudden change in mental status and behavior is called a *seizure*. A seizure is not a disease but a sign of an underlying condition. Seizures can cause both a change in mental status and uncontrolled muscular movements known as **convulsions** (Figure 16.5).

Convulsions can appear as stiffening of the entire body, including the arms and legs. This is referred to as **tonic muscle activity**. There may also be jerking movements of the arms and legs, referred to as **clonic muscle activity**. Many **generalized seizures** are characterized by both tonic and clonic muscle activity. When a seizure causes the entire body to convulse, it is referred to as a generalized seizure. (An older term for a generalized seizure is *grand mal*.)

Seizures characterized by no loss of awareness with a localized area of convulsion are known as **partial seizures**. (An older term for a partial seizure is *petit mal*).

Seizures that occur in young children (between infancy and age 5) that are triggered by fever are called **febrile seizures**.

convulsions ▶ uncontrolled muscular contractions.

tonic muscle activity ▶ stiffening of the muscles during a generalized seizure; most evident in the arms and legs.

clonic muscle activity ▶ violent jerking of the muscles during a seizure; most evident during a generalized seizure.

generalized seizure ▶ seizure characterized by loss of consciousness and generalized muscle contractions.

partial seizure ▶ seizure characterized by a localized area of muscle contractions

febrile seizure ▶ seizure in a young child triggered by a fever.

Seizures can be very frightening for a patient's family, friends, and others who may witness them. Even though most seizures last less than a minute, it can seem much longer to the observer. Talk to witnesses to determine what the patient was doing prior to the seizure and if the patient has a history of seizure activity. Although some people have seizures on a regular basis, someone with advanced medical training should evaluate most people experiencing seizures.

Approximately 2 million people in the United States have some form of epilepsy.[1] **Epilepsy** is a disorder of the brain that causes seizures. Common causes of seizures are:

- Epilepsy
- Ingestion of drugs, alcohol, or poisons
- Alcohol withdrawal
- Brain tumors
- High fever
- Complications of diabetes
- Stroke
- Heat stroke
- Head trauma
- Hypoxia

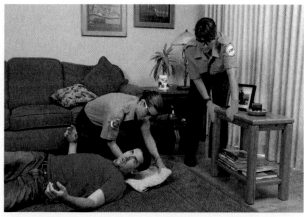

Figure 16.5 In situations in which the patient may be having a seizure, protect the patient from injury.

epilepsy ▶ disorder of the brain that causes seizures.

In cases of generalized seizure, any or all of the following may be present:

- Sudden loss of responsiveness
- Patient may report seeing a bright light or bright colors or the sensation of a strong odor prior to losing responsiveness
- Convulsions
- Loss of bladder and/or bowel control
- Labored breathing and possible frothing at the mouth
- Patient may complain of a headache prior to or following a seizure
- Following the seizure, the patient's body completely relaxes

Basic care for a generalized seizure includes the following steps:

1. Take BSI precautions and perform a primary assessment.
2. During the seizure, protect the patient from further injury. Move objects away from the patient and place something soft under their head if necessary.
3. Do not attempt to restrain the patient or force anything into their mouth.
4. Loosen restrictive clothing.
5. After convulsions have stopped, place the patient in the recovery position.
6. Perform a primary assessment.
7. Administer oxygen per local protocols.
8. Provide care for any injuries that may have occurred as a result of the seizure.

Protect the patient from embarrassment both during and after the seizure by asking onlookers to step away and give the patient some privacy. Patients with a history of seizures will often refuse care when they regain consciousness. If they refuse care, suggest that they contact a friend or family member so they can be observed following the seizure. After a seizure, the patient will generally feel tired and weak and may not be fully alert. This is called the **postictal** stage of a seizure. Talk to the patient, and provide reassurance as they gradually become more responsive. Provide emotional support to the patient and family members until additional medical help arrives.

postictal ▶ phase of a seizure following convulsions.

Do not attempt to restrain a patient who is actively convulsing.[2] Restraining the arms, legs, or head could result in injury to muscles and bones. Instead, protect the patient by moving objects that they might strike and provide padding of the ground beneath their arms, legs, and head with anything soft.

Do not attempt to open or place anything inside the mouth of a seizing patient.[3] It could cause broken teeth or aspiration of blood or a foreign object. The patient may stop breathing and become hypoxic during a seizure, but this can be normal. Attempting to force open an airway of a convulsing patient can do more harm.

Monitor the patient's mouth and airway closely. If you notice an accumulation of secretions or blood in the mouth, consider placing them in the recovery position to assist in clearing the airway.

Most seizures are not life threatening. Some patients may experience a life-threatening condition that occurs when they have very long seizures or seizures that repeat one after another. This is a condition known as **status epilepticus**, which is an extreme emergency. Prolonged seizures can cause the brain to become dangerously hypoxic. Ensure that an ALS ambulance, if available, is called for immediate transport to the hospital.

status epilepticus ▶ life-threatening condition that occurs when an individual has very long seizures or seizures that occur in quick succession.

Stroke

LO7 Describe the signs and symptoms of a patient experiencing a stroke.

LO8 Explain the appropriate assessment and care for a patient experiencing a stroke.

stroke ▶ medical emergency that occurs when an area of the brain does not receive an adequate blood supply, leading to death of brain cells.

One potentially serious cause of altered mental status is a **stroke**, or cerebrovascular accident (CVA), also known as a *brain attack*. A stroke occurs when blood flow to a portion of the brain is disrupted. Common causes of stroke include obstruction of a blood vessel, typically from a clot, or a ruptured blood vessel. During a stroke, a portion of the brain does not receive an adequate supply of oxygenated blood, and brain cells begin to die. In some cases, this damage is so great that it can lead to death (Key Skill 16.1).

Common signs and symptoms of a stroke are:

- Facial droop (on one side)
- Hemiparesis (weakness on one side of the body)
- Difficulty with speech or vision

KEY SKILL 16.1

Emergency Care for Patients Experiencing a Stroke

Causes of cerebrovascular accident stroke

Blockage (cerebrovascular occlusion)

Diseased artery ruptures

Cerebral Thrombosis (Clot)

Blockage in arteries supplying oxygenated blood will result in damage to affected parts of the brain.

Cerebral Hemorrhage (Rupture)

An aneurysm or other weakened area of an artery ruptures. This has two effects:

- An area of the brain is deprived of oxygenated blood.
- The accumulation of blood around the brain puts pressure on the brain, displacing tissue and interfering with function. Cerebral hemorrhage is often associated with artery disease and hypertension (high blood pressure).

Signs and Symptoms of Stroke

- Headache
- Syncope (fainting)
- Altered mental status
- Numbness/tingling of the hands/feet
- Hemiparesis (weakness on one side of the body)
- Difficulty with speech or vision
- Confusion
- Dizziness
- Seizures
- Altered breathing patterns
- Unequal pupils

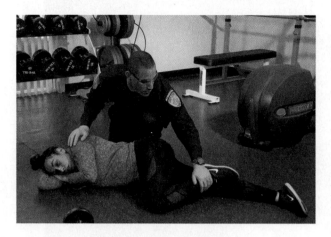

- Loss of bowel and/or bladder control
- Hypertension (high blood pressure)

Emergency Care for Patients Experiencing a Stroke

1. Take BSI precautions and perform a primary assessment.
2. Reassure the patient while performing a secondary assessment.
3. Obtain baseline vital signs.
4. Administer oxygen per local protocols.
5. Position the patient for comfort and airway protection.
6. Perform frequent reassessments.

- Altered mental status
- Severe headache
- Confusion

Less common signs and symptoms of a stroke are:

- Syncope (fainting)
- Numbness/tingling of the hands/feet
- Dizziness
- Seizures
- Altered breathing patterns
- Unequal pupils
- Loss of bowel and/or bladder control
- Hypertension (high blood pressure)

Several assessment tools can be helpful when assessing a responsive patient suspected of having a stroke. One of the most common is the Cincinnati Prehospital Stroke Scale (CPSS). The CPSS uses three assessment characteristics, and the presence of an abnormality in any one of the three areas indicates a strong likelihood of a stroke. The three areas are:

- *Facial droop.* A stroke may involve the area of the brain that controls the facial muscles, causing them to droop or sag on one side. To assess for facial droop, have the patient look directly at you and smile or show their teeth. Observe if the facial muscles do not move equally on both sides or if there is facial droop on one side or the other (Figure 16.6).

> **REMEMBER**
>
> A stroke is similar to a myocardial infarction (heart attack) in that the time it takes for the patient to receive definitive care is critical. For every minute a stroke is left untreated, an estimated 1.9 million neurons (nerve cells) are destroyed. For this reason, any patient suspected of having a stroke should be considered the highest priority for rapid transport.

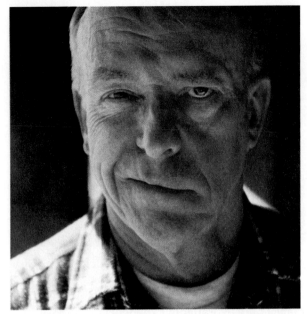

Figure 16.6 A patient having a stroke may exhibit facial droop on one side or the other.

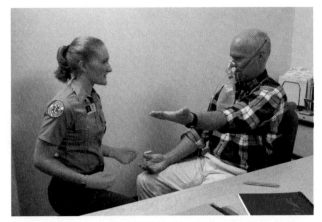

Figure 16.7 An inability to hold both arms up may be a sign of possible stroke.

- *Arm drift.* A stroke will often cause mild to severe weakness to one side of the body, resulting in poor function of the arms and legs on one side. To assess for this, have the patient close their eyes and hold both arms straight out in front of them with palms turned upward. Observe for arm drift, which means that one arm drops down while the other remains up. It is also significant if the patient cannot bring both arms up together (Figure 16.7).
- *Abnormal speech.* Often a stroke will affect the part of the brain that controls the tongue and other muscles required for speech. To assess for normal speech function, ask the patient to say a simple, common phrase such as, "You can't teach an old dog new tricks." Observe for slurred speech, inappropriate words, or an inability to respond verbally.

FAST is another tool that can be used to evaluate a patient for the possible presence of a stroke. The FAST acronym stands for:

F — Facial droop
A — Arm weakness
S — Speech difficulty
T — Time to call 911

If any of these signs are present, you should activate 911 or the closest ALS resource for transport to a designated stroke hospital, if available.

Time plays a very important role when a stroke is suspected. The sooner the patient can get to the hospital, the sooner they can begin receiving definitive care and the better the outcome. A key question to ask the patient when stroke is suspected is, "What time did the symptoms first appear?" This is often referred to as the patient's "last known normal."

When providing emergency care for a patient when stroke is suspected, you should:

1. Take BSI precautions and perform a primary assessment.
2. Reassure the patient while performing a secondary assessment.
3. Obtain a thorough history related to onset of signs and symptoms.
4. Obtain baseline vital signs.
5. Administer oxygen per local protocols.
6. Position the patient for comfort and airway protection.
7. Perform frequent reassessments.

Prompt recognition is important when dealing with patients who exhibit signs and symptoms of stroke. Medications called *thrombolytics* are commonly given in the hospital setting to patients experiencing a stroke.[4] If these medications are given soon enough, they can greatly decrease the long-term effects of the stroke.

FIRST ON SCENE (continued)

The girl is convulsing on the dorm room's dirty carpet. Her arms and legs are pulling and pushing slowly in all directions, her back is arched severely, and her head is snapping rhythmically from side to side, sending foamy splatters of saliva onto the carpet.

"What did you guys give her?" Jordan demands of the small group of terrified young men.

"Nothing!" Kaden shouts, holding his palms out to show that he didn't possess anything that would have had this effect on the girl. "We were just drinking some beer and playing video games! We didn't do anything!"

Jordan looks down at the girl and sees that her lips are bluish and her breathing is coming in gasps as she convulses. "How long has she been like this?" he asks.

"Since just before I knocked on your door." Kaden keeps looking from the girl to his friends and then back to Jordan. "Just a couple of minutes."

Jordan suddenly feels useless. The freshmen had the sense to pull furniture away so the girl wouldn't crash into anything, and one of them put a sweatshirt under her head, but as long as she is seizing, there is nothing he can do.

"Kaden," Jordan says, pointing to the cowering young man. "Bring me a phone right now. She needs an ambulance, and I have to let campus security know what's going on."

Diabetic Emergency

LO9 Describe the signs and symptoms of a patient experiencing a diabetic emergency.

LO10 Differentiate between the signs and symptoms of hyperglycemia and hypoglycemia.

LO11 Explain the appropriate assessment and care for a patient experiencing a diabetic emergency.

Glucose, a simple sugar, is the main source of energy for the body's cells. It is carried to the cells via the bloodstream. However, for glucose to enter the cells, insulin (a hormone secreted by the pancreas) must be present. Once inside the cell, glucose is used to create the energy required for the cell to function.

Diabetes is a disease in which the body either cannot produce enough insulin or cannot use insulin effectively. Although some patients can manage their condition with a specific diet, others require the administration of oral medications or must inject themselves with insulin (Key Skill 16.2).

Hyperglycemia High blood sugar, or **hyperglycemia**, is usually a gradual event, taking many hours to several days to develop. It can occur when the patient eats normally but fails to take a normal dose of insulin or eats too much for the amount of insulin being taken. The onset of signs and symptoms is gradual. If left untreated, hyperglycemia can lead to unresponsiveness and a condition known as *diabetic coma*.

Signs and symptoms of hyperglycemia include:

- Extreme thirst
- Frequent urination
- Abdominal pain
- Rapid, weak pulse
- Sweet or fruity odor on the patient's breath, called *ketone breath* (ketones smell like acetone, a compound found in nail polish remover)
- Dry mouth
- Restlessness
- Altered mental status, including unresponsiveness

diabetes ▶ refers to diabetes mellitus, a disease in which individuals either do not produce enough insulin or their body cannot use insulin effectively.

hyperglycemia ▶ abnormally high blood sugar level.

Emergency Care for Patients Experiencing a Diabetic Emergency

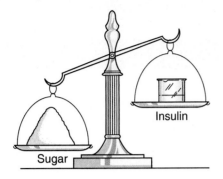

Hyperglycemia

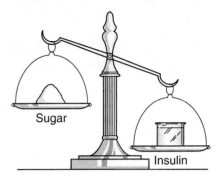

Hypoglycemia

Hyperglycemia
Causes

- A new onset of diabetes that has not been diagnosed or treated
- Failure to take diabetic medications as prescribed
- Eating more food than the supply of insulin can manage
- The presence of an infection or other stress that disrupts the glucose/insulin balance

Signs and Symptoms

- Gradual onset of signs and symptoms over hours or days
- Dry mouth and intense thirst
- Abdominal pain and vomiting
- Gradually increasing restlessness and confusion
- Unresponsiveness with these signs: deep, sighing respirations; weak, rapid pulse; dry, red, warm skin; eyes that appear sunken; breath smelling of acetone (sickly sweet, similar to nail-polish remover)

Emergency Care

1. Take BSI precautions and perform a primary assessment.
2. Reassure the patient while performing a secondary assessment.
3. Obtain baseline vital signs.
4. Administer oxygen per local protocols.
5. Position the patient for comfort and airway protection.
6. Perform frequent reassessments.

Hypoglycemia
Causes

- Taking too much insulin
- Not eating enough
- Overexertion
- Inability to keep food down (vomiting)

Signs and Symptoms

The following signs and symptoms are commonly seen in the patient experiencing hypoglycemia and may appear more rapidly than those related to hyperglycemia:

- Dizziness and headache
- Altered mental status
- Agitated or aggressive behavior
- Convulsions
- Rapid, weak pulse
- Hunger
- Pale, cool, moist skin

Emergency Care

- For a responsive patient who can manage their own airway and swallow without difficulty, administer oral glucose or a substitute such as honey, candy, soft drink, or orange juice. Administering anything by mouth to a patient without a gag reflex risks the potential of choking.
- For an unresponsive patient, place them in the recovery position, administer oxygen per local protocols, and consider oral glucose per local protocols and medical direction.

hypoglycemia ▶ abnormally low blood sugar level.

Hypoglycemia   An individual with diabetes who has taken too much insulin, eaten too little sugar, overexerted themselves, or experienced excessive emotional stress—or any combination of these—may develop **hypoglycemia** (low blood sugar). The signs and symptoms of hypoglycemia usually come on over a period of several minutes to a few hours.

Signs and symptoms of hypoglycemia include:

- Dizziness and headache
- Altered mental status
- Agitated or aggressive behavior
- Convulsions

- Rapid, weak pulse
- Hunger
- Pale, cool, moist skin

Emergency Care Sometimes a patient with hyperglycemia or hypoglycemia may appear to be drunk. Always check for underlying conditions—such as diabetic complications—when caring for someone who appears to be intoxicated.

When faced with a patient who has either hyperglycemia or hypoglycemia:

- Determine if the patient has diabetes. Look for medical identification jewelry. Question the patient and family members.
- If the patient is known to have diabetes or is suspected of having the disease and they are responsive, administer oral glucose.

Emergency care for a diabetic emergency consists of the following steps:

1. Take BSI precautions and perform a primary assessment.
2. Perform a secondary assessment. Obtain a medical history, and determine if the patient has diabetes. Find out if the patient has taken insulin and/or has eaten recently.
3. Obtain baseline vital signs.
4. Administer oxygen per local protocols.
5. Make certain that the patient can swallow without difficulty before giving anything by mouth. If the patient can swallow without choking and you are not certain if the problem is too much sugar (hyperglycemia) or too little sugar (hypoglycemia), administer oral glucose per local protocol. Check local protocols and always call for medical direction before assisting a patient with medications.

> **REMEMBER**
>
> Be very cautious about giving a patient anything by mouth. Carefully evaluate their level of responsiveness and their ability to swallow. If they are responsive, able to follow simple commands, and can swallow without difficulty, they may be able to accept liquids or solids without risk of choking. *Always follow your local protocols.*

FIRST ON SCENE (*continued*)

As Jordan hangs up the cell phone and tosses it onto the couch, he turns to Kaden. "Go down to the front of the building and wait for the ambulance."

As the young man runs from the room, the girl's shaking tapers off and then stops. She is still unconscious but is now snoring loudly. Jordan squats next to her and gently opens her airway by placing one hand on her cool, moist forehead and the

other under her jaw. The girl's snoring stops, and her lip color changes from blue to the same paleness as the rest of her face.

With the help of the two remaining students, Jordan is able to roll the girl into the recovery position. It is then that he notices something shiny inside the collar of her denim jacket. He reaches down and pulls out a MedicAlert necklace indicating that the girl has epilepsy.

Poisoning and Overdose

A poison is any substance that can be harmful to the body. Every day in the United States, an average of 87 people die from unintentional poisoning, and more than 2,000 are treated in emergency departments.[5]

An **overdose** is an excessive and potentially dangerous dose of a drug or prescribed medication. An overdose can be either intentional or accidental. Rates of overdose deaths involving synthetic opioids, which include fentanyl and fentanyl analogs, increased more than 56 percent from 2019 to 2020.[6] In 2020, more than 56,000 people in the United States died from overdoses involving synthetic opioids, which was more than 18 times the number of such deaths in 2013.

overdose ▶ excessive and potentially dangerous dose of a drug or prescribed medication.

Routes of Exposure

We usually think of a poison as a liquid or solid chemical that has been ingested (swallowed), but there are actually four routes of exposure, or ways that a substance can enter the body. They are ingestion, inhalation, absorption, and injection:

- *Ingestion.* Substances taken into the body by way of the mouth enter the bloodstream through the digestive system.

- *Inhalation.* Substances breathed in during normal respiration enter the bloodstream through the respiratory system. The poison enters the lungs and can pass into the bloodstream by way of the alveoli. Inhaled poisons take the form of gases, vapors, and sprays, including carbon monoxide, ammonia, chlorine, volatile liquid chemicals, and pesticides.
- *Absorption.* Substances enter the bloodstream through the skin and body tissues. Many such poisons damage the skin and are slowly absorbed into the bloodstream.
- *Injection.* Substances are delivered directly into the bloodstream by some kind of puncture. Insects, spiders, snakes, and certain marine life can inject poisons into the body. Injection may also be self-induced by a hypodermic needle.

Poison Control Centers

LO12 State when it is most appropriate to contact the poison control center.

There are more than 55 regional poison control centers in the United States, most of which are staffed 24 hours a day. The staff at each center is trained to advise you on what should be done for most cases of poisoning. There are several ways the Emergency Medical Responder can access a poison control center. The first is by calling the national poison control center number at 1-800-222-1222 (Figure 16.8). Another way is by contacting the EMS dispatcher who, in most cases, can put you in direct contact with the poison control center. The dispatcher will typically stay on the line and dispatch the appropriate resources, if necessary.

To aid the poison control center or medical direction, gather any containers at the scene of the emergency. Let them know if the patient has vomited and describe the vomit. Check the vomit for evidence of what may have been ingested, such as pill fragments. When possible, and if it can be done quickly, gather information from the patient or from bystanders before you call the center.

Ingested Poisons

LO13 Describe the signs and symptoms of a patient experiencing an overdose or poisoning.

LO14 Explain the appropriate assessment and care for a patient experiencing an overdose or poisoning.

In cases of possible ingested poisoning, you must gather information quickly. If possible, do so while you are conducting the primary assessment. Note any containers at the scene that may hold poisonous substances (Figure 16.9). Question the patient and any bystanders.

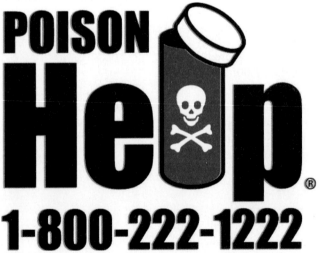

Figure 16.8 The American Association of Poison Control Centers maintains an easy-to-remember 800 number. *(American Association of Poison Control Centers)*

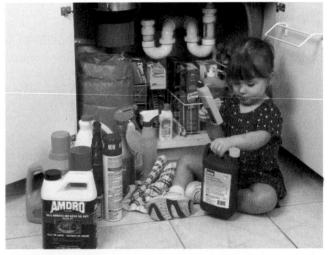

Figure 16.9 Poisons come in colorful containers that are often appealing to children.

The signs and symptoms of ingested poisons can be gathered during the scene size-up and primary assessment. They may include any number of the following:

- Burns or stains around the patient's mouth
- Unusual breath odors or odors on the patient's clothing
- Abnormal vital signs
- Sweating
- Dilated or constricted pupils
- Excessive saliva formation or foaming at the mouth
- Burning in the mouth or throat or painful swallowing
- Abdominal pain
- Nausea, vomiting, diarrhea
- Convulsions
- Altered mental status, including unresponsiveness

Contact your local poison control center to obtain advice on appropriate care for specific poisons. But do not provide any care, other than for the ABCs to ensure control of life-threatening situations, until you have contacted medical direction.

Do not give anything by mouth unless specifically instructed to do so by poison control or medical direction. Never attempt to dilute the poison or give activated charcoal unless instructed to do so by poison control or medical direction. The patient who is unresponsive may not have an intact gag reflex. Follow your local guidelines and the instructions given by the poison control center.

Emergency care for responsive patients is as follows:

1. Take BSI precautions and perform a primary assessment.
2. Ensure an open airway and adequate breathing.
3. Perform a secondary assessment. Obtain as much information as possible about the specific substance ingested, and call the poison control center or medical direction for instructions.
4. Do not give anything by mouth unless directed by a health care provider or the poison control center.
5. Administer oxygen or assist ventilations as necessary.
6. If supplies are available and you are directed to do so, give activated charcoal. For an adult, give 25 to 50 grams. For a child, give 12.5 to 25 grams.
7. In case of vomiting, position the patient so no vomit will be aspirated (inhaled). Place them in the recovery position or in a semi-sitting position with their head turned to the side.
8. If possible, save vomit for later analysis by hospital staff.

In addition to the usual risks, if the patient has ingested a highly concentrated dose of certain poisons, such as arsenic or cyanide, and if deposits remain on the patient's lips, there is a chance the rescuer may be exposed. Your best protection is to utilize proper body substance isolation precautions such as gloves, mask with eye shield, and protective gown, if necessary.

Inhaled Poisons

LO15 Describe the signs and symptoms of a patient experiencing carbon monoxide poisoning.

Poisons that are inhaled can reach the circulatory system directly through the lungs. Gases, fumes, vapors, and dust are all forms of inhaled poisons. Be especially alert for possible exposure as you enter the scene. If the scene is not safe, do not enter.

Gather information from the patient and bystanders as quickly as possible. Look for indications of inhaled poisons. Possible sources include automobile exhaust systems, stoves, charcoal grills, industrial solvents, and spray cans.

Signs and symptoms of inhaled poisons vary depending on the source of the poison. Shortness of breath and coughing are common indicators. Often, the patient's eyes will appear to be irritated.

REMEMBER

In your jurisdiction, Emergency Medical Responder care for ingested poisons may include giving the patient activated charcoal. Check local protocols and always call for medical direction before administering activated charcoal.

REMEMBER

Providing liquids by mouth to patients who have ingested a poison may be dangerous. This is especially true if the patient has been convulsing or if the source of the poison is a strong acid, alkali, or petroleum product such as gasoline or diesel fuel. Included in those groups of substances are oven cleaners, drain cleaners, toilet bowl cleaners, lye, ammonia, bleach, and kerosene. Always check for burns around the patient's mouth and for unusual odors on the patient's breath. Follow the poison control center's instructions.

Emergency care consists of safely removing the patient from the source of the inhaled poison, maintaining an open airway, administering oxygen, providing life-support measures, contacting the poison control center or medical direction, and making certain the EMS system has been activated. Remember to gather information from the patient and bystanders such as substance inhaled, length of time exposed, early care measures, and the patient's initial reactions and appearance.

Smoke Inhalation   Responding to a fire presents problems other than just burns. One such problem is smoke inhalation. The smoke from any fire source contains hot air and poisonous substances. Modern building materials and furnishings often contain plastics and other synthetics that release toxic fumes when they burn or overheat. It is possible for substances in smoke to burn the skin and the airway, irritate the eyes, and cause breathing problems. Do not attempt to rescue a victim unless you have been trained to do so and have all the required personnel and equipment.

You will probably see irritation to the skin, eyes, and airway associated with smoke. Look for signs of soot or singed hair around the nose and/or mouth. These may be signs of smoke inhalation, along with inhalation of the hot gases from the combustion process of fire.

Irritation to the skin and eyes may be cared for by flushing with water. But your first priority will be the patient's airway. In cases of smoke inhalation, you should:

1. Move the patient to a safe, smoke-free area.
2. Perform a primary assessment and assist with breathing as necessary.
3. Administer oxygen, if allowed to do so.
4. If the patient is responsive, let them assume a position of comfort.
5. Obtain baseline vital signs.
6. Closely monitor the airway and breathing status.

Carbon Monoxide   Carbon monoxide poisoning may occur at fire scenes. When carbon monoxide enters the bloodstream, it attaches to molecules within red blood cells called *hemoglobin*. This iron-containing molecule normally binds to oxygen but, due to carbon monoxide's high affinity for hemoglobin, oxygen is displaced. The patient will complain of headache and dizziness and may experience confusion, seizures, and coma. Proper care requires moving the patient away from the carbon monoxide source and following the same basic procedures as would be provided for any victim of smoke inhalation or inhaled poison.

Absorbed Poisons

Absorbed poisons usually irritate or damage the skin or eyes. However, there are cases in which a poison can be absorbed with little or no damage to the skin. The patient, bystanders, and other clues at the scene will help you determine if you are dealing with such cases.

Signs and symptoms of absorbed poisoning include any or all of the following:

- Skin reactions, ranging from mild irritations to severe burns
- Hives
- Itching
- Eye irritation
- Headache

Emergency care for absorbed poisons includes moving the patient from the source of the poison when it is safe to do so. Brush any powdered chemicals off the skin with a gloved hand, and avoid inhaling the powder as it is being removed. Flush the exposed area with water. Carefully remove all contaminated clothing from the patient, including shoes and jewelry. Be certain to have someone contact the poison control center or medical direction and activate the EMS system.

Injected Poisons

Bites and stings are common ways poisons can be injected into our bodies. Common sources include insects, spiders, snakes, marine life, and other animals. Some of these poisons cause very serious emergencies for anyone exposed. Others cause problems for only those patients who are sensitive to the poison. In all cases of injected poisons, be alert for signs of anaphylactic shock, a life-threatening allergic reaction, and manage the patient's airway, breathing, and circulation very closely.

Poisons can also be injected into the body by a hypodermic needle. Gather information from the patient, bystanders, and the scene. Signs and symptoms of injected poisoning include:

- Noticeable sting, bite, or puncture mark on the skin
- Pain at or around the wound site
- Itching
- Altered mental status
- Difficulty breathing and abnormal pulse rate
- Headache
- Nausea
- Anaphylactic shock

Emergency care for bites and stings includes the following steps:

1. Take BSI precautions and perform a primary assessment.
2. Perform a secondary assessment.
3. Administer oxygen per local protocols.
4. Scrape away insect stingers and venom sacs. Do not pull out stingers. Always scrape them from the patient's skin. A plastic credit card works well as a scraper.
5. Flush the injury site with clean water.
6. Place a wrapped cold pack over the injury site for comfort.

Some patients sensitive to stings or bites carry medication such as epinephrine (EpiPen). Assist these patients with taking their medications. Your Emergency Medical Responder course may include training in how to administer medications by injection when the patient cannot do this on their own. Do only what you have been trained to do.

In cases of snakebite on an extremity, flush the injury site with water and apply a pressure dressing; this has been shown to slow the spread of the toxin in a poisonous snakebite. Wrap a bandage around the limb beginning at the top and wind it down toward the hand or foot. Apply with firm, snug pressure, but use caution to avoid making the bandage too tight. Proper application of the bandage should allow for a finger to be easily inserted between the bandage and the skin. Closely monitor the distal circulation, sensation, and motor function in the extremity. Transport should not be delayed for application of the pressure bandage. Should the bite occur on the head, neck, or torso, flush the area with water and expedite transport to a hospital.

Alcohol Intoxication/Abuse

In the United States, the most commonly abused substance is alcohol (ethanol). In addition to its direct effects, alcohol is often mixed with other abused substances, worsening effects on the body. Alcohol is classified as a drug. The letters *ETOH* are a commonly used shorthand for ethanol, which is the chemical name for drinking alcohol. As with any other drug, acute and chronic alcohol abuse can lead to illness, poisoning of the body, abnormal behavior, and even death. A patient under the influence of alcohol is at risk for causing harm to themselves and others.

As an Emergency Medical Responder, try to provide care to the patient experiencing alcohol intoxication as you would any other patient. It is often difficult to determine if the patient's problem has been caused by alcohol and if alcohol abuse is the only problem. If the patient allows you to do so, conduct a secondary assessment that includes a thorough history. In some cases, you will have to depend on bystanders for meaningful information. Also, remember that diabetes, epilepsy, head injuries, high fevers, and other medical problems can make a patient appear to be drunk.

For all situations involving patients with alcohol or other drug emergencies, perform a thorough scene size-up and remain alert for changes in mental status. Once you can approach the patient, let them know who you are and what you are going to do before you start the assessment. You may have to modify your approach and communication techniques as you try to determine whether the situation also involves a medical or a trauma problem. It may be difficult to perform a physical exam or any care procedures until you can calm the patient and gain their confidence.

Signs of alcohol intoxication include the following:

- Odor of alcohol on the patient's breath or clothing
- Unsteady, uncoordinated movements
- Slurred speech and the inability to carry on a conversation
- Flushed appearance, often with sweating and complaining of being warm
- Nausea and vomiting

A patient with a long history of alcohol abuse who suddenly stops ingesting alcohol may experience withdrawal symptoms. Common signs and symptoms of alcohol withdrawal include:

- High blood pressure and rapid heart rate
- Confusion and restlessness
- Abnormal behavior
- Hallucinations
- Tremors (shaking) of the hands
- Convulsions

Some of the signs displayed in alcohol intoxication and withdrawal are similar to those found in other medical emergencies. Do your best to obtain a good medical history to rule out other possible medical problems. Remember, people who abuse alcohol may also be injured or ill. The effects of the alcohol might mask the typical signs and symptoms observed during assessment. Also, be on the alert for other signs, such as abnormal vital signs.

Basic care for the patient showing signs of alcohol intoxication consists of the following:

1. Take appropriate BSI precautions, and perform a primary assessment.
2. Ensure a clear airway and adequate breathing.
3. Perform a thorough secondary assessment to detect any signs of illness or injury. Remember that alcohol may mask pain. Look carefully for mechanisms of injury and signs of illness.
4. Monitor vital signs, staying alert for respiratory problems.
5. Help the patient when they are vomiting, so the vomit will not be aspirated (inhaled).
6. Protect the patient from further injury.

Delirium tremens (DTs) may occur in severe cases of alcohol withdrawal. Signs and symptoms of DTs include nightmares, severe agitation, disorientation, confusion, hallucinations, abnormal vital signs, and convulsions. These signs and symptoms may appear 3 to 10 days following the cessation of alcohol.

Drug Abuse/Overdose

Commonly abused drugs include opioids, stimulants, depressants, and hallucinogens (Table 16.1). Stimulants affect the nervous system to excite the user. Depressants affect the central nervous system to relax the user. Narcotics/opioids affect the nervous system and change many of the normal activities of the body. Often, they produce an intense state of relaxation and feelings of well-being. Hallucinogens (mind-altering drugs) act on the nervous system to produce an intense state of excitement or distortion of the user's surroundings.

The signs and symptoms of drug abuse and overdose can vary from patient to patient, even for the same drug. You need to assess the scene, bystanders, and the patient to determine if you are dealing with drug abuse and to identify the substance. When questioning the patient and bystanders, you may get better results if you ask if the patient has been taking any "medications or recreational drugs," rather than using the term "illegal drugs." If you have any doubts, then ask if the patient has taken drugs or is "using anything." Patients may be reluctant to give information about their drug use.

TABLE 16.1	Drug Use During the Past Year as Reported in the National Survey on Drug Use and Health, 2021
Drug	**Percentage Age 12 and Older Reporting Use in Past Year**
Marijuana	18.7
Marijuana plus other illicit drugs	8.3
Prescription psychotherapeutics	5.1
Opioids	3.3
Central nervous system stimulants	3.3
Pain relievers	3.1
Hallucinogens	2.6
Cocaine	1.7
Tranquilizers	1.5
Benzodiazepines (central nervous system depressants)	1.4
Stimulants	1.3
Methamphetamine	.9
Inhalants	.8
Crack cocaine	.4
Heroin	.4
Sedatives	.3

(Adapted from: SAMHSA, Center for Behavioral Health Statistics and Quality, National Survey on Drug Use and Health, 2021.)

Signs and Symptoms Signs and symptoms of drug use have a lot in common with many medical emergencies. Never just assume drug abuse by itself.

Signs and symptoms related to specific categories of drugs include the following:

- *Stimulants.* These cause excitement, increased pulse and breathing rates, rapid speech, dry mouth, dilated pupils, sweating, and the complaint of having gone without sleep for long periods. The most common stimulants are cocaine, amphetamines, and methamphetamine.
- *Depressants.* These can cause the patient to be sluggish or sleepy, lack normal coordination of body movements, and have slurred speech. Pulse and breathing rates are low, often to the point of a true emergency. Common depressants include Xanax, Valium, Klonopin, and Ativan.
- *Hallucinogens.* These can cause a fast pulse rate, dilated pupils, and a flushed face. The patient often sees things and hears voices or sounds that do not exist, has little concept of real time, and may not be aware of the actual environment. Often, the patient makes no sense when speaking. Many show signs of anxiety, fearfulness, and paranoia. Some patients become aggressive. Others tend to withdraw. Common hallucinogens include LSD, psilocybin, and peyote.
- *Narcotics/opioids.* Reduced pulse and breathing rates and a lowered skin temperature are often seen in the patient who is abusing narcotics. The pupils are constricted, muscles are relaxed, and sweating is heavy. The patient is very sleepy and does not wish to do anything. In overdoses, coma is a common event. Respiratory arrest may occur. Common narcotics include codeine, heroin, hydrocodone, oxycodone, morphine, and fentanyl.

- *Volatile chemicals.* The user may seem dazed or show temporary loss of contact with reality. This patient may go into a coma. The inside of the nose and mouth may show swollen membranes. The patient may complain of numbness or tingling inside the head or a headache. The face may be flushed and the pulse rate accelerated. There may be a chemical odor to the patient's breath, skin, or clothing. Common chemicals include aerosol sprays, cleaning fluids, glue, paint, paint thinner, and nail polish remover.

Withdrawal from drugs varies from patient to patient and from drug to drug. In most cases of withdrawal, you will see shaking, anxiety, nausea, confusion, irritability, sweating, and increased pulse and breathing rates.

CREW RESOURCE MANAGEMENT

When working at the scene of a possible overdose or poisoning, make sure that everyone on the team is keeping an eye out for evidence of what the person may have inhaled, ingested, or injected. Look for drug paraphernalia or pill containers anywhere at the scene.

Emergency Care When providing care for overdose patients, you should:

1. Take BSI precautions and perform a primary assessment.
2. Maintain an open airway and ensure adequate breathing.
3. Perform a secondary assessment.
4. Obtain baseline vital signs.
5. Administer oxygen per local protocols.
6. Be alert for vomiting and the need to manage the airway and breathing.
7. Continue to reassure the patient throughout all phases of care.

As a rescuer you must remain aware of the risk of being exposed to drugs that may be on or around the patient. Exposure to small amounts of very potent drugs such as fentanyl can cause signs and symptoms for the rescuer. It should be noted that many recreational drugs are being laced with fentanyl, causing an epidemic of accidental overdoses. Always wear gloves and use an appropriate barrier device when providing rescue breaths.

For all cases of possible drug overdose, it is good practice to contact medical direction and the regional poison control center. Also, be sure to locate any drug or pill containers and give them to the EMS crew when they arrive.

Naloxone (brand name Narcan®) is a drug administered to patients who have overdosed on an opioid. It is a widely distributed lifesaving tool that quickly reverses the effects of the opioid. This drug is available in pharmacies without a prescription but is stored behind the counter so a pharmacist must assist in its purchase. Pharmacies, hospitals, EMS systems, and many community-based organizations are making naloxone available to anyone who wants it. It is usually dispensed as a nasal atomizer (Figure 16.10).

Once the drug has been administered (Figure 16.11), you will need to monitor the patient closely as they may become more awake and agitated. Be alert for vomiting and be prepared to help manage their airway and breathing until EMS arrives. In some cases, it may be necessary to administer two doses. If the patient does not appear to be waking up or breathing normally within 3 minutes of the first dose, administer a second dose. Always follow local protocols. (See Appendix 2 for more information on naloxone.)

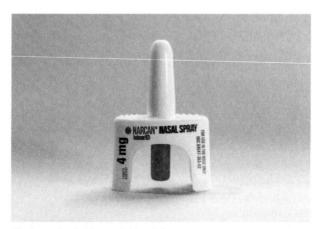

Figure 16.10 Narcan® Nasal Spray.
(Hanson L/Shutterstock)

REMEMBER

Do your best to be nonjudgmental of the patient with drug or alcohol addiction. Your view of the patient may cloud your ability to treat them appropriately. Regardless of the addiction, the patient has an acute emergency that requires immediate and often lifesaving intervention.

REMEMBER

At the time of publication, a growing number of states have passed laws permitting Emergency Medical Responders to administer naloxone (Narcan), a drug that functions as an antidote to all narcotics. Naloxone is administered by either a spray into the nose or an autoinjector similar to the EpiPen. Follow the local protocols approved by your medical director.

Sepsis

LO16 Describe the signs and symptoms of a patient experiencing sepsis.

LO17 Explain the appropriate assessment and care for a patient experiencing sepsis.

Everyone gets an infection from time to time, such as a respiratory infection or an infection that arises from a cut or scrape on the skin. **Sepsis** is an extreme and overactive response to an infection. It is most often associated with infections of the lungs (pneumonia), abdomen, or urinary tract. When the body's immune system overreacts to the infection, it can set up a chain of events and widespread inflammation that can damage multiple organ systems. Sepsis can progress to *septic shock*, which is a severe and dangerous drop in blood pressure.[7] Without treatment, sepsis can result in tissue damage, organ failure, and death.

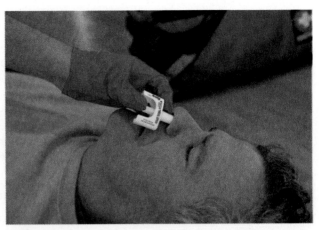

Figure 16.11 Narcan® is administered by placing the tip of the atomizer in one nostril and pressing the plunger firmly to release the medication into the patient's nose.
(Edward T. Dickinson, MD)

Signs and symptoms of sepsis include:

- Fever
- Chills
- Rapid breathing
- Rapid heart rate
- Low blood pressure
- Altered mental status

sepsis ▶ potentially life-threatening condition caused by the body producing an extreme and damaging response to an infection.

Although sepsis can have numerous causes, patients in the following groups are more susceptible:

- Infants and older adults
- Patients who have undergone a tissue or organ transplant
- Patients who have undergone radiation or chemotherapy
- Patients with burns
- Patients with diabetes
- Patients with HIV or AIDS

General care for a patient with signs and symptoms of sepsis is as follows:

1. Take appropriate BSI precautions, and perform a primary assessment.
2. Perform a secondary assessment.
3. Obtain baseline vital signs.
4. Administer oxygen per local protocols.
5. Perform reassessments as necessary.

Allergic Reactions

LO18 Describe the signs and symptoms of an allergic reaction.

LO19 Explain the appropriate assessment and care for a patient experiencing anaphylaxis (severe allergic reaction).

Allergic reactions occur when people come in contact with a substance to which they are allergic. Substances that cause an allergic response are called *allergens*. The body's immune system considers the allergen an invader and attempts to fight it. In minor reactions, there may be only mild swelling of the skin and itching. **Anaphylaxis**, also called anaphylactic shock, is a severe and potentially life-threatening allergic reaction.

There is no way of knowing if patients will stabilize, grow worse slowly or rapidly, or overcome the reaction on their own. Many patients rapidly become worse. For some,

anaphylaxis ▶ severe and potentially life-threatening allergic reaction.

the allergic response can be fatal unless special care is provided quickly. Anaphylaxis causes the air passages to constrict, making it difficult for the patient to breathe. It also causes the blood vessels to dilate, resulting in a dangerously low blood pressure.[8]

Anaphylaxis has many different causes, such as insect bites and stings; foods (e.g., nuts, spices, shellfish); inhaled substances, including dust and pollens; chemicals, inhaled or when in contact with the skin; and medications, injected or taken by mouth.

Signs and symptoms of anaphylaxis are:

- Burning, itching, or breaking out of the skin (hives or some type of rash)
- Restlessness and anxiety
- Breathing difficulty
- Altered mental status
- Rapid, weak pulse
- Swelling of the tongue and throat
- Abnormally low blood pressure

When you interview a patient you suspect may be having an allergic reaction, ask if they are allergic to anything and if they have been in contact with that substance. If unresponsive, look for medical identification jewelry, which might indicate a history of allergies.

Some people who have known allergies carry prescribed medications to take in case of an emergency. Those medications (usually an epinephrine autoinjector such as an EpiPen) are intended to be self-administered by the patient (see Appendix 2). Your jurisdiction may allow Emergency Medical Responders to assist with an epinephrine autoinjector. Epinephrine is a form of adrenaline that helps to open the air passages and constrict the blood vessels.

Your local protocols will determine if you can assist the patient in administering the medication. Your instructor will inform you of local policies for the care of these patients.

Emergency care for anaphylaxis:

1. Take appropriate BSI precautions, and perform a primary assessment.
2. Ensure a clear airway and adequate breathing.
3. Perform a secondary assessment.
4. Administer oxygen per local protocols.
5. Assist the patient with their prescribed epinephrine autoinjector as indicated by local protocols.
6. Perform reassessments as necessary and closely monitor vital signs and ABCs until EMS arrives.

<aside>
REMEMBER

Minor allergic reactions are generally limited to one body system, such as the skin. Anaphylaxis is a severe allergic reaction that affects multiple body systems. This usually includes the respiratory system—with severe wheezing and hoarseness. Breathing may also be hampered by a swollen tongue. The release of histamine causes dilation of capillaries, which results in hives. When the arteries dilate, the patient becomes hypotensive.
</aside>

Kidney (Renal) Failure

LO20 Describe the signs and symptoms of a patient experiencing an emergency related to renal failure.

LO21 Explain the special considerations that apply to caring for a patient undergoing hemodialysis.

Kidney failure, also called renal failure, occurs when the kidneys fail to function normally. The kidneys serve as complex filters for the blood and are essential for the removal of excess water and waste products from the blood. The kidneys can fail for a wide variety of reasons, including injury, blood loss, disease, and reactions to medications.

Patients most at risk for renal failure include adults older than 60 and those with a history of diabetes, high blood pressure, or heart disease, and those with a family member with kidney failure.

Common signs and symptoms of renal failure include:

- Weakness
- Altered mental status
- Edema (swelling) in the lower extremities, abdomen, face, or other areas of the body

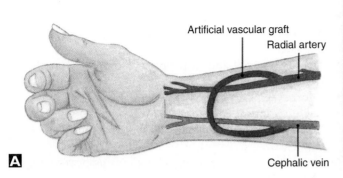

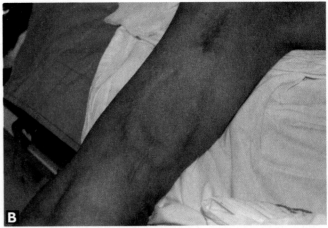

Figure 16.12 (A) During hemodialysis, the dialysis machine is connected to an access site, such as a shunt, beneath the skin. (B) A shunt can be clearly seen beneath the skin.
(© Edward T. Dickinson, MD)

- Increased heart rate
- Increased blood pressure
- Decreased urine output

Hemodialysis is the process of using a machine to filter excess water, salts, and waste products from the blood when the kidneys are no longer able to do this properly. A patient with advanced renal failure must undergo hemodialysis at frequent intervals, usually at a specialty dialysis center. The dialysis machine is connected to the patient via a surgically implanted access point (shunt or fistula) beneath the skin of the arm (Figure 16.12A and B). The patient's blood is run through the dialysis machine, where it is filtered and then returned to the body by way of the shunt or fistula.

Emergency care of the patient with renal failure is as follows:

1. Take appropriate BSI precautions, and perform a primary assessment.
2. Perform a secondary assessment.
3. Control any bleeding from the access point with direct pressure.
4. Administer oxygen per local protocols.
5. Perform reassessments as necessary.

Behavioral Emergencies

LO22 Describe the signs and symptoms of a patient experiencing a suspected behavioral emergency.

LO23 Explain the appropriate assessment and care for a patient experiencing a suspected behavioral emergency.

Behavior is the manner in which an individual acts or conducts themselves. "Normal" behavior is behavior that is considered typical and that aligns with the expectations of family members, friends, and society in general. It does not interfere with the daily activities of life. Behavior that is unacceptable or intolerable to others is known as abnormal (atypical) behavior. Although caring for a patient with a behavioral emergency might be challenging, it is crucial that you remain professional and provide appropriate care.

A situation in which the patient exhibits abnormal behavior that is unacceptable or intolerable to the patient, family, or community is considered a **behavioral emergency**. Such behavior may occur because of extremes of emotion or a psychological or medical condition. Other causes of behavioral changes include situational stress (a patient reacting to events at the scene), mind-altering substances, psychiatric disorders, and psychological crises such as a panic attack.

hemodialysis ▶ process of mechanically filtering the blood to remove wastes and excess fluid.

REMEMBER

Hemodialysis replaces the function of the kidneys. Therefore, if the patient misses an appointment for dialysis, they will develop the signs and symptoms of renal failure. Patients miss their appointments for many reasons, including their financial situation, lack of transportation, inconvenience, and noncompliance with medical advice.

SCENE SAFETY

Responding to a behavioral emergency can present many risks for responders. Although most patients want your care, patients experiencing a behavioral emergency may not want any part of it. Consider the need for law enforcement early in the call, and do not allow yourself to be cornered in a room with the patient.

behavioral emergency ▶ situation in which an individual exhibits abnormal behavior that is unacceptable or intolerable to the patient, family, or community.

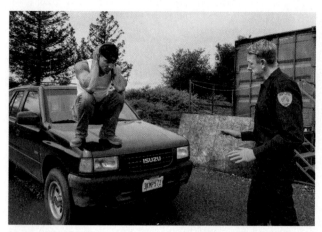

Figure 16.13 Be aware of your body language and avoid sudden movements so the person you are approaching doesn't perceive you as a threat.

Assessment and Emergency Care

Follow these guidelines when performing an assessment of a patient who may be experiencing a behavioral emergency:

- Approach with caution and observe for signs of agitation or violence. Do not approach the patient if it is not safe.
- Identify yourself and let the patient know you are there to help.
- Inform the patient of what you are doing at all times.
- Ask questions in a calm reassuring voice.
- Without being judgmental, allow the patient to tell what happened.
- Show that you are listening by rephrasing or repeating part of what is said.
- Be aware of your posture and body language to ensure that they aren't perceived as threatening by the patient (Figure 16.13).
- Assess the patient's mental status: appearance, activity, speech, and their orientation to person (self), place, time, and event.
- Always consider the need for law enforcement.

Emergency care of a patient with a behavioral emergency includes the following:

- Perform a scene size-up and consider the need for law enforcement.
- Perform a primary assessment by observing the patient from a safe distance.
- Acknowledge that the patient seems to be upset and restate that you are there to help.
- Inform the patient of what you are doing and ask questions in a calm reassuring voice.
- Encourage the patient to state what is troubling them.
- Answer questions honestly and do not threaten, challenge, or argue.
- Involve trusted family members or friends if appropriate.
- Do not make quick moves.
- Do not "play along" with hallucinations or auditory disturbances.
- Leave yourself a way out. Never let a potentially violent patient come between you and your exit.

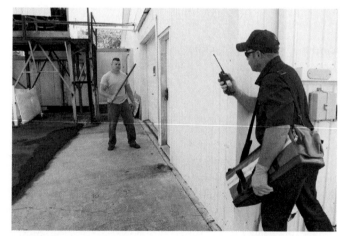

Figure 16.14 Law enforcement officers may be needed to approach and control a patient experiencing a behavioral emergency.

Assessing the Potential for Violence

Sometimes patients experience conditions that cause them to become violent and uncooperative. As an Emergency Medical Responder, your priority is to prevent the patient from harming themselves or others while also protecting yourself. Consider contacting law enforcement (Figure 16.14), and note the following:

- *Scene size-up.* Use caution when approaching a scene. Observe the patient and the surroundings for any indication that they might be a danger to themselves or others. Remain alert to the presence of weapons or anything that may be used as a weapon.
- *History.* Often, patients who have exhibited violent behavior in the past will repeat it. Take such a history into consideration during your assessment.

- *Posture.* How is the patient standing? Are they in an offensive stance? What does their body language tell you? Are you positioned at a safe distance?
- *Verbal communication.* Often, verbal abuse is a precursor to violence. If a patient continues to use foul language or raise their voice, consider such action as a possible warning sign of violent behavior.
- *Physical activity.* Patients may begin to pace or wave their arms in the air. Such movements may escalate into more violent behavior.

CREW RESOURCE MANAGEMENT

It is especially important to plan out your approach when dealing with a potentially aggressive or violent patient. Discuss the approach as a team and make sure that everyone knows the plan. Every team member must be focused on the safety of the team and the patient.

Restraining Patients

In some cases, patients experiencing a behavioral emergency might become violent to the point that it is necessary to physically restrain them. An attempt should be made to verbally deescalate the patient's anger or aggression. When this fails, physical restraint may be necessary to protect the patient, yourself, and others. Do not attempt to restrain a patient except as a last resort. Make certain you have enough resources and a coordinated plan of action (Figure 16.15). Review the section on patient restraint in Chapter 6.

In situations when restraint may be necessary, follow your local guidelines for contacting police and consulting medical direction. Remember, the emotional disturbance may be caused by an underlying medical condition that the patient is not aware of, does not understand, or cannot control. Because of this, emotionally disturbed patients may threaten those who are trying to help and will often resist emergency care.

You cannot provide emergency care to a patient without proper consent, so you must have a reasonable belief that the patient will harm themselves or others and would want help if they were able to understand and consent to it. Contact medical direction for guidance before attempting to provide care to a patient without consent. Local protocols may require you to contact law enforcement for assistance.

Do not approach a violent or potentially violent patient alone. While waiting for assistance, try the following:

- Sit or stand passively, but remain alert to the patient's actions and responses.
- Talk and listen to the patient to divert their focus and keep them from harming themselves and/or others.
- Restate what the person is saying. This will demonstrate that you understand what they are saying.
- Redirect the conversation to keep it focused on the situation at hand.
- Show empathy by reassuring the patient that you understand.

REMEMBER

Physically restraining a patient should be the last resort, done only when it is clear that without doing so the patient may harm themselves or others. Your personal safety is paramount. If you are injured, the number of patients on the scene is doubled. Use the least amount of restraint necessary to protect the patient and others from harm, and do not be afraid to stop and evaluate whether your actions are making things better or worse. There is nothing wrong with a tactical retreat and reassessment of the situation. It may be better to wait until additional help arrives.

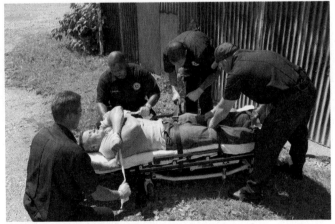

Figure 16.15 Use restraint only as a last resort.

- Avoid any action that may alarm the patient and cause them to react violently.
- Wait for law enforcement assistance to arrive if restraining the patient is necessary. Allow police officers to take the lead in restraining the patient.
- Use reasonable force only to defend yourself against attack.

FIRST ON SCENE WRAP-UP

The small room is bustling with firefighters, ambulance personnel, campus security, and two city police officers. Jordan describes the patient's seizure and points out the medical identification necklace to the firefighters who are the first on scene.

"Who took care of this patient before we got here?" the paramedic from the ambulance asks, as he starts an IV on the unconscious girl. A firefighter points at Jordan.

"You did a great job." The paramedic administers a clear fluid into the IV line with a huge syringe. "You kept her airway open by rolling her onto her side. I couldn't have asked you to do better than that."

Jordan smiles and feels his face get hot at the compliment. Before he walks from the room, he is happy to see the girl blink her eyes several times and begin to ask questions of the paramedic.

Summary

- Medical emergencies involve conditions that threaten an individual's life and are caused by some type of illness. One of the most common signs of a medical emergency is an altered mental status.
- Several conditions can cause a patient to experience an altered mental status, including seizures, strokes, diabetic emergencies, poisonings, breathing problems, and cardiac events.
- Altered mental status can present with a wide range of signs and symptoms, from confusion and dizziness to seizures and syncope (fainting).
- The assessment and care of a patient with an altered mental status is dependent on the Emergency Medical Responder observing the patient's environment and asking questions.
- A sudden loss of consciousness and convulsions characterize a generalized seizure. It is most important to protect the patient from harm while waiting for the seizure to subside.
- Following a generalized seizure, the patient will be unresponsive. This is referred to as the postictal stage. Monitor the patient's airway and breathing status closely until they regain consciousness.
- A stroke occurs when there is a disruption in blood flow to the brain caused by a clot or a ruptured artery.
- Common signs and symptoms of a stroke include headache, altered mental status, confusion, difficulty speaking or swallowing, and paresis (weakness) on one side of the body.
- Patients experiencing a stroke should be closely monitored since they may experience airway compromise, breathing difficulty, or cardiac arrest.
- Diabetes is a disease in which the pancreas does not produce adequate amounts of the hormone insulin or when the body cannot properly process insulin.
- Diabetic emergencies can present with altered mental status, abnormal breathing, abdominal pain, seizures, extreme thirst, fruity breath odor, and unresponsiveness.
- When it cannot be determined if the diabetic emergency is caused by hypoglycemia or hyperglycemia, the care for both should be the same. Administer oral glucose (if appropriate), provide oxygen, and activate the EMS system. Monitor the patient's ABCs and place them in the recovery position if they are unresponsive.
- Common signs and symptoms of poisoning are altered mental status, vomiting, abdominal pain, sweating, abnormal pulse and/or breathing, unresponsiveness, pain when breathing or swallowing, dilated or constricted pupils, and weakness or dizziness.

- Patients experiencing carbon monoxide poisoning may present with headaches, dizziness, confusion, seizures, and even coma. If a patient presents with these signs and symptoms and has been near any source of combustion (e.g., fire, automobile, heater), you should suspect carbon monoxide poisoning.
- Caring for the patient who has been exposed to poison or has overdosed is primarily about protecting the airway, administering oxygen (if allowed), activating the EMS system, and monitoring the ABCs.
- A local, regional, or national poison control center should be contacted (per local protocols) once you have established that the patient has been exposed to poison and you have determined the type of poison encountered.
- A patient who already has a serious infection can develop sepsis, which is the body's extreme overreaction to the infection. Untreated sepsis can cause tissue damage, organ failure, and death. Fever, chills, confusion, unresponsiveness, rapid breathing, rapid heart rate, and low blood pressure are common signs and symptoms.
- Patients with sepsis must be treated at a hospital as soon as possible. The Emergency Medical Responder should ensure activation of the EMS system, provide oxygen (if allowed), and monitor the patient's ABCs closely while awaiting advanced care.
- Anaphylaxis is a life-threatening allergic reaction characterized by altered mental status, difficulty breathing, and swelling of the tongue and throat. Support the ABCs and assist with the prescribed epinephrine autoinjector (per local protocols), if available.
- Renal failure occurs when the kidneys no longer function normally. Hemodialysis is the process of mechanically filtering the blood and removing excess water, salts, and waste products.
- Any time a patient is behaving in a manner that is dangerous to themselves, family members, or the community, they are said to be having a behavioral emergency. Emergency Medical Responders should first and foremost ensure their own safety and the safety of others near the patient. Then they should clearly and calmly identify themselves to the patient, ensure that the EMS system is activated, and engage the patient with clear, effective communication until assistance arrives.

Take Action

20 Questions

Assessing a medical patient, especially one with an altered mental status, can be very challenging—especially if the patient is unable to provide any clues to what may be going on. Getting some practice with asking questions when you do not know what is wrong will be very helpful when you encounter your first real patient.

Pair up with another student in your class. One of you will serve as the patient and use this chapter as a reference while the other one asks the questions. Select a specific medical problem such as stroke or hyperglycemia. As the individual playing the role of the patient, take a few minutes to refer to the specific signs and symptoms of the complaint. When you are ready, instruct the individual acting as the Emergency Medical Responder to begin asking questions. The goal is to identify the specific medical condition in as few questions as possible.

First on Scene Patient Handoff

I arrived on scene to find an approximately 18-year-old female convulsing on the floor. According to bystanders, the patient had been convulsing for approximately 1 minute prior to my arrival. The convulsions lasted for approximately 90 seconds. Once the convulsions stopped, I checked her airway. Patient was breathing, but her airway was obstructed as evidenced by a snoring sound. I tilted her head back, the snoring disappeared, and her breathing returned to normal depth and tidal volume. I placed the patient into the recovery position and monitored her airway until EMS arrived.

First on Scene Run Review

Recall the events of the First on Scene scenario in this chapter, and answer the following questions related to the call. Rationales are offered in the Answer Key at the back of the book.

1. When an individual has had a seizure, what information should you get from them and/or bystanders?
2. What should your treatment be after an individual has had a seizure?
3. If an individual has no prior history of seizures, do they still need to go to the hospital?

Quick Quiz

To check your understanding of the chapter, answer the following questions. Then compare your answers to those in the Answer Key at the back of the book.

1. A patient with altered mental status is best defined as one who:
   a. is unresponsive.
   b. cannot speak properly.
   c. can only speak in short sentences.
   d. is not alert or responsive to surroundings.

2. A patient who is unresponsive and having generalized muscle contractions is likely experiencing a(n):
   a. stroke.
   b. seizure.
   c. heart attack.
   d. overdose.

3. Which of the following is the best example of appropriate care for a patient experiencing a seizure?
   a. Protect the patient from injury, and place them in the recovery position following the seizure.
   b. Place them in a semi-sitting position, and apply oxygen following the seizure.
   c. Place them in a prone position, and provide oxygen by nasal cannula.
   d. Restrain them and assist ventilations with a bag-mask device.

4. A patient who presents with abnormal behavior that is unacceptable to family members and others is said to be experiencing a(n):
   a. psychosis.
   b. mental breakdown.
   c. altered behavioral state.
   d. behavioral emergency.

5. One of the best techniques for dealing with a patient experiencing a behavioral emergency is to:

a. not let the patient know what you are doing.

b. not believe a thing the patient says.

c. speak in a calm and reassuring voice.

d. acknowledge the "voices" he is hearing.

6. Which of the following is NOT evaluated as part of the Cincinnati Prehospital Stroke Scale?

a. Abnormal speech

b. Equal circulation

c. Facial droop

d. Arm drift

7. Your patient is presenting with an altered mental status and a history of diabetes. He states that he took his normal dose of insulin this morning but has not had anything to eat. His most likely problem is:

a. hyperglycemia.

b. anaphylaxis.

c. hypoglycemia.

d. a stroke.

8. You are caring for a 16-year-old who intentionally ingested a large number of Tylenol pills approximately 30 minutes ago. You should:

a. place them in the recovery position.

b. contact poison control.

c. obtain baseline vital signs.

d. give large amounts of water.

9. You have responded to a call for a possible overdose, and you should first:

a. assess the patient's vital signs.

b. determine if the patient is experiencing any hallucinations.

c. gently restrain the patient.

d. ensure that the scene is safe.

10. What is the most commonly abused substance in the United States?

a. Arsenic

b. Amyl nitrate

c. Butane

d. Alcohol

11. Compared to hyperglycemia, hypoglycemia has an onset that is:

a. usually slower.

b. the same.

c. usually faster.

d. unpredictable.

12. Which medical emergency is caused by a disruption of blood flow to the brain?

a. Diabetic coma

b. Overdose

c. Stroke

d. Heart attack

13. Once a seizure has ended, the patient is said to be in the _____ state.

a. REM

b. postictal

c. syncopal

d. recovery

14. The process of sending a patient's blood through a machine-based filter is referred to as:

a. photodialysis.

b. syncope.

c. hemodialysis.

d. autodialysis.

15. All of the following are common causes of renal failure EXCEPT:

a. heart attack.

b. injury to the kidneys.

c. diabetes.

d. kidney infection.

16. You are caring for a 10-year-old boy who was stung by a bee. He is crying in pain and is able to breathe and swallow without difficulty. You observe a small red dot where the sting occurred, and he states that it itches. This is most likely a:

a. severe reaction requiring immediate transport.

b. mild reaction requiring immediate transport.

c. mild reaction that may not require transport.

d. severe reaction that does not require transport.

17. A severe allergic reaction causes the air passages:

a. and blood vessels to dilate.

b. and blood vessels to constrict.

c. to dilate and the blood vessels to constrict.

d. to constrict and the blood vessels to dilate.

Endnotes

1. GBD 2015 Disease and Injury Incidence and Prevalence Collaborators. "Global, regional, and national incidence, prevalence, and years lived with disability for 310 diseases and injuries, 1990–2015: a systematic analysis for the Global Burden of Disease Study 2015," *The Lancet*, Vol.388, No.10053 (October 2016): 1545–1602.

2. David Markenson, J.D. Ferguson, L. Chameides, P. Cassan, K.L. Chung, J. Epstein, L. Gonzales, R.A. Herrington, J.L. Pellegrino, N. Ratcliff, and A. Singer, "2015 American Heart Association and American Red Cross Guidelines for First Aid," *Circulation*, Vol.132 (2015): S269–S311, originally published October 14, 2015.

3. Ibid.

4. Wanda L. Rivera-Bou, Jose G. Cabanas, and Salvador E. Villanueva, "Thrombolytic Therapy for Acute Ischemic Stroke," Medscape website, updated August 4, 2021. Accessed September 22, 2022 at https://emedicine.medscape.com/article/811234-overview#aw2aab6b8

5. Gummin, D.D., Mowry, J.B., Spyker, D.A., Brooks, D.E., Fraser, M.O., Banner W. 2016 annual report of the American Association of Poison Control Centers' National Poison Data System (NPDS): 34th annual report. *Clinical Toxicology*, Vol.55, No.10 (2016): 1072–1254. doi:10.1080/15563650.2017.1388-87.

6. https://www.cdc.gov/opioids/basics/fentanyl.html

7. Mahapatra, S., Heffner, A.C. Septic Shock. [Updated 2022 Jun 21]. In: StatPearls [Internet]. Treasure Island (FL): StatPearls Publishing; 2022 Jan–. Available from: https://www.ncbi.nlm.nih.gov/books/NBK430939/

8. McLendon, K., Sternard, B.T. Anaphylaxis. [Updated 2022 May 15]. In: StatPearls [Internet]. Treasure Island (FL): StatPearls Publishing; 2022 Jan–. Available from: https://www.ncbi.nlm.nih.gov/books/NBK482124/

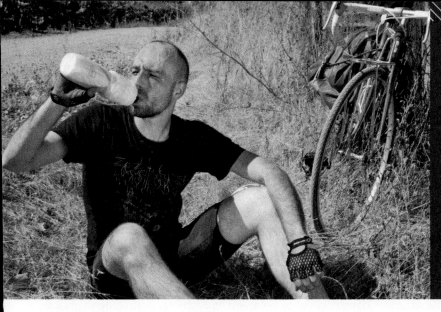

17

Caring for Environmental Emergencies

Education Standards

Trauma—Environmental Emergencies

Medicine—Toxicology

Competencies

Recognizes and manages life threats based on assessment findings for an acutely injured patient while awaiting additional emergency medical response.

Recognizes and manages life threats based on assessment findings of a patient with a medical emergency while awaiting additional emergency response.

LEARNING OBJECTIVES

Upon successful completion of this chapter, the student should be able to:

Cognitive

1. Define the chapter key terms.

2. Explain the five ways the body loses excess heat.

3. Describe the signs and symptoms of a patient experiencing hyperthermia.

4. Explain the appropriate assessment and care for a patient experiencing a heat-related emergency.

5. Differentiate the signs and symptoms of heat exhaustion and heat stroke.

6. Describe the signs and symptoms of a cold-related emergency.

7. Explain the appropriate assessment and care for a patient experiencing a cold-related emergency.

8. Describe the signs and symptoms of emergencies related to bites and stings.

9. Explain the appropriate assessment and care for a patient experiencing an emergency related to a bite or sting.

10. Describe common factors leading to submersion injuries.

11. Describe common methods used for water rescue.

12. Explain the hazards related to water rescue.

13. Describe the signs and symptoms of a submersion injury.

14. Explain the appropriate care for a patient with a submersion injury.

15. Describe the safety concerns involving ice-related incidents.

Psychomotor

16. Demonstrate the ability to appropriately assess and care for a patient experiencing a heat-related emergency.

17. Demonstrate the ability to appropriately assess and care for a patient experiencing a cold-related emergency.

18. Demonstrate the ability to appropriately assess and care for a patient experiencing an emergency secondary to a bite or sting.

Affective

19. Value the importance of proper training when attempting to conduct a water rescue.

KEY TERMS

conduction (*p. 344*)
convection (*p. 344*)
core temperature (*p. 344*)
drowning (*p. 355*)
evaporation (*p. 344*)
frostbite (*p. 350*)

heat cramps (*p. 346*)
heat exhaustion (*p. 347*)
heat stroke (*p. 347*)
hyperthermia (*p. 344*)
hypothermia (*p. 344*)
radiation (*p. 344*)

This chapter provides an overview of some of the more common environmental emergencies that you are likely to encounter as an Emergency Medical Responder. They include a wide variety of conditions such as exposure to extremes of heat and cold as well as bites, stings, and water- and cold-related emergencies.

FIRST ON SCENE

It's got to be coming from over here, Anastasia thinks as she makes her way toward the sound of sobbing coming from somewhere on the hiking path. The day is unseasonably hot, and Anastasia squints in the bright sunlight that beats against the dirt and rock, creating thick, watery-looking waves against the ground.

"Help, somebody!" a raspy voice calls out to Anastasia's immediate left. In the shade she sees a man lying semiconscious on the ground. The woman who called out is standing over him. She says her name is Aubree.

"What's wrong?" Anastasia asks, although she is pretty sure she knows what is happening. She unzips her backpack and pulls out three water bottles.

"We were hiking, and Juan said he was getting too hot. He started breathing funny and saying funny things. He was sweating so much. We both are."

Anastasia looks down and feels Juan's forehead, which is burning hot. She checks his neck and core area, but he doesn't seem to be sweating anymore. "I think he might be overheating." As soon as the words leave her mouth, Juan's body starts to convulse.

"What's going on?" shrieks his companion.

Temperature and the Body

LO2 Explain the five ways the body loses excess heat.

core temperature ► temperature of the internal organs of the body's core.

The human body operates within a very narrow temperature range. It is capable of efficiently regulating its own **core temperature** in many different environmental conditions. The body's "core" refers to the torso. (The head, arms, and legs are not part of the body's core.) Core temperature is the temperature of the internal organs of the body's core. Normal core temperature is 98.6 degrees Fahrenheit or 37 degrees Celsius. The process of temperature regulation is controlled by the brain through various mechanisms.

hypothermia ► abnormally low core body temperature.

hyperthermia ► abnormally high core body temperature.

Hypothermia (abnormally low core body temperature) and **hyperthermia** (abnormally high core body temperature) may result when the body is not able to regulate temperature effectively. Hypothermia can occur when the body loses heat faster than it can produce it. Hyperthermia can occur when the body gains heat faster than it can shed it.

The body loses heat through several means (Figure 17.1):

radiation ► loss of body heat to the atmosphere.

- *Radiation.* With **radiation**, heat is emitted into the environment. This is the heat lost to the surrounding air as it dissipates off the body.

conduction ► loss of body heat through direct contact with an object or the ground.

- *Conduction.* Body heat is transferred to an object with which the body is in contact. For instance, **conduction** occurs when our bodies are in contact with a cool or cold surface such as the ground or when immersed in water.

convection ► loss of body heat when air that is close to the skin moves away, taking body heat with it.

- *Convection.* With **convection**, body heat is lost to surrounding air that becomes warmer, rises, and is replaced with cooler air. This occurs when cool air is warmed by our bodies then moves away. That air is replaced by cooler air, and the cycle continues. Wind can greatly increase the effects of convection.

evaporation ► loss of body heat when perspiration (sweat) on the skin turns from liquid to vapor.

- *Evaporation.* Body heat is lost when perspiration is changed from liquid to vapor. Sweating is a normal body function used to shed heat. As the sweat on our skin evaporates, it carries heat with it. Wind can also greatly increase the effectiveness of **evaporation**.
- *Respiration.* Heat leaves the body with each breath. Our breath contains a considerable amount of moisture. As we breathe out, we expel warm, moist air from within our bodies.

You must consider each of these methods of heat loss when you are caring for patients with emergencies related to heat or cold.

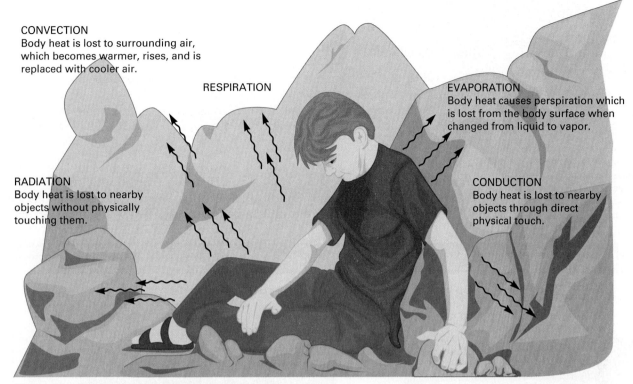

CONVECTION
Body heat is lost to surrounding air, which becomes warmer, rises, and is replaced with cooler air.

RESPIRATION

EVAPORATION
Body heat causes perspiration which is lost from the body surface when changed from liquid to vapor.

RADIATION
Body heat is lost to nearby objects without physically touching them.

CONDUCTION
Body heat is lost to nearby objects through direct physical touch.

Figure 17.1 Mechanisms of heat loss for the body.

Heat Emergencies

LO3 Describe the signs and symptoms of a patient experiencing hyperthermia.

LO4 Explain the appropriate assessment and care for a patient experiencing a heat-related emergency.

The human body can maintain an ideal core temperature in a wide variety of environments. Overexposure to hot and humid environments can cause the body to retain too much heat, which can create an abnormally high core temperature known as *hyperthermia*. Hyperthermia can result from a patient being outside on a hot, humid afternoon for a prolonged period of time or from exposure to excessive heat while indoors, such as in a sauna or steam room. Left unchecked, hyperthermia can lead to a serious emergency and even death.

The body generates heat in many ways. Some of the body's normal processes, such as digestion, metabolism, and movement, generate heat. The entire process is controlled by a structure deep in the brain called the hypothalamus. The hypothalamus serves as the body's thermostat, carefully regulating all processes to maintain a normal core body temperature.

Sweating, also called perspiring, is one of the body's most effective ways of ridding itself of excess heat. On a really hot day, you can lose up to 1 liter (about 2 pints) of sweat per hour. Sweat evaporates from the skin, taking with it excess heat. The effects of heat loss through evaporation are greatly reduced when the humidity is high, as the ambient air is already saturated with moisture.

A dry-heat (low-humidity) environment can often fool individuals, causing them to continue to work in or be exposed to heat far beyond the point that can be managed by their bodies. For this reason, exposure to a hot, dry environment can be worse than exposure to a hot, humid environment.

Signs and symptoms of hyperthermia include:

- Feeling hot
- Feeling dizzy/lightheaded
- Flushed skin
- Skin that is hot to the touch
- Nausea/vomiting

> **SCENE SAFETY**
>
> Extreme environments (overly hot or cold) can be dangerous for emergency personnel as well as for patients. When working in these environments, make sure that you have appropriate clothing, sufficient food and water, and consider carrying some type of two-way satellite communication device.

- Muscle cramps
- Headache
- Sweating
- Altered mental status

When dealing with problems created by exposure to excessive heat, you must perform a thorough history and physical exam. A previous history of medical problems may make the effects of heat exposure much worse. The very young, very old, and those with chronic illnesses are especially susceptible to the effects of heat and cold exposure (Key Skill 17.1).

heat cramps ▶ muscle cramps, most often in the lower limbs and abdomen, associated with the loss of fluids and electrolytes while active in a hot environment.

Heat Cramps

Heat cramps are painful muscle spasms following strenuous activity in a hot environment. Heat cramps are usually caused by an electrolyte imbalance and typically occur in the muscles of the calves, arms, abdomen, and/or back. In most cases, the patient will be fully alert and

---

KEY SKILL 17.1

Providing Care for Heat-Related Emergencies

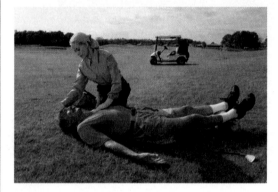
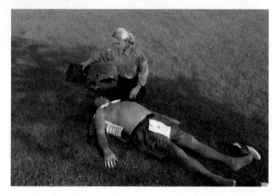

Heat Cramps/Exhaustion

Heat cramps may be an early sign of a true heat emergency.

Signs and Symptoms

- Mild to severe muscle cramps in legs, arms, abdomen, or back
- Exhaustion, dizziness, and light-headedness
- Weak pulse and rapid, shallow breathing
- Heavy perspiration
- Normal to pale skin color

Emergency Care

- Move the patient to a nearby cool place. Loosen or remove their clothing. Spray them with a water mist if possible and fan them. Be careful not to overcool the patient. If the patient begins to shiver, stop the cooling.
- Give water or a balanced electrolyte drink to the responsive patient.
- Position the responsive patient on their back with legs elevated; position the unresponsive patient on their left side, monitoring airway and breathing.
- Help ease cramps by applying moist towels over cramped muscles or, if the patient has no history of circulatory problems, apply gentle but firm pressure on the cramped muscle.

Heat Stroke

Heat stroke is a life-threatening emergency.

Signs and Symptoms

- Altered mental status
- Skin that is hot to the touch
- Rapid, shallow breathing
- Strong, rapid pulse
- Weakness, dizziness
- Little to no perspiration
- Seizures or muscular twitching

Emergency Care

- Rapidly cool the patient in any manner. Move the patient to a cool place and remove their clothing. Keep the skin wet by applying wet towels. Fan the patient.
- Wrap cold packs or ice bags, if available, and place them at the neck, armpits, wrists, and groin. Fan the patient to increase heat loss.
- Find a tub or other container and immerse patient in cool water, if practical.
- Monitor the patient's vital signs continuously.
- Provide oxygen at 15 liters per minute via nonrebreather mask if permitted by local protocols.

sweaty, with normal to warm skin temperature. Emergency care includes having the patient stop any activity and moving them to a cool location. It may be appropriate to allow the patient to drink an electrolyte-carbohydrate mixture, such as juice, milk, or a commercial electrolyte drink.[1] The symptoms of heat cramps are usually short lived and are relieved with rest and hydration.

Heat Exhaustion

| LO5 | Differentiate the signs and symptoms of heat exhaustion and heat stroke.

Heat exhaustion is most often caused by a combination of exercise-induced heat, typically in a hot environment, and fluid and electrolyte loss through excessive sweating. The body's normal cooling mechanisms become overworked and begin to fail. Heat exhaustion occurs when the body is barely able to shed as much heat as it is generating. The problem will typically resolve on its own once the patient stops the activity, is moved to a cool place, and allowed to replace fluids.

The signs and symptoms of heat exhaustion may last several minutes to a couple of hours. These include:

- Mild to moderate perspiration
- Warm to cool skin temperature
- Normal to pale skin color
- Weakness, exhaustion, or dizziness
- Nausea and vomiting
- Muscle cramps (usually in legs and abdomen)
- Rapid, weak pulse
- Normal to rapid breathing

Emergency care for heat exhaustion includes:

1. Take appropriate BSI precautions.
2. Perform a primary assessment and ensure an open airway and adequate breathing.
3. Move the patient to a cool area and allow them to lie down.
4. Loosen or remove excess clothing.
5. Cool the patient with a cool water spray and by fanning.[2] Be careful not to overcool the patient.
6. Consider giving the patient small sips of water, juice, or a sports drink if allowed by local protocol.

heat exhaustion ▶ the body's response to overheating, which may include heavy sweating, rapid pulse, and moist, pale skin that may feel normal or cool to the touch.

REMEMBER

Severe cases of hyperthermia may result in permanent damage to organs with the highest metabolic activity, such as the brain and heart. As the body's temperature climbs, every organ attempts to compensate by eliminating more waste, which generates acids that build up in the system. Eventually, the organs fail to compensate and permanent damage, or even death, occurs.

Heat Stroke

| LO5 | Differentiate the signs and symptoms of heat exhaustion and heat stroke.

Heat stroke is the most severe form of hyperthermia. It is a life-threatening emergency in which the body temperature may increase to 105°F (40.5°C) or higher. Prolonged exposure to heat raises the core temperature to dangerous levels. This condition is thought of as "hot and dry" because the body's sweating mechanism has stopped working, and skin feels warm or hot to the touch. Heatstroke can lead to organ failure, brain damage, and death.

The patient with heat stroke will almost always present with an altered mental status. They may be sleepy or confused and unsure of what is happening. If you are caring for a patient with a heat emergency and they have an altered mental status, assume it is heat stroke and provide care accordingly.

heat stroke ▶ life-threatening emergency that results from prolonged exposure to heat.

Signs and symptoms of heat stroke include:

- Altered mental status
- Skin that is hot to the touch
- Skin that is slightly moist to dry
- Rapid, shallow breathing
- Rapid pulse
- Weakness, exhaustion, or dizziness
- Nausea and vomiting
- Convulsions

Emergency care for heat stroke includes:

1. Take appropriate BSI precautions.
2. Perform a primary assessment and ensure an open airway and adequate breathing.
3. Move the patient to a cool area and lie them down.
4. Remove excess clothing and cool the patient by dowsing with cool water or immersing them in cool water. Be careful not to overcool the patient.
5. Place wrapped cold packs or ice bags, if available, under the armpits, on the groin, and on each side of the neck. Follow your local protocols.
6. Place the patient in the recovery position.
7. Provide oxygen per local protocols.
8. Monitor vital signs.

Cold Emergencies

Several emergencies can occur when the body is exposed to a cold environment and is unable to generate heat faster than it sheds it. Hypothermia is an abnormally low core temperature. Localized injury (frostbite) most commonly causes damage to toes, fingers, ears, and the nose.

Hypothermia

LO6 Describe the signs and symptoms of a cold-related emergency.

LO7 Explain the appropriate assessment and care for a patient experiencing a cold-related emergency.

When the body loses heat faster than it can be generated and the core temperature drops below normal, a condition known as *hypothermia* may result. Hypothermia may be mild, moderate, or severe (Table 17.1). When in a cold environment, the body will attempt to generate its own heat by increasing muscle activity (shivering). If the core temperature continues to drop, shivering will eventually stop, and the body can no longer warm itself (Figure 17.2).

As with heat exposure, young children and older adults are more susceptible to the effects of cold exposure. Patients with medical conditions that affect perfusion, such as diabetes, are also at greater risk for the effects of hypothermia. The risk for hypothermia is sometimes obvious, such as an individual who is working or playing outside in a cold environment. In other cases, the risk for hypothermia can be much less obvious. For example, older adults on tight budgets who keep their thermostat at a lower-than-comfortable setting during the winter are often affected by prolonged exposure to a moderately cold environment.

The temperature of the extremities is not a reliable indicator of the patient's core temperature. As the body cools, the extremities will cool first, but the body will preserve heat in the core (abdomen and thorax) for the proper functioning of vital organs.

The patient experiencing hypothermia will often present with a cool or cold abdominal skin temperature. Place the back of your ungloved hand against the patient's abdomen to assess general temperature. In healthy adults, the abdomen should be warm.

Signs and symptoms of hypothermia include:

- Altered mental status
- Shivering (early sign)

REMEMBER

Children are particularly vulnerable to temperature extremes. One reason for this is that their internal thermostat is not fully developed and cannot compensate as well as that of an adult. Young children are often not able to make changes to adjust for temperature extremes. They may not be able to get themselves out of a hot car or add layers of clothing when the environment is cold.

SCENE SAFETY

Do not give the patient with an altered mental status anything by mouth. They may not be able to manage their own airway and may vomit or aspirate.

REMEMBER

The environmental temperature does not have to be below freezing for hypothermia to occur.

TABLE 17.1　Stages of Hypothermia

SEVERITY	PRESENTATION	APPROXIMATE CORE TEMPERATURE
Mild	Alert but may be confused, shivering	Below 95°F (35°C)
Moderate	Drowsy, decreased level of responsiveness, not shivering	86°–93.2°F (30°–34°C)
Severe	Unresponsive, vital signs may be undetectable	Below 86°F (<30°C)

Source: National Ski Patrol, Edward C. McNamara, David H. Johe, and Deborah A. Endly, Outdoor Emergency Care, 5th Edition (Upper Saddle River, NJ: Pearson Publishing, 2012), p. 825. *(Reprinted and electronically reproduced by permission of Pearson Education, Inc., New York, NY)*

- Absence of shivering (late sign)
- Cool or cold skin temperature
- Abnormal pulse (initially rapid, then slow)
- Lack of coordination
- Muscle rigidity
- Impaired judgment
- Complaints of joint/muscle stiffness

A patient experiencing the signs of hypothermia should be transported to an appropriate hospital as soon as is practical. Just because they are removed from the cold environment does not mean the risk of further heat loss is over.

REMEMBER

Do not allow the patient with hypothermia to drink alcohol or caffeine. These substances may affect blood vessels and worsen the patient's condition.

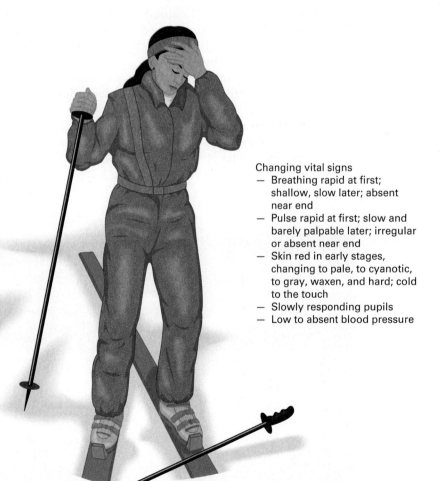

Decreasing mental status
— Amnesia, memory lapses, and incoherence
— Mood changes
— Impaired judgment
— Reduced ability to communicate
— Dizziness
— Vague, slow, slurred, or thick speech
— Drowsiness progressing even to unresponsiveness

Decreasing motor and sensory function
— Stiffness, rigidity
— Lack of coordination
— Exhaustion
— Shivering at first, little or no shivering later
— Loss of sensation

Changing vital signs
— Breathing rapid at first; shallow, slow later; absent near end
— Pulse rapid at first; slow and barely palpable later; irregular or absent near end
— Skin red in early stages, changing to pale, to cyanotic, to gray, waxen, and hard; cold to the touch
— Slowly responding pupils
— Low to absent blood pressure

Figure 17.2 Signs and symptoms of hypothermia.

Emergency care for hypothermia includes:

1. Take appropriate BSI precautions.
2. Perform a primary assessment and ensure an open airway and adequate breathing.
3. Remove the patient from the cold environment, but do not allow the patient to walk or exert themselves in any way.
4. Protect the patient from further heat loss.
5. Remove any wet clothing and place a blanket over and under the patient. Remember to handle the patient gently.
6. Administer oxygen per local protocols.
7. Monitor vital signs.
8. Do not give the patient anything to eat or drink.

REMEMBER

If you are providing care to a patient with frostbite in a remote area where there is a long delay in getting the patient to a hospital, you should avoid rewarming if there is any chance the injury might refreeze.

If the patient with hypothermia is far from a medical facility where they can receive definitive care, begin active rewarming.[3] Active rewarming includes placing the patient in or near a heat source and placing wrapped heat packs around the core, armpits, neck, and groin. Do not delay transport to provide active rewarming.

Some cases of hypothermia are extreme. The patient might be unresponsive, with skin that is cold to the touch and show no vital signs. You cannot assume this patient is dead. Assess the pulse for at least 30 to 45 seconds. If there is no pulse, begin CPR at once and arrange for immediate transport. In most instances, a patient will not be pronounced dead until the hospital team can bring the patient's core temperature to within a normal range.

Localized Cold Injury

frostbite ▶ localized cold injury in which the skin and underlying tissues are frozen.

Frostbite, also called a localized cold injury, is the freezing of the skin and underlying tissues (Figure 17.3). It is caused by a significant exposure to cold temperature (below 32°F or 0°C). It mainly occurs in the extremities and most commonly affects the fingers, toes, ears, face, and nose.

A typical situation in which a localized cold injury can occur is when a person spends a prolonged period of time outdoors during the winter without proper clothing/gear to protect the extremities (e.g., scarf, gloves, boots). The core of the body remains warm, but the exposed extremities are susceptible to the impact of cold and wind. Most patients will describe a localized cold injury as starting with a cold sensation in the extremities that leads to pain, followed by numbness. This is the classic progression of symptoms (Key Skill 17.2).

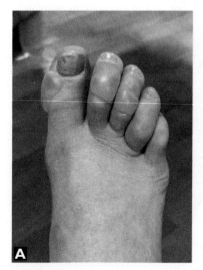
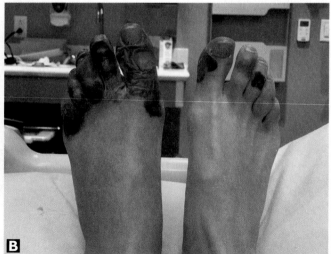

Figure 17.3 (A) Moderate frostbite of the toes. (B) Severe frostbite of the toes.
(Chris Le Baudour)

Providing Care for Localized Cold Injury

CONDITION	SKIN SURFACE	TISSUE UNDER SKIN	SKIN COLOR
Early, superficial	Soft	Soft	Pale
Late, deep	Hard	Initially soft, progressing to hard	Pale and waxy, progressing to blotchy, then to yellow-gray to blue-gray

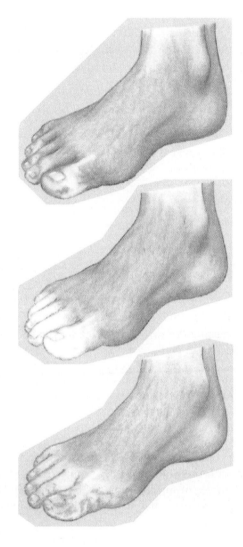

Early, Superficial

Slow onset with numbing of affected area. Have the patient rewarm the area with their own body heat. Tingling and burning sensations are common during rewarming.

Late, Deep

Tissues below the surface will initially have their normal bounce. Protect the entire limb. Handle gently. Keep the patient at rest and provide external warmth to the injury site. Untreated, this will progress to where the tissue below the surface will feel hard. Provide the same care you would for early superficial cold injury. Immediate EMS transport is recommended.

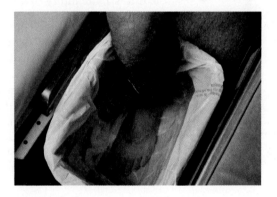

Rewarming

Do not attempt to rewarm the body part if there is any chance it could refreeze, or if you are close to a medical facility.[4] Begin rewarming of the body part only if transport is delayed. In cases of late or deep frostbite and if medical direction allows, rewarm the affected part by immersing it in warm water (100°F to 105°F [37.7°C to 40°C]) for 20 to 30 minutes. After rewarming, gently dry the body part and pad between fingers or toes. Dress the affected area, cover and elevate the limb, and keep the patient warm. Chemical warmers should not be placed directly on frostbitten tissue as they may cause burns.

Signs and symptoms of a localized cold injury include:

Early Signs

- Numbness and tingling in the exposed area
- Slow or absent capillary refill
- Skin is cool to the touch but remains soft.
- If thawed, tingling and pain are present.

Late Signs

- White, waxy skin in patients with light skin. Inspect the palms of the hands and soles of the feet in patients with darker skin.
- The skin of the affected area is firm to hard.
- Swelling may be present.
- Blisters may be present.
- If thawed, skin may appear flushed with areas of purple and blanching.

Emergency care for a localized cold injury is as follows:

1. Take appropriate BSI precautions.
2. Perform a primary assessment and ensure an open airway and adequate breathing.
3. Remove the patient from the cold environment and protect them from further cold exposure.
4. Remove any wet or constrictive clothing.
5. If it is an early injury:

   - Manually stabilize the extremity or affected part.
   - Remove any jewelry.
   - Cover the affected part with a loose-fitting gauze wrap.
   - Do not rub or massage the affected parts as this may cause damage if ice crystals have already formed in the tissues.
   - Do not re-expose the injured area to cold.

6. If it is a late injury (deep frostbite):

   - Attempt to remove jewelry from the injured area.
   - Cover the injured area with dry, sterile dressings. Place dressings between fingers and toes prior to covering.
   - Do not break blisters.
   - Do not rub or massage the injured part.
   - Consider rewarming. (Some jurisdictions allow rewarming. Check local protocols.)
   - If legs are affected, do not allow the patient to walk.

It is not recommended to attempt to rewarm a frozen part if there is any chance that the part could refreeze before reaching advanced care.

Bites and Stings

Regardless of where we live, our environment contains many insects and animals that can pose a threat when people come in contact with them. Insect stings, spider bites, stings from marine life, and snakebites can all be sources of injected poisons (see Chapter 16). Some of those poisons cause very serious emergencies, while others cause only a minor local reaction such as redness and swelling.

FIRST ON SCENE (*continued*)

Aubree asks Anastasia, "My friend . . . did he just have some kind of seizure?"

"I think he might have heat stroke," Anastasia replies.

Anastasia gently rolls Juan into the recovery position. She checks his breathing and pulse, both of which are rapid. Juan has already removed most of his clothing, which is piled nearby. Anastasia opens two of the water bottles and soaks his remaining clothes and skin.

"I think I'm going to throw up," Aubree says as she sits down by Juan. Her coloring is becoming pale as she begins fanning herself.

"Here," Anastasia says, passing her the last water bottle. "Slowly drink some of this and stay right there in the shade. Help will be here soon, and you can help me keep Juan cool."

Assessment of a patient who has sustained a bite or sting involves an inspection of the injury site. Look for redness and swelling directly at the site (Figure 17.4). The patient will usually report pain, itching, or discomfort at the site. Localized redness and swelling are quite normal. If you observe the area of redness expanding, producing hives or increased swelling—especially involving the face, neck, and chest—the patient may be developing a severe reaction called anaphylaxis. Be alert for other indications of anaphylaxis, such as difficulty breathing and/or swallowing, hoarseness, wheezing, and altered mental status.

It will be important to determine if the patient has a history of past allergic reactions to similar bites or stings. In the event the patient has a history of severe allergic reactions, remain alert for anaphylaxis.

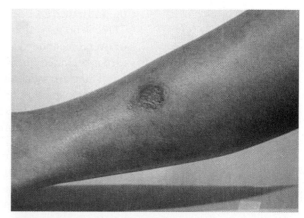

Figure 17.4 The local reaction caused by a brown recluse spider several days after the initial bite.
(Centers for Disease Control and Prevention)

Assessment of and Emergency Care for Bites and Stings

LO8 Describe the signs and symptoms of emergencies related to bites and stings.

LO9 Explain the appropriate assessment and care for a patient experiencing an emergency related to a bite or sting.

Gather information from the patient, bystanders, and the scene. Attempt to identify the insect or animal that may have caused the bite or sting.

Signs and symptoms of a reaction to a bite or sting include:

- Noticeable puncture marks on the skin
- Pain at or around the injury site
- Redness and itching at the injury site
- Weakness, dizziness
- Difficulty breathing
- Headache
- Nausea
- Altered mental status

Emergency care for a localized reaction is as follows:

1. Take appropriate BSI precautions.
2. Perform a scene size-up, and ensure that the scene is safe for both you and the patient.
3. Perform a primary assessment, and ensure an open airway and adequate breathing.
4. Scrape away noticeable bee or wasp stingers and venom sacs. Do not attempt to pinch or pull out stingers because it may force more venom into the wound. A plastic credit card works well as a scraper (Figure 17.5).
5. Flush the area with water.
6. After flushing, place a clean dressing over the site.
7. Closely monitor the patient for difficulty swallowing or difficulty breathing that may indicate a severe reaction.

Anaphylaxis

Recall from Chapter 16 that *anaphylaxis* (also called anaphylactic shock), occurs when people come into contact with substances to which they are severely allergic. The immune system considers

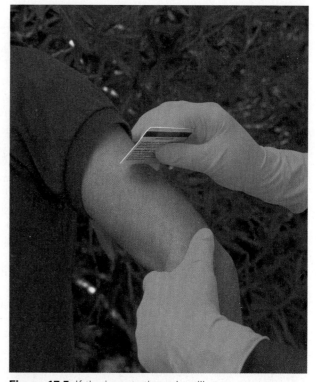

Figure 17.5 If the insect stinger is still present, remove it by scraping it away with the edge of a credit card or similar object.

the substance an invader and reacts to counteract it. This is a life-threatening emergency. There is no way of knowing if a patient will remain stable, grow worse slowly or rapidly, or overcome the reaction on their own. For some, death is a certain outcome unless special care is provided quickly.

There are many different causes of anaphylaxis, such as insect bites and stings, foods (e.g., nuts, spices, shellfish), inhaled substances (including dust and pollen), and certain chemicals and medications.

Signs and symptoms of anaphylaxis include:

- Moderate to severe difficulty breathing
- Swelling of the throat
- Difficulty swallowing
- Altered mental status
- Burning, itching, or breaking out of the skin (hives or other type of rash)
- Pulse that is rapid, very weak, or not detected
- Lips that turn blue (cyanosis)
- Swelling of the face and tongue
- Restlessness

As you perform your primary assessment, ask if the patient is allergic to anything and, if so, whether they have been in contact with that substance. Remember to always look for medical identification jewelry, which may indicate history of an allergy.

To provide emergency care to patients with anaphylaxis, follow the same procedures used for shock (see Chapters 16 and 19). In some jurisdictions, EMTs and Emergency Medical Responders are authorized to carry and administer an epinephrine autoinjector for anaphylaxis. Check local protocols, and always call for medical direction before assisting a patient with medications.

You may have to support a patient's breathing by providing ventilations with a bag-mask device. If available, use supplemental oxygen as well. Rapid transport to an appropriate hospital is essential.

Snake Bites

Between 7,000 and 8,000 people in the United States are bitten by venomous snakes each year, with fewer than 20 deaths being reported annually.[5] (In the United States, more people die each year from bee and wasp stings than from snake bites.) Signs and symptoms of a snake bite may take several hours to develop. Death from a snake bite is usually not a rapidly occurring event unless anaphylactic shock also occurs. Keeping the patient calm will be an important part of your care. There is usually time to activate the EMS system and to provide care for the patient.

Until proven otherwise, consider all snake bites to be from venomous snakes. The patient or bystanders may indicate that the snake was not venomous. They could be mistaken. If you see the live snake, do not approach it to determine its species. Only if safe to do so from a distance, note its size and coloration and snap a picture if you can do so safely.

Signs and symptoms of snake bite may include:

- Noticeable bite to the skin. This may appear as nothing more than a discoloration.
- Pain and swelling in the area of the bite. This may be slow to develop, taking 30 minutes to several hours.
- Rapid pulse and labored breathing
- Weakness
- Vision problems
- Nausea and vomiting

Emergency care for a snake bite includes:

1. Take appropriate BSI precautions.
2. Perform a scene size-up and ensure that the scene is safe for you and the patient.
3. Perform a primary assessment and ensure an open airway and adequate breathing.
4. Clean the site with soap and water.
5. Remove any rings, bracelets, and other constricting items from the affected extremity.
6. If the bite is on an arm or leg, apply a pressure bandage around the entire length of the limb.
7. Provide supplemental oxygen, if available.
8. Provide care for shock and monitor vital signs.

For snake bites on an arm or leg, it is recommended that you place a pressure bandage around the entire length of the extremity. An ACE™ or similar-style bandage is ideal for this application. This is a safe and effective way to slow the movement of the venom by slowing flow through the lymph system.[6]

The bandage should be comfortably tight and allow for a finger to be slipped under it. Do not place it so tight that it cuts off arterial flow. Monitor for a distal pulse at the wrist or ankle, depending on the extremity involved. Check with your instructor regarding your local protocols.

Do not place an ice bag or cold pack on the bite unless you are directed to do so by a health care provider or the poison control center.

Jellyfish Stings

Jellyfish are often found floating in shallow water near beaches. While most jellyfish do not pose serious danger, they can inflict a very painful sting when they come in contact with human skin. A nematocyst—a threadlike stinger—is released when the tentacles of the jellyfish come in contact with the skin. When the stinger penetrates the skin, a small amount of venom is released, causing moderate to severe pain, swelling, and redness.

Emergency care for jellyfish stings involves preventing additional venom discharge and providing pain relief. The application of vinegar (4% to 6% acetic acid solution) over the injury site will deactivate the needles that remain in the skin. This should be applied as soon as possible and for at least 30 seconds.[7]

For pain relief, the injury site should be rinsed with hot water (113°F/45°C or as hot as can be tolerated by the patient). If hot water is not readily available, wrapped hot packs may be used. Use caution when applying hot packs to avoid burning the skin.

Water-Related Incidents

LO10 Describe common factors leading to submersion injuries.

LO11 Describe common methods used for water rescue.

LO12 Explain the hazards related to water rescue.

When people think of water-related incidents, they tend to think only of **drowning**. However, a variety of injuries occur on, in, and near the water. Boating, water skiing, and diving into shallow water can all produce airway obstructions, fractures, bleeding, and soft-tissue injuries. Other types of incidents, such as falls from bridges and watercraft collisions, also occur. In these cases, the patients sustain injuries associated with the underlying mechanism of injury plus the effects of the water hazard (drowning, hypothermia, delayed care due to complicated rescue, and so on).

Sometimes, the mishap or drowning may have been caused by a medical emergency such as a seizure or heart attack that took place while the patient was in the water or on a boat. Knowing how the incident occurred may give you clues to detecting the medical emergency. As with all aspects of care, consider the mechanism of injury or nature of illness

drowning ▶ respiratory impairment due to submersion in water or other liquid.

and perform a thorough patient assessment. They may be critical in deciding the procedures to follow when caring for a patient.

Take special care to look for the following when your patient is the victim of a water-related emergency:

- Airway obstruction may be from water, foreign matter in the airway, or a swollen airway. Spasms along the airway are common in cases of submersion in water.
- Cardiac arrest is usually related to respiratory arrest.
- Injuries to the head and neck are to be expected in boating, water-skiing, and diving incidents.
- While performing a patient assessment, be alert for suspected fractures, soft-tissue injuries, and internal bleeding.
- The water does not have to be very cold, and the length of stay in the water does not have to be very long for hypothermia to occur.

CREW RESOURCE MANAGEMENT

Water rescue operations are inherently dangerous. Each and every team member must remain vigilant for changing and unsafe conditions. Everyone must be comfortable with speaking up and letting the others know if they see anything unsafe.

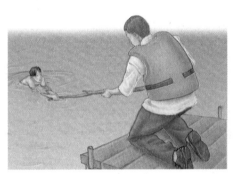

Reach

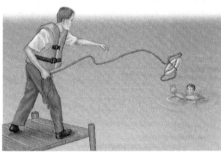

Throw

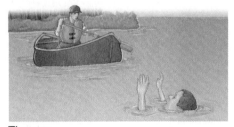

Then go

Figure 17.6 Reach for the victim. Throw an object to them. If necessary, go to the individual if you are trained to do so.

Reaching the Victim

The U.S. Coast Guard, the American Red Cross, and the YMCA are three organizations that offer water safety and rescue courses. Unless you are trained in water rescue, do not go into the water to save someone.

If the patient is close to shore or poolside, attempt to reach and pull the patient from the water. If unable to reach the individual with your hand, attempt to use a branch, fishing pole, stick, an oar, or other such object. A towel, shirt, or an article of your own clothing may work as well. In cases where there is no object nearby or conditions are such that you may only have one opportunity to grab the individual (such as strong currents), lie down flat on your stomach, and extend your arm or leg (not recommended for the nonswimmer). In all cases, make sure your position is secure and you will not be pulled into the water. This is critical if you are extending an arm or leg to the individual.

If the individual is alert but too far away to be pulled from the water, then you must carefully throw an object that will float. A personal flotation device (PFD), life jacket, or ring buoy (life preserver) is ideal, but those objects may not be at the scene. If that is the case, then the best course of action is to throw anything that will float. Objects you might use include inflated automobile tubes, foam cushions, plastic jugs, logs, boards, plastic picnic containers, surfboards, pieces of wood, large balls, and plastic toys. Two empty, capped plastic milk jugs can keep an adult afloat for hours. It is best to tie rope to the objects so they can be retrieved if they do not land near the patient. You may have to add some water to lightweight plastic jugs so you can throw them the required distance.

Once you are sure that the individual has a flotation device or floating object to hold on to, try to find a way to tow the patient to shore. Throw the patient a line or another flotation device attached to a line. Make sure your own position is a safe one. If you must reduce the distance for throwing the line, and if conditions are safe and you are a strong swimmer, wade no deeper than your waist.

Again, in water-rescue situations (Figure 17.6), begin by trying to pull the patient from the water. If this cannot be done, throw objects that will float and try to tow the patient from the water. Unless you are a good swimmer and trained in water rescue and lifesaving, do not swim to the patient. Even so, wear a personal flotation device.

Care for the Patient

The appropriate steps for patient care depend on whether any type of neck or spine injury has occurred.

Patient with No Neck or Spine Injuries   Once the patient is safely removed from the water, you should:

1. Manage the patient, being mindful of possible neck or back injuries.
2. Perform a primary assessment and ensure an open airway and adequate breathing.
3. If needed, provide mouth-to-mask resuscitation as quickly as possible. Check for airway obstruction.
4. Provide CPR if needed. Make certain that someone has activated the EMS system.
5. If there is breathing and a pulse, perform a secondary assessment. But first cover the patient to conserve body heat. Uncover only those areas of the body involved in assessment. If hypothermia is suspected, remove excess wet clothing to minimize heat loss.
6. If the patient can be moved, take them to a warm place. Do not allow the patient to walk. Handle the patient gently at all times.
7. Provide care for shock.

You may encounter water in the airway of a patient who was pulled from the water. Turn the patient on their side and allow excess water to exit the mouth. Watch the patient's chest rise and fall with each breath.

Often a patient with water in the airway will also have water in the stomach. Current American Heart Association and American Red Cross guidelines indicate that you should not attempt to relieve water or air from the patient's stomach (unless immediate suctioning is available) due to the risk of forcing material from the stomach into the patient's airway, even to the point of entering the lungs. When gastric distention occurs, reposition the airway and continue with resuscitation, making sure each breath is just enough to make the chest begin to rise.

Humans have a reaction in cold water that is similar to other mammals. This reaction is called the *mammalian diving reflex*. When the face of an individual or other mammal is submerged in cold water, the mammalian diving reflex slows down the body's metabolism, which results in a decrease in oxygen consumption. At the same time, the reflex causes a redistribution of blood to more vital organs—the brain, heart, and lungs. The diving reflex is more pronounced in infants and children, and they may fare better in cold-water drowning than adults. Start CPR on all drowning victims as soon as they are pulled from the water. Cases have been reported in which cold-water drowning victims, especially children, were revived and fully recovered after being in the water for longer than 30 minutes.

> **REMEMBER**
>
> Drowning victims who are resuscitated are very likely to vomit. Rescuers should have suction ready and be prepared to clear the airway when this occurs. Consider placing the patient in the recovery position to help manage the airway.

Patient with Neck or Spine Injuries   Injuries to the neck and spinal column can occur during many water-related incidents. The Emergency Medical Responder is not expected to know how to use long spine boards and other floating, rigid devices for rescue situations.

When a patient with possible neck and spine injuries is responsive and you are in shallow, warm water, stabilize the patient until the EMS system responds with personnel trained to remove the patient from the water. Keep the patient floating in a face-up position while you support the back and stabilize the head and neck.

If a patient is unresponsive, neck and spine injuries may not be easily detected. In such a situation, assume the patient has these injuries and provide care accordingly. Also assume neck and spine injuries whenever you find a patient with head injuries.

If you arrive at the scene and find the unresponsive patient has already been removed from the water, have someone activate the EMS system and begin your primary assessment. Provide life support care as needed, using the jaw-thrust maneuver rather than the head-tilt/chin-lift maneuver. After breathing and circulation are ensured, and bleeding is cared for, perform a secondary assessment, providing care as needed. Keep the patient warm and provide care for shock.

If the patient is still in the water, do not attempt a rescue unless you are a good swimmer, are trained to do so, and have others at hand who can help you. Providing care for the patient with a possible spinal injury who is still in the water requires you to do the following (Key Skill 17.3):

Water Rescue

Stand at side of patient. . .grasp right arm with your right hand and left arm with your left hand . . .float arms gently above head.

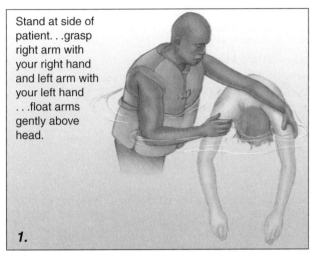

1.

Clasp patient's arms firmly against head. . .this braces the neck and keeps the head in line with the body. . . move forward so patient glides to surface.

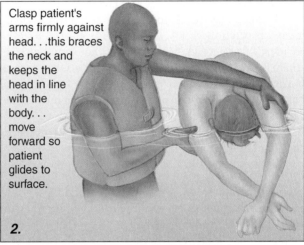

2.

Rotate patient toward you by pushing near arm down and pulling far arm toward you until patient is face up. . .keep patient's head firmly braced between his or her arms.

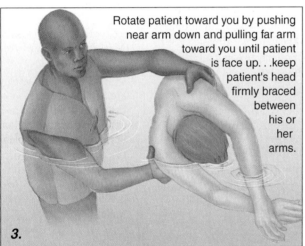

3.

Maintain pressure on patient's arms to brace head. . . move slowly to keep patient afloat. . . if necessary, begin rescue breathing in water. . . wait for help to remove patient from water.

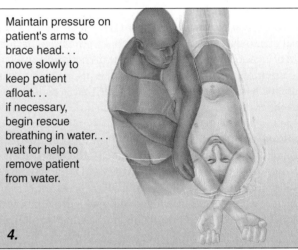

4.

If necessary to keep patient afloat, use one arm to brace head and arms and the other to support hips. . .

if necessary, begin rescue breathing in water. . .wait for assistance to remove patient from water.

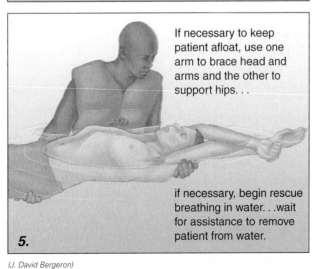

5.

Only specially trained personnel, using a backboard and cervical collar, should remove a patient with a neck or spinal injury from the water.

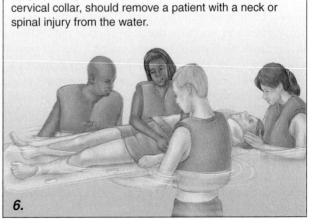

6.

(J. David Bergeron)

358

1. Turn the patient face up in the water. This should be done while you are in the water and wearing a personal flotation device. To turn the patient, you should:
   a. Position yourself at the patient's side. Grasp the patient's arms midway between the elbow and shoulder, and gently float them above the patient's head.
   b. Clasp the patient's arms firmly against their head to brace the neck and keep the head in line. Move forward in the water to bring the patient's body to the surface and in line.
   c. Rotate the patient by pushing down on the near arm and pulling the far arm toward you, making sure you brace the patient's head firmly with their arms. Do not lift the patient.
   d. Once the patient is face up, maintain pressure on the patient's arms to brace the head.
   e. In shallow water, you can hold the patient's arms with one hand and support the hips with the other.
   f. In deeper water, continue to move toward shallow water where you can stand or be supported by someone else.
2. If necessary, begin your primary assessment while the patient is still in the water.
3. If needed, provide rescue breathing as soon as possible. Use the jaw-thrust maneuver to protect the patient's neck and spine. CPR will not be effective while the patient is in the water.
4. If someone is there to help you, have that individual support the patient along the midline of the back while you provide support to the patient's head and neck. Float the patient to shore and continue to provide back and neck support. Wait for trained rescue personnel equipped with a backboard and cervical collar to remove the patient from the water.
5. Once the patient is out of the water, attempts at resuscitation can begin. In some cases, depending on the boat's stability and water conditions, you may be able to provide effective CPR in the boat until other rescuers arrive.
6. If the patient is breathing, cover them to conserve body heat and perform a secondary assessment, caring for any injuries you may find.

> **REMEMBER**
>
> Attempt to remove the patient from the water yourself *only* if trained rescue personnel will not arrive soon and the patient has problems with the ABCs. You must make every effort to maintain in-line stabilization of the patient's body.

Submersion Injuries

LO13 | Describe the signs and symptoms of a submersion injury.

LO14 | Explain the appropriate care for a patient with a submersion injury.

Other injuries related to submersion in water are commonly associated with the sport of scuba diving. Incidents involving scuba diving can produce a variety of injuries resulting in a temporary loss of consciousness or even death. A common problem seen in submersion incidents related to scuba diving is decompression sickness.

Decompression sickness occurs when small bubbles of nitrogen gas form in the blood and tissues when a diver ascends from a depth too quickly. These bubbles can form an air embolism that will obstruct blood flow wherever they form and cause severe pain and even death. The most common symptom of decompression sickness is a dull, aching pain in the joints. This is referred to as "the bends." The onset of the bends is usually slow for scuba divers, taking up to 48 hours to appear.

Decompression sickness can be mild to severe. In severe cases, an air embolism can develop in the bloodstream. The onset is rapid, with signs of personality changes and distorted senses sometimes giving the impression of drunkenness. The patient may have convulsions and rapidly become unresponsive. You should suspect possible air embolism when the patient has any of the following signs or symptoms:

- Personality changes
- Distorted senses; blurred vision is most common
- Chest pain
- Numbness and tingling sensations in the arms and/or legs
- General weakness or weakness of one or more limbs
- Frothy blood in the mouth or nose
- Convulsions

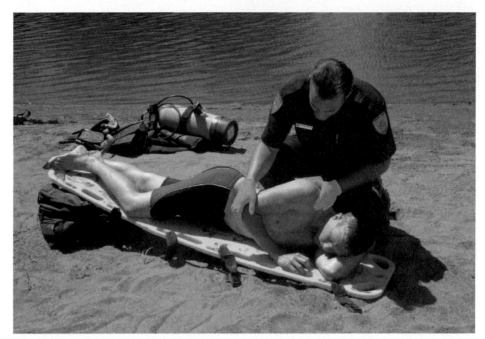

Figure 17.7 For scuba accidents, position the patient head down.

Signs and symptoms of decompression sickness include:

- Fatigue
- Pain in the muscles and joints
- Numbness or paralysis
- Choking, coughing, and/or labored breathing
- Chest pain
- Collapse and unresponsiveness
- Blotches on the skin (mottling); sometimes these rashes keep changing appearance

If you think a patient has decompression sickness due to a dive, be certain that the dispatcher is aware of the problem. Dispatch may wish to direct the transport team to take the patient to a special facility (hyperbaric trauma center) where a patient is exposed to oxygen under greatly increased pressure conditions. This procedure is done in a sealed hyperbaric chamber.

While waiting for the transport team, provide care for shock and constantly monitor the patient. Positioning of the patient is critical to avoid gas bubbles in the blood reaching the brain. Place the patient on their left side. The patient may also be placed in a slight head-down position (Figure 17.7). Provide oxygen per local protocols.

Ice-Related Incidents

LO15 Describe the safety concerns involving ice-related incidents.

Ice rescues require special training. Unless you are trained specifically to work on ice, do not attempt a rescue. You may walk on an undetected thin spot, fall through the ice, and quickly drown. All rescuers who are on or at the edge of the ice must wear personal flotation devices.

The major problem faced in ice rescue is reaching the victim. Never walk out to the individual or attempt to enter the water through a hole in the ice to find the victim. Never attempt an ice rescue by yourself unless you have some basic equipment, such as a personal flotation device and a ladder, and you are specifically trained in single-rescuer techniques. Never go onto ice that is rapidly breaking up. Your best course of action will be to work with others from a safe ice surface or the shore (Figure 17.8).

> **REMEMBER**
>
> Scuba divers increase the risk of decompression sickness if they fly within 12 hours following a dive.

> **REMEMBER**
>
> When a diver ascends too quickly while holding their breath or does not allow air to freely escape their lungs, a condition called *barotrauma* occurs. As the diver ascends, the air in the lungs, the sinuses, and middle ear expands. If the pressure is not gradually released, the expanding air can result in trauma to the lungs, such as a pneumothorax. Expanding air in the sinuses and middle ear produces severe pain.

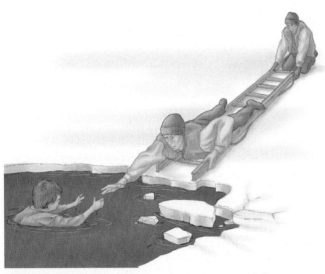

Figure 17.8 A safe ice rescue requires teamwork from specially trained responders.

First, throw a line to the individual or reach out with a stick or a pole. If the victim is not holding on to the ice but trying to keep afloat in open water, throw anything that will float. Do not try to go onto the ice to rescue the individual. Call for help immediately. Ice rescues require special training, protective clothing, and rescue equipment.

If you have had specialized training, have the necessary equipment and personnel, and must go onto the ice to get the patient, it is strongly recommended that you work with other trained help. Pushing a long ladder out onto the ice and crawling along the ladder is a very effective method of safe rescue, providing someone is holding the ladder from a safe position. If enough people are on hand, a human chain can be formed to reach the patient; however, these rescuers should be trained and wearing PFDs.

Expect to find injuries with any patient who has fallen through the ice. Hypothermia is often a problem and should always be considered. Do not attempt to actively rewarm a severely hypothermic patient. Simply get them to a warm environment, remove wet clothing, and cover them with blankets to minimize further heat loss.

FIRST ON SCENE WRAP-UP

A team of trained responders arrives quickly with response bags and a basket stretcher to help get Juan down the side of the rocky path.

"We've kept him cool and we've been fanning him," Anastasia reports as the team surrounds Juan, swiftly attaching an oxygen mask and pulling out ice packs. "He had what looked like a seizure about 8 minutes ago, and he's been in and out of consciousness since then, only muttering every once in a while."

"You two look pretty exhausted yourself," one of the responders says as he pulls out a few water bottles, glistening with condensation. "Drink these and soak your shirts as we make our way down with your friend, okay? There are air-conditioned vehicles at the bottom of the trail waiting for you."

Aubree takes a drink of water then grabs Anastasia's hand and shakes it. "Thank you so much for helping us. I don't know what would have happened if you weren't out here to find us."

"No problem," Anastasia says, sounding relieved. "Just make sure to check the weather forecast next time and bring enough water."

Summary

- The body loses heat in five ways: radiation, conduction, convection, evaporation, and respiration.
- A hot and humid environment may cause the body to generate too much heat, which can create an abnormally high body temperature, known as hyperthermia.
- Early signs and symptoms of hyperthermia include cramps; excessive sweating; rapid, weak pulse; and weakness.
- Heat cramps are sudden and sometimes severe muscle cramps, most often occurring in the legs, arms, abdomen, and/or back.
- Heat exhaustion results from prolonged exposure to heat, which creates moist, pale skin that may feel normal or cool to the touch.
- Heat stroke is the most severe form of hyperthermia and a life-threatening emergency. It results from prolonged exposure to heat and causes hot, dry, or moist skin; altered mental status; and rapid breathing.
- Emergency care for heat emergencies includes removing patients from the hot environment, cooling them with water, and fanning them.
- In cold environments, body heat may be lost faster than it can be generated. Rapid heat loss creates a state of low body temperature known as hypothermia.
- Patients who have hypothermia will have cool skin temperature, shivering, decreased mental status, stiff or rigid posture, and poor judgment. The environmental temperature does not have to be below freezing for hypothermia to occur.
- Frostbite is characterized by the freezing or near freezing of skin and underlying tissues. Patients with frostbite will experience a feeling of cold followed by pain and, finally, numbness or tingling.
- Emergency care for frostbite includes removing the patient from the cold environment, removing any wet clothes, keeping the patient calm and warm, and stabilizing any cold extremity.
- When providing care for injected venoms other than from a snake bite, care for shock, scrape away stingers and venom sacs, and place an ice bag or cold pack over the area.
- For snakebite, keep the patient calm and lying down, clean the site, apply a pressure bandage on the affected extremity, and provide care for shock.
- Anaphylaxis, also called anaphylactic shock, is a life-threatening emergency. It is a severe and potentially life-threatening allergic reaction to bee stings, insect bites, and substances such as chemicals, foods, dust, pollen, and drugs.
- Signs of anaphylaxis include burning or itching skin; hives; difficulty breathing; rapid, weak pulse; swelling of the face and tongue; cyanosis; and altered mental status.
- Care for anaphylaxis is the same as for shock. Transport the patient to a hospital as soon as possible, and care for the patient according to local protocols. Ask the patient about allergies, and look for medical identification jewelry.
- Emergency care for a drowning victim includes safely removing them from the water, performing a primary assessment, and providing rescue breaths or CPR as indicated.
- Always be mindful of the potential for neck or back injuries with a drowning victim.
- Many submersion injuries are related to scuba diving and result when an individual ascends too quickly.
- Decompression sickness, also known as "the bends," results when tiny gas bubbles form in the blood and tissues, causing pain.
- In severe cases, these bubbles can form an air embolism that can obstruct blood flow, resulting in death.

Take Action

Stings and Bites

Environments vary widely. In addition to differences in climate and weather, there are differences in the types of creatures that can pose a threat to humans who inhabit the area. In this activity, identify at least two creatures that are common to your environment or region. They should be animals that sting or bite and are venomous to some degree.

1. Identify two creatures commonly found in your area. They can be animals, spiders, or insects that are venomous.
2. Using the internet, research the common signs and symptoms that result when someone is bitten or stung.
3. Research the most appropriate care that the Emergency Medical Responder can provide for a bite/sting. How does the care differ once the patient is in the hands of more advanced medical personnel?
4. Share your results with your fellow classmates to learn about other creatures that you did not research. When you chose the same creatures, did your results match what your fellow classmates found?

First on Scene Patient Handoff

Juan is a 34-year-old male who had been hiking for several hours when he started to become confused. According to his companion, she helped him to the shade where they have been for the past hour. On our arrival Juan was A&O × 2 and his vitals were respirations 30 rapid and shallow, heart rate 140 and weak. Skin was pink, hot, and dry. We immediately began cooling him with water and fanning him. It appears he had a mild generalized seizure lasting about 45 seconds and has been mostly unresponsive since. We have been monitoring his breathing and pulse the whole time.

First on Scene Run Review

Recall the events of the First on Scene scenario in this chapter, and answer the following questions related to the call. Rationales are offered in the Answer Key at the back of the book.

1. What are the signs that might indicate a patient has heat stroke?
2. Does Anastasia need to ask permission before helping Juan? Why or why not?
3. What information does Anastasia need to give to the EMS responders?

Quick Quiz

To check your understanding of the chapter, answer the following questions. Then compare your answers to those in the Answer Key at the back of the book.

1. Which of the following is an example of heat loss through conduction?

   a. A 66-year-old man found lying on the frozen ground without a coat
   b. A 14-year-old boy wearing thin clothing in cold temperatures
   c. A 23-year-old woman outside in cool, windy weather
   d. An older woman standing in the cool night air

2. More serious heat-related injuries should be suspected when the patient presents with:

   a. dizziness
   b. muscle cramps
   c. hot, dry skin
   d. weakness

3. Your patient is a 38-year-old man who has been working outside in a hot, humid climate. He is alert and oriented, complaining of feeling weak and dizzy. His skin is warm and moist, and he has respirations of 16, a heart rate of 104, and a blood pressure of 110/70. You should FIRST:

   a. place cold packs at the groin, armpits, and neck
   b. move the patient to a cool area in the shade
   c. offer the patient some salt tablets
   d. wet the skin, turn the air conditioning on high, and vigorously fan the patient

4. A patient who is experiencing an abnormally low core body temperature is said to be:

   a. hyperthermic
   b. cyanotic
   c. hypothermic
   d. hyperglycemic

5. An injury characterized by the freezing or near freezing of skin and underlying tissues is known as:

   a. frostbite
   b. frostnip
   c. hypothermia
   d. cold bite

6. All of the following are appropriate steps in the management of a patient with hypothermia, EXCEPT:

   a. removing the patient from the cold environment
   b. protecting them from further heat loss
   c. providing warm liquids to drink
   d. monitoring their vital signs

7. A patient who presents with warm, moist skin; weakness; and nausea is likely experiencing:

   a. heat exhaustion
   b. heat stroke
   c. heat cramps
   d. mild heat stroke

8. Your patient was hiking and was bitten on the ankle by a rattlesnake. When caring for this patient, you should:

   a. keep the foot lower than the level of the patient's heart
   b. apply a pressure bandage around the entire extremity
   c. apply a tourniquet above the bite
   d. apply ice to the area of the bite

9. It is late winter, and you respond to an alley to find what appears to be a homeless man lying on the ground. Your patient presents with confusion, shivering, and muscle stiffness. Based on his presentation, this man's likely problem is:

   a. a localized cold injury
   b. frostnip
   c. frostbite
   d. hypothermia

10. You are caring for an individual who fell from a rope swing, landed in the water, and is now unresponsive. She has a large laceration on the top of her head. You should:

    a. suspect spine injury

    b. begin CPR in the water

    c. drag her by one arm to shore

    d. wait for EMS before beginning care

11. You are caring for a marathon runner who has collapsed at the finish line. She presents with altered mental status, hot and dry skin, and is vomiting. You should first:

    a. ensure she has a clear airway

    b. soak her down with cool water

    c. obtain baseline vital signs

    d. request an ALS ambulance

12. It is a cold winter night, and you are caring for an older man who was found several hours after wandering away from a memory care facility. He is alert to verbal stimuli, cold to the touch, and has a weak carotid pulse. You are 60 minutes from the nearest hospital. You should first:

    a. take spinal precautions

    b. begin CPR

    c. administer supplemental oxygen

    d. begin active rewarming

13. You are caring for a young woman who was playing with her dog outdoors when she began having difficulty breathing. She states that she felt a sharp sting on the back of her neck and now is dizzy and is having trouble swallowing. You suspect she may be experiencing:

    a. an anaphylactic reaction

    b. a mild allergic reaction

    c. an acute asthma attack

    d. extreme hay fever

14. You are caring for a man who states that he was bitten on the foot by a snake about 20 minutes ago. He is alert and oriented but is complaining of severe pain at the site. You should FIRST:

    a. wash the wound with soap and water

    b. wrap the limb with a pressure bandage

    c. place a splint on the leg and foot

    d. wait for EMS before beginning care

15. You are caring for a young girl whose mother states that she came in contact with what looked like a jellyfish while playing in the water. The child is in extreme pain and crying. To help relieve some of the pain, you should:

    a. wrap the wound with a dry sterile dressing

    b. rinse the wound with hot water

    c. flush the wound with salt water

    d. wrap the wound with wet dressings

Endnotes

1. David Markenson, J.D. Ferguson, L. Chameides, P. Cassan, K.L. Chung, J. Epstein, L. Gonzales, R.A. Herrington, J.L. Pellegrino, N. Ratcliff, and A. Singer, "2015 American Heart Association and American Red Cross Guidelines for First Aid," *Circulation*, Vol. 132 (2015): S269–S311, originally published October 14, 2015.
2. Ibid.
3. Ibid.
4. E.M. Singletary, N.P. Charlton, J.L. Epstein, J.D. Ferguson, J.L. Jensen, A.I. MacPherson, J.L. Pellegrino, W.R. Smith, J.M. Swain, L.F. Lojero-Wheatley, and D.A. Zideman "Part 15: First Aid: 2015 American Heart Association and American Red Cross Guidelines Update for First Aid," *Circulation*, Vol. 132, Suppl. 2 (2015): S574–S589.
5. Ibid.
6. Ibid.
7. Ibid.

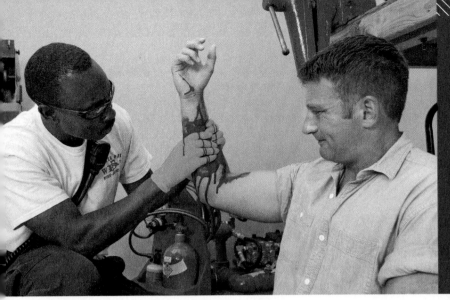

18

Caring for Soft Tissue Injuries and Bleeding

LEARNING OBJECTIVES

Upon successful completion of this chapter, the student should be able to:

Cognitive

1. Define the chapter key terms.

2. Explain the importance of using appropriate body substance isolation (BSI) precautions when caring for a patient with external bleeding.

3. Differentiate the characteristics of arterial, venous, and capillary bleeding.

4. Explain the proper care for a patient with active external bleeding.

5. Explain the purpose of a dressing.

6. Explain the purpose of a bandage.

7. Describe the signs and symptoms of internal bleeding.

8. Explain the proper care of a patient with suspected internal bleeding.

9. Identify the characteristics of multisystem trauma.

10. Describe common types of external soft tissue injuries.

11. Explain proper emergency care for a patient with an open wound.

12. Explain the proper care for a patient with an impaled object.

13. Explain the proper care for an amputation injury.

14. Explain the proper care for an injury to the eye.

15. Explain the proper care for a nosebleed.

16. Differentiate superficial, partial-thickness, and full-thickness burns.

17. Explain the process for determining percentage of body surface area affected by a burn.

18. Explain the proper care for patients with superficial, partial-thickness, and full-thickness burns.

19. Differentiate the care for thermal, chemical, and electrical burns.

Psychomotor

20. Demonstrate the proper care for a patient with suspected internal bleeding.

21. Demonstrate the proper techniques for controlling external bleeding.

22. Demonstrate the proper care of a patient with an impaled object.

23. Demonstrate the proper care of a patient with an amputation injury.

24. Demonstrate the proper care of a patient with a burn injury.

Affective

25. Value the importance of proper body substance isolation (BSI) precautions when caring for patients with soft tissue injuries.

Education Standards

Trauma—Bleeding, Soft Tissue Trauma

Competencies

Recognize and manage life threats based on assessment findings for an acutely injured patient while awaiting additional emergency medical response.

In the United States, unintentional injuries are the fourth leading cause of death for all ages.[1] As an Emergency Medical Responder, you will provide emergency care to patients with injuries that range from minor to life threatening. Early assessment and intervention is crucial to the proper care of these patients. You must be familiar with the care of soft tissue injuries and how to help keep bleeding under control. This chapter introduces many of the most common types of soft tissue injuries, including burns, as well as how to manage the bleeding that is so often associated with these injuries.

As with patients who experience a heart attack or stroke, the effects of a traumatic injury can be very time-sensitive. The sooner these patients reach the definitive care offered by a hospital, the greater their chances for survival. It is vitally important that you perform a fast and efficient assessment of patients with traumatic injuries and do what you can to expedite transport.

FIRST ON SCENE

"This darn fifth wheel lock is sticking," Casey shouts to his partner Taine as he crouches with his left arm under the trailer. "Rock the tractor a little."

Sitting in the driver's seat of the big rig watching his partner in the side mirror, Taine slips the transmission into reverse and eases off the clutch. The semi lurches backward, thundering into the empty trailer as Casey pulls on the handle to unlock it. Taine then pulls the stick down into a low forward gear and eases the clutch again.

The truck bounces forward this time, and the fifth wheel lock snaps free. Taine pulls the tractor forward about 10 feet, puts it in neutral, and sets the noisy parking brake. As he climbs down out of the cab, he notices Casey rolling around on the ground, holding his left hand close to his body. It takes Taine a second before he sees the blood. There is a lot of it.

"What happened, Casey?" He runs over to his friend, careful not to step in the pool of bright red blood.

Casey, his face contorted in pain, keeps cursing under his breath and rolling from side to side in the parking lot.

"Let me see your hand." Taine demands. Casey holds his left hand up for a moment, long enough for Taine to see that all of the skin and most of the flesh is gone from the ring finger. From the tip to where it meets the hand is now nothing more than a spindly red bone. Casey then buries his hand back close to his body and curses through clenched teeth.

Heart, Blood, and Blood Vessels

The Heart

The heart is the center of the circulatory system. It is responsible for pumping blood through the many miles of vessels and to all the body's tissues and organs. When an injury occurs and the soft tissues are damaged, blood will be forced out of the circulatory system with each beat of the heart (Figure 18.1). Review Chapter 14 for more details related to the circulatory system.

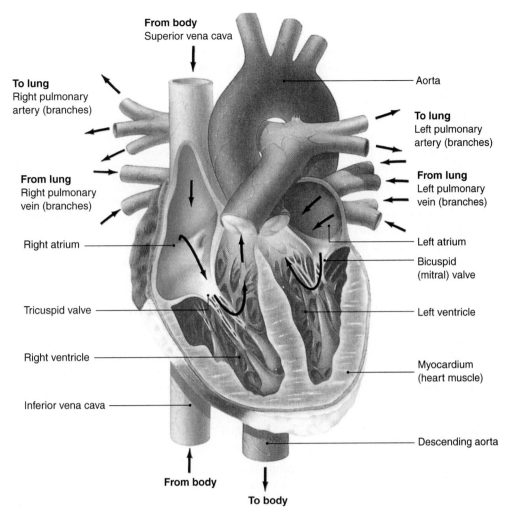

From body
Superior vena cava

To lung
Right pulmonary
artery (branches)

From lung
Right pulmonary
vein (branches)

Right atrium

Tricuspid valve

Right ventricle

Inferior vena cava

Aorta

To lung
Left pulmonary
artery (branches)

From lung
Left pulmonary
vein (branches)

Left atrium

Bicuspid
(mitral) valve

Left ventricle

Myocardium
(heart muscle)

Descending aorta

From body

To body

Figure 18.1 Structures of the heart and flow of blood.

Blood

Blood performs many functions necessary to sustain life. Blood carries oxygen to the body's cells and carries away carbon dioxide (Figure 18.2). It transports nutrients to the cells and carries away waste products. The blood contains cells that destroy bacteria and produce substances that help resist infection. Elements in the blood act to combine blood cells, forming sticky clots at the site of cuts to help control bleeding. Without an adequate supply of blood circulating through your body, vital organs begin to starve for oxygen and nutrients and will eventually shut down. When organ systems begin to fail, death will soon follow.

The functions of blood are to:

- transport oxygen and carbon dioxide.
- transport nutrients to the tissues.
- transport wastes from the tissues to the organs of excretion: kidneys, lungs, and liver.
- transport hormones, water, salts, and other compounds needed to keep the body's functions in balance (body regulation).
- protect against disease-causing organisms (defense).

Blood contains red blood cells, white blood cells, platelets, and other elements involved in forming blood clots. These are carried by a watery, salty fluid called *plasma*. The volume of blood in the typical adult body is approximately 6 liters (1.5 gallons). When bleeding occurs, the body not only loses

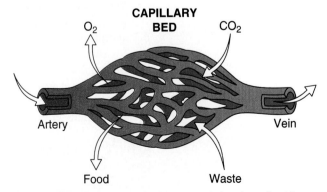

**CAPILLARY
BED**

O_2 CO_2

Artery   Vein

Food   Waste

Figure 18.2 The exchange of oxygen and carbon dioxide occurs at the capillary level.

blood cells and clotting elements, but it also loses plasma and total fluid volume. This loss can be significant because blood volume must be maintained at a certain level to ensure good perfusion and nutrient exchange for the cells and vital organs. The body has more blood than is needed to produce minimum circulation. During bleeding, once this reserve is gone, the patient experiences circulatory system failure, followed very quickly by death.

Blood Vessels

arteries ▶ vessels that carry blood away from the heart (typically oxygenated blood).

Arteries carry blood away from the heart and to the tissues and organs. The largest artery is the *aorta*. The smallest arteries are called *arterioles*. At certain points in the body, where arteries are close to the skin surface, you can feel the blood pumping through an artery. These are the *pulse points*, places where you can feel the pulsations caused by the pumping heart.

veins ▶ vessels that return blood to the heart, (typically deoxygenated blood).

Veins carry blood from the tissues, organs, and systems of the body back to the heart. The largest veins are the superior and inferior *vena cava*. The smallest veins are called *venules*. On some parts of the body, you can see the blue of veins showing through skin where they are close to the surface.

capillaries ▶ smallest blood vessels in the body.

The oxygen and nutrients carried by arteries are passed off to the body's cells when the blood reaches a small system of vessels called **capillaries**. Capillaries have thin walls that eventually become a single cell thick, allowing for the exchange of nutrients and wastes. Some organs, such as the kidneys and liver, act as disposal and maintenance organs. The heart is the organ that works with the lungs to replenish oxygen. Once the blood has dropped off its supply of oxygen for the body's cells to use, it travels from the capillary system into the veins and back to the heart, through the lungs to pick up oxygen, and back to the heart again to be pumped through vessels to the body (see Figure 18.1). By the time blood reaches the capillaries, pressure and speed are greatly reduced and the beating action of the heart no longer causes palpable pulsations. Recall that the adequate supply of well-oxygenated blood to the vital organs and tissues is called *perfusion*. Good perfusion is essential to life.

Bleeding

LO2 Explain the importance of using appropriate body substance isolation (BSI) precautions when caring for a patient with external bleeding.

Understanding the circulatory system and how it functions will assist you in assessing and caring for patients with soft tissue injuries. Uncontrolled bleeding should always be taken seriously. If not stopped, it will lead to shock and eventually death.

Keep the following general considerations in mind while you learn how to provide emergency care for patients with soft tissue injuries:

- *Body substance isolation (BSI) precautions.* The risk of infectious disease should always be assessed and minimized when caring for patients who are bleeding. BSI precautions must be taken routinely to avoid direct contact with blood and other potentially infectious body fluids. Gloves should be worn during every patient encounter. Additional equipment such as goggles, gowns, and a mask should also be used when there is an increased risk of contact with blood or other body fluids, as in cases of childbirth or when a patient is spitting or vomiting blood.
- *Severity of blood loss.* Determining the severity of blood loss should be based on the patient's signs and symptoms and an estimation of visible blood loss. If signs and symptoms of shock are present, bleeding should be considered serious. (Treatment for shock is discussed in more detail in Chapter 19.)
- *Body's normal response to bleeding.* The body's automatic response to bleeding is blood vessel constriction and clotting. However, in cases of major bleeding, clotting may not occur because the flow of blood from the wound is too great to allow for the formation of a clot.

CREW RESOURCE MANAGEMENT

Keep your team safe by minimizing the number of crew members who may be exposed to the patient's blood. Use only those crew members who are needed to provide proper care for the patient.

External Bleeding

LO3 Differentiate the characteristics of arterial, venous, and capillary bleeding.

Bleeding can be classified as external or internal. External bleeding may be classified into the following types (Figure 18.3):

- *Arterial bleeding.* Arterial bleeding occurs when the arteries carrying blood away from the heart are damaged. The bleeding is often characterized by a spurting action with each beat of the heart. The color of arterial blood is bright red because it contains oxygen. Depending on the size of the artery that has been damaged, a great deal of blood can be lost in a short amount of time.
- *Venous bleeding.* Venous bleeding occurs when veins that return blood to the heart have been damaged. Veins often lie close to the surface of the skin. A steady flow of dark red blood characterizes venous bleeding. Depending on the size of the vein affected, venous bleeding can also be serious.
- *Capillary bleeding.* Capillary bleeding is characterized by a slow oozing of bright red blood from tissues. Capillary bleeding is common with minor scrapes and abrasions to the skin.

Evaluating External Bleeding

Studies have shown that it is extremely difficult to estimate the amount of blood loss by the area covered in blood or the amount of clothing soaked in blood. Instead of spending time making poor estimates, your priority should be assessment of the patient's signs and symptoms. They are a much better predictor of the amount of blood loss.

Of the three types of external bleeding, arterial bleeding is usually the most serious. This is because blood within the arteries is under much higher pressure than that within the veins or capillaries. The pressure created with each beat of the heart can prevent the blood from clotting in the wound. Arterial bleeding can take several minutes or more to clot. Because arteries are typically located deep within body structures, capillary and venous bleeding are seen more often than arterial bleeding.

Venous bleeding can range from very minor to very severe. Some veins are located near the surface of the body, and many are large enough to be seen through the skin. Other veins are deep in the body and can be as large as arteries. Bleeding from a deep vein can produce rapid blood loss. Surface bleeding from a vein can be profuse, but blood loss is not as rapid as that seen from arteries and deep veins because of their smaller diameters and lower pressure. Veins tend to collapse as soon as they are cut. This often reduces the severity of venous bleeding.

Most individuals experience little difficulty with capillary bleeding. The blood oozes slowly, and clotting is very likely to occur within a few minutes. However, the larger the

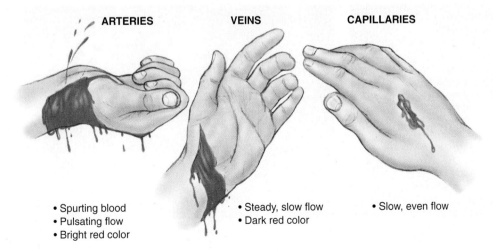

ARTERIES   **VEINS**   **CAPILLARIES**

- Spurting blood
- Pulsating flow
- Bright red color

- Steady, slow flow
- Dark red color

- Slow, even flow

Figure 18.3 Three types of bleeding.

bandage ▶ material used to hold a dressing in place on the body.

area of the wound, the higher the likelihood of infection. Capillary bleeding requires care to stop blood flow and reduce contamination.

If bleeding is severe, bleeding control must begin during the primary assessment. Even though it may prove challenging, an Emergency Medical Responder may be faced with the task of controlling severe bleeding while also evaluating airway and breathing. Some of these tasks should be delegated to others at the scene when appropriate.

Controlling External Bleeding

LO4 Explain the proper care for a patient with active external bleeding.

LO5 Explain the purpose of a dressing.

LO6 Explain the purpose of a bandage.

The three steps to controlling external bleeding of an extremity are: direct pressure; use of a pressure **bandage**; and the **tourniquet**, which may be used when all other bleeding control steps have failed (Key Skill 18.1).

KEY SKILL 18.1

Controlling External Bleeding

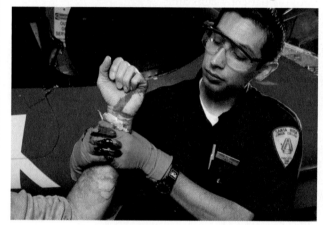

1. Use BSI precautions.

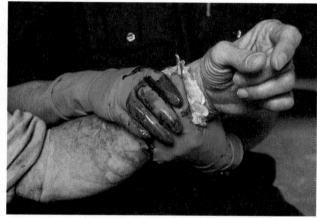

2. Apply direct pressure with a clean dressing and apply a pressure bandage.

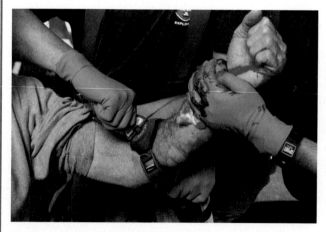

3. If the bleeding does not stop, apply a tourniquet.

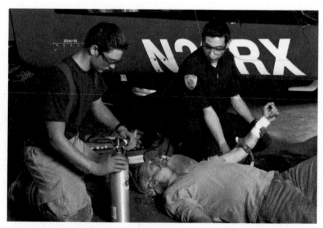

4. Care for shock. Administer oxygen and monitor the ABCs.

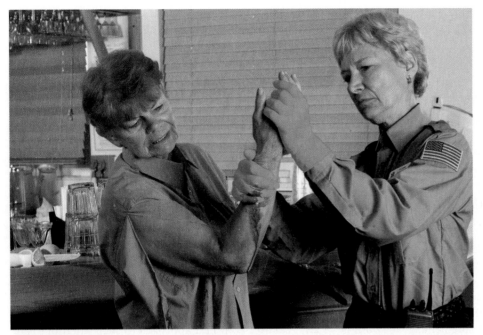

Figure 18.4 In cases of profuse bleeding, use your gloved hand to apply pressure to the wound. Do not waste time hunting for a dressing.

Direct Pressure Most cases of external bleeding can be controlled by applying direct pressure to the site of the wound.[2] The amount of pressure should be firm and held in place long enough to control the bleeding. Ideally, a clean **dressing** should be placed over the wound. If profuse bleeding is found during the primary assessment and you do not have dressings immediately available:

dressing ▶ material used to cover an open wound, typically made of absorbent gauze that may be sterile or nonsterile.

1. Place your gloved hand(s) directly over the wound and apply pressure (Figure 18.4).
2. Keep applying steady, firm pressure.

If dressings are immediately available, then do the following (Figure 18.5):

1. Apply firm pressure using clean dressings or a clean cloth.
2. Apply pressure until the bleeding is controlled. In some cases, this may take several minutes. Resist the temptation to remove pressure repeatedly to determine if the bleeding has stopped. Assume it has stopped only when you do not see bleeding through or around the dressing and bandage.
3. Secure the dressing in place with a tight bandage to create a pressure bandage.

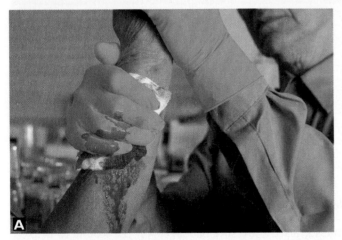
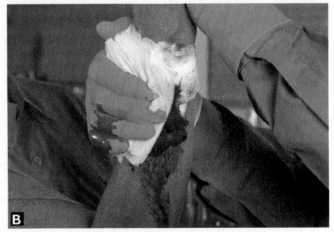

Figure 18.5 (A) To control bleeding, place a clean dressing on the wound and apply direct pressure. (B) If the wound bleeds through the dressings, apply several more over the initial dressing.

Resist the temptation to remove or replace any dressing that has been applied directly to the wound. To do so may interrupt clot formation and restart bleeding. If an outer dressing becomes soaked with blood, replace it with another dressing. Make sure you do not disturb the dressing that is immediately against the wound.

The application of a pressure bandage can be helpful during the early stages of attempting to control bleeding. To apply a pressure bandage, follow these steps:

1. Place several layers of clean dressings directly on the wound. Maintain pressure with your gloved hands.
2. Use a roller bandage or cravat (folded triangular bandage) to secure the dressings in place. It should be wrapped firmly over the dressing and above and below the wound.
3. Tightly wrap the bandage around the dressing and the limb.
4. Check for a distal pulse to be certain the pressure has not restricted circulation beyond the wound.

A pressure bandage should not be removed once it is in place. If bleeding continues, add more pressure by using the palm of your gloved hand or applying more dressing pads, and continue the process of bandaging. (Do not remove the bandage to add more pads.) You may also apply more bandages to increase the direct pressure.

If you are dealing with bleeding from the chest, abdomen, or neck, attempting to apply a pressure bandage may not be of any real use. Your best approach to such situations is to maintain direct pressure on the wound using a dressing held in place by your gloved hand.

Elevation   Elevation alone has not been shown to help control bleeding.[3] However, it may be used in combination with direct pressure when dealing with bleeding from an arm or leg. Elevating the extremity can make it easier to apply direct pressure and place a pressure bandage. Do not elevate if you suspect fractures to the extremity or possible spinal injury.

Tourniquet   Sometimes bleeding is so severe that no amount of direct pressure will control it. When this occurs, do not wait too long to move to the next step. If, while using direct pressure, you are unable to control the bleeding within 2 to 3 minutes, or if bleeding is very severe from the beginning, your best course of action is to place a **tourniquet** just above the injury site. A partial amputation of the arm or leg may leave you with no other choice but to use a tourniquet. In cases in which there is profuse bleeding from an arm or leg wound, a tourniquet should be applied to stop life-threatening bleeding after direct pressure and elevation have failed.[4]

tourniquet ▸ device used to cut off all blood supply past the point of application.

REMEMBER

Recent research by the U.S. military suggests that a tourniquet can be an effective tool for controlling severe bleeding and ultimately saving lives. The use of a tourniquet does not necessarily mean the individual will lose the injured limb. In the vast majority of cases, the patient will get to the hospital in time to save the limb.

FIRST ON SCENE (continued)

Taine runs across the busy parking lot and slams through the doors of the truck stop. He is breathing too heavily to say anything and, as the store's tinny overhead speakers play an upbeat tune, all eyes turn toward him. He catches his breath and shouts, "Somebody call an ambulance! My friend just tore his finger off out back."

He turns and heads back out the door and across the parking lot. A woman standing in line at the register sets a soft drink down on a counter and runs out the door after him. They reach the semi at the same time.

The woman kneels and puts her hand on Casey's shoulder. "My name is Gina, and I'm an Emergency Medical Responder," she says. "May I help you?"

"Oh, God." Casey is still squeezing his left hand, trying to make the overwhelming pain go away. "Only if you can knock me out!"

If all other methods have failed and you must apply a tourniquet, carefully follow these steps:

1. If you have not already done so, place a pressure bandage over the wound to help control bleeding while you apply the tourniquet.
2. Place the tourniquet 2 to 3 inches proximal to the wound.

3. Secure the tourniquet in place and tighten until you no longer feel a distal pulse.
4. Once the tourniquet is in place, do not loosen it.
5. Record the time the tourniquet was applied.
6. Provide care for shock, but do not cover the tourniquet.

Hemostatic Dressings and Agents Specialized dressings called **hemostatic dressings** are commonly used for the management of bleeding wounds (Figure 18.6). Typically, they are traditional gauze dressings treated with chemicals called hemostatic agents, which may help promote the formation of clots directly at the wound site. These dressings are a good resource when the wound cannot be managed by a tourniquet, such as a wound that is very proximal on a limb or a wound on the torso. The dressing is designed to be packed deep into a wound so that the treated material can get as close to the site of bleeding as possible. Be sure to follow local protocols.

hemostatic dressing ▶ dressing that has been treated with a specialized chemical that when placed onto a wound promotes clotting.

CREW RESOURCE MANAGEMENT

Sometimes it can be helpful to involve the patient in their own care. Asking them to hold a dressing in place while you apply the bandage can distract them from their pain.

Dressing and Bandaging One of the most basic skills an Emergency Medical Responder must learn is properly dressing and bandaging a wound. If you follow the basic principles of dressing and bandaging, you will provide effective emergency care for the patient.

Dressings, whenever possible, should be sterile. Commercially prepared dressings come in a variety of sizes. The most common size is 4 inches square. Dressings are referred to according to size, such as 2 × 2s, 4 × 4s, 5 × 9s, and 10 × 30s.

Throughout this text, you will find reference to *bulky dressings*, or *multi-trauma dressings*. Often large enough to allow for the complete covering of large wounds, these thick dressings are used to help control very serious bleeding and to stabilize impaled objects.

To be most effective, dressings must be secured in place over the wound. In most instances, the dressing should be secured to the wound using a bandage (Figure 18.7). Common bandages include roller gauze, cravats, and elastic bandages. Use extra caution when applying elastic bandages because it is possible to inadvertently apply them too tightly, cutting off circulation to the distal extremity.

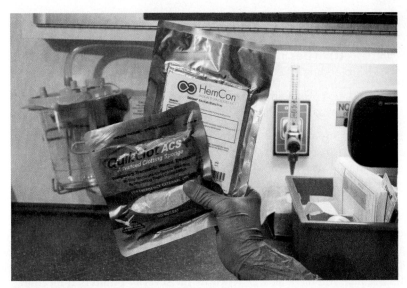

Figure 18.6 Examples of hemostatic dressings.

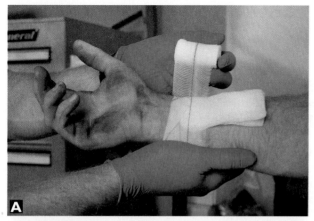

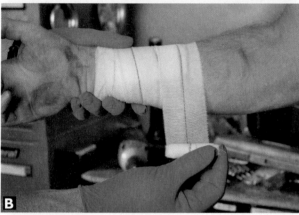

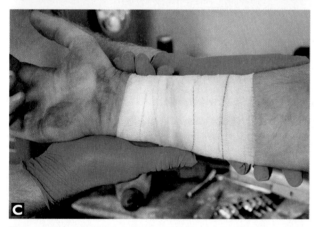

Figure 18.7 (A) Begin by securing the end of the bandage with several overlapping wraps. (B) Continue to wrap so the entire dressing is covered. (C) Secure the end of the bandage with tape.

The following rules apply to dressing wounds:

- A dressing and bandage are of little value if they do not help control bleeding. Continue to apply dressing material and pressure as needed to control the bleeding.
- Use sterile or clean materials when available. Avoid touching dressings in the area that will come into contact with the wound.
- Cover the entire surface of the wound and, if possible, the immediate area surrounding the wound.
- Once a dressing is applied to a wound, it must remain in place. Add new dressings on top of blood-soaked dressings. When a dressing is removed from a wound, bleeding may restart or increase in rate.

The following rules apply to bandaging:

- Do not bandage too tightly. It should hold the dressing snugly in place but not restrict blood supply to the distal extremity.
- Do not bandage too loosely. The dressing must not be allowed to slip from the wound or move while on the wound.
- Do not leave loose ends. Loose ends of tape, dressing, or cloth might get caught on objects when the patient is being moved.
- Do not cover fingers or toes unless they are injured. These areas must be left exposed for you to watch for color changes that indicate a change in circulation. Blue skin; pale skin; and complaints of numbness, pain, and tingling sensations all indicate that the bandage may be too tight.
- Wrap the bandage around the limb, starting at its distal (far) end and working toward its proximal end.
- Always check distal circulation, sensation, and motor function before and after bandaging.
- See Key Skill 18.2 for examples of dressing and bandaging techniques.

Internal Bleeding

LO7 Describe the signs and symptoms of internal bleeding.

LO8 Explain the proper care of a patient with suspected internal bleeding.

Internal bleeding can range from a minor bruise to a damaged internal organ, resulting in a life-threatening problem. Most small bruises are examples of minor internal bleeding that occurs beneath the skin. However, these seemingly simple bruises may be a sign of more serious underlying bleeding. Of primary concern to Emergency Medical Responders is internal bleeding that brings about signs of shock. Some cases of internal bleeding are so severe that the patient dies in a matter of seconds. Other cases take minutes to hours before becoming life threatening. Your ability to recognize the potential for serious internal bleeding and the signs of shock is critical for victims of trauma.

The care you provide for internal bleeding, even when the bleeding is not severe, may save the patient's life. Because you have no way to know the severity of internal bleeding, always assume it is severe and care for the patient aggressively.

Understanding Types of Dressing and Bandaging

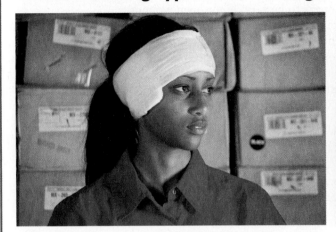

1. Typical dressing and bandage for an injured ear.

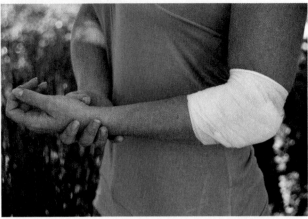

2. Typical dressing and bandage for an injured elbow.

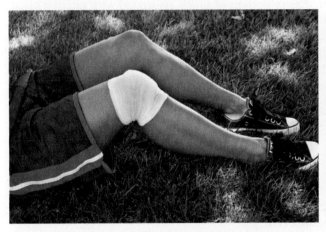

3. Typical dressing and bandage for an injured knee.

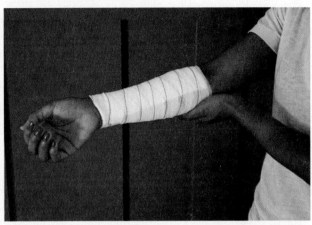

4. Typical dressing and bandage for an injured forearm.

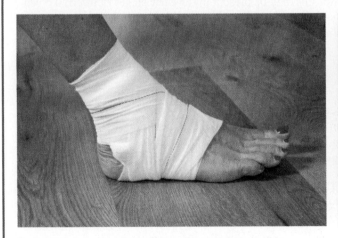

5. Typical dressing and bandage for an injured ankle.

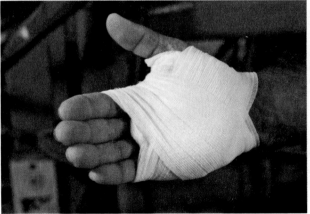

6. Typical dressing and bandage for an injured hand.

Detecting Internal Bleeding   One of the most common causes of internal bleeding is **blunt trauma**, also called blunt force trauma. Blunt trauma can cause injuries to vessels and organs deep within the chest and/or abdomen. It can cause serious internal damage with little or no external evidence. Penetrating injuries can also cause significant internal damage while leaving what appear to be very minor open wounds.

Pay special attention to bruises on the neck, chest, and abdomen. Severe injury with internal bleeding may show no more than a bruise at first, to be followed by the rapid decline of the patient's condition. Bruise detection can be particularly important in assessing possible internal bleeding when the patient is unresponsive and thus unable to complain of pain that would clearly indicate the problem.

Suspect internal bleeding whenever you detect any of the following signs:

- Evidence of blunt trauma
- Vomiting or coughing up blood
- Presence of bruises
- Penetrating wounds to the abdomen
- Pain, rigidity, or distension of the abdomen
- Bleeding from the rectum or vagina

Always suspect internal bleeding if the patient has been injured and the signs and symptoms of shock are present. The symptoms of shock associated with internal bleeding are restlessness or anxiety, increased pulse rate, thirst, feeling cold, and rapid breathing. However, during the early stages of internal bleeding, there may not yet be signs or symptoms. Do not wait for signs and symptoms to develop. Treat the patient based on the mechanism of injury (MOI) and/or history.

The signs of shock associated with internal bleeding include:

- Decreasing level of responsiveness
- Restlessness or combativeness
- Shallow, rapid breathing
- Rapid, weak pulse
- Pale, cool, moist skin
- Delayed capillary refill (>2 seconds)
- Dilated pupils, which may respond sluggishly
- Abnormally low blood pressure (late sign)

None of these signs or symptoms may be present in the early stages of internal bleeding. If the mechanism of injury is severe enough to make you think that there may be internal bleeding, assume that there is such bleeding and provide the necessary care.

Managing Internal Bleeding   The steps in the emergency care of patients with suspected internal bleeding include:

1. Take appropriate BSI precautions.
2. Perform a primary assessment. Ensure an open airway and adequate breathing.
3. Provide high-flow oxygen if allowed. Follow local protocols.
4. Perform a thorough secondary assessment, looking for evidence of trauma.
5. Provide care for shock.
6. Reassure the patient and keep them calm.
7. Facilitate rapid transport to an appropriate trauma center.

Multisystem Trauma

LO9 Identify the characteristics of multisystem trauma.

Isolated trauma, also called *isolated injury*, is trauma that is restricted to a specific part of the body, such as an arm or leg. It is fairly easy to tell when these areas are injured. The damage is isolated to muscle, bone, and soft tissue and does not affect any major organ systems.

In contrast, with **multisystem trauma**, the patient has sustained a significant MOI to the torso such as from an automobile collision, a fall from a height, or a gunshot wound. In this case, you should assume numerous body organ systems have been impacted. Blunt trauma sustained from a vehicle collision can result in damage to the heart, lungs, brain, and the organ systems within the abdomen.

multisystem trauma ▶ trauma to the body that affects multiple organ systems.

Multisystem trauma creates a critical situation for the patient because a combination of injuries to multiple body systems can quickly overwhelm the patient's ability to compensate, leading to shock and death.

The best way to anticipate multisystem trauma is to evaluate the MOI and assume that the patient has sustained all possible injuries. Proper treatment involves activation of the EMS system, supporting the ABCs, and treating each life threat as you identify it. It is necessary to understand the importance of rapid transport to an appropriate trauma center for victims of multisystem trauma. Be sure to request transport as soon as possible and consider the need for air medical transport if available.

 FIRST ON SCENE *(continued)*

Gina looks at Casey's bloody hand and notices that it isn't actively bleeding. She turns to Taine, who is still trying to catch his breath, and asks if there is a first-aid kit in the truck. Taine thinks for a moment and brightens, "Oh, yeah! We have one in the side box!"

He turns and hurries to the truck. As he digs out the first-aid kit, he sees the skin of Casey's finger hanging limply from the fifth wheel lock handle. It is dangling from something that flickers like gold, so he steps closer. It is Casey's wedding ring. It got caught on the lock handle and, when it finally popped open, the action of the lock handle must have pulled off the skin and flesh, leaving the bone still attached to the hand.

Taine turns, feeling queasy, and hurries back over with the first-aid kit. Casey is now extremely pale, and Taine can see that he has thrown up on the pavement.

"Quick," Gina says, grabbing the kit from Taine's shaking hands. "I need you to cover him with your jacket and keep him from getting cold."

Soft Tissue Injuries

The soft tissues of the body include the skin, muscles, nerves, blood vessels, and all the connective tissues that hold these structures together (Figure 18.8). Growing up, most of us experienced soft tissue injuries such as bruises, scratches, and cuts. These minor injuries are relatively easy to care for and rarely end up as life threatening. As an Emergency Medical Responder, you are likely to respond to people with much more serious injuries.

Except for cases of spine injury and certain types of internal injury, most adults can tell if there is an injury. Your training will build on this ability so you will not miss detectable injuries. This is the reason there has been so much emphasis on patient assessment. As you progress through this course, you will be trained to determine the extent of an injury and the emergency procedures needed to care for it.

Types of Injuries

LO10 Describe common types of external soft tissue injuries.

Soft tissue injuries can be categorized as closed wounds or open wounds.

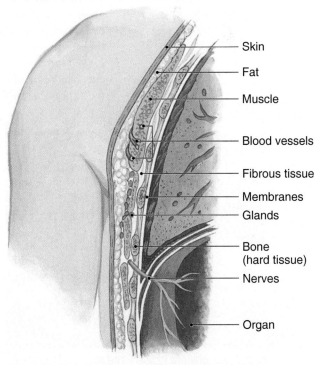

Figure 18.8 Soft tissues and associated underlying structures.

- Skin
- Fat
- Muscle
- Blood vessels
- Fibrous tissue
- Membranes
- Glands
- Bone (hard tissue)
- Nerves
- Organ

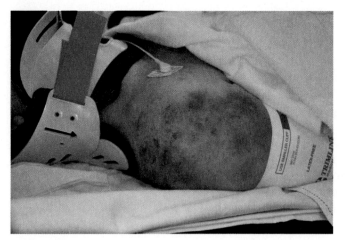

Figure 18.9 Bruises are the most common form of closed wounds.
(© Edward T. Dickinson, MD)

REMEMBER

Many patients may not bruise immediately following an injury. Do not dismiss the possibility of injury due to the absence of bruising. For many patients, bruising can take several hours to appear.

Closed Wounds   A *closed wound* is an injury in which the skin is not broken. The impact of a blunt object usually causes such injuries. Internal bleeding can range from minor to major, while the extent of injury can range from a simple *bruise* to the rupturing of internal organs.

One of the most obvious signs of a closed wound is the presence of swelling and/or bruises (Figure 18.9). There is always some internal bleeding associated with a bruise. Because the outer skin is not broken, the blood leaks between tissues, causing discoloration over time ranging from black and blue to a brownish yellow. Keep in mind that large bruises can mean serious blood loss and may be evidence of extensive tissue damage under the site of the bruise.

Open Wounds   In the case of an *open wound*, the skin is damaged and there is obvious bleeding. The extent of injury can range from a mild abrasion (scrape) to a laceration (tearing or cutting open of the skin). Simple scraping of the skin may produce no bleeding, while more severe open wounds may be associated with minor to life-threatening bleeding.

Open wounds may be classified as:

- *Abrasions.* Wounds such as skinned elbows and knees, "road rash," and "rug burns," are minor open wounds known as abrasions (Figure 18.10). Although these injuries may be painful, tissue injury is usually not serious because the skin is not fully penetrated and the force causing the injury does not crush or rupture underlying structures. Wound infection tends to be the most serious problem faced when caring for abrasions to the skin.
- *Lacerations.* With lacerations, the skin is fully penetrated, with injury also occurring to tissues lying under the skin. Lacerations may be classified as:
  - *Smooth cuts, or incisions* (Figure 18.11). These types of lacerations are produced by very sharp objects, such as razor blades, knives, and broken glass. The edges of a smooth cut appear straight, with no apparent tears or jagged areas. Deep incisions can cause severe tissue damage and life-threatening bleeding.
  - *Jagged cuts.* These are tears with rough edges (Figure 18.12). Sometimes jagged cuts can be produced from the impact of a blunt object. Usually they occur when the skin is cut by an object that does not have a very sharp edge.

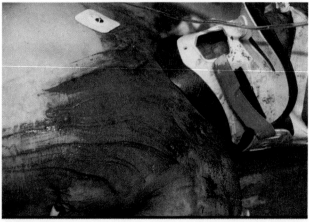

Figure 18.10 Abrasions are typically the least serious form of open wound.
(© Edward T. Dickinson, MD)

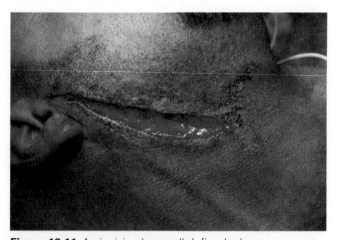

Figure 18.11 An incision has well-defined edges.
(© Edward T. Dickinson, MD)

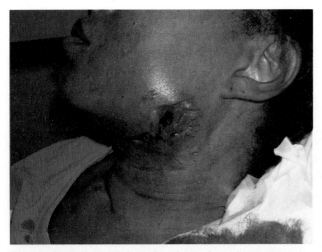

Figure 18.12 A laceration often has edges that are irregular and jagged.
(© Edward T. Dickinson, MD)

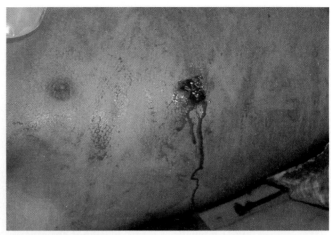

Figure 18.13 Often a puncture wound has very little external bleeding.
(© Edward T. Dickinson, MD)

- *Punctures.* Objects such as knives, nails, and ice picks can produce puncture wounds, also known as **penetrating trauma**. An object puncturing the body will tear through the skin and usually proceed in a straight line, damaging tissues in its path. A puncture wound can range from shallow to deep (Figure 18.13). It may also have both an entrance and an exit wound, created when the object, such as a bullet, passes through the body. Often, the exit wound is the larger and more serious of the two wounds (Figure 18.14).
- *Avulsions.* These wounds most frequently involve the tearing loose or tearing off of large flaps of skin (Figure 18.15). A torn ear, an eyeball removed from its socket, and the loss of a tooth are examples of **avulsions**.
- *Amputations.* These wounds involve the cutting or tearing off of the fingers, toes, hands, feet, arms, or legs (Figure 18.16). Because the word **amputation** can also refer to a surgical procedure, this injury is often called a *traumatic amputation*.

penetrating trauma ▸ injury to the body caused by any object that punctures the skin.

avulsion ▸ tearing loose of skin or other soft tissues.

amputation ▸ cutting or tearing off of a body part.

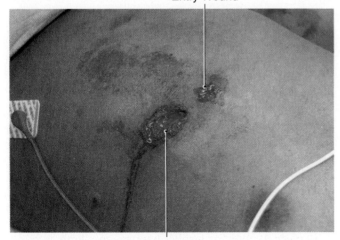

Entry Wound

Exit Wound

Figure 18.14 A penetrating wound can have both an entrance wound and an exit wound. Often the exit wound is the larger of the two.
(© Edward T. Dickinson, MD)

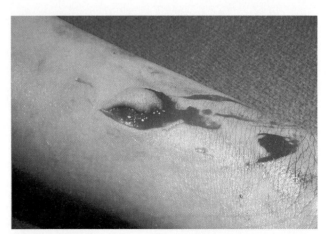

Figure 18.15 An avulsion typically results in a flap of skin that is torn away.
(© Dr. Bryan E. Bledsoe)

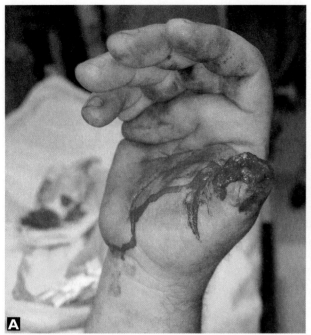
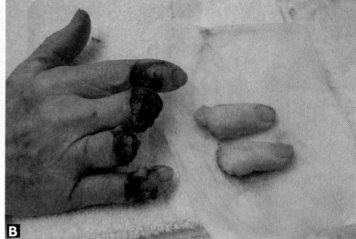

Figure 18.16 Amputations (A) of the thumb and (B) of the fingers.
(© Edward T. Dickinson, MD)

- *Crush injuries.* Crush injuries occur when a body part is pressed between two surfaces. The greater the force, the greater the damage. Soft tissues and internal organs may be crushed, often rupturing (Figure 18.17). Both external and internal bleeding can be profuse.

Emergency Care of Open Wounds

LO11 Explain proper emergency care for a patient with an open wound.

To provide emergency care for open wounds, follow these steps:

1. Don the appropriate protective equipment for the situation. Gloves and eye protection are the minimum level of protection for managing open wounds.
2. Perform a primary assessment and ensure an open airway and adequate breathing. Do not let the unpleasant sight of an open wound distract you from more important priorities.

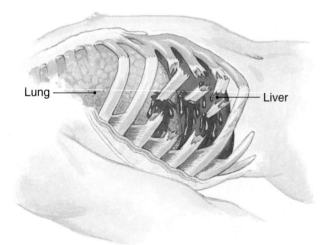

Figure 18.17 Crush injuries often result in significant damage to the underlying soft tissue and organs.

3. Expose the wound. Cut away clothing over and around an open wound. When doing this, avoid cutting directly through holes made by knives or bullets. They may serve as valuable evidence if the patient is a victim of a crime.
4. Remove superficial foreign matter from the surface of the wound with a sterile gauze pad.
5. Control the bleeding with direct pressure. A tourniquet should be used if direct pressure and a pressure bandage do not control the bleeding.
6. Administer oxygen per local protocols.
7. Prevent further contamination by using a sterile dressing or clean cloth to cover the wound. After the bleeding has been controlled, bandage the dressing in place. If applying a roller bandage to a limb, it is standard practice to begin at the distal side of the wound and wrap to the proximal end.
8. Keep the patient lying still, and care for shock.
9. Reassure the patient and initiate transport as appropriate.

Emergency Care of Puncture Wounds

LO12 Explain the proper care for a patient with an impaled object.

When dealing with any puncture wound, assume that there is extensive internal injury and internal bleeding. Always check for an exit wound, realizing that exit wounds can be more serious than entrance wounds (in the case of gunshot injury). Care for entrance and exit wounds as you would any open wound.

When the puncture wound involves an impaled object, in most instances you will want to stabilize the impaled object in place and NOT remove it. There is a good chance that the object is sealing the wound, plugging holes in open vessels deep in the wound. Removing the object could allow those wounds to bleed freely. The object must be stabilized with bulky dressings or pads. Begin by placing these materials on opposite sides of the object. Use tape or cravats to hold all dressings and pads in place (Key Skill 18.3).

To care for a patient whose puncture wound contains an impaled object (such as glass, a knife, wood, metal, or plastic), do the following (Figures 18.18 and 18.19):

1. Take appropriate BSI precautions.
2. Expose the wound without disturbing the impaled object.
3. Do not remove an impaled object.

KEY SKILL 18.3

Caring for a Patient with an Impaled Object

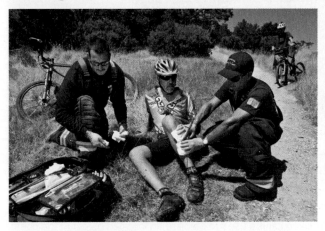

1. Control any obvious bleeding.

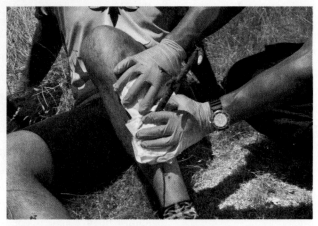

2. Manually stabilize the impaled object.

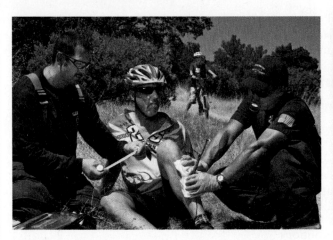

3. Add bulky dressings to help stabilize the object.

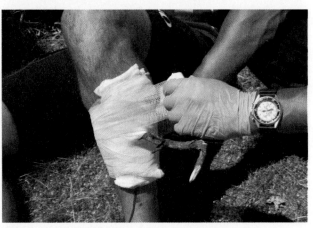

4. Use a bandage to secure the dressings in place.

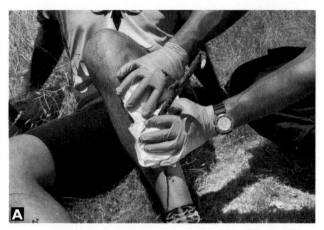 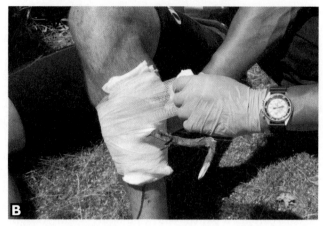

Figure 18.18 Emergency care for a wound with an impaled object. (A) Stabilize the object with bulky dressings. (B) Secure the dressings with an appropriate bandage.

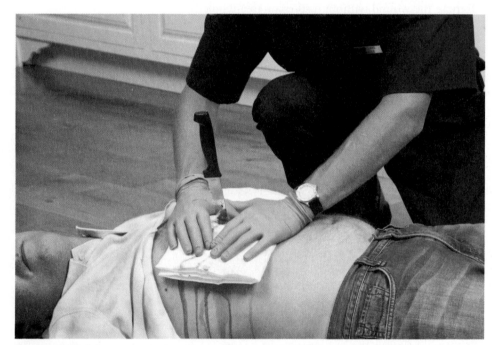

Figure 18.19 A large trauma dressing can be used to stabilize an impaled object in the chest.

REMEMBER

Take special care to avoid cutting your gloves or hands on an impaled object. Spread your fingers around the object and apply pressure to the wound site. Do not put any pressure on the object or the tissues that are up against the edge of a sharp impaled object.

4. Control the bleeding. Administer oxygen per local protocols.
5. Stabilize the impaled object by using bulky dressings.
6. Keep the patient at rest and provide care for shock.

Avulsions and Amputations

LO13 Explain the proper care for an amputation injury.

LO14 Explain the proper care for an injury to the eye.

LO15 Explain the proper care for nosebleed.

Emergency care for avulsions and amputations are the same. If skin or another body part is torn from the body, or if a flap of skin has been torn loose, care for the wound with bulky dressings and direct pressure. Follow these steps:

1. Take appropriate BSI precautions.
2. Expose the wound.
3. Control bleeding and provide care as you would for any open wound.

4. If the wound is an avulsion, gently fold the skin back to its normal position prior to applying direct pressure. Follow local protocols.

5. Provide care for shock. Administer oxygen per local protocols.

Save and preserve an avulsed or amputated part. This is best done by wrapping the body part in a sterile dressing and placing it into a plastic bag or wrapping it in plastic wrap. If possible, keep the part cool (not cold; avoid freezing). Do not place the avulsed or amputated part in water or in direct contact with ice.[5] Direct contact with ice can damage the skin, especially tissue that may already have compromised circulation. Be certain the bag with the part in it is transported with the patient. Label the bag with the patient's name.

In most cases of avulsion or amputation, bleeding can be controlled by direct pressure and a pressure bandage secured firmly over the stump or area of avulsion. Apply a tourniquet if the bleeding continues.

Protruding Organs   A deep, open wound to the abdomen can cause organs such as the intestines to protrude through the wound opening. This is known as an *evisceration*. Follow these guidelines when caring for an open abdominal wound:

- Do not try to push protruding organ(s) back into the body cavity.
- Place a thick, moist dressing over the protruding organs and cover the dressing with a plastic covering to contain the moisture and heat.
- Provide care for shock. Do not give the patient anything by mouth.

Scalp Injuries   Injuries to the scalp can be difficult to care for because of the numerous blood vessels found there. Many of these vessels are close to the surface of the skin, producing profuse bleeding from even minor wounds. Additional problems arise if the bones of the skull are involved.

Injuries to the scalp (and face) require an extra effort on the part of the Emergency Medical Responder to provide emotional support for patients. The injuries tend to be very painful, produce bleeding that frightens many patients, and are in a body region where people have concern for their appearance.

The procedures for the emergency care of soft tissue injuries previously discussed in this chapter apply to injuries to the soft tissues of the scalp. Use caution when applying direct pressure to a scalp wound. If there is the possibility of a skull fracture, you do not want to push the broken pieces into the skull.

Emergency care of scalp wounds includes the following:

- Control bleeding with a dressing held in place with gentle pressure. Avoid exerting excessive pressure if there are signs of a fractured skull or the injury site feels spongy.
- A roller bandage or gauze can be wrapped around the patient's head to hold dressings in place once the bleeding has been controlled. If there is any indication of neck or spinal injuries, use caution to keep the patient's head immobilized when applying the bandage.
- If there are no signs of skull fracture or injuries to the spine, neck, or chest, you may position the patient so the head and shoulders are elevated.

Facial Wounds   The first concern when caring for facial injuries is to make certain that the patient's airway is open and breathing is adequate. Even though bleeding may appear to be external only, check the airway and ensure that blood is not causing an obstruction. Continue to watch the patient to be sure the airway remains open and clear of fluids and obstructions.

When caring for patients with facial injuries, you should:

1. Ensure an open and clear airway, being careful to note and properly care for neck and spinal injuries.

2. Control bleeding by direct pressure, being careful not to press too hard because many facial fractures are not obvious.

3. Apply a dressing and bandage.

REMEMBER

Facial injuries, even minor ones, may cause significant fear and anxiety, particularly in young patients who may be very concerned about disfigurement. By speaking in a calm and reassuring voice, you can help your patient remain calm. Do not make promises such as, "It will heal fine." Instead, say something like, "Let's get you taken care of, okay?"

If an object has passed through the cheek wall and is sticking into the mouth, you may have to remove it. It is also appropriate to remove an impaled object if it interferes with your ability to perform proper CPR. Do so only if the object blocks the airway or is loose and could fall into the airway. To remove an impaled object from the cheek, follow these steps:

1. Look into the mouth to see if the object has passed through the cheek wall.
2. If you find penetration, carefully pull or push the object out of the cheek wall, back in the direction from which the object entered.
3. If you remove an impaled object, place the dressing material between the wound and the patient's teeth, leaving some of the dressing outside the mouth so it can be held to prevent swallowing it. Watch closely to be sure the dressing does not work its way loose and into the airway.
4. Position the patient so blood will drain from the mouth. Use dressing material packed against the inside wound to control the flow of blood. If bleeding is difficult to control and you suspect neck or spinal injuries, roll the patient while maintaining manual stabilization of the head and neck.
5. Dress and bandage the outside of the wound.
6. Provide care for shock.

Eye Injuries   Injuries to the eyes are rarely life threatening, but they can be emotionally traumatic. The prospect of losing one's sight can be overwhelming. Following are a few important points that must be emphasized when caring for an injury to the eye:

- Do not remove any impaled objects.
- Do not try to put the eye back into its socket.
- Do not apply pressure directly to an injured eyeball.

Problems resulting from foreign objects in the eyes are common. These problems can range from minor irritations to permanent injury. If the patient's own tears do not wash away a foreign object, use running water to remove it (Figure 18.20). Do not apply the wash if there are impaled objects or cuts in the eye. Apply the flow of water at the corner of the eye socket closest to the patient's nose. You may have to help the patient hold open the eyelids. As you pour the water, direct the patient to look from side to side and up and down. Before completing the wash, have the patient blink several times. When possible, continue the wash for at least 20 minutes or for the time recommended by medical direction.

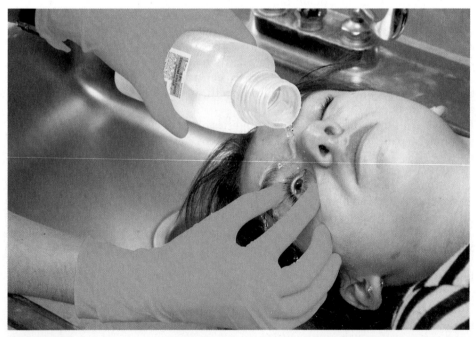

Figure 18.20 For foreign objects in the eye, flush with water from a medial to lateral direction.

If there are sharp objects in the patient's eye, do not direct the patient to move the eyes during the wash. After the wash, cover both eyes with dry dressings (Figure 18.21).

Whenever you are caring for a patient with eye injuries, you will have to cover both of the patient's eyes. In most cases, only one eye will actually be injured. However, when one eye moves, the other eye also will move (sympathetic movement). If you cover the injured eye and leave the uninjured eye uncovered, the uninjured eye will continue to react to activities and movement. Each time the uninjured eye moves, so will the injured one. Having both eyes covered reduces eye movements.

Having both eyes covered can cause fear and anxiety in the patient. Tell them why you are covering the uninjured eye. Keep close to the patient or have someone else stay close. Try to maintain contact with them through conversation and touch.

Burns to the eye must always be considered serious, requiring special in-hospital care. As an Emergency Medical Responder, you may have to provide emergency care for burns to the eyes caused by heat, light, or chemicals. The following are guidelines to follow when caring for the various types of burns to the eyes:

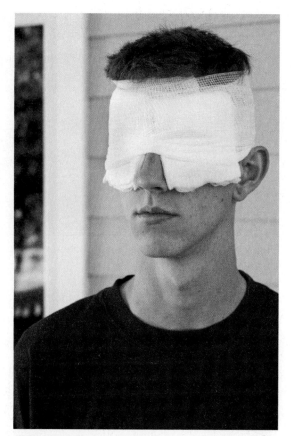

Figure 18.21 When caring for an eye injury, cover both eyes to minimize movement of the injured eye.

- *Thermal (heat) burns.* Do not try to inspect the eyes if there are signs of thermal burns to the eyelids. With the patient's eyelids closed, cover the eyes with loose, moist dressings. If you have no means to moisten the dressings, apply dry dressings. Do not apply any burn ointment to the eyelids.
- *Light burns.* "Snow blindness" and "welder's blindness" are two examples of light burns. Close the patient's eyelids and apply dark patches over both eyes. If you do not have dark patches, use thick dressings or dressings followed with a layer of an opaque material such as dark plastic.
- *Chemical burns.* Many chemicals cause rapid, severe damage to the eyes. Flush the eyes with water. Do not delay emergency care by trying to locate sterile water. Use any source of clean drinking water. If possible, continue the washing flow for at least 20 minutes. After washing the patient's eyes, close the eyelids and apply loose, moist dressings.

If you find an object impaled in the globe of a patient's eye, you should:

1. Use several layers of dressing or small rolls of gauze to make thick pads. Place them on the sides of the object (Figure 18.22A). If you only have enough material for one thick pad, cut a hole equal to the size of the eye opening in the center of the pad. Set the pad over the patient's eye, allowing the impaled object to stick out through the opening cut into the pad.
2. Fit a disposable cardboard drinking cup or paper cone over the impaled object (Figure 18.22B). This will serve as a protective shield. Rest the cup or cone on the thick dressing pad, but do not allow this protective shield to come in contact with the impaled object.
3. Hold the pad and protective shield in place with a roller bandage or with a wrapping of gauze or other cloth material.
4. Use dressing material to cover the uninjured eye and bandage this dressing in place. This will reduce sympathetic eye movements.
5. Provide care for shock.
6. Provide emotional support to the patient.

Wrapping a paper cup or cone with gauze is tricky and cannot be done easily unless you practice. Ideally, you should wrap around the cup and then continue around the patient's head and wrap around the cup again. This procedure is repeated until the cup is stable. Take great care not to push the cup down onto the impaled object or pull the cup out of place.

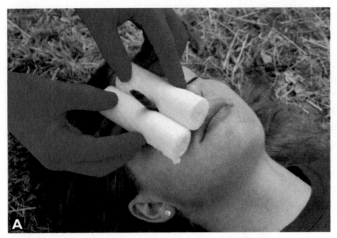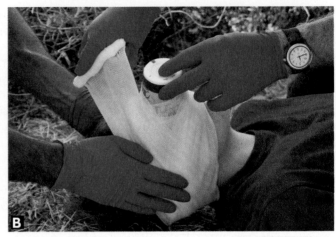

Figure 18.22 Emergency care for a patient with an object impaled in the eye includes (A) stabilizing and protecting the object and (B) securing it in place.

If the eye is pulled out of the socket (avulsed eye), the care provided is the same as for an object impaled in the eye.

Ear Injuries   Emergency care for external ear injuries includes the following:

- *Cuts.* Apply dressings and bandage in place.
- *Tears.* Apply bulky dressings, beginning with several layers behind the torn tissue.
- *Avulsions.* Use bulky dressings bandaged into place. Save the avulsed part in a plastic bag or plastic wrap. Keep the part dry and cool. If no plastic is available, then wrap in dressing material. Be certain to label the bag, wrap, or dressing with the patient's name.

Internal ear injuries may appear as bleeding from the ears. Any such bleeding must be considered a sign of serious head injury. Bloody or clear fluids draining from the ear may indicate the presence of skull fracture. For such cases, assume there is serious injury and provide the necessary care. (See Chapter 21 for more information about head injuries.)

Do not pack the external ear canal. If there is bleeding or clear fluid leaking from the ears, apply external dressings—sterile if possible—and hold them in place with bandages. Report this bleeding to the transport crew.

Do not attempt to remove foreign objects from inside the ear. Apply external dressings, if necessary, and provide emotional support to the patient.

If the patient tells you that it feels like their ears are "clogged" or "stopped up," suspect possible damage to the eardrum, fluids in the middle ear, or objects in the ear canal. These conditions must be treated in a medical facility.

Nose Injuries   When dealing with injuries to the nose—when there are no suspected skull fractures or spinal injuries—you will have two duties: maintain an open airway and control bleeding.

For a nosebleed in a responsive patient, maintain an open airway. Have the patient assume a seated position, leaning slightly forward. This position will help prevent blood and mucus from obstructing the airway or draining down the throat and into the stomach, which can cause nausea and vomiting. Next, have the patient pinch the nostrils. Bleeding is usually controlled when the nostrils are pinched shut. If the patient cannot pinch them shut, you will have to do so. Do not pack the patient's nostrils. Do not allow the patient to blow their nose (Figure 18.23).

For a nosebleed in an unresponsive patient or in a patient injured in such a way that they cannot be placed in a seated position, place them on one side with the head turned to provide drainage from the nose and mouth. Attempt to control bleeding by pinching the nostrils shut. Do not pack the nose. Do not remove objects or probe into the nose.

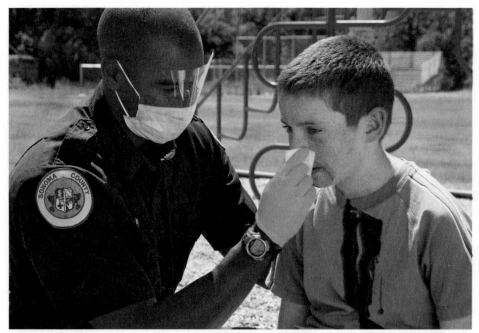

Figure 18.23 For a nosebleed, have the patient lean forward and squeeze both nostrils with a clean dressing.

For an avulsion of the nose, apply a pressure bandage to the site. Save the avulsed part in a plastic bag, wrapped in plastic wrap, or a sterile or clean dressing. Keep the body part cool.

Injury to the Mouth　As with all injuries that occur in or around the airway, your first concern will be to ensure an open airway. If there are no suspected skull, neck, or spinal injuries, assist the patient to a seated position with the head tilted slightly forward to allow for drainage. If the patient cannot be placed in a seated position, position them on one side with the head turned slightly downward to provide some drainage for blood and other fluids.

For cut lips, use a rolled or folded dressing. Place the dressing between the patient's lip and gum. Take great care that the patient does not swallow the dressing.

For avulsed lips, apply a pressure bandage to the site of injury. Save the avulsed part in a plastic bag or wrap, or wrap with a sterile or clean dressing. Keep the avulsed part cool.

For cuts to the internal cheek, position a dressing between the patient's cheek and gum. (Do not pack the mouth with dressings.) Hold the dressing in place with a gloved hand. Always leave 3 to 4 inches of dressing material outside the patient's mouth to allow for quick removal. This is necessary to prevent the patient from swallowing the dressing. If possible, position the patient's head to allow drainage.

Neck Wounds　Be aware of the following signs that indicate soft tissue wounds to the neck:

- Difficulty speaking, loss of voice
- Difficulty swallowing
- Obvious swelling or bruising of the neck
- Pain on swallowing or speaking
- Obvious cuts or puncture wounds

Follow these steps when caring for an open wound to the neck (Figure 18.24):

1. Immediately apply direct pressure to the wound, using the palm of your gloved hand.
2. Apply an occlusive dressing or some type of plastic over the wound. Use tape to seal the dressing on all sides. This will minimize the possibility that air can be drawn into the wound, causing an air embolism.
3. Provide care for shock and provide oxygen if allowed. Follow local protocols.

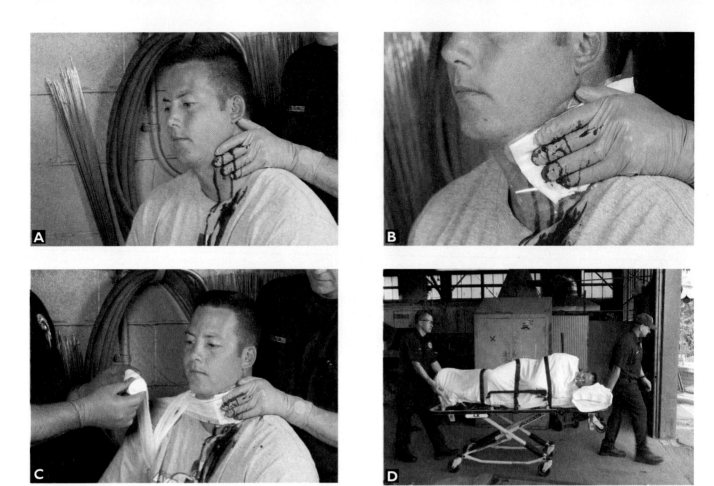

Figure 18.24 Use a gloved hand to help control bleeding from the neck. (A) Apply direct pressure. (B) The dressing should extend beyond all sides of the wound. (C) Secure the dressing with a figure-eight wrap, using a roller bandage. (D) If no spinal injury is suspected, place the patient on their left side and care for shock.

Injury to the Genitalia   Because of the location, the genitalia are not a common site of injury. The pelvis and the thighs usually prevent injury to these organs, which are known as the *external genitalia*. When injury does occur, two types of soft tissue injuries are commonly seen:

- *Blunt trauma.* Such an injury is very painful, but little can be done by the Emergency Medical Responder. An ice pack, if available, can help.
- *Cuts.* Direct pressure should control bleeding. A sterile dressing or a sanitary pad should be used. If these are not available, then use any clean, bulky dressing.

The emergency care for all soft tissue injuries applies when caring for injuries to the genitalia: Do not remove impaled objects. Save avulsed parts, wrapping them in plastic, sterile dressings, or any clean dressing.

You must perform your duties in a manner that will reduce embarrassment for the patient. Tell the patient what you are going to do. Tell them why you must examine and care for the genitalia. Protect the patient from the sight of onlookers by having them leave the scene. Conduct all procedures in the same manner as you would care for an injury to any other part of the body.

In cases where there is known or suspected sexual violence, take extra care to make the patient feel safe and in control of their body. Maintain the patient's privacy, and do not touch them or expose their genitalia without their consent. Allow them to be with someone they know and trust if that's what they want. If there are no immediate life threats, allow the patient to place the bandages over their genital region. The patient should be transported by EMS to the emergency department. If possible, the caregiver should be of the same sex as the patient to lessen any fears the patient may have.

Some genital injuries are self-inflicted or are the result of abuse. Whatever the cause, the patient will need emotional support and understanding. For cases of suspected abuse, remember that you are mandated to report your suspicions to law enforcement.

Burns

LO16 Differentiate superficial, partial-thickness, and full-thickness burns.

Emergency Medical Responders should consider burns to be complex soft tissue injuries that can range from a superficial burn to the epidermis (outermost layer of skin) to a serious, deep injury that involves nerves, blood vessels, muscles, and bones. Careful patient assessment is necessary to avoid missing injuries or medical problems that may be far more serious than the obvious burns.

Classification of Burns

Burns are classified in several ways. One way is to categorize burns based on the agent that caused the injury (source of the burn). This information should be gathered and forwarded to more highly trained personnel during transfer of care. Categories of burns based on source include:

- *Thermal (heat) burns*, which may be caused by fire, steam, or hot objects
- *Chemical burns*, which may be caused by caustic substances, such as acids and alkalis
- *Electrical burns*, which originate from outlets, frayed wires, and faulty circuits
- *Lightning burns*, which occur during electrical storms
- *Light burns*, which occur with intense light. Light from an arc welder or industrial laser will damage unprotected eyes. Also, ultraviolet light (including sunlight) can burn the eyes and skin.
- *Radiation burns*, which usually result from nuclear sources

Most often burns are categorized according to the depth of the injury (Figure 18.25).

- *Superficial burns* involve the epidermis, the outermost layer of skin. Signs and symptoms include reddening of the skin and pain at the site. A common example is sunburn.
- *Partial-thickness burns* involve the epidermis and the dermis, the top two layers of skin (Figure 18.26). These burns present with intense pain, white to red skin that is moist and mottled (in light-skinned patients), and blisters. A classic example is a steam burn.
- *Full-thickness burns* extend through all skin layers (epidermis, dermis, and hypodermis) and may involve subcutaneous layers, muscle, bone, or organs (Figure 18.27). Full-thickness burns can be dry and leathery and may appear white, dark brown, or charred. Because there is often nerve damage present, there may be little to no sensation of pain.

Severity of Burns

LO17 Explain the process for determining percentage of body surface area affected by a burn.

An important aspect of emergency care is being able to assess the severity of a burn, or extent of the damage. Defining the severity of a burn will involve evaluating the depth of the

JEDI

In the United States, certain population groups are known to be more at risk of experiencing sexual violence. These include but are not limited to individuals who are homeless, disabled, or who work in the sex trade. Do not allow biases you may have to get in the way of providing the absolute best and most empathetic care you can to all patients.

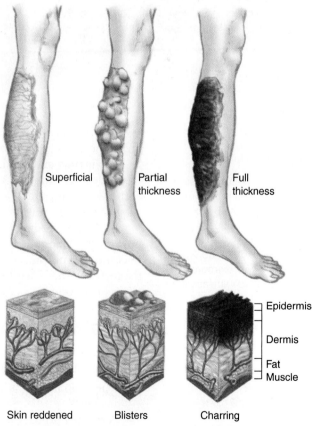

Superficial   Partial thickness   Full thickness

Skin reddened   Blisters   Charring

Epidermis
Dermis
Fat
Muscle

Figure 18.25 Burns are classified by depth of injury.

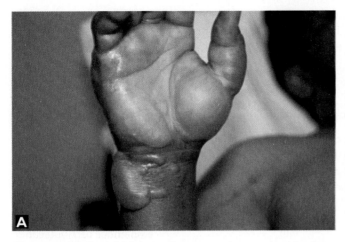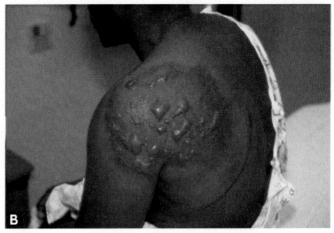

Figure 18.26 Partial-thickness burns are characterized by the presence of redness and blisters.
(© Edward T. Dickinson, MD)

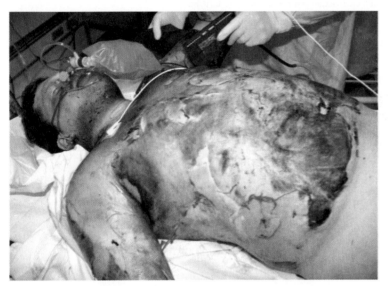

Figure 18.27 Full-thickness burns involve all layers of the skin.
(© Edward T. Dickinson, MD)

burn as well as the total body surface area (BSA) affected. A superficial or partial-thickness burn that involves less than 9% of the patient's total BSA is considered a minor burn. The exceptions are if the burn involves the respiratory system, face, hands, feet, groin, buttocks, or a major joint.

Any burn to the face (other than sunburn) should be considered a serious burn. Other serious burns include any partial-thickness burns covering a large area of the body or burns involving the feet, hands, groin, buttocks, or major joints.

One of the tasks you will need to perform when caring for a patient with a burn injury is to estimate the amount of BSA affected by the burn. A common system used for this purpose is called the *rule of nines* (Figure 18.28). For adults, the head and neck, chest, abdomen, each arm, the front of each leg, the back of each leg, the upper back, and the lower back and buttocks are each considered equal to 9% of the total body surface area. This gives a total of 99%. The remaining 1% is assigned to the genital area.

For infants and children, a simple approach assigns 18% to the head and neck, 9% to each upper limb, 18% to the chest and abdomen, 18% to the entire back, 14% to each lower limb, and 1% to the genital area. This method adds up to a total of 101% but provides an easy way to make approximate determinations.

By using the rule of nines, you can add up the areas affected by burns to determine how much of the patient's body has been injured. For example, if an adult patient has full-thickness thermal burns to the chest and front of one leg, this 9% plus 9% means 18% of the total BSA has been burned. Note that burns often overlap different body regions. So, when in doubt, always estimate to the higher percentage.

Emergency Care of Burns

LO18 Explain the proper care for patients with superficial, partial-thickness, and full-thickness burns.

Regardless of the system used to evaluate burns, follow these guidelines:

- Perform a primary assessment and ensure an open airway and adequate breathing.
- Provide care for all burns, even the most minor or superficial ones.

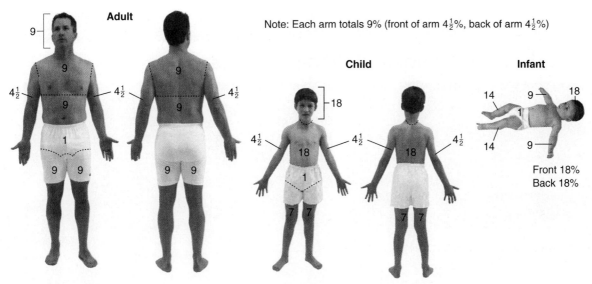

Figure 18.28 The rule of nines for estimating body surface area affected by burns.

- The following partial- or full-thickness burns should be considered serious and should be evaluated by a health care provider:
  - Burns to the hands, feet, face, groin, buttocks, thighs, and major joints
  - Any burn that encircles a body part
  - Burns estimated at greater than 15% of the patient's body surface area
  - Burns that include respiratory system involvement
- When in doubt, overestimate the amount of area affected.
- Always consider the effects of a burn to be more serious if the patient is a child, older adult, or a person with a medical condition (such as respiratory disease) or who has other injuries.

For emergency care of a patient with burns, take BSI precautions and follow these steps:

1. Stop the burning process immediately. This may require the patient to stop, drop, and roll to extinguish the flames. You might also have to smother the flames and wet down or remove smoldering clothing.
2. Flush superficial burns with water (or saline) for several minutes. For partial- or full-thickness burns, do not flush with water unless they involve an area of less than 15% of the total BSA. Flushing large burn areas may cause the patient to become chilled. Follow local protocols.
3. Remove smoldering clothing and jewelry. Do not remove any clothing that is melted onto the skin.
4. Continually monitor the airway. Any burns to the face or exposure to smoke may cause airway problems. Administer oxygen per local protocols.
5. Prevent further contamination. Keep the burned area clean by covering it with a dressing. Infection is common with burns.
6. Cover partial- and full-thickness burns with dry, sterile dressings if available. In some EMS systems, you may be instructed to moisten dressings before placing them on the patient. Otherwise, place dry, sterile dressings onto the burned area. Follow local protocols.
7. If the eyes or eyelids have been burned, place clean dressings or pads over them. Moisten these pads with sterile water if possible.
8. If a serious burn involves the hands or feet, always place a clean pad between toes or fingers before completing the dressing.
9. Provide oxygen and care for shock.

Specialized commercial dressings are designed specifically for burn injuries (Key Skill 18.4). These dressings are typically sterile and come presoaked in a special solution that promotes cooling. These are used widely by the military and are becoming more commonplace in many EMS systems.

> **REMEMBER**
>
> Burns are some of the most disturbing injuries. Severe burns often smell foul, and the amount of tissue destruction can be nauseating for both you and your patient. Caring for these patients will require you to steel your nerves and concentrate on providing the proper treatment. Being prepared for this is half the battle.

Using Premoistened Commercial Burn Dressings

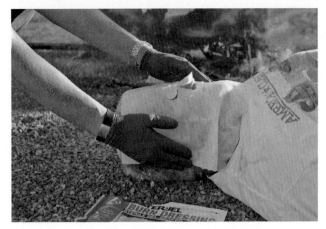

1. Burns to the face covered with premoistened commercial dressing (WaterJel® Burn Dressing).

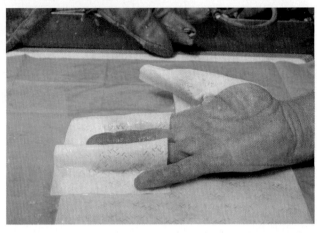

2. Premoistened commercial dressing used to care for a burn to the hand. Separate the fingers.

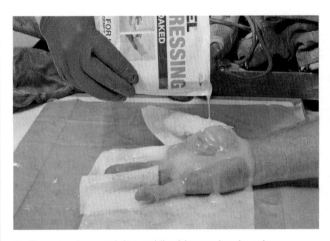

3. Then apply remaining gel liquid over the dressing.

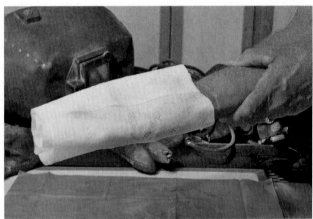

4. Wrap the entire hand.

Thermal Burns

LO19 Differentiate the care for thermal, chemical, and electrical burns.

See Key Skill 18.5 for a summary of caring for thermal burns.

Chemical Burns

LO19 Differentiate the care for thermal, chemical, and electrical burns.

Many chemicals are harmless if they are used properly or remain contained. However, if those chemicals come in contact with the human body, they can cause harm. Some irritate the skin and create burns very quickly. Others create a slow, painful burning process. In either case, it is crucial to stop the burning process and remove the irritant (Figure 18.29).

Scenes involving patients with chemical burns can be very dangerous. Thus, completing a scene size-up and ensuring scene safety is important. If you believe there are hazards at the scene that will place you in danger, do not attempt a rescue unless you have been trained to do so and have the necessary equipment.

Assessment and Care of Thermal Burns

DEPTH OF BURN	TISSUE BURNED			COLOR CHANGES	PAIN	BLISTERS
	EPIDERMIS	DERMIS	SUBCUTANEOUS			
Superficial	Yes	No	No	Red	Yes	No
Partial-thickness	Yes	Yes	No	Deep red	Yes	Yes
Full-thickness	Yes	Yes	Yes	Charred black or white	Yes	Yes

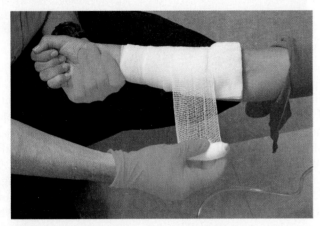

SERIOUS BURNS: Partial-thickness and full-thickness burns

- Stop the burning process.
- Support the ABCs.
- Wrap the area with dry, clean dressings.
- Provide care for shock.
- Moisten the dressing only if the burn is less than 9% of the skin surface. Follow local protocols.

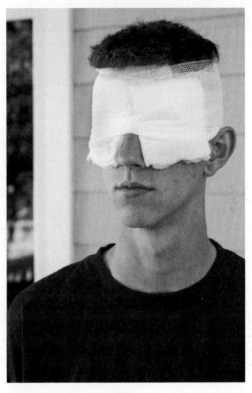

Burns to the eyes:

- Do not open the eyelids if they are burned.
- Be certain the burn is thermal, not chemical.
- Apply moist, clean gauze pads to both eyes.

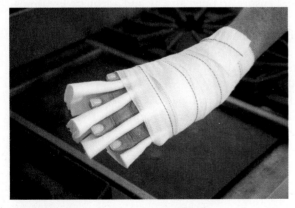

If hands or toes are burned:

- Separate digits with clean gauze pads. Do not pull them apart if they are stuck together.

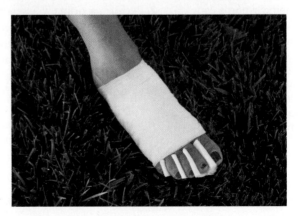

- When appropriate, elevate the extremity.

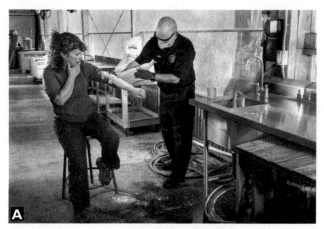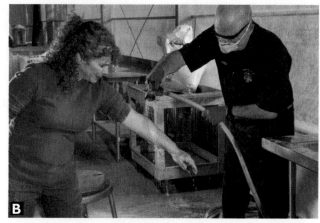

Figure 18.29 Chemical burns: (A) Brush away dried powders, then (B) flush the skin with water.

The primary method of caring for most chemical burns is to wash away the chemical with water. First, you must verify what the chemical is and/or ask those at the scene who may know the proper method for dealing with the chemical. In most cases, a simple wetting of the burned area is not enough. Flush the area of the patient's body that has been exposed. Continue to flush the area for at least 20 minutes. Be sure to remove all contaminated clothing, shoes, socks, and jewelry from the patient during the wash.

Once you have flushed the area for at least 20 minutes, apply a dry sterile dressing, care for shock, and make sure EMS has been notified. If the patient begins to complain of increased burning or irritation once a dressing is in place, remove the dressing and flush the burned area with water for several minutes more. Then apply a new dry dressing.

When providing emergency care for chemical burns:

1. Flush the burned area for at least 20 minutes. If possible and if it can be done quickly, try to identify any chemical powders before applying water.
2. Apply a dry sterile dressing.
3. If burning continues, remove the dressing and flush again.

If dry lime is the agent causing the burn, *do not* begin by flushing with water. Instead, use a *dry* dressing to *brush* the substance off the patient's skin, hair, and clothing. Also have the patient remove any contaminated clothing or jewelry. Once this is done, you may flush the area with water.

Chemical burns to the eyes require immediate attention. Assume that both eyes are involved. When caring for chemical burns to the eyes, you should:

1. Take appropriate BSI precautions.
2. Perform a primary assessment and ensure an open airway and adequate breathing.
3. Immediately flush the eyes with clean water.
4. Keep the water flowing from a faucet, bucket, or other source into the eyes. Use caution not to contaminate the good eye, if one eye is not affected, as you flush. Keep the good eye up and the injured eye down to prevent cross-contamination.
5. Continue flushing for at least 20 minutes.
6. After flushing the eyes, cover both with moistened pads.
7. Remove the pads and flush again if the patient begins to complain about increased burning sensations or irritation.

Electrical Burns

LO19 Differentiate the care for thermal, chemical, and electrical burns.

On the scene of an electrical injury, electrical burns (Figure 18.30) are not usually the most serious problem a patient sustains. Cardiac arrest, nervous system damage, fractures, and injury to internal organs may occur with these incidents

SCENE SAFETY

Scenes involving patients with chemical burns can be very dangerous. If there are hazards at the scene that will place you in danger, do not attempt a rescue unless you have been trained to do so and have the necessary equipment.

The scene of an electrical injury is often very hazardous. Make sure the source of electricity has been turned off before caring for the patient. If the electricity is still active, do not attempt a rescue unless you have been trained to do so and have the necessary equipment.

To provide emergency care for a patient with an electrical burn, you should:

1. Perform a scene size-up and take appropriate BSI precautions.
2. Perform a primary assessment and ensure an open airway and adequate breathing.
3. Evaluate the burn. Look for two burn sites: an entrance and an exit wound. The entrance wound (often the hand) is where the electricity entered the body. The exit wound is where the electricity came into contact with a ground (often a foot). The entrance wound may be small, and you may need to look very carefully for it. The exit wound may be large and obvious.
4. Apply dry, clean dressings to the burn sites. You may apply moistened dressings if transport is delayed, the burn involves less than 9% of the body surface area, and the patient will not be in a cold environment.
5. Provide oxygen and care for shock.

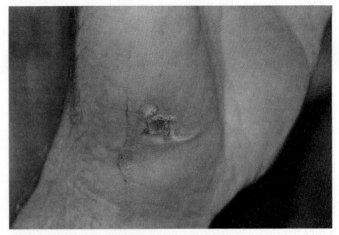
Figure 18.30 Electrical burn to the hand.
(© Edward T. Dickinson, MD)

Infants and Children

Children are frequently the victims of accidental burns, but it is all too common that burns are used by adults as a form of discipline or punishment. As an advocate for the patient, carefully evaluate the injuries and the story provided by the caregivers. Remain objective and focus on caring for the child. Consider the possibility of child abuse when the injuries and the explanation provided are not consistent. If the burns are suspicious, document your findings carefully. Report your suspicion to the appropriate authorities.

FIRST ON SCENE WRAP-UP

Gina has just finished dressing and bandaging Casey's finger when an ambulance arrives with sirens blaring. Casey has regained some of his color and says the nausea is pretty much gone but that the pain is understandably still "10 out of 10."

The EMTs thank Taine for activating the EMS system and Gina for caring for Casey appropriately when he started to go into shock.

The ambulance pulls out of the parking lot to transport Casey to the nearest trauma center. Gina takes several deep breaths as she walks back into the truck stop. She smiles, knowing that Casey will be okay.

Summary

- To prevent possible exposure to infectious diseases while caring for patients who are bleeding, BSI precautions and personal protective equipment (PPE) such as gloves and eye protection should be used.
- Arterial bleeding is characterized by blood that spurts or sprays from a wound. Venous bleeding can be heavy but flows steadily from a wound. Capillary bleeding will slowly ooze from a wound.
- If a patient is bleeding from an open wound, you should apply direct pressure and a pressure bandage to control bleeding. If these techniques don't work, consider applying a tourniquet.
- Dressings are made of clean or sterile cloth. They help control bleeding and protect wounds from contamination. Bandages are used to hold dressings in place.
- Bruising, swelling, abdominal rigidity or guarding, vomiting blood, bleeding from the rectum or vagina, or the onset of shock following blunt trauma can all indicate internal bleeding from a closed wound. Emergency care for internal bleeding involves recognition, activating the EMS system, keeping the patient still and comfortable, being alert for vomiting, and treating for shock.
- Open wounds include abrasions, lacerations (incisions and jagged cuts), avulsions, punctures, and amputations.
- Impaled objects should be stabilized in place using bulky dressings or improvised materials. Never remove an impaled object unless it is interfering with the patient's airway.
- Multisystem trauma occurs when a patient has sustained a significant mechanism of injury that has caused trauma to multiple body systems, such as the skin, muscles, circulation, and nerves. It is often characterized by the signs and symptoms of internal and external bleeding, pain in numerous locations, altered levels of consciousness, and the rapid onset of shock.
- Amputations should initially be cared for with direct pressure or tourniquets to control bleeding. The patient should then be treated for shock and transported by ambulance (with the amputated part) as soon as possible.
- Eye injuries can be very serious and must be treated carefully to prevent permanent damage and blindness. Although it is important to cover the uninjured eye to prevent movement of the injured eye, this can be frightening to the patient. Constantly reassure these patients by speaking to them and touching them gently.
- Nosebleeds should be cared for by pinching the nostrils together and having the patient lean forward. Activate the EMS system if the bleeding cannot be controlled or grows worse.
- The three burn classifications based on depth of the injury are superficial, partial thickness, and full thickness. Superficial burns can be red and painful but are not generally serious because they affect only the top layer of the skin. Partial-thickness burns are more severe, with the damage reaching into the dermis and presenting with pain, swelling, and blisters. Full-thickness burns cause damage down to the bone, killing affected nerves and tissues and presenting with white, rigid skin and very little pain.
- The rule of nines is a widely accepted method of determining the body surface area affected by a burn. It divides the body into sections valued in 9% increments and allows for easy estimation of the burned area.
- Burns are treated by first stopping the burning process and removing any affected clothing or jewelry. For chemical burns, the chemicals should be flushed thoroughly with large amounts of water (after first brushing off any dry chemicals). Dry lime should be brushed away before flushing with water. For electrical burns, the source must be determined and shut off immediately. Burned areas should then be covered with dry, sterile gauze while awaiting the arrival of EMS personnel. For severe burns, you should constantly monitor the patient's airway and treat for shock.

Take Action

The Spill Drill

This activity will help you to become better at estimating external blood loss. Like any other skill you will learn, it will take practice to acquire and to remain proficient at it. You will need a fellow student, a metric measuring cup, and some red food coloring.

1. Without letting your partner know the amount, add water to the measuring cup and put in a few drops of red food coloring to simulate blood.
2. Find a hard floor surface onto which you can pour the water without creating a hazard or a stain.
3. Have your partner examine the spill and estimate the amount of liquid spilled onto the floor.

Take turns and use different amounts of water and see how closely you can come to estimating the fluid amounts. Once you and your partner get more proficient at guessing, try putting the water onto some old clothing. Since clothing absorbs fluid, it becomes much more of a challenge to guess the amount.

Guess the BSA

This is an easy yet practical way to quickly learn the skill of estimating body surface area (BSA). Estimating BSA is commonly done for burn patients because some facilities can manage only small burns and some patients may need to be transported to burn centers for immediate care.

1. Working in groups of three or four, have one person determine a body part or area of the body to be affected and describe it to the others.
2. The others must then estimate the percentage of BSA affected according to the description given.
3. Everyone then compares answers to see if they all agree. If they do not, find out why.

The activity should continue until all in the group have had the opportunity to choose an injury.

First on Scene Patient Handoff

I arrived on scene to find a 35-year-old male in the fetal position clutching his left hand. The patient's chief complaint was 10/10 pain to the left ring finger. Upon exposing the injury, the flesh on the finger was removed. The patient was showing signs and symptoms of shock, so treatment of warming the patient and making him more comfortable were implemented. The patient was A&O × 4, his skin was pale, cool, and clammy. This was improved to pink, warm, and clammy by giving the patient layers. The patient vomited one time prior to EMS arrival. The patient's medication and emergency information is saved on his phone.

First on Scene Run Review

Recall the events of the First on Scene scenario in this chapter and answer the following questions related to the call. Rationales are offered in the Answer Key at the back of the book.

1. Given the type of injury that Casey sustained, what type of bleeding is most likely?
2. Since the wound was not actively bleeding, what should be your next priority?
3. Could the skin from the finger be reattached, and how would you transport it?
4. Once the wound is cared for, what additional treatment is appropriate for Casey?

Quick Quiz

To check your understanding of the chapter, answer the following questions. Then compare your answers to those in the Answer Key at the back of the book.

1. Which of the following is NOT a typical characteristic of arterial bleeding?

   a. Blood spurts from the wound.
   b. Blood flows slowly from the wound.
   c. The color of the blood is bright red.
   d. Blood loss is often profuse in a short period of time.

2. Which of the following describes the appropriate body substance isolation (BSI) precautions to use when caring for a patient with external bleeding?

   a. Sterile gloves
   b. Face shield and gown
   c. Gloves and goggles
   d. N95 mask and safety goggles

3. Most cases of external bleeding can be controlled by:

   a. applying direct pressure.
   b. using a tourniquet.
   c. securing a pressure bandage.
   d. applying a clotting agent.

4. The material placed directly over a wound to help control bleeding is called a(n):

   a. bandage.
   b. elastic bandage.
   c. occlusive dressing.
   d. dressing.

5. A wound in which the top layers of skin have been scraped off, commonly seen in falls, can best be described as a(n):

   a. abrasion.
   b. amputation.
   c. laceration.
   d. avulsion.

6. You are caring for a patient with a severe soft tissue injury to the lower leg. You have exposed the wound, and it is bleeding. What should you do?

   a. Apply direct pressure.
   b. Remove debris from the wound.
   c. Care for shock.
   d. Elevate the extremity.

7. A 37-year-old female has cut her arm while using a circular saw. The wound continues to bleed heavily despite the direct pressure and bandage you have applied. You should:

   a. reapply the pressure bandage.
   b. apply a tourniquet.
   c. have the patient hold her arm above her head.
   d. check her blood pressure.

8. A patient has a small wooden splinter impaled in their eye. You should:

   a. remove the splinter.
   b. instruct the patient to look down and to the left.
   c. gently bandage both eyes.
   d. bandage only the injured eye.

9. Which of the following patients is most at risk for multisystem trauma?

   a. 16-year-old girl who fell 4 feet from a ladder
   b. 66-year-old woman ejected from a vehicle rollover
   c. 44-year-old man whose foot was crushed by a forklift
   d. 27-year-old man struck in the head by a baseball bat

10. Your patient has burned his hand. The skin is red and blistered, and the burn is extremely painful. You would classify this burn as:

    a. superficial.
    b. partial thickness.
    c. full thickness.
    d. severe.

11. Your patient shows signs of shock, and you suspect she is bleeding internally. You should:

    a. facilitate immediate transport.
    b. allow her to take sips of water.
    c. withhold oxygen.
    d. elevate her feet.

12. Which of the following mechanisms would most likely cause serious internal bleeding?

    a. Ground-level fall
    b. Thermal burn
    c. Blunt force trauma
    d. Low-speed vehicle collision

13. Which of the following best describes the appropriate care for an amputated body part?

    a. Wrap it with clean gauze and place it on ice.
    b. Apply a tourniquet to the exposed end of the part.
    c. Bandage the part back onto the body.
    d. Place the part in sterile water.

14. A 33-year-old male cut himself with a hunting knife. He has a large flap of skin partially hanging off his arm. This wound would best be described as a(n):

    a. laceration.
    b. abrasion.
    c. amputation.
    d. avulsion.

15. A 23-year-old woman has been kicked in the abdomen by a horse. She is alert and oriented and complaining of pain to her lower abdomen. You should suspect:

    a. a flail chest.
    b. internal bleeding.
    c. a fractured pelvis.
    d. an ectopic pregnancy.

16. Your patient has been impaled through the right thigh by a long piece of metal bar. You should:

    a. carefully remove the object.
    b. tie both legs together.
    c. stabilize the object with bulky dressings.
    d. cut both ends of the bar to make it shorter.

17. A 22-year-old female splashed a chemical into her eye during a chemistry lab. She states repeatedly that her eye is "burning." You should first:

    a. cover both eyes with dry dressings.
    b. instruct her to blink rapidly.
    c. wipe her eyes with moist dressings.
    d. flush both eyes with water for 20 minutes.

18. You arrive on the scene to find a young girl with an active nosebleed. She is crying and the sight of the blood is scaring her. You should:

    a. position her on her side while holding pressure on the nose.
    b. have her lean forward while you pinch the nostrils.
    c. have her lean backward as far as possible while holding the nose.
    d. pack both nostrils with sterile gauze.

19. You are caring for a burn victim who has partial-thickness burns covering his right arm and the front of his entire torso. What is the estimated BSA affected?

    a. 18%
    b. 25%
    c. 27%
    d. 36%

20. You are caring for a burn victim with both partial- and full-thickness burns over 40% of her body. You should first:

    a. cover her with sterile burn sheets.
    b. ensure that the burning process has stopped.
    c. apply moist dressings over the burns.
    d. not cover the burns, but you should arrange transport.

Endnotes

1. Mortality in the United States, 2021. Centers for Disease Control and Prevention, National Center for Health Statistics, NCHS Data Brief No. 456, December 2022, accessed April 12, 2023. https://www.cdc.gov/nchs/data/databriefs/db456.pdf

2. D. Markenson, J.D. Ferguson, L. Chameides, P. Cassan, K.L. Chung, J. Epstein, L. Gonzales, R.A. Herrington, J.L. Pellegrino, N. Ratcliff, and A. Singer, "2015 American Heart Association and American Red Cross Guidelines for First Aid," *Circulation*, Vol. 132 (2015): S269–S311, originally published October 14, 2015.

3. Ibid.

4. C. Beaucreux, B. Vivien, E. Miles, S. Ausset, and P. Pasquier, "Application of Tourniquet in Civilian Trauma: Systematic Review of the Literature," *Anaesthesia Critical Care and Pain Medicine* (January 2018) pii: S2352-5568(17)30265-5. doi: 10.1016/j.accpm.2017.11.017.

5. D. Markenson, J. D. Ferguson, L. Chameides, P. Cassan, K.L. Chung, J. Epstein, L. Gonzales, R.A. Herrington, J.L. Pellegrino, N. Ratcliff, and A. Singer, "2015 American Heart Association and American Red Cross Guidelines for First Aid," *Circulation*, Vol. 132 (2015): S269–S311, originally published October 14, 2015.

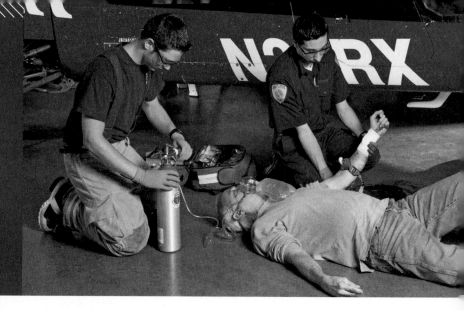

19

Recognition and Care of Shock

Education Standards

Shock and Resuscitation

Trauma—Bleeding, Multisystem Trauma

Competencies

Uses assessment information to recognize shock based on assessment findings and manages the emergency while awaiting additional emergency response.

LEARNING OBJECTIVES

Upon successful completion of this chapter, the student should be able to:

Cognitive

1. Define the chapter key terms.
2. Explain the pathophysiology of shock.
3. Describe the four categories of shock.
4. List the six main types of shock and their causes.
5. Describe the signs and symptoms of shock.
6. Explain the proper care of a patient presenting with signs and symptoms of shock.

Psychomotor

7. Demonstrate the proper techniques for caring for a patient at risk for shock.

Affective

8. Value the importance of proper body substance isolation (BSI) precautions when caring for a patient with suspected shock.

KEY TERMS

anaphylactic shock (*p. 403*)
cardiogenic shock (*p. 401*)
compensated shock (*p. 404*)
decompensated shock (*p. 404*)
hemorrhagic shock (*p. 403*)
hypotension (*p. 401*)
hypovolemic shock (*p. 402*)

neurogenic shock (*p. 403*)
psychogenic shock (*p. 404*)
pericardial tamponade (*p. 402*)
pulmonary embolism (*p. 402*)
septic shock (*p. 404*)
tension pneumothorax (*p. 402*)

According to the Centers for Disease Control and Prevention (CDC), unintentional injuries are the fourth leading cause of death in the United States.[1] Many of those deaths can be directly attributed to the shock that almost always develops secondary to injury. This is why it is so critical for Emergency Medical Responders to understand the process of shock and know how to anticipate it, recognize it, and most importantly, how to care for patients who experience it. Early identification, appropriate care, and coordinating rapid transport contribute greatly to the patient's chance of survival. This chapter covers the four primary categories of shock and common types of shock and provides guidance on how to recognize and care for patients experiencing this life-threatening condition.

Irv, an Emergency Medical Responder and firefighter, has just finished washing the engine parked in the driveway of Station 4 when the radio buzzes to life.

"Engine 4, ready to copy?" The dispatcher pauses briefly and then continues. "You're going to 9-1-4-4 Founders Parkway, the Smith Cabinet Shop, for a power saw injury."

"Engine 4 responding from the station." Irv keys the portable radio. Another firefighter appears in the truck bay, followed closely by one more, and they all climb up into the glistening red truck while Irv starts the engine.

"Wow," Cass, the last one into the truck, says as he bounces into the passenger seat. "I hope it's not like that last call we had out there. Remember? That guy with the amputated hand."

"I remember." Irv frowns. The road dust the tires are kicking up is already settling on the truck, which is still wet from washing.

Perfusion and Shock

| LO2 | Explain the pathophysiology of shock. |
| LO3 | Describe the four categories of shock. |

Recall from Chapter 4 that *perfusion* is the adequate delivery of well-oxygenated blood and nutrients to the cells of the body and the proper elimination of waste products. During normal perfusion, oxygen, carbon dioxide, nutrients, and waste products are all exchanged properly.

Shock (defined in Chapter 5), also known as *hypoperfusion*, results when one or more of these processes fails (Figure 19.1). The development of shock is progressive and can occur rapidly or slowly. For instance, a patient with severe bleeding will begin showing the signs of shock within minutes. In contrast, a patient with a slow bleed that goes undetected or uncared for may display the signs of shock slowly over several hours or even days.

Categories of Shock

Shock is a very complex process affecting many body systems. This chapter aims to provide a level of understanding that will allow you to deliver the best care quickly and efficiently while waiting for more advanced care to arrive and transport the patient. The first thing you need to know is that there are different types of shock, each of which falls into one of the following four categories:

- *Cardiogenic shock.* The heart must be functioning properly to maintain a proper blood pressure to circulate blood adequately. If the heart fails to pump an adequate volume of blood, the result can be **hypotension**, an abnormally low blood pressure. **Cardiogenic shock** is sometimes referred to as *pump failure* (Figure 19.2).
- *Distributive shock.* Blood circulates throughout the body via a closed system of vessels. The vessels are made up of smooth muscle and can dilate and constrict, depending on the needs of the body. Certain conditions can cause the vessels to dilate excessively, resulting in a much larger space than the available blood supply can fill. When there is more space within the system than blood to fill it, blood pressure drops and shock results (Figure 19.3).
- *Hypovolemic shock.* The term *hypovolemic* means low fluid volume. **Hypovolemic shock** includes all types of shock caused by a lack of adequate fluid in the body. This lack of fluid can be

hypotension ▸ abnormally low blood pressure.

cardiogenic shock ▸ form of shock caused when the heart is unable to pump blood efficiently.

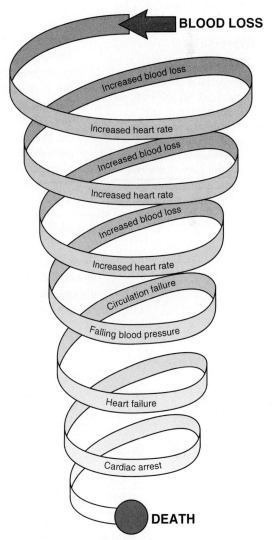

Figure 19.1 If left untreated, blood loss will lead to shock and eventually death.

hypovolemic shock ▶ category of shock caused by an abnormally low fluid volume (blood or plasma) in the body.

pulmonary embolism ▶ blockage of an artery in the lungs.

pericardial tamponade ▶ accumulation of fluid in the sac surrounding the heart, restricting the heart's ability to expand and contract.

tension pneumothorax ▶ accumulation of air in the pleural space, increasing pressure in the chest and reducing the amount of blood returned to the heart.

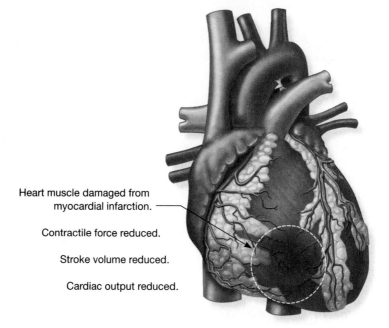

Heart muscle damaged from myocardial infarction.

Contractile force reduced.

Stroke volume reduced.

Cardiac output reduced.

Figure 19.2 Heart attack as a cause of cardiogenic shock: Damaged heart muscle results in reduced force of contractions and reduced cardiac output.

caused by such things as bleeding, burns, vomiting, diarrhea, and severe dehydration. There must be an adequate amount of fluid within the body and circulatory system at all times. If there is a significant loss of fluid volume, blood pressure will drop, and this may lead to the onset of signs and symptoms of shock (Figure 19.4).

- *Obstructive shock.* This is sometimes referred to as a category and a type of shock. The adequate flow of blood can be disrupted due to a variety of obstructions to the heart, lungs, and great vessels. Conditions such as **pulmonary embolism**, **pericardial tamponade**, **tension pneumothorax**, and trauma can all lead to obstructive shock. The obstruction of blood flow reduces perfusion, which can lead to shock (Figure 19.5).

CREW RESOURCE MANAGEMENT

Trauma scenes often involve multiple patients. Every member of the rescue team must be looking for evidence of shock in the patients they are evaluating and must communicate that information to the team leader. Teamwork and constant communication will ensure that the most critical patients get cared for and transported first.

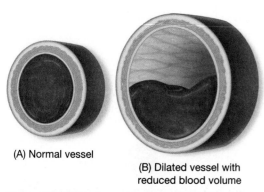

(A) Normal vessel

(B) Dilated vessel with reduced blood volume

Figure 19.3 Shock can be caused by an uncontrolled dilation of the blood vessels.

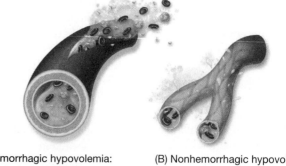

(A) Hemorrhagic hypovolemia: loss of whole blood (plasma and formed elements)

(B) Nonhemorrhagic hypovolemia: loss of plasma

Figure 19.4 (A) Hemorrhagic hypovolemia: loss of blood. (B) Non-hemorrhagic hypovolemia: loss of plasma and other fluids.

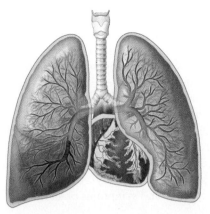
(A) Pulmonary embolism

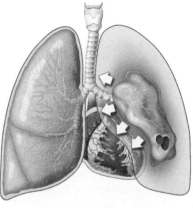
(B) Tension pneumothorax

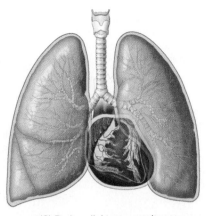
(C) Pericardial tamponade

Figure 19.5 Causes of obstructive shock: (A) pulmonary embolism—blocked artery in a lung, (B) tension pneumothorax—buildup of air inside the chest, (C) pericardial tamponade—accumulation of fluid in the sac around the heart.

 FIRST ON SCENE *(continued)*

As the fire engine pulls up to the large, roll-up door leading to the main cabinet workshop, the crew is greeted by a nervous-looking man with blood soaking the front of his denim apron.

"He's just inside," the man tells them. "A broken saw blade hit his arm, and he's bleedin' like a stuck pig."

The patient, a 28-year-old carpenter named Parker, is holding a blood-soaked towel tightly around his left forearm and leaning unsteadily against a workbench. Cass immediately notices that Parker's clothes are soaked with blood, and he is very pale.

"Tell you what," Irv says as he wraps both of his gloved hands tightly around the bleeding limb. "Let's get you down on the floor and more comfortable."

"I was . . . I was working on a hinge cutout . . . and . . . and . . ." The man's voice trails off and sweat begins to accumulate on his forehead.

"Quick," Cass says. "Lay him down. Someone get me a blanket or some jackets."

Types of Shock

LO4 List the six main types of shock and their causes.

There are six main types of shock. Most of these fall into one of the four categories described in the previous section. A patient may experience one or more of the following types of shock:

- *Hemorrhagic shock.* A form of hypovolemic shock, **hemorrhagic shock** occurs when the body loses a significant amount of whole blood from the circulatory system. It can be caused by uncontrolled internal or external bleeding. When the body loses significant amounts of blood, it can no longer maintain an adequate blood pressure or carry oxygen to the vital organs

- *Cardiogenic shock.* **Cardiogenic shock** is both a category and specific type of shock that results when the heart is unable to pump enough blood at a consistent pressure to the vital organs. The heart can become damaged due to trauma or from a heart attack, making it unable to pump blood efficiently.

- *Neurogenic shock.* A form of distributive shock, **neurogenic shock** occurs when the spinal cord is damaged and is unable to control the tone (size) of the blood vessels by way of the sympathetic nervous system. The vessels dilate uncontrollably, causing an increase in the space within the circulatory system, which in turn causes a drop in blood pressure. This results in inadequate perfusion and shock.

- *Anaphylactic shock.* A form of distributive shock, **anaphylactic shock** is caused when the body experiences anaphylaxis, a severe and potentially life-threatening allergic reaction. This extreme reaction causes the blood vessels to dilate uncontrollably, resulting in a loss of blood pressure and, thus, perfusion.

hemorrhagic shock ▶ form of hypovolemic shock that occurs when the body loses a significant amount of blood.

neurogenic shock ▶ form of distributive shock resulting from spinal-cord injury.

anaphylactic shock ▶ form of distributive shock caused by a severe allergic reaction.

- *Psychogenic shock.* A form of distributive shock, **psychogenic shock** often causes fainting. It usually occurs when an emotional factor, such as fear, causes the nervous system to react and rapidly dilate the blood vessels. This rapid dilation of the vessels is followed by a sudden drop in blood pressure, which disrupts the flow of blood to the brain. In most cases, this is a self-correcting form of shock. Once the patient lies down, the situation will correct itself and the blood pressure should return to normal.

- *Septic shock.* A form of distributive shock, **septic shock** is a life-threatening drop in blood pressure caused by sepsis, the body's extreme overreaction to an infection that can damage multiple organ systems (see Chapter 16). Symptoms include low blood pressure, pale and cool arms and legs, chills, difficulty breathing, and decreased urine output. Mental confusion and disorientation may also develop quickly. As in other cases of shock, perfusion is compromised, leading to signs and symptoms of shock.

The Body's Response During Shock

The human body has an amazing ability to adjust and compensate when things go wrong. In the case of shock, sophisticated pressure receptors called *baroreceptors* throughout the circulatory system can detect the slightest change in blood pressure long before any outward signs of shock appear.

In the early stages of shock, the sympathetic nervous system is activated and causes changes that include increased heart rate, constriction of the blood vessels, and increased contraction of the heart. These changes work together to help maintain an adequate blood pressure, which is necessary for perfusion. A process called **compensated shock** is the body's attempt to compensate for a drop in blood pressure.

As the body detects the slightest drop in pressure within the circulatory system, it releases hormones such as epinephrine that will increase heart rate in an attempt to maintain blood pressure. If the increase in heart rate alone is not enough to maintain a good blood pressure, additional hormones are released that will constrict the blood vessels in the nonessential areas, such as the skin and intestinal tract.[2] The constriction of these vessels will redirect the blood to the vital organs, where it is needed.

If the root cause of the shock is not corrected soon enough, the body's compensatory mechanisms will begin to fail because they, too, are not receiving adequate perfusion. When this happens, the heart rate begins to slow, breathing slows, and blood pressure drops to a dangerous level. This failure of the normal compensatory mechanisms is **decompensated shock**. If the root cause of the shock is not cared for soon enough, the patient will eventually enter irreversible shock and will die.

Signs and Symptoms of Shock

LO5 Describe the signs and symptoms of shock.

As previously noted, shock is a progressive process that the body uses to compensate for poor perfusion, and the signs and symptoms typically develop over time. Depending on the severity of the situation, the signs of shock can appear over several minutes to several hours.

The early signs and symptoms of shock are restlessness, anxiety, altered mental status, increased heart rate, normal to slightly low blood pressure, and mildly increased breathing rate. As shock progresses, the patient's skin may become pale, cool, and moist, and they may experience nausea and vomiting. Pupils become sluggish and dilated.

Those signs and symptoms follow the order in which they may be detected during the primary assessment. However, all signs and symptoms of shock may not present at once, and they do not necessarily occur in the order listed. Look for the following signs:

- *Restlessness or combativeness.* The patient is reacting to the body's loss of adequate perfusion. They feel that something is wrong and may be afraid. In some cases, this behavioral change may be the first sign of developing shock.

- *Changes in mental status.* As adequate circulation to the brain continues to fail, the patient will become confused, disoriented, sleepy, or unresponsive. Changes in mental status are some of the most sensitive and predictable signs of shock.

- *Increased pulse rate.* The body is trying to compensate for a drop in blood pressure and poor perfusion.
- *Pale, cool, moist skin.* As blood is redirected to the vital organs from the skin, the skin will become pale and feel cool to the touch. Capillary refill will be much slower than normal. Stimulation from the sympathetic nervous system also causes sweating.
- *Respiratory and cardiac arrest.* As the body's ability to compensate weakens, respiratory and cardiac arrest are inevitable.

If the cause of shock is not stopped, the compensatory mechanisms will begin to fail, resulting in decompensated shock. The late signs and symptoms that appear as the patient enters decompensated shock are unresponsiveness, decreasing heart rate, very low blood pressure, slow and shallow respirations, skin that is pale, cool, and moist, and pupils that are sluggish and dilated.

Mechanism of Injury and Shock

LO6 Explain the proper care of a patient presenting with signs and symptoms of shock.

One of the keys to the successful care of trauma patients is to operate on the assumption that internal bleeding is likely based on the mechanism of injury (MOI). Do not wait for signs and symptoms to develop before you begin caring for shock. In cases of trauma or injury, examine and consider the MOI carefully. If there is any chance that the patient may have sustained blunt trauma to the head, chest, abdomen, or pelvis, suspect that internal bleeding exists and care for the patient accordingly. Of course, you must also identify and stop all external bleeding immediately upon discovery.

Caring for Shock

In most cases, the patient will require more advanced care both in the field and in the hospital. However, if shock is recognized early on, the Emergency Medical Responder can provide care that will minimize its progression and ensure prompt transport to the hospital.

Help delay the progression of shock by doing the following:

1. Perform a primary assessment and ensure an open airway and adequate breathing.
2. Control all major external bleeding.
3. Administer oxygen per local protocols.
4. Keep the patient in a supine position.
5. Calm and reassure the patient and maintain a normal body temperature by covering them with a blanket.
6. Continue to monitor and support the ABCs.
7. Do not give the patient anything by mouth. Even if the patient expresses serious thirst, do not give any fluids or food, and be alert for vomiting.
8. Monitor the patient's vital signs. This must be done at least every 5 minutes.
9. Expedite transport to a trauma center if available.

You will not be able to reverse shock, but you may be able to delay its progression by following the procedures described. If you are trained to do so and your state laws allow, oxygen can be significant in the care of patients experiencing shock. Administer oxygen per local protocols.

Fainting

Fainting, also known as syncope, is a brief loss of consciousness because of a reduction in blood flow to the brain. It most often is a self-correcting form of mild temporary shock, also called *psychogenic shock*. It's important to consider that the patient may have been injured in a fall due to fainting. Be certain to examine the patient who has fainted for injury. Even if no other problems are apparent, keep them lying down and at rest for several minutes.

JEDI

One sign of shock is pale skin as blood moves away from the extremities toward the vital organs. Since there is such a wide range of variation in skin pigmentation, you must look for as many signs and symptoms as possible. You can look at mucous membranes and/or capillary refill to help you assess for adequate perfusion.

REMEMBER

Lack of perfusion results in shock, and the organ that depends most on perfusion is the brain. That is why an altered mental status is the most sensitive indicator for the presence of shock. Therefore, any patient with an altered mental status should be suspected of being in shock until it is proved otherwise.

REMEMBER

Provide care for all injured patients as if shock will develop. Carefully monitor all patients for early signs of shock.

REMEMBER

Even after finding success with using tourniquets for bleeding injuries, the U.S. military continued to lose patients to shock. Research found that hypothermia was the cause. Keep your patients warm because they are unable to maintain normal body temperature when they are in shock.

Fainting can also be a warning of a serious underlying condition such as a brain tumor, heart disease, or diabetes. Always recommend that the patient see a health care provider as soon as possible if they experience a fainting spell.

FIRST ON SCENE WRAP-UP

Parker is carefully lowered to the floor in a supine position and covered with a blanket. Irv controls the bleeding with a pressure bandage and tourniquet and places a nonrebreather mask at 15 LPM of oxygen. Within a few minutes, an ambulance arrives and rapidly transports Parker to the trauma center, where he is treated for shock, blood loss, and a deep laceration on his left forearm.

Parker is released from the hospital the next morning and, except for some weakness in one finger, makes a full recovery. He has since returned to work and is proudly working on a new set of cabinets that his company is donating to the Station 4 kitchen.

Summary

- Perfusion is the adequate delivery of well-oxygenated blood and nutrients to the cells of the body and the proper elimination of waste products.
- Shock, also known as hypoperfusion, is the failure of the body's circulatory system to provide enough oxygenated blood and nutrients to the cells of the body.
- The signs and symptoms of shock include increased pulse; increased breathing rate; restlessness or combativeness; pale, cool, and moist skin; nausea and vomiting; and loss of responsiveness.
- There are several types of shock, each falling into one of four main categories. The four categories of shock are cardiogenic shock, hypovolemic shock, distributive shock, and obstructive shock.
- It is important to begin caring for shock if the mechanism of injury suggests internal injury or bleeding.
- Do not wait for the signs and symptoms to appear before caring for shock.
- Care for shock includes supporting the ABCs, keeping the patient lying flat, controlling all external bleeding, administering oxygen if allowed, maintaining a normal body temperature, and expediting transport.

Take Action

You Can Run, But you Cannot Hide

This activity will help you become better at taking repeated sets of vital signs, an important skill when monitoring patients for shock. You will need a blood pressure cuff, a stethoscope, and another student to act as your patient. Then follow these steps:

1. To begin, take a complete set of baseline vital signs on your partner, and record them on a piece of paper.
2. Now have your partner run a predetermined course. It can be several hundred yards or up and down several flights of stairs. The goal is to get the pulse well above the resting rate.
3. Once your partner returns, have them immediately lie down, and obtain their blood pressure, pulse, and respirations. Record them on the same paper.
4. Wait 5 minutes (as your "patient" relaxes) and repeat the vitals.
5. Obtain the vital signs at least 3 times or until they have returned to normal.

This activity will allow you to get practice taking vital signs on someone other than a resting simulated patient. It will also give you more practice taking vitals quickly and comparing each set with the previous set—just as you would when monitoring a patient for shock.

First on Scene Patient Handoff

Parker is a 28-year-old male who sustained a large open wound to his left forearm caused by a broken saw blade. We observed a 6-inch open wound and have controlled the bleeding with a pressure bandage and tourniquet. We estimate the patient lost 1 liter of blood. Parker is A&O × 4 and vitals are respirations 24, good tidal volume and unlabored, pulse 104 and regular, the last BP was 136/86, skin is pale, cool, and moist. We have him on 15 LPM by nonrebreather mask, and patient states the only medical history is insulin-controlled diabetes.

First on Scene Run Review

Recall the events of the First on Scene scenario in this chapter, and answer the following questions related to the call. Rationales are offered in the Answer Key at the back of the book.

1. What information would you want from dispatch en route to the call?
2. Why did Irv place the patient down on the floor?
3. How would you control the bleeding?

Quick Quiz

To check your understanding of the chapter, answer the following questions. Then compare your answers to those in the Answer Key at the back of the book.

1. All of the following are signs of shock EXCEPT:
   a. increased pulse rate.
   b. decreasing blood pressure.
   c. pink, warm, moist skin.
   d. altered mental status.

2. When the body sustains a significant loss of blood, which type of shock is most likely to occur?
   a. Anaphylactic
   b. Cardiogenic
   c. Hemorrhagic
   d. Septic

3. The four categories of shock are:
   a. psychogenic, respiratory, hypoglycemic, neurogenic.
   b. cardiogenic, hypovolemic, distributive, obstructive.
   c. obstructive, anemic, hypoxic, cardiogenic.
   d. hypoxic, ventricular, diabetic, distributive.

4. Psychogenic shock can present as:
   a. hyperperfusion.
   b. a stress reaction.
   c. decompensation.
   d. fainting.

5. Which of the following does NOT describe a common pathophysiology of shock?
   a. Dilated blood vessels
   b. Obstruction of blood flow
   c. Severe fluid loss
   d. Increased total blood volume

6. You arrive at the scene of an unresponsive man who crashed his motorcycle into a tree at a high rate of speed. His skin is pale and clammy, pulse is 44 and weak, and you are unable to obtain a blood pressure. This patient is most likely experiencing _____ shock.
   a. psychogenic
   b. compensated
   c. decompensated
   d. respiratory

7. Which of the following interventions is most important to the survival of a patient showing signs of shock?
   a. Splinting fractures
   b. Immediate transport
   c. Spinal immobilization
   d. Bandaging wounds

8. When injury to the spinal cord causes systemic dilation of the blood vessels, _____ shock develops.
   a. psychogenic
   b. hemorrhagic
   c. compensated
   d. neurogenic

9. You arrive at the scene of a small child who was involved in a car accident. Her only apparent injury is a deformity to her right arm. Which of the following best describes the appropriate care for this child?
   a. Splint the arm and suggest that her parents take her to the hospital.
   b. Assume that she has internal injuries and treat for shock.
   c. Provide oxygen and splint the arm.
   d. Place her on a long backboard and transport.

10. Why does a patient's pulse rate increase as shock develops?
    a. To force oxygenated blood out of the patient's body core
    b. To counteract the high blood pressure
    c. To maintain adequate perfusion
    d. To create more blood to compensate for fluid loss

Endnotes

1. *Mortality in the United States, 2021.* Centers for Disease Control and Prevention, National Center for Health Statistics, NCHS Data Brief No. 456, December 2022, accessed April 12, 2023. https://www.cdc.gov/nchs/data/databriefs/db456.pdf

2. Fabrizio Giuseppe Bonanno, "Physiopathology of Shock," *Journal of Emergencies, Trauma, and Shock*, Vol. 4, No. 2 (2011): 222–232, doi:10.4103/0974-2700.82210.

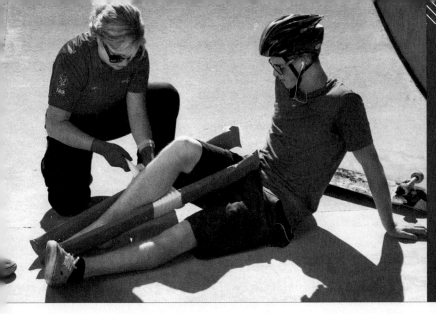

20

Caring for Muscle and Bone Injuries

LEARNING OBJECTIVES

Upon successful completion of this chapter, the student should be able to:

Cognitive

1. Define the chapter key terms.

2. Describe the components that make up the musculoskeletal system.

3. Identify the major bones of the skeletal system.

4. Explain the functions of the musculoskeletal system.

5. Differentiate between direct and indirect forces and the injuries they cause.

6. Differentiate between an open and a closed skeletal injury.

7. Differentiate between a strain, sprain, fracture, and dislocation.

8. Describe the signs and symptoms of a musculoskeletal injury.

9. Explain the importance of an appropriate assessment of the distal extremities.

10. Describe the appropriate care for a patient with a musculoskeletal injury.

11. Explain the priority of care for a patient with a suspected open skeletal injury.

12. Explain the purpose and methods for manual stabilization of a skeletal injury.

13. Explain the criteria for placing an angulated extremity injury into anatomical position.

14. Explain the priority of care for a patient with multisystem trauma.

Psychomotor

15. Demonstrate the appropriate assessment of a skeletal injury.

16. Demonstrate the appropriate care for a patient with a long bone injury.

17. Demonstrate the appropriate care for a patient with a joint injury.

18. Demonstrate the appropriate technique for manual stabilization of a skeletal injury.

19. Demonstrate the proper placement of an angulated extremity injury into an anatomical position.

20. Demonstrate the proper placement of an arm sling.

21. Demonstrate the ability to place the hand/foot in the position of function during immobilization of an extremity.

Affective

22. Value the importance of proper body substance isolation (BSI) precautions when caring for patients with musculoskeletal injuries.

Education Standards

Trauma—Orthopedic Trauma

Competencies

Uses assessment information to recognize shock, respiratory failure or arrest, and cardiac arrest based on assessment findings and manages the emergency while awaiting additional emergency response.

angulated (*p. 416*)

closed fracture (*p. 421*)

cravat (*p. 422*)

dislocation (*p. 415*)

fracture (*p. 415*)

manual stabilization (*p. 420*)

open fracture (*p. 417*)

position of function (*p. 427*)

sling (*p. 424*)

splint (*p. 420*)

sprain (*p. 415*)

strain (*p. 415*)

swathe (*p. 419*)

Bones are the foundation of the body. Like the steel girders that provide the strength and structure for buildings, bones provide the tough, internal structure and support for the demanding activities we put our bodies through on a daily basis. Unlike steel girders, bones are made of living tissue. Bones are able to move and bend by the action of muscles and other tissues, controlled by messages received from the brain via the nervous system.

In your role as an Emergency Medical Responder, you will assist many patients with muscle and bone injuries. This chapter covers the general causes and types of these injuries, signs and symptoms, and the care that should be provided.

FIRST ON SCENE

Ron reaches down, pushes a brightly colored golf tee into the soft ground facing the fairway, and balances his ball on it. "Okay," he says to his wife, Annie, after standing back up. "I'll bet you lunch that I get a birdie on this hole."

"You're on," she says, smiling from her seat in the golf cart. He repositions his feet several times, draws the club back over his shoulder, and swings it in surprisingly good form, considering how the rest of his game has been going. The ball flies high and straight, moving in sharp contrast to the royal blue of the early morning sky. Annie steps from the cart, mouth agape. Using the scorecard to shield her eyes, she follows the ball's descent to the distant green.

"Annie! The cart!" Ron yells, forgetting about the nearly perfect drive.

Annie turns and sees the golf cart rolling slowly backward, gaining speed as it heads for a nearby sand trap. She jogs over to it and tries to step back into the driver's seat but, just as she reaches it, there is a loud snap and her right leg folds underneath her.

She falls to the ground, clutching her badly bent leg. The cart continues down the slope and overturns into the trap, sending a spray of sand onto the fairway.

The Musculoskeletal System

LO2 Describe the components that make up the musculoskeletal system.

LO3 Identify the major bones of the skeletal system.

LO4 Explain the functions of the musculoskeletal system.

The musculoskeletal system is made up of many muscles, bones, joints, and connective tissues. Trauma, whether minor or major, can cause a variety of injuries to the structures and tissues that make up the musculoskeletal system. When assessing those injuries,

Emergency Medical Responders are not expected to determine whether an injury is a fractured bone, a dislocated joint, a ligament sprain, or a muscle strain. Instead, the EMR's job is to carefully assess the patient, looking for signs and symptoms of injury such as pain, swelling, deformity, and discoloration. Sometimes injuries can be easily identified as fractures, dislocations, or both, simply due to the amount of deformity. However, most musculoskeletal injuries are not that obvious, and often pain is the only symptom.

The extremities include the many bones and joints of the arms and legs. Surrounding the bones and joints are muscles and other soft tissues such as ligaments and tendons. Blood vessels and nerves run through and along these structures and tissues. Figure 20.1 shows the major blood vessels and a few of the major nerves in the arms and legs. You do not need to remember every vessel and nerve, but you must remember that a large network of both is woven throughout the skeletal system. Vessels supply bones and muscles with blood and nutrients, and nerves carry signals that control movement. Injuries to blood vessels and nerves can cause swelling, loss of movement, and significant pain. Careful assessment and management is important for minimizing pain, further damage to vessels and nerves, and blood loss.

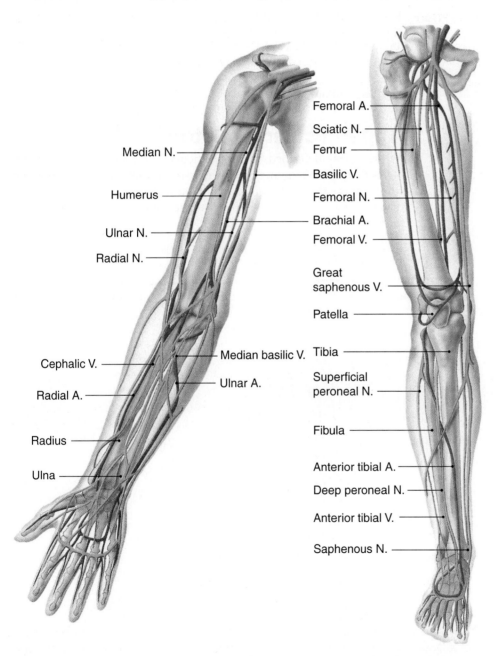

Figure 20.1 Nerves and vessels of the extremities. (A = artery; N = nerve; V = vein.)

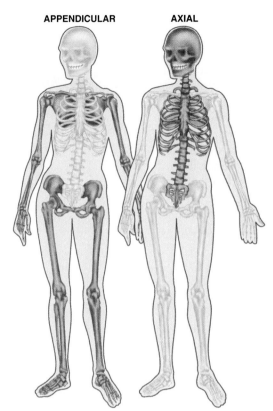

APPENDICULAR   AXIAL

Figure 20.2 The two major divisions of the skeletal system are the appendicular skeleton (left figure) and the axial skeleton (right figure).

The musculoskeletal system has four major functions:

1. *Support.* Bones support the soft tissues of the body, acting as a framework that provides a rigid structure for the attachment of muscles and other body parts.
2. *Movement.* Muscles, bones, and joints act together to produce movement.
3. *Protection.* Many bones in the body provide protection for vital organs: the skull protects the brain; the spine protects the spinal cord; the ribs protect the heart, lungs, liver, stomach, and spleen; and the pelvis protects the urinary bladder and internal reproductive organs.
4. *Cell production.* Some bones have the special function of producing blood cells.

The two major divisions of the skeletal system are the *axial skeleton* and the *appendicular skeleton* (Figure 20.2). The bones that form the upright axis of the body, including the skull, spinal column, sternum (breastbone), and ribs make up the axial skeleton. The appendicular skeleton consists of the bones that form the upper and lower extremities, including the clavicles and scapulae and bones of the arms, wrists, hands, hips, legs, ankles, and feet.

Appendicular Skeleton

As previously described, the appendicular skeleton is made up of the bones that form the upper and lower extremities. The upper extremities consist of the shoulder girdle and both arms, down to and including the fingers (Figure 20.3). Table 20.1 lists the common and medical names for bones of the upper extremities.

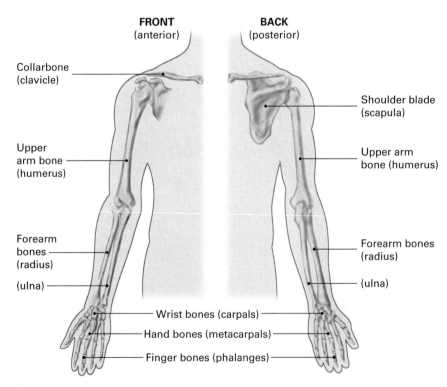

Figure 20.3 Bones of the upper extremities.

TABLE 20.1 Bones of the Upper Extremities

Common Name	Medical Name
Collarbone	Clavicle
Shoulder blade	Scapula
Upper arm	Humerus
Forearm bones	Ulna (medial), radius (lateral)
Wrist bones	Carpals
Hand bones	Metacarpals
Fingers	Phalanges

The lower extremities consist of the pelvis and both legs, down to and including the toes (Figure 20.4). Table 20.2 lists the common and medical names for bones of the lower extremities.

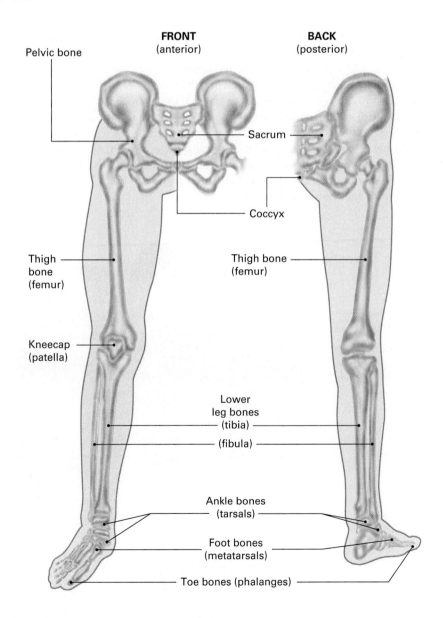

FRONT
(anterior)

BACK
(posterior)

Pelvic bone

Sacrum

Coccyx

Thigh bone (femur)

Thigh bone (femur)

Kneecap (patella)

Lower leg bones (tibia)

(fibula)

Ankle bones (tarsals)

Foot bones (metatarsals)

Toe bones (phalanges)

Figure 20.4 Bones of the lower extremities.

TABLE 20.2 Bones of the Lower Extremities

Common Name	Medical Name
Pelvic girdle (pelvis and hips)	Innominate or os coxae
Thigh	Femur
Kneecap	Patella
Lower leg bones	Tibia (medial), fibula (lateral)
Ankle bones	Tarsals
Foot bones	Metatarsals
Toes	Phalanges

Causes of Extremity Injuries

SCENE SAFETY

Scene safety is especially important at emergency scenes that involve trauma. The conditions that caused the injury to the patient may still exist after you arrive on the scene. Once on scene, keep an eye out for both obvious and not-so-obvious hazards.

LO5 Differentiate between direct and indirect forces and the injuries they cause.

Three primary forces cause musculoskeletal injuries. They are *direct force, indirect force*, and *twisting force* (Figure 20.5). Extremities often are injured because of the direct force applied to a bone when an individual falls and strikes an object or when an object strikes an individual. Sometimes the energy of a force may be transferred up or down the extremity, which can result in an injury farther along the extremity. Such indirect force injuries can occur, for instance, when one puts out a hand to break a fall and dislocates the shoulder instead of, or in addition to, breaking their wrist.

An example of an injury caused by a twisting force is when someone gets a hand or foot caught in a wheel or gear. The body remains stationary while the hand or foot turns in the wheel. Twisting injuries can also be caused when the body keeps moving forward while the hand or foot remains trapped.

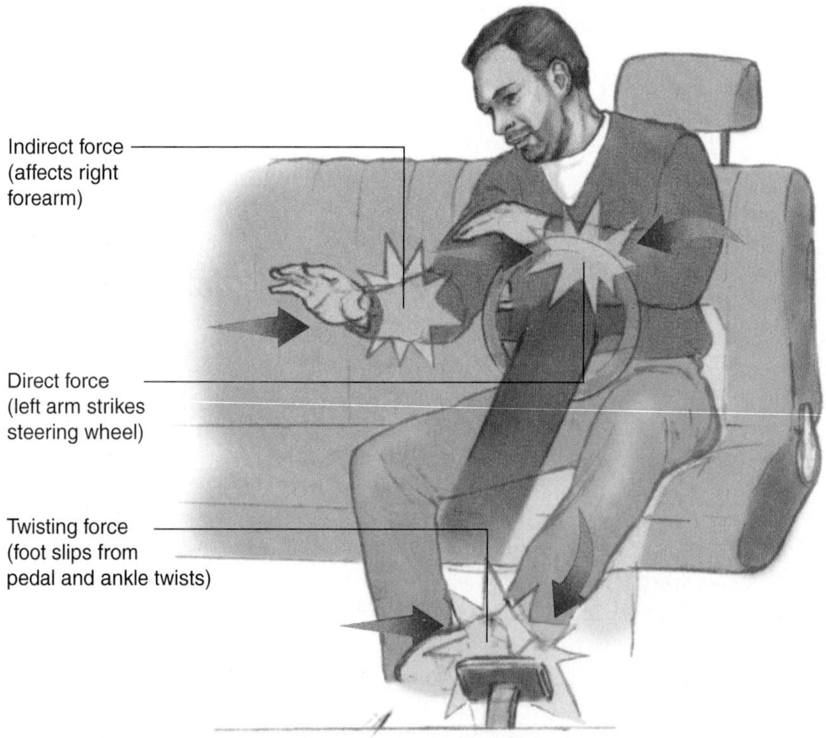
Indirect force (affects right forearm)
Direct force (left arm strikes steering wheel)
Twisting force (foot slips from pedal and ankle twists)

Figure 20.5 Three forces that cause musculoskeletal injury.

Types of Injuries

| LO6 | Differentiate between an open and closed skeletal injury. |

| LO7 | Differentiate between a strain, sprain, fracture, and dislocation. |

Skeletal injuries can be placed into one of two basic categories: closed or open (Figure 20.6). An injury is considered *closed* when there is no break in the skin. In some cases, the bones and surrounding soft tissue can be damaged extensively even though the skin is unbroken. An exception to the term "closed injury" is an injury to the head. A closed head injury may, indeed, have an open wound to the scalp but, because the cranium remains intact, it is referred to as a closed head injury.

An injury is considered *open* when the soft tissues adjacent to an injury are damaged and open. The mechanism of injury causes the bone ends or pieces of bone to tear through the skin from inside out or, in some cases, something enters and opens the skin from the outside and also breaks the bone underneath (for example, a gunshot wound).

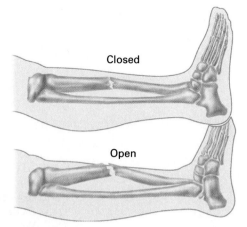

Closed

Open

Figure 20.6 Examples of a closed and open fracture of the lower leg.

Any strong force to the extremities, such as blunt force trauma, can cause damage to bones and the surrounding tissues (Key Skill 20.1). Most musculoskeletal injuries will present with pain. In more severe injuries, swelling, discoloration, and deformity may also be present. Do not be concerned with identifying the injury as a **fracture**, **dislocation**, **sprain**, or **strain**. In most cases, the true extent of the injury cannot be determined until X-rays are obtained and examined by a health care provider. Instead, you should assess the mechanism of injury and provide care for the injury based on the presenting signs and symptoms.

Although you will not diagnose specific types of musculoskeletal injuries, you should know something about each one:

fracture ▶ bone that is broken, chipped, cracked, or splintered.

dislocation ▶ pulling or pushing of a bone end partially or completely free of a joint.

sprain ▶ partial or complete tearing of the ligaments and tendons that support a joint.

strain ▶ overstretching or tearing of a muscle.

- *Fracture.* Any time a bone is broken, chipped, cracked, or splintered, it results in what is commonly referred to as a fracture.
- *Dislocation.* This occurs when one end of a bone that is part of a joint is pulled or pushed out of place. Dislocations often result in serious damage to tendons, ligaments, nerves, and blood vessels because of the way they hold a joint together or weave in and around a joint. Sometimes the force that caused a dislocation of a bone will also cause it or an adjoining bone to fracture, resulting in what is referred to as a *fracture-dislocation.*
- *Sprain.* Ligaments are tough, fibrous tissues that hold bones together at the joints. Tendons attach muscle to bone. Excessive twisting forces can cause ligaments and tendons to stretch or tear, resulting in a sprain injury.
- *Strain.* A strain is caused by overexerting, overworking, overstretching, or tearing of a muscle.

KEY SKILL 20.1

Understanding Select Mechanisms Of Extremity Injury

MECHANISM OF INJURY The force or forces that may have caused the patient's injury

DIRECT FORCE Energy transmitted directly to an extremity, causing an injury at the site of impact

INDIRECT FORCE Energy from a direct-force blow that is transferred along the axis of a bone and causes an injury farther along the extremity

TWISTING FORCE The force caused when an extremity or part of an extremity is caught in a twisting or circular mechanism while the rest of the extremity or the body is stationary or moving in another direction

DOWNWARD BLOW Clavicle and scapula

LATERAL BLOW Clavicle, scapula, humerus

LATERAL BLOW Knee, hip, femur (very forceful)

INDIRECT FORCE Pelvis, hip, knee, leg bones, shoulder, humerus, elbow, forearm bones

TWISTING FORCE Hip, femur, knee, leg bones, ankle, shoulder, elbow, forearm, wrist

FORCED FLEXION OR HYPEREXTENSION Elbow, wrist, fingers, femur, knee, foot

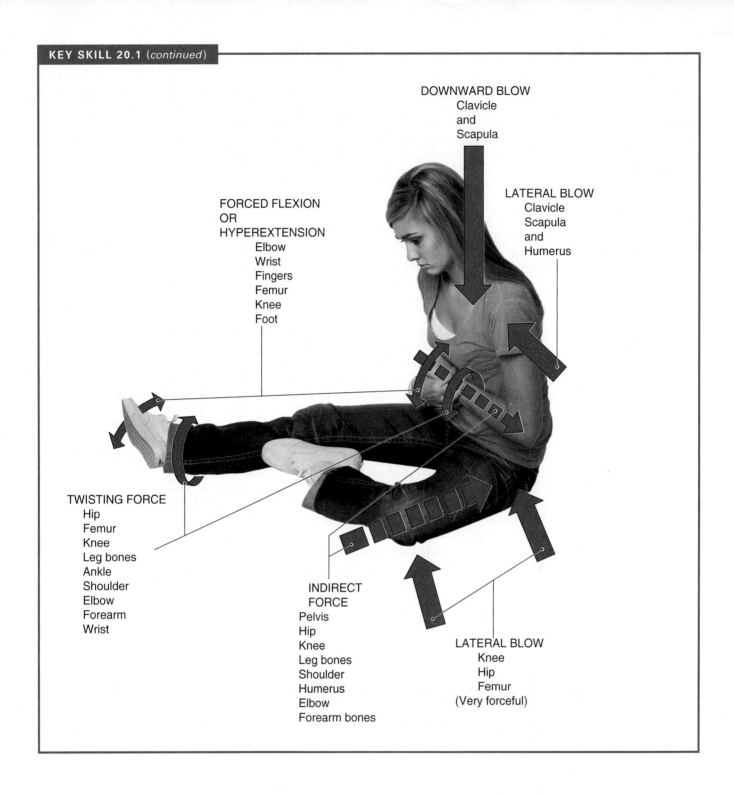

DOWNWARD BLOW
Clavicle
and
Scapula

LATERAL BLOW
Clavicle
Scapula
and
Humerus

FORCED FLEXION
OR
HYPEREXTENSION
Elbow
Wrist
Fingers
Femur
Knee
Foot

TWISTING FORCE
Hip
Femur
Knee
Leg bones
Ankle
Shoulder
Elbow
Forearm
Wrist

INDIRECT
FORCE
Pelvis
Hip
Knee
Leg bones
Shoulder
Humerus
Elbow
Forearm bones

LATERAL BLOW
Knee
Hip
Femur
(Very forceful)

angulated ▸ refers to an injured limb that is deformed and out of normal alignment.

    A sign commonly seen in serious bone injuries is angulation. **Angulated** (deformed) injuries occur when an extremity is bent where it normally should be straight. Such injuries may be relatively minor, which means that the vessels and nerves that serve the extremity are likely to still be intact. In those cases, you will most likely be able to feel a distal pulse, and the patient will have normal sensation (able to feel your touch) and motor function (able to move the hand or foot). If angulated injuries are extreme, they can cause damage to blood vessels, disrupting blood flow, and damage to nerves, affecting sensation. You may not feel a distal pulse, and the patient may experience a change in sensation and/or motor function. Deformed injuries may be open or closed.

Signs and Symptoms of Extremity Injuries

LO8 Describe the signs and symptoms of a musculoskeletal injury.

LO9 Explain the importance of an appropriate assessment of the distal extremities.

The main signs and symptoms to look for in an extremity injury are:

- *Pain.* Pain occurs when nerves surrounding the injury have been injured and are being pressed by swelling tissue or broken bone ends. Tissues near the injury site will be very tender. The patient can usually tell you where it hurts. As part of your secondary assessment, gently palpate the areas above and below the injury site to help determine the exact location of the primary area of pain.
- *Swelling.* The area around the injury will begin to swell because blood from ruptured blood vessels is collecting inside the tissues.
- *Discoloration.* Blood trapped under the skin may cause it to look reddish or discolored. Later, as these blood cells die, they cause the typical black and blue bruising, which may take 24 hours or longer to develop.
- *Deformity.* When deformity occurs, a part of a limb appears different in size or shape than the same part on the opposite side of the patient's body. (Always compare both arms and legs to one another.) If a bone appears to have an unusual angle, bulge, or swelling, consider this deformity to be a sign of possible fracture or dislocation. Feel gently along the patient's limbs, noting any lumps, swelling, discoloration, and/or ends of bones protruding through the skin.

Other common signs and symptoms of an extremity injury include:

- *Inability to move a joint or limb.* Sometimes movement is possible but very painful. Ask the patient if they are able to move the affected joint, even if they can move it only very little. Any amount of movement is a good sign. Then ask the patient to move the fingers or toes on the affected limb. Again, any amount of movement is a good sign. Do not force any movement.
- *Numbness or tingling sensation.* This can be caused from pressure on nerves or blood vessels due to swelling or damage.
- *Loss of distal pulse.* Bone ends or bone fragments may be pressing against or cutting through an artery. Swelling from internal bleeding around the fracture may be pressing against an artery. The extremity may be pale and cold because of restricted blood flow then turn bluish (cyanotic) because of lack of oxygen.
- *Slow capillary refill.* A decrease in perfusion may be indicated by an increase in capillary refill time (explained further later in this section.)
- *Grating.* When the ends of fractured bones rub together making a grating sound, also called *crepitus.* Do not ask a patient to move to confirm or reproduce this sound.
- *Sound described as cracking or snapping at the time of injury.* If the patient or bystanders tell you they heard this sound, suspect that a fracture has occurred.
- *Exposed bone.* In cases of **open fracture**, the fragments or ends of broken bones may be visible where they break through the skin.

open fracture ▶ broken bone in which bone ends or fragments protrude through the skin.

Assessment All injured extremities should be assessed for adequate circulation, sensation, and motor function (CSM) before and after immobilization. Check circulation by assessing distal pulses and capillary refill. In the absence of a pulse, good color can be interpreted as good circulation. If possible, compare the injured side to the uninjured side. A warm extremity may also be a sign that circulation is intact.

To assess for normal sensation of the distal extremity, squeeze the fingers or toes of the injured extremity and ask the patient to tell you if they can feel your touch and where you are touching. Ask the patient if your touch feels normal or if they feel any numbness or a tingling sensation. Checking for sensation and motor function gives you information about the status of the nerves that supply the injured extremity. A lack of feeling or the inability to move may indicate damage to a nerve. This nerve damage may be the result of injury to the spinal cord and not just an injury to the extremity.

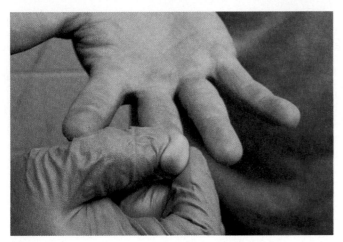

Figure 20.7 Assessing capillary refill in the fingers.

To evaluate motor function, begin by asking the patient to wiggle their fingers or toes. Next, you can check the strength of the extremity. For the hands, place your thumbs in the patient's hands and ask them to squeeze. For the feet, place your hands at the bottom of the patient's feet and ask them to press down on your hands. In either case, note the strength and compare the good side with the injured side. In most instances, you will notice a weakness on the injured side, which is usually due to pain. Ask the patient if it causes pain when they squeeze or press on your hands.

Several important signs will tell you the state of circulation to the extremity:

- If the injury site is swollen and discolored, there is bleeding in the tissues.
- If there is no distal pulse and the extremity is pale and cool, circulation to the extremity may be compromised.
- If the extremity is pale or bluish (cyanotic), there is lack of circulation and, thus, a lack of oxygen in the limb.

Capillary Refill Time   Another tool for assessing the circulation or perfusion status of a distal extremity is capillary refill time. To assess capillary refill time, press the nail bed or pad of a finger or toe on the injured extremity between your finger and thumb. The pressure forces blood out of the tissues, causing them to blanch (turn white). When you release pressure, the blood should flow back into the tissues in less than 2 seconds. If it takes longer than 2 seconds for the tissues to refill with blood, it may be a sign of compromised circulation to the extremity. For dark-skinned individuals, capillary refill time may be assessed using the palm of the hand, as this area is typically lighter in color. Capillary refill time may be affected by factors such as the temperature of the environment, medications, and preexisting medical conditions. When possible, capillary refill should be assessed on both the injured and uninjured extremities for comparison (Figure 20.7).

Assessing and Managing Musculoskeletal Injuries

LO10 Describe the appropriate care for a patient with a musculoskeletal injury.

LO11 Explain the priority of care for a patient with a suspected open skeletal injury.

In the scene size-up, quickly determine scene safety and don all appropriate personal protective equipment. Note the mechanism of injury and the total number of patients. Then determine what additional assistance you may need. If the mechanism of injury suggests a possible spinal injury and the scene is safe to enter, immediately stabilize your patient's head and neck (discussed further in Chapter 21).

During your primary assessment, get an impression of the environment and the patient, and determine how quickly the patient needs to be moved and transported. Do not focus on obvious injuries until you have assessed the ABCs and mental status. Detect and correct life-threatening problems as quickly as possible. Look for and control all major bleeding.

Caring for injuries follows a certain order. If there is time after correcting and stabilizing life-threatening injuries, checking for and stabilizing neck and spinal injuries, and providing care for shock, then you can focus on any extremity injuries. Always be sure to note the mechanism of injury because this will give you an idea of the possible extent, type, and location of injuries.

JEDI

It is important to preserve the patient's dignity while examining for injuries. If you must expose a woman's chest or remove anyone's pants, delegate rescuers to hold up a sheet or form a "human shield" from onlookers. It is rarely necessary to completely undress a patient.

"Don't touch it, Ron. Don't touch it!" Annie shouts as he tries to gently straighten her deformed leg. It is already beginning to swell and grow purple deep below the skin, halfway between her knee and ankle.

"Listen, Annie," Ron says, trying to maintain eye contact. "I can't feel a pulse in your foot, so I have to try to straighten your leg. It's going to hurt, but I've got to do it."

"Is everything okay?" A course groundskeeper pulls up in an electric cart stacked high with plastic bags full of freshly cut grass. At the sight of Annie's leg, he immediately grows pale and looks away.

"Can you please call 911?" Ron asks. The man nods, still looking away, and pulls out his cell phone.

When caring for skeletal injuries, the first priority is given to possible injury to the spine. Next, care for possible injuries to the following:

- Head injuries can disrupt normal breathing and may cause airway problems in some patients.
- The rib cage protects the heart and lungs. Trauma to the chest can damage internal organs and interfere with adequate breathing.
- The pelvis protects reproductive and urinary organs, major nerves, and blood vessels.
- It takes major trauma to injure the femur, the largest, strongest bone in the body, which is surrounded by major nerves and blood vessels. Blood loss from a fractured femur can be life threatening.
- Trauma to an extremity can disrupt blood flow through the limb and damage important nerve pathways.

Always evaluate the mechanism of injury and be concerned with major bleeding and possible shock whenever there are injuries to the chest, pelvis, or femur. A significant amount of blood can be lost internally in those areas. Monitor the patient's signs and symptoms carefully for changes. A rapid, weak pulse; pale skin color; an altered mental status; and cold extremities are signs and symptoms that should alert you to manage and transport the patient as soon as possible.

Follow these steps in caring for skeletal injuries:

1. Always take proper BSI precautions, and perform a scene size-up before focusing on a particular injury.
   - Perform a primary assessment and ensure an open airway and adequate breathing.
   - Manage life-threatening problems first.
   - Prioritize and manage other injuries second.
2. Carefully cut away clothing to expose the injury site. Control bleeding if there is an open wound. Check for distal circulation, sensation, and motor function in the affected extremity.
3. Immobilize the extremity using manual stabilization.
   - Immobilize the suspected fracture site.
   - Immobilize the joints above and below the suspected fracture site. For an arm, use a sling and secure it to the body with a **swathe** to keep it elevated across the chest. Splinted, immobilized legs may be propped up on a folded blanket or pillow if there is no indication of spinal injury.
   - Recheck distal circulation, sensation, and motor function often.
4. Apply a cold pack to the injury site to help reduce the pain and swelling. Never put a cold pack directly on the skin. Wrap it in gauze or a towel then place it gently over the injury site. If the patient experiences pain from this extra pressure on the injury, place the cold pack just above the site.

swathe ▶ bandage or cloth folded into a narrow band used to secure a sling or splint to the body.

SCENE SAFETY

You may be called on to help lift or move a patient with a musculoskeletal injury. Doing so can put great stress on your back if you do not use good body mechanics. Use caution when lifting patients or heavy objects, and do not attempt a lift unless you have enough people to assist.

5. Administer oxygen as soon as possible per local protocols.
6. Monitor the patient's vital signs. Maintain a comfortable body temperature to help minimize the effects of shock.

Emotional support is important when caring for a patient with musculoskeletal injuries. Tell the patient exactly what you intend to do before doing it. Keep them informed as much as possible all along the way. Minimizing surprises such as a sudden increase in pain or sudden movement gives them confidence and relieves anxiety.

CREW RESOURCE MANAGEMENT

Managing multiple skeletal injuries can be challenging. It may be more efficient to have different crew members working on different injuries at the same time. This will reduce the time on scene, allowing the patient to be transported sooner.

Splinting

LO12 Explain the purpose and methods for manual stabilization of a skeletal injury.

splint ▶ any device used to immobilize an injured extremity.

manual stabilization ▶ restricting the movement of an injured individual or body part by using one's hands.

Splinting is the process of immobilizing an injury, using a commercial **splint** or an improvised device such as a piece of wood, cardboard, or a folded blanket. Any object that can be used to restrict the movement of an injury is called a splint. **Manual stabilization** is the process of using your hands to restrict the movement of an injured individual or body part.

Why Splint?

The application of splints reduces pain and minimizes further injury.[1] Splinting also allows emergency care providers to reposition and transfer the patient while minimizing movement of the injured area. Moving a patient who has musculoskeletal injuries prior to splinting can cause damage to soft tissues, leading to complications and prolonging recovery (Figure 20.8). Complications include:

- *Pain.* A splint can reduce much of the patient's pain because it secures the broken or dislocated bones in place and prevents them from compressing or damaging surrounding nerves and tissues.
- *Damage to soft tissues.* The movement of an injured extremity may cause blood vessels, nerves, and muscles to be crushed, ruptured, pinched, or compressed.

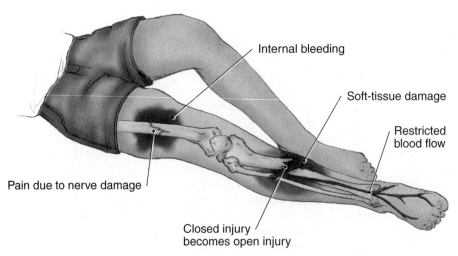

Internal bleeding

Soft-tissue damage

Restricted blood flow

Pain due to nerve damage

Closed injury becomes open injury

Figure 20.8 Complications associated with extremity injuries can be prevented or decreased with splinting.

Splinting reduces movement of the injured part, the possibility of further damage to soft tissues, and the accompanying pain, internal bleeding, and swelling.

- *Bleeding.* The initial force of injury may have caused bone ends to damage soft tissues and blood vessels. Splinting will stabilize the injury and apply a steady pressure that can reduce and control bleeding.
- *Restricted blood flow.* Dislocated joints, fractured bones, and bone fragments can press against blood vessels and restrict blood flow. Splinting can help relieve the pressure against blood vessels.
- *Closed injuries become open injuries.* The sharp edge of a broken bone can rip through skin to produce an open wound. Immobilizing the injured extremity by splinting it will minimize movement of the broken part and help prevent a **closed fracture** from becoming an open one.

closed fracture ▶ broken bone that does not have an associated break in the outer layers of the skin.

General Rules for Splinting

For all cases of splinting, you will (Key Skill 20.2):

- Assess and reassure the patient, and explain what you plan to do.
- Expose the injury site. Cut away clothing if it cannot be easily removed or folded back. Remove jewelry from the injured limb if it can be done without using force, causing pain, or repositioning the patient or the limb.
- Control all major bleeding. If necessary, use direct pressure. Avoid applying pressure directly over exposed bone ends. To control major bleeding, use bulky dressings secured snugly with a bandage.
- Dress open wounds. Do not push bone ends back into the wound. Do not try to pick bone fragments from the wound. If the bone ends withdraw into the wound as you care for it, report this to personnel who take over patient care.
- Check distal circulation, sensation, and motor function before and after splinting.
- Splint injuries before moving the patient. Move the patient before splinting only if another injury or the environment is life threatening.
- Have all materials ready and at hand before splinting. Use padded splints for patient comfort and improved contact between limb and splint. Wrap unpadded splints in dressings before applying them.
- If distal circulation is absent and local protocols allow, gently attempt to realign an angulated limb in the anatomical position before splinting. Attempt to reposition the limb to regain a pulse if the limb has no pulse and is cold and blue.

KEY SKILL 20.2

Splinting an Upper Extremity

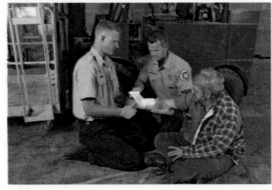

1. After controlling bleeding, dress and bandage open wounds to the injured extremity.

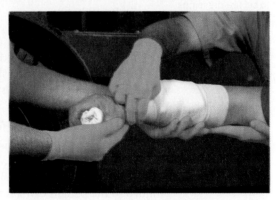

2. Check distal circulation, sensation, and motor function before splinting.

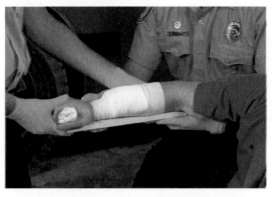

3. Select an appropriate-size splint for the injury and pad the splint thoroughly.

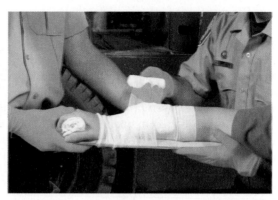

4. Firmly secure the splint, leaving fingertips or toes exposed so you can monitor distal circulation, sensation, and motor function.

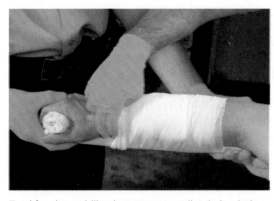

5. After immobilization, reassess distal circulation, sensation, and motor function.

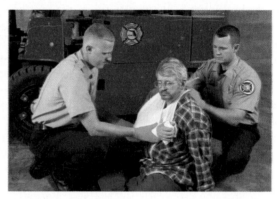

6. Elevate the extremity. For an arm, use the sling to immobilize it against the chest. For a leg, prop it on a pillow or rolled blanket (if there is no indication of spinal injury).

- Immobilize the suspected fracture site and the joints above and below the injury site. Secure upper extremities to the torso with a sling and swathe. If the injury is to the thigh, secure the lower extremities to each other.
- Secure splints with **cravats** or roller gauze, starting at the distal end of the extremity. Leave fingertips and toes exposed so you can monitor circulation, sensation, and motor function.
- Elevate the extremity. For an arm, use a sling and swathe. For a leg, prop it on a pillow or rolled blanket if there is no indication of spinal injury. If there is indication of a spinal injury, keep the patient lying supine.
- Minimize the effects of shock by maintaining body temperature and providing oxygen if local protocols allow.

cravat ▶ triangular bandage folded to a width of 2 to 3 inches used to secure dressings and splints in place.

Manual Stabilization

Manual stabilization involves using your hands to keep an injured extremity from moving. In most instances, when you arrive you will find the patient using their hands to attempt to stabilize their own injury. It may be appropriate to take over manual stabilization of the injury so the patient can assume a more comfortable position, such as lying down. In the case of arm injuries, the patient may be holding the arm tight against the body to keep it from moving. This may be the best position for the patient, so do not be in too much of a hurry to take control of the extremity. You can still evaluate distal circulation, sensation, and motor function while they hold the arm securely (Figure 20.9).

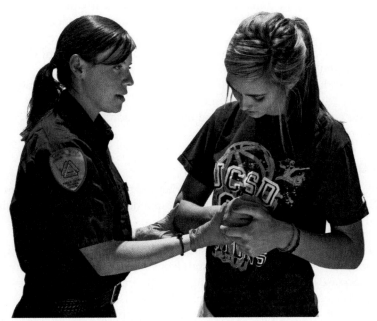

Figure 20.9 Manual stabilization of an injured limb.

When caring for leg injuries, it is best to take over manual stabilization. Assign one individual for this purpose, and have that individual maintain manual stabilization throughout the splinting process. You may find that even the slightest amount of movement is very painful for the patient. In those instances, consider just maintaining manual stabilization until the ambulance arrives.

CREW RESOURCE MANAGEMENT

When caring for patients with multisystem trauma, the team must work together to prioritize injuries and ensure rapid transport. Share your findings out loud as you find issues during the assessment. This will keep the entire team informed and aware as priorities change.

Managing Angulated Injuries

LO13 Explain the criteria for placing an angulated extremity injury into anatomical position.

The main reason for straightening closed deformed injuries is to restore circulation, but straight limbs also make it easier for you to apply a splint. If the limb cannot be straightened or if you are not allowed to straighten it, immobilize the limb in the position found. Do only what you have been trained to do and what is allowed in your EMS system. If you are unable to find a distal pulse and the skin in the distal extremity is pale or blue and cold, act immediately to minimize potential permanent damage. You may be directed to gently align the limb in an attempt to restore a distal pulse. Do not force the limb if you meet resistance or if the patient complains of too much pain. If unable to straighten the limb, immobilize it as best you can in the position you find it.

Follow these steps to attempt to straighten an injured limb when a pulse cannot be detected:

1. Carefully explain to the patient what you plan to do and why.
2. Support the extremity with both hands to minimize movement of the injury site. Use additional rescuers if needed.

3. While supporting the limb proximal to the injury, gently pull traction from the distal end as you carefully straighten the extremity. Traction is achieved by grasping the hand or foot and gently pulling straight out with a steady force.
4. Move slowly until you bring the extremity into a natural position similar to the uninjured limb.
5. To prevent the injury from returning to its angulated position, apply a splint to the extremity while maintaining gentle traction.
6. Reassess circulation, sensation, and motor function.
7. Reassure the patient as best you can.

Types of Splints

There are many types of splints on the market today. The two main types of splints are: soft and rigid. As an Emergency Medical Responder, you should be familiar with those commonly used by your agency or in your region.

Soft Splints   When properly applied, soft splints such as pillows, blankets, towels, slings, and dressings may be very effective in stabilizing injuries. Soft splints can provide support and help decrease both pain and swelling.

A **sling** is a common type of soft splint that is fashioned from a triangular bandage. It is used to stabilize an upper extremity injury. A properly placed sling will adequately immobilize the elbow and provide support to the lower arm. Once the arm is placed in a sling, a swathe is used to hold the arm against the side of the chest and restrict movement of the shoulder. A swathe is made from a triangular bandage, which is folded to a width of 2 to 4 inches. Together, the sling and swathe work well to immobilize both the elbow and shoulder joints, which is necessary when caring for suspected fractures of the arm.

The sling and swathe are generally effective for injuries to the shoulder, upper arm, elbow, lower arm, and wrist. To make and apply a sling and swathe, follow these steps (Key Skill 20.3):

1. Use a commercial sling or make one from a piece of cloth or sheet. Fold or cut this material into the shape of a triangle. The ideal sling should be about 50 to 60 inches long at its base and 36 to 40 inches long on each of its sides.
2. Position the triangular material over the patient's chest. The top of the triangle should point toward the patient's injured arm and extend beyond the elbow. The top end should be draped over the uninjured shoulder. Have the patient position their arm so the hand is higher than the elbow. If the patient cannot hold their arm, have your partner or a bystander support the arm while you prepare and secure the sling.
3. Bring the bottom end of the triangle up and over the patient's arm and shoulder on the injured side.
4. Draw up on the ends of the sling so the patient's hand on the injured side is about 4 inches above the elbow. Tie the two ends together. Be sure to position the knot so it does not rest on the back of the patient's neck. Place a flat layer of cloth (gauze pads or handkerchief) under the knot for comfort. Leave the patient's fingertips exposed so you can check for circulation, sensation, and motor function.
5. Take the point of the sling at the patient's elbow and fold it forward. Then tuck it in, pin it in place, or twist and tie the point. It may be easier to tie the point before the sling is placed on the patient. This will form a pocket for the patient's elbow.
6. Take a second piece of triangular cloth and fold it into a 2- to 4-inch width. Center it on the widest part of the patient's injured arm. Take one end across the patient's back and one end across the chest and tie on the opposite side under the other arm. Be sure the swathe is placed as low over the injured arm as possible. This will ensure that it stays close to the body and minimizes movement of the shoulder.

sling ▶ large, triangular bandage or other cloth device used to immobilize the elbow and support the forearm.

Sling and Swathe

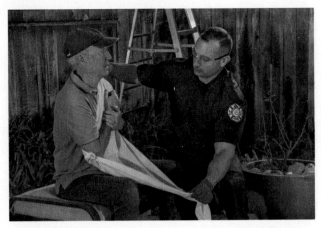

1. Place one end of the base of the triangular bandage over the uninjured shoulder. Ensure that the top of the triangle is pointed toward the injured arm.

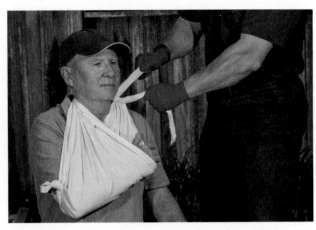

2. Bring the lower end of the bandage up and over the shoulder on the injured side. Tie a knot at the side of the neck.

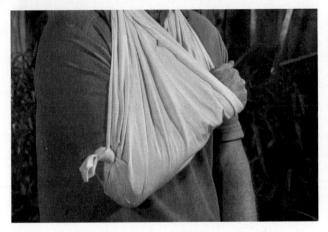

3. Pin or tape the apex to form a pocket at the elbow.

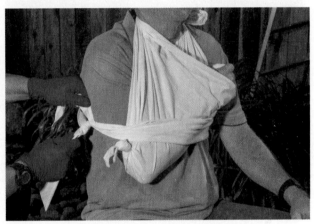

4. Secure the arm to the body with a swathe.

Rigid Splints Rigid splints have very little flexibility. They can be made of plastic, metal, wood, compressed cardboard, or even rolled-up newspapers or magazines. They are applied along an injured extremity to immobilize the suspected fracture site and, if possible, the joints directly above and below the injury site.

Commercial Splints A wide variety of commercial splints are available for emergency care. They are made of wood, aluminum, cardboard, foam, wire, or plastic. Some come with their own washable pads, and others require padding to be applied before being secured. Most splints are either solid rigid pieces or inflatable plastic splints. They include air splints, vacuum splints, board-and-wire ladder splints, heavy-duty cardboard splints, and flexible aluminum splints. All EMTs and many Emergency Medical Responders carry traction splints for splinting and stabilizing isolated femur injuries. (Key Skill 20.4 shows examples of commercial splints for upper- and lower-extremity immobilization.)

Inflatable Splints Inflatable splints, also called *air splints*, are not carried by all Emergency Medical Responder units. If you carry them and your jurisdiction allows their use, your instructor will teach you their application. Typically, air splints are used for patients with injuries to the arms or lower legs.

> **REMEMBER**
>
> When applying a rigid splint to an extremity, fill the space between the patient and the splint with soft cushioning material or bandages. Do this whether or not the injury is angulated.

Understanding Various SAM® Splint Applications

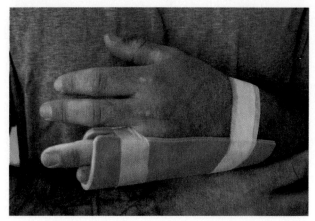

1. SAM® Splint configured to immobilize an injured finger.

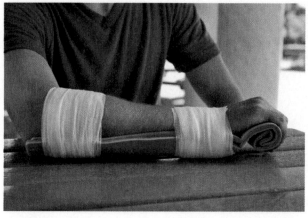

2. SAM® Splint configured to immobilize an injured forearm.

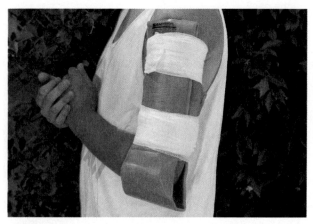

3. SAM® Splint configured to immobilize an injured humerus.

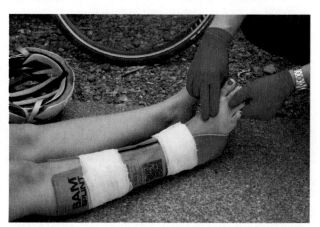

4. SAM® Splint configured to immobilize an injured lower leg.

REMEMBER

If performed correctly, the application of a splint will provide great comfort to the patient. However, an ill-fitting splint or a sloppy splinting job can cause great pain and discomfort. Be sure to practice your splinting skills regularly so they will be fresh and ready when you need them.

When using an air splint on the arm, slip it uninflated over your forearm. Then grasp the patient's hand and pull gentle traction while you slip the air splint from your arm onto the patient's arm. Smooth out the splint and inflate it. It will be important to follow the manufacturer's recommendations for inflation pressure to ensure the correct amount of pressure is used.

After inflating the splint, you must monitor the limb for changes in circulation, sensation, and motor function. Monitor the splint for changes in pressure. If the patient is moved to a warmer or colder location, the air in the splint will expand or contract with the temperature change. You will have to recheck the pressure in the splint. You may have to remove increased pressure by deflating the splint slightly. The pressure in the splint also will change if the patient is moved to a different altitude, which can be a concern when patients are flown or transported down from mountain accident scenes. Frequently monitor the pressure in the splint.

Once an air splint is applied, you may not be able to assess the distal pulse. Instead, evaluate capillary refill, skin color, sensation, and motor function.

Improvised Splints Emergency Medical Responders may arrive at the scene of an emergency without any splints, or they may use their supply of splints on one patient and have none for another patient. So, it is helpful to know how to make splints from materials found at the scene. Such an improvised splint may be soft or rigid and may be made from a variety of materials.

Rigid splints can be made from pieces of lumber, plywood, compressed wood products, cardboard, rolled newspapers or magazines, umbrellas, canes, broom or shovel handles, sporting equipment (e.g., shin guards), and tongue depressors for fingers. Soft splints can be made from towels, blankets, pillows, and bulky clothing such as sweaters and coats. Most of these items can be found at the scene.

FIRST ON SCENE (continued)

After carefully straightening Annie's leg, Ron is able to find a strong pulse in her foot. "Now we need to splint it in this position," he says, looking at a stand of small trees that line the course. Perhaps the branches are strong enough for a splint.

"Why don't you use the golf clubs," Annie whispers as she tries to breathe deeply through the pain. Ron grins and shakes his head slightly, imagining his buddies at the volunteer fire station finding out that he was prepared to break down a tree to make a splint when golf clubs were at hand.

"That's a great idea," he says and jogs over to the overturned golf cart. He grabs several clubs and the shoulder straps from both bags.

Management of Specific Extremity Injuries

Usually, the mechanism of injury and the patient's signs and symptoms indicate possible injuries that require splints. In general, apply rigid splints for injuries to the arms and the lower leg. Rigid splints also may be used for injuries to the thigh, but traction splints are more effective. (Follow local protocols.) Use soft splints (blanket, towel, pillow, or sling and swathe) if rigid splints are not available. Provide further rigid support by securing upper extremities to the torso with a swathe and lower extremities to each other.

Upper Extremity Injuries

Methods for splinting each type of upper extremity injury are summarized in Key Skill 20.5. For injuries to the upper extremities, be sure to place the hand in a **position of function**, in which the fingers are slightly flexed and the wrist is cocked slightly upward. The position of function is a normal and comfortable position for the patient, especially

position of function ▶ refers to placement of a hand or foot; the natural position of the body at rest.

KEY SKILL 20.5

Upper Extremity Splinting

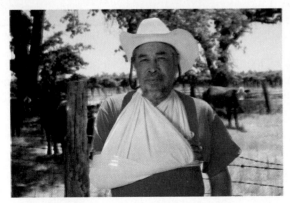

1. Shoulder. Apply a sling and swathe. Ensure that the hand is higher than the elbow, and secure the entire arm with a swathe.

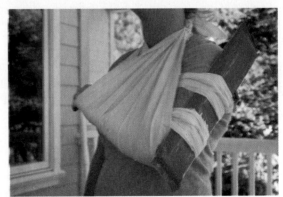

2. Upper arm. Immobilize with a rigid splint from the shoulder to the elbow. Apply a sling and swathe that will elevate and support the limb.

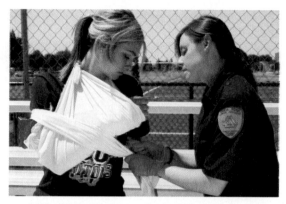

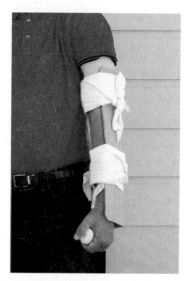

3. Elbow (bent). Secure short rigid splints on either side of the arm, and apply a sling and swathe to elevate and support the limb.

4. Elbow (straight). Pad the armpit. The splint should extend from the armpit beyond the fingertips. Use roller bandages to secure the splint to the arm starting at the distal end. Secure the arm to the body with cravats.

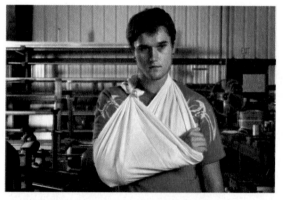

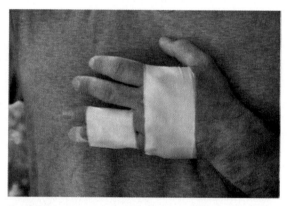

5. Forearm, wrist, hand. The splint should extend from the elbow to beyond the fingertips. Use a sling and swathe for elevation and support.

6. Finger. Use a tongue depressor as a splint or tape the finger to an uninjured finger.

Note: Place a roll of dressing in the hand to maintain position of function.

if the extremity from forearm to hand is secured against a rigid splint. You may easily secure the hand in its position of function by placing a roll of gauze in the patient's hand before immobilizing or simply by allowing the fingers of the hand to extend over the end of the splint.

Injuries to the Shoulder   A common sign of shoulder injury is deformity, usually indicating a dislocation injury (Figure 20.10). Injuries to the shoulder joint often produce what is known as an *anterior dislocation*. (Remember that anterior means "to the front.") The proximal end of the humerus (upper arm bone) can be seen as a bulge under the skin at the anterior side of the shoulder.

It is not practical to use a rigid splint for injuries to the collarbone, shoulder blade, or shoulder joint. Place padding between the patient's injured arm and chest, use a cravat to secure the padding in place, and use a sling and swathe to secure the arm to the chest.

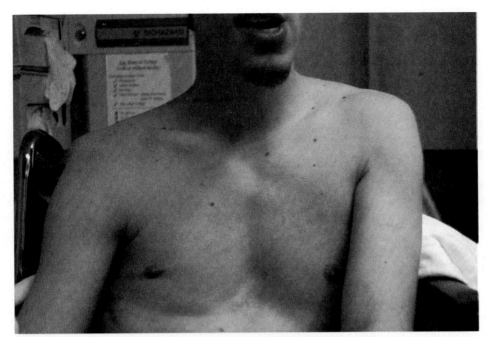

Figure 20.10 Deformity caused by dislocation of the shoulder joint (left).
(© Edward T. Dickinson, MD)

Remember to check for distal circulation, sensation, and motor function before and after splinting. If there is no pulse, attempt to reposition to regain a pulse, but do not force the arm. Do not attempt to straighten injuries that involve the joint. Joint injuries should be immobilized in the position in which they are found.

When you provide care for patients with shoulder injuries, follow these steps:

1. Take appropriate BSI precautions.
2. Assess and provide support for the ABCs.
3. Check distal circulation. If there is no pulse, arrange to transport as soon as possible. Note the time that you observed the absence of the distal pulse.
4. Check for sensation and motor function of the fingers on the injured arm. If the patient has no feeling or cannot move, they will need transport as soon as possible.
5. Apply a sling and swathe. If necessary, place padding (pillow, blanket, or towel) to fill any space between the patient's arm and chest on the injured side before applying the sling and swathe.
6. Reassess the distal pulse. If the pulse is absent, you may have to gently reposition the injured arm and reapply the sling and swathe. In such cases, follow your local protocols. Sometimes a dislocated shoulder will correct itself. If this happens, check the distal circulation, sensation, and motor function, and apply a sling and swathe. This patient still must see a health care provider.

Injuries to the Upper Arm   When possible, secure a rigid splint to the limb to help stabilize the injury site. Next, apply a sling and swathe to ensure that the extremity is fully immobilized. If you use a sling and swathe on an injury that seems very close to the elbow, modify the full sling to minimize pressure on the elbow.

If the upper arm is angulated, check for a distal pulse. If it is present and the patient can tolerate movement, gently move the arm to the splinting position (bend the elbow with the hand elevated above the level of the elbow) and splint it. Do not force the arm to this position, and do not try to straighten the angulation. Recheck for a distal pulse.

If you do not feel a pulse, attempt to straighten the angulation in the upper arm bone if your EMS system allows you to do so. Do not force the arm. You should attempt to straighten the angulation only once and stop if there is resistance or severe pain. If straightening the limb fails to restore a distal pulse, arrange to transport the patient as soon as possible. If the pulse is restored, splint the arm and recheck the distal pulse.

If you use a rigid splint, secure it to the outer side of the arm with roller gauze or cravats. Next, apply a sling and swathe. The swathe will secure the injured arm to the body and immobilize the joints above and below the injury site.

When you apply a splint to an upper arm injury, work with a partner. One of you will maintain manual stabilization, while the other applies the splint and the sling and swathe. To apply a splint for injuries to the upper arm, follow these steps:

1. Check for distal circulation, sensation, and motor function.
2. Select a padded splint long enough for the area between the shoulder and elbow.
3. Apply manual stabilization to the injured extremity. If there is angulation or no distal pulse, gently realign and recheck for pulse.
4. Place the splint against the injured extremity.
5. Secure the splint to the patient with a roller bandage or cravats. Begin securing at the distal end of the splint.
6. Maintain the hand in the position of function and apply a sling and swathe. Recheck distal circulation, sensation, and motor function.
7. Provide oxygen as soon as possible and maintain body temperature to prevent the effects of developing shock.

Injuries to the Elbow The elbow is a joint formed by the lower, or distal, end of the humerus (upper arm bone) and the proximal (upper) end of the forearm bones, the radius and ulna. When possible ask the patient to position an injured arm into a flexed (bent) position at approximately 90 degrees. This will permit the application of a sling and allow for the most comfortable position. If the patient is unable to bend the elbow, you must immobilize the arm in the position in which it is found. Have your partner stabilize the arm while you apply and secure the splint. Check circulation, sensation, and motor function before and after splinting.

The following methods can be used in caring for a patient with an elbow injury (Key Skill 20.6):

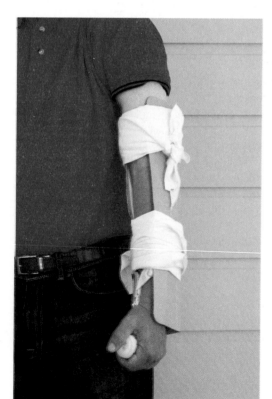

Figure 20.11 An injured elbow immobilized in a straight position using a cardboard splint.

- If the elbow is found in a flexed position natural for the joint, rigid splinting is preferred. However, a simple sling and a swathe may be effective.
- If the elbow is found in a straight position and cannot be placed in the natural flexed position, immobilize it in the straight position (Figure 20.11). Rigid splinting is preferred, but body splinting is effective. This is done by tying the injured arm along the side of the patient's torso. If you use a rigid splint, select a padded splint that will extend from the patient's armpit past the fingertips. Place a roll of dressing in the patient's hand to maintain it in the position of function, and secure the splint with roller gauze or folded cravats starting at the distal end of the arm (fingertips).
- If the elbow appears to be dislocated and it is in an unnatural or awkward position and cannot be repositioned, place padding around the arm and between the arm and chest, if necessary. If possible, secure the arm to the body with a sling and swathe.

Injuries to the Forearm, Wrist, and Hand The approach you take for an injured forearm, wrist, or hand will depend on the severity of the injury and what materials you have on hand. In some instances, a simple sling and swathe or pillow may be sufficient (Figure 20.12). You may have to get more creative with injuries that are dislocated or angulated. Be sure to check distal circulation, sensation, and motor function before and after splinting.

To use a rigid splint for an injury to the forearm, wrist, or hand, select a padded rigid splint that extends from beyond the elbow to past the fingertips. Place a roll of dressing in the patient's hand to maintain the hand in the position of function. The steps for splinting the forearm, wrist, and hand are the same as steps 3 to 7 for the upper arm (described previously). An alternative method for maintaining the position of function in the hand is to allow the fingers to curve over the end of the rigid splint.

Immobilizing a Bent Elbow

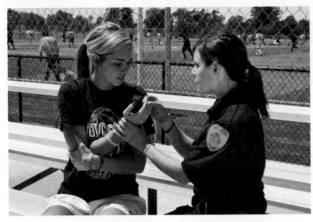

1. Check circulation, sensation, and motor function prior to splinting.

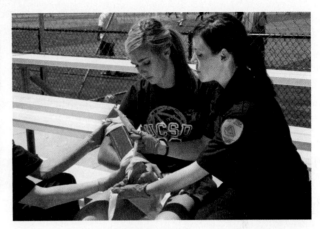

2. Secure rigid splint(s) to the arm.

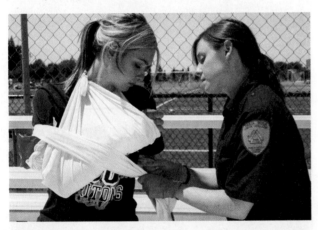

3. Apply a sling and swathe.

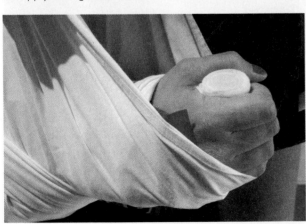

4. Recheck circulation, sensation, and motor function.

5. Ensure that the hand is in the position of function.

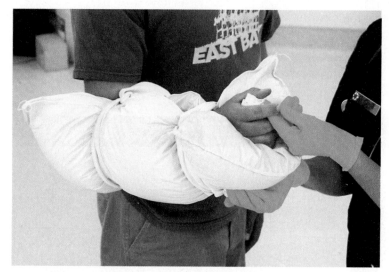

Figure 20.12 A pillow makes a good soft splint for wrist and hand injuries.

Rolled newspapers or magazines and folded cardboard make effective rigid splints for injuries to the forearm or wrist, but they still should be padded. Apply a sling after splinting to keep the forearm elevated. Add a swathe to secure the forearm to the chest, and immobilize the joint above and below the injury site (Key Skill 20.7).

Injuries to the Fingers Not all injuries to the fingers require rigid splinting. You can immobilize an injured finger by taping the finger to an adjacent, uninjured finger. You can tape the finger to a tongue depressor, an aluminum splint, or a pen or pencil. You can also make a soft splint by placing a roll of gauze in the patient's hand and wrapping more gauze around the hand and dressing. This soft-splint method immobilizes the hand and fingers and keeps them in the position of function.

KEY SKILL 20.7

Immobilizing a Forearm

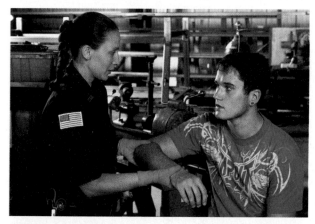

1. Manually stabilize the limb prior to splinting.

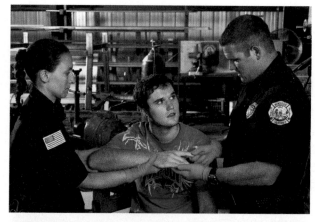

2. Check circulation, sensation, and motor function.

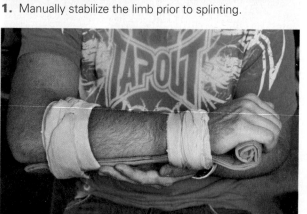

3. Apply a rigid splint to the limb.

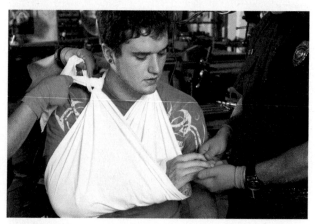

4. Place the limb in a sling, and recheck circulation, sensation, and motor function.

Apply a sling to keep the forearm elevated. Apply a swathe to immobilize the joints above the injury site, as well as to improve circulation and patient comfort.

Do not attempt to "pop" dislocated fingers back into place. Immobilize dislocated fingers as you would an injured hand.

Lower Extremity Injuries

LO14 Explain the priority of care for a patient with multisystem trauma.

When the patient has multiple injuries or has sustained multisystem trauma, it is usually best to totally immobilize them on a long board or scoop stretcher rather than to try to immobilize each individual injury. Valuable time can be lost trying to immobilize individual injuries. If you suspect multisystem trauma, immobilization on a long board and rapid transport are essential.

Before moving or rolling a patient with suspected spinal injury or with lower extremity injuries, be sure you have the proper equipment ready and a sufficient number of rescue personnel on hand to assist.

Injuries to the Pelvic Girdle   The patient may have injuries to the pelvic girdle (pelvis and hip joints) if the:

- patient complains of pain in the pelvis, hips, or groin.
- patient complains of pain when gentle pressure is applied to the sides of the hips or to the hip bones.
- patient cannot lift their legs while lying supine (face up). The patient will usually tell you that "It hurts" or "I can't move my legs."
- foot on the injured side turns laterally (outward) or medially (inward) more than the foot on the uninjured side.
- injured extremity appears shorter than the one on the uninjured side.
- pelvis or hip joint has noticeable deformity.

Pelvic injuries are serious because they can damage major blood vessels and internal organs. Injuries to these soft tissues can cause profuse internal bleeding, and the force that caused the pelvic injury may also have caused spinal injuries. Because of all these critical factors, it may be best to wait for more advanced care to arrive before attempting to immobilize a patient with a pelvic injury. In the meantime, provide oxygen as soon as possible and maintain body temperature to delay the onset of shock. Note the mechanism of injury so you can report it to the transport team.

Pelvic girdle injuries may be best managed using a specialized commercial splint. One such device is the SAM® Sling (Key Skill 20.8). If you do not carry this equipment, you may continue patient assessment while you are waiting for more advanced care to arrive.

When the transport team arrives, you can help them place the stabilized patient on a scoop stretcher or spine board. Provide oxygen to the patient as soon as possible and cover them to maintain body temperature and to help reduce the chance of developing shock. If you suspect spinal injury, do not attempt to move the patient until you have additional help. In the meantime, stabilize the patient's head and neck and continue to reassure them.

Because the signs and symptoms of musculoskeletal injuries are similar, you will not be trying to determine which type of injury the patient has sustained. Even so, there are certain signs that indicate a possible hip dislocation. Look for them because you do not want to attempt to move an injured leg if there is a possible hip dislocation. If you suspect a hip dislocation, there may also be injury to the femur (thigh bone). Do not try to straighten an angulated femur if the hip appears to be dislocated.

REMEMBER

The term *pelvic girdle* refers to the entire area of the pelvis and hips. Pelvic fractures can result in significant bleeding because the arteries that supply the legs with blood are tightly bound to the pelvic bones. Commercial devices called pelvic slings or binders can be tightened around the pelvis to serve as a splint and help reduce bleeding.

Applying the SAM® Sling Pelvic Splint

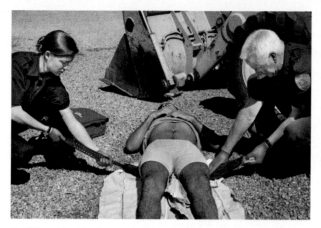

1. Place the device under the patient at the level of the pelvis.

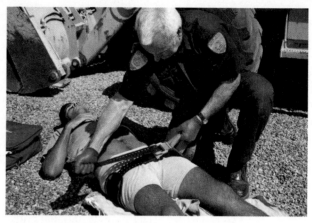

2. Wrap the device over the top and pull until you hear the buckle click. This signifies the appropriate amount of pressure.

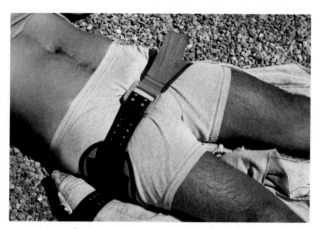

3. The SAM® Sling applied to an injured pelvis.

There are two types of hip dislocation:

- *Anterior hip dislocation.* The leg from hip to foot is rotated laterally (outward) farther than the leg on the uninjured side. Leg rotation may also be an indication of hip fracture. With hip fracture, the injured leg may appear to be shorter than the other leg. You will probably see or feel the bony end of the femur under the skin at the front or side of the leg where it joins the torso.
- *Posterior hip dislocation.* This is the most common type. The leg is rotated medially (inward), and the knee is usually bent. You may see or feel the bony end of the femur under the skin at the back of the leg where it joins the buttocks.

If you suspect a dislocated hip, wait for more advanced care to arrive. While waiting, provide oxygen as soon as possible, and cover the patient to maintain body temperature and help prevent shock. You can immobilize the injured leg by securing pillows or folded blankets or towels around the injured leg to support the leg and provide comfort to the patient. Do not reposition or move the patient's leg while securing pillows or blankets.

Injuries to the Upper Leg Injuries to the femur can be life threatening even when the injury is closed because bleeding inside the tissues can be severe. There may be a severe and obvious deformity with femur fractures. The leg below the injury site may be bent where there is no joint, or it will appear twisted.

Consider the use of a rigid splint or a device called a *traction splint* for injuries to the femur. Traction splints allow for the application of constant traction to the injured extremity. This is helpful to reduce pain, swelling, and movement. Traction splints should be considered only for suspected isolated mid-shaft femur fractures when the injury does not involve the knee or the hip/pelvis. They should also not be used if there are injuries to the lower leg or ankle.

Emergency Medical Responder units may carry traction splints, and you may be trained and allowed to use them. (Your instructor will advise you if traction splints are part of your local protocols.) Soft splints are not as effective as rigid or traction splints, but they will stabilize the injury and provide some pain relief.

While waiting for the transport team, provide the patient some relief from pain by securing a rolled-up blanket between the legs in the same way you would for injuries to the pelvic girdle. This is effective once the patient is secured to a spine board or scoop stretcher (a form of rigid splinting). Provide oxygen as soon as possible and cover the patient to maintain body warmth to help prevent shock.

Injuries to the Knee In most cases, you will not be able to tell if the knee is fractured, dislocated, or both. Because of the many nerves and blood vessels and the possibility that soft tissues were damaged, immobilize an injured knee in the position in which it is found. Do not attempt to reposition or straighten an injured knee. Some EMS systems allow Emergency Medical Responders to make one attempt at straightening the limb if there is no distal pulse. Your instructor will let you know the requirements of your local protocols.

Rigid splinting is the most effective method to use when immobilizing an injured knee, but you can provide support to the leg and comfort to the patient with soft splints. Secure pillows or folded blankets around the knee, especially if it is found in the bent position. Do not reposition or move the patient's legs to place or secure pillows or blankets. If the injured knee is found in the straight position, you can effectively immobilize it with a rolled-up blanket placed between both legs and secured with cravats, just as you would for a femur injury.

To immobilize an injured knee in the straight position, secure a long splint behind the leg from the patient's buttocks to beyond the foot. You also may use the method described for splinting the lower leg (described in the following section). In cases in which the patient's leg will remain flexed at the knee, you may secure one or two shorter splints at an angle across the thigh and lower leg (A-frame) with cravats (Key Skill 20.9).

KEY SKILL 20.9

Immobilizing a Bent Knee

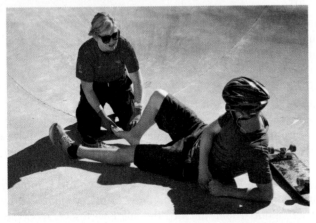

1. Assess distal circulation, sensation, and motor function.

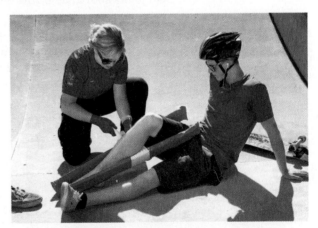

2. Apply rigid splints on either side of the limb.

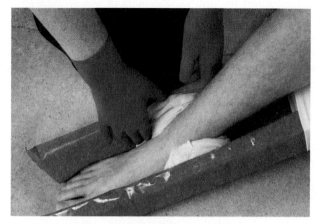

3. Pad the splints on both sides of the ankle.

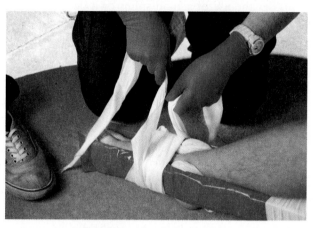

4. Secure the distal ends of the splints.

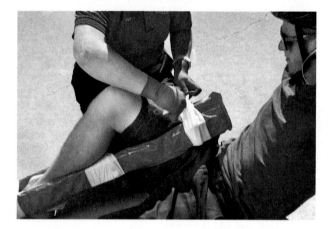

5. Secure the proximal end of the splints.

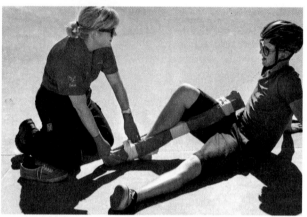

6. Reassess distal circulation, sensation, and motor function.

Injuries to the Lower Leg   You can provide care for injuries to the lower leg with either rigid or soft splints. A blanket roll between the legs is an effective soft splint. Secure it in the same manner as for pelvic, thigh, and knee injuries. Once you have placed the patient on the spine board or scoop stretcher (rigid splinting), you have completed immobilizing all joints above and below the injury site (Key Skill 20.10).

If you use a rigid splint, you will need assistance. One individual must maintain manual stabilization while you apply the splint. A single-splint method also may be used to immobilize lower leg injuries.

Injuries to the Ankle or Foot   Rigid splints may be used for injuries to the ankle or foot, but the soft splint is probably the most comfortable for the patient and the quickest to apply. If you apply a rigid splint, use one that extends from above the patient's knee to beyond the foot as described for the single-splint method for the lower leg.

When soft-splinting an injury to the foot or ankle, immobilize it in the position found with a pillow or folded blanket. Secure the soft splint around the foot and ankle with several cravats or with roller gauze (Figure 20.13) and elevate it by propping it on a blanket roll or pillow.

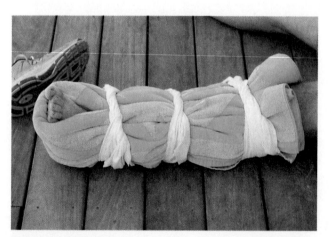

Figure 20.13 Immobilization of the lower leg using a towel.

Immobilizing the Lower Leg

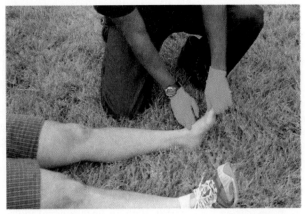

1. Assess circulation, sensation, and motor function prior to splinting the extremity.

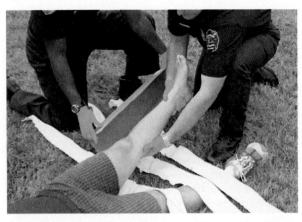

2. Choose a splint that extends from the heel to well above the knee.

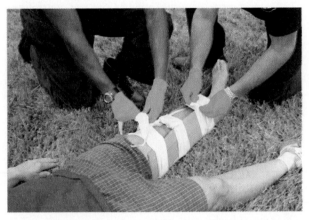

3. Secure the splint above and below the knee and at the ankle.

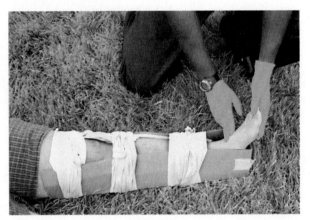

4. Reassess circulation, sensation, and motor function after the splint is secure.

FIRST ON SCENE WRAP-UP

Ron has just finished splinting Annie's leg with a putter and a sand wedge when the ambulance approaches, moving slowly across the grass. The EMTs compliment Ron on straightening and splinting Annie's injured leg, and they decide to transport her with the makeshift splint. Just before the ambulance crew shuts the doors, Ron pats Annie's uninjured leg and says, "Let me get this golf cart figured out, and I'll meet you over at the ER."

"Ron!" She looks at him sternly, her voice muffled by the oxygen mask. "Don't you dare finish the game without me!"

Summary

- The musculoskeletal system is made up of muscles, bones, joints, connective tissues, blood vessels, and nerves.
- Support, movement, protection, and cell production are the primary functions of the musculoskeletal system.
- The bones of the axial skeleton (skull, spine, ribs, and sternum) and appendicular skeleton (upper and lower extremities) make up the skeletal system.
- The signs and symptoms of musculoskeletal injury include pain, swelling, discoloration, and deformity.
- A strain is the stretching or tearing of a muscle, and a sprain is the partial or complete tearing of a ligament. A fracture is the cracking or breaking of a bone, and a dislocation is when the end of a bone is pulled partially or completely away from a joint.
- An open skeletal injury is when a broken bone end or bone fragments tear through the skin.
- Proper care for a musculoskeletal injury includes assessment and monitoring of the patient's ABCs and appropriate immobilization of the injury.
- It is critical to assess the circulation, sensation, and motor function of extremities distal to an injury to determine if blood vessels or nerves may have been damaged.
- Direct force causes injury at the point where there was impact to the body, but an indirect-force injury is caused when energy is transmitted from the point of contact to a different area of the body where it causes injury.
- If an injured extremity is angulated, it should be splinted in place unless there is no distal circulation and the limb can be placed back into correct anatomical position with ease and without causing pain for the patient.
- Skeletal injuries should be stabilized to prevent them from worsening, such as a closed fracture becoming an open fracture.
- When caring for a patient with an open skeletal injury, it is important to begin with a primary assessment to evaluate for life threats and determine if other injuries are present. It is important to expose the injury site and control excessive bleeding. The injury should also be properly immobilized and splinted. Administer oxygen if allowed and monitor the patient's vital signs until transport.
- When caring for a patient with multisystem trauma, it is critical to assess and monitor the ABCs, assume and care for spinal injury, control any severe bleeding, and treat for shock while coordinating rapid transport.

Take Action

Practice Makes Perfect

When it comes to developing long-bone and joint-splinting skills, there is nothing better than good, old-fashioned practice. This activity allows you to practice these skills using only the most basic of materials. You will need a small assortment of easy-to-gather supplies: newspaper, a couple of magazines, some short and long pieces of cardboard, and several triangular bandages. You will need another student to play the role of patient.

Using the following four "rules," take turns with your partner splinting various simulated injuries. Alternate back and forth and change the injury from upper to lower extremity and from long-bone to joint injuries.

1. Check circulation, sensation, and motor function before moving the injury.
2. Immobilize the suspected fracture site.
3. Immobilize the joints above and below the suspected fracture site.
4. Reevaluate circulation, sensation, and motor function.

Refer to these rules as you progress through the splinting process. Carefully evaluate each step of the way to see if what you are doing is really meeting the objective. Since bone injuries are relatively low in the priority list of a busy emergency department, be sure to make comfort a high priority as you apply the splints. Pad all potential pressure points and fill all voids. If you are playing patient, be sure to let the "Emergency Medical Responder" know if they touch or move your injury in a way that might cause pain.

First on Scene Patient Handoff

Annie is a 63-year-old female with an injury to her left lower leg following a fall trying to stop a runaway golf cart. The limb was initially found angulated, and the distal pulse was absent. After carefully straightening the limb the pulse quickly returned. CSM in the foot is normal, and an improvised splint was applied to the limb. Vital signs are within normal limits. The patient denies hitting her head or losing consciousness.

First on Scene Run Review

Recall the events of the First on Scene scenario in this chapter, and answer the following questions related to the call. Rationales are offered in the Answer Key at the back of the book.

1. Should Ron have straightened out the leg? Why or why not?
2. Did Ron do the right thing by splinting the leg? Explain your reasoning.
3. What information should Ron give the ambulance crew?

Quick Quiz

To check your understanding of the chapter, answer the following questions. Then compare your answers to those in the Answer Key at the back of the book.

1. All of the following are functions of the musculoskeletal system EXCEPT:
   a. hormone production.
   b. support.
   c. protection.
   d. cell production.

2. An injury that is characterized by broken skin above the site of fracture is commonly described as a(n) _____ fracture.
   a. open
   b. closed
   c. complex
   d. superficial

3. Which of the following would NOT be considered appropriate when caring for a suspected fracture?
   a. Cut away clothing to expose the injury site.
   b. Put possible dislocations back into place.
   c. Assess circulation, sensation, and motor function.
   d. Immobilize the joint above and below the injury site.

4. A boy fell off a slide and dislocated his shoulder when he threw out his hand to break his fall. This injury was caused by:
   a. direct force.
   b. blunt force trauma.
   c. indirect force.
   d. penetrating trauma.

5. A _____ occurs when a bone end is moved partially or completely away from a joint.
   a. fracture
   b. dislocation
   c. concussion
   d. rotation

6. When assessing a patient with a musculoskeletal injury, it is important to check:
   a. circulation, sensation, and motor function.
   b. grip strength, range of motion, and pain level.
   c. color, range of motion, and capillary refill.
   d. circulation, grip strength, and weight-bearing ability.

7. All of the following are common signs and symptoms of an extremity injury EXCEPT:
   a. pain.
   b. swelling.
   c. deformity.
   d. lengthening.

8. The partial or complete tearing of ligaments and tendons that support a joint is called a:
   a. strain.
   b. sprain.
   c. fracture.
   d. dislocation.

9. You are caring for a patient who has an injury characterized by an open wound, severe deformity, and bleeding. Your highest priority is:
   a. straightening the deformity.
   b. covering the open wound.
   c. splinting the extremity.
   d. controlling bleeding.

10. In which of the following situations would it be appropriate to place an angulated extremity back into anatomical position?

    a. The distal pulse is absent.
    b. There is an open wound.
    c. A splint is unavailable.
    d. The patient is in significant pain.

11. A triangular bandage used to stabilize the elbow and arm is called a:

    a. cravat.
    b. dressing.
    c. bandage.
    d. sling.

12. When properly applied, a sling and swathe will adequately immobilize all of the following EXCEPT the:

    a. elbow.
    b. forearm.
    c. shoulder.
    d. knee.

13. It is important to maintain the hand and foot of an injured extremity in a normal and comfortable position during splinting. This position is called the:

    a. recumbent position.
    b. position of function.
    c. position of comfort.
    d. resting position.

14. A young girl has a deformed right arm after her brother accidentally hit her with a bat. This injury was caused by:

    a. direct force.
    b. twisting force.
    c. indirect force.
    d. referred pain.

15. You have just finished applying a splint to a patient's injured leg. You should:

    a. ask the patient to try and move his or her leg.
    b. recheck circulation, sensation, and motor function.
    c. obtain a blood pressure.
    d. immobilize using a soft stretcher.

16. You are caring for a patient who has one leg that is shortened with the foot rotated to one side. These are likely signs of a possible:

    a. spinal injury.
    b. dislocated hip.
    c. fractured knee.
    d. sprained ankle.

17. A woman has injured her ankle. It is swollen and very painful. Which of the following materials would be appropriate to use to immobilize the injured ankle?

    a. Short spine board
    b. Traction splint
    c. Sling and swathe
    d. Folded blanket

18. You are caring for an angulated injury to the lower leg and you find severe bleeding from the wound. You should:

    a. place the patient on oxygen.
    b. use direct pressure to control the bleeding.
    c. attempt to straighten the leg.
    d. check distal CSM before anything else.

19. You are caring for a 10-year-old boy who has fallen 12 feet. He has angulated injuries to both legs and is unresponsive. He is breathing adequately, and you find no bleeding. You should first:

    a. hold manual stabilization of his head and neck.
    b. straighten the angulated legs.
    c. check distal CSM in both legs.
    d. place him on a long board.

20. You are caring for a woman with a badly injured ankle. You should:

    a. leave the shoe in place.
    b. carefully remove the shoe.
    c. wait for EMTs to decide what to do.
    d. just loosen the shoelaces.

Endnote

1. David Markenson, J.D., Ferguson, L., Chameides, P., Cassan, K.L., Chung, J., Epstein, L., Gonzales, R.A., Herrington, J.L., Pellegrino, N., Ratcliff, and Singer, A. "2015 American Heart Association and American Red Cross Guidelines for First Aid," *Circulation*, Vol. 132 (2015): S269–S311, originally published October 14, 2015.

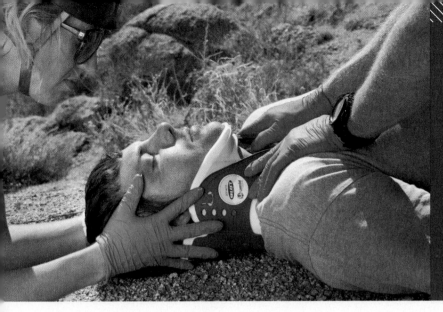

21

Caring for Head and Spinal Injuries

LEARNING OBJECTIVES

Upon successful completion of this chapter, the student should be able to:

Cognitive

1. Define the chapter key terms.
2. Describe the major components of the nervous system.
3. Describe the major components of the cranium.
4. Describe the major components of the spinal column.
5. Explain how the mechanism of injury relates to the potential for spinal injury.
6. Differentiate between an open and closed head injury.
7. Describe the signs and symptoms of a head injury.
8. Explain the appropriate assessment and care for a patient with a head injury.
9. Describe the signs and symptoms of a spinal injury.
10. Explain the appropriate assessment and care for a patient with a suspected spinal injury.
11. Explain the special considerations of airway management for a patient with suspected cervical spine injury.

Psychomotor

12. Demonstrate the appropriate assessment and care for a patient with a head injury.

13. Demonstrate the appropriate assessment and care for a patient with a suspected spinal injury.
14. Demonstrate the appropriate airway management for a patient with a suspected cervical spine injury.
15. Demonstrate the appropriate technique for manual stabilization of the cervical spine.
16. Demonstrate the appropriate sizing and application of a cervical collar.
17. Demonstrate the proper technique for log-rolling a patient.
18. Demonstrate the proper technique for immobilization of a supine patient.
19. Demonstrate the proper technique for immobilization of a seated patient.
20. Demonstrate the proper technique for removing a helmet from a patient with a suspected spinal injury.

Affective

21. Value the importance of proper body substance isolation (BSI) precautions when caring for patients with head and spinal injuries.

Education Standards

Trauma—Head, Facial, Neck, and Spine Trauma

Competencies

Uses assessment information to recognize and manage life threats based on assessment findings for an acutely injured patient while awaiting additional emergency response.

central nervous system (*p. 442*)

concussion (*p. 445*)

cranium (*p. 442*)

distracting injury (*p. 451*)

paralysis (*p. 448*)

peripheral nervous system (*p. 442*)

spinal motion restriction (*p. 450*)

traumatic brain injury (TBI) (*p. 445*)

Injuries to the head and spine are very common and can lead to significant disability and even death if not identified and managed appropriately. This chapter discusses the common causes of head and spinal injuries and the proper techniques for assessment and care of patients with suspected head or spinal injuries.

FIRST ON SCENE

"Safety officer to the ground stage." Shelby hears the call as she makes her way to the auditorium where the stage is being set for the concert that night. A small crowd has gathered at the west side of the stage.

"He fell!" a booming voice says as Shelby enters the scene. It is the stage manager. "Marc did exactly what I told him not to do, and he fell!"

"Marc," Shelby says, setting her equipment down beside a young man lying beside the 10-foot-tall stage. A young stage technician is holding Marc's head still and straight. "My name is Shelby, and I'm going to help you until the medics arrive, okay?"

"Okay," Marc says softly, his eyes moving back and forth among the faces huddled nearby. "I'm so sorry. I didn't think I was that close to the edge. I should be fine, boss," he says as he starts to move his arms to get up.

"Don't move just yet," Shelby says, noticing a small stream of blood dripping from his scalp. "You fell from a pretty decent height onto this concrete, and I don't want you compromising your neck or spine."

"Oh my God," Marc says, panicked. "I can't feel my legs."

Anatomy of the Head and Spine

LO2 Describe the major components of the nervous system.

LO3 Describe the major components of the cranium.

LO4 Describe the major components of the spinal column.

cranium ▶ the skull.

central nervous system ▶ composed of the brain and spinal cord; responsible for voluntary and involuntary control of all bodily functions.

peripheral nervous system ▶ nerves that extend from the spinal cord throughout the body; transmits signals between the brain and the rest of the body.

The adult **cranium**, or skull, consists of 22 bones. It is divided into two regions, the cranial vault (bones that encase the brain) and the facial bones (Figure 21.1). The cranium sits at the top of the spinal column and can twist and move in many directions. It is this position and ability to move in all directions that makes the head and neck so susceptible to injury.

The face is made up of several strong, irregularly shaped bones. The facial bones include bones of the cheeks, the upper part of the nose, upper jaw, lower jaw, and part of the eye sockets. These bones are fused into immovable joints except for the mandible (lower jawbone), which is the only movable bone in the head.

The brain and the spinal cord make up the **central nervous system**, which is responsible for processing the information it receives from all parts of the body and coordinating responses. These include conscious thought, memory, and reasoning as well as the voluntary control of muscles and involuntary control of heart rate, respirations, and temperature regulation.

The **peripheral nervous system** consists of the many nerves that extend from the spinal cord throughout the body. These nerves carry messages from the brain to the body and from the body back to the brain. Injury to the spine can damage the spinal cord and prevent it from carrying messages to or from parts of the body. When nerves are damaged, the affected part of the body no longer has contact with the brain and is unable to function normally. The damage could be temporary, caused by pressure or swelling that may be corrected with proper care, or the damage could be permanent. In addition, the spinal cord controls several types of reflexes, which allow us to react quickly to such things as pain and heat.

The brain is surrounded by three protective layers of tissue called *meninges* (Figure 21.2). In addition, the brain and spinal cord are surrounded by a clear fluid called *cerebrospinal fluid*. This fluid serves as a protective cushion in the event of injury. When the brain becomes injured, some or all of these structures can be compromised.

The spinal column begins at the base of the skull and extends down into the pelvis. It consists of approximately 33 bones called vertebrae (Figure 21.3). The spinal cord extends down the center of these bones.

Mechanism of Injury

LO5 Explain how the mechanism of injury relates to the potential for spinal injury.

Injuries to the head and spine may not always be obvious. It is essential that you carefully evaluate your patient to determine the mechanism of injury (MOI) (Key Skill 21.1).

Figure 21.1 Bones of the skull.

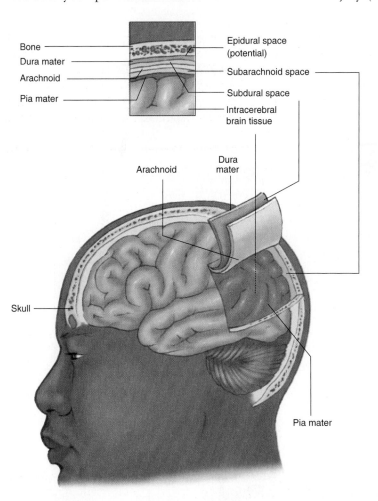

Figure 21.2 The brain is protected by three layers of membranes called meninges. The inner layer is the pia mater, the middle is the arachnoid, and the outer layer is the dura mater.

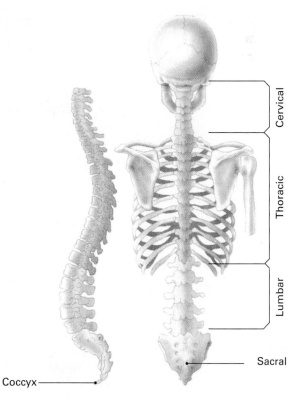

Figure 21.3 Segments of the spinal column.

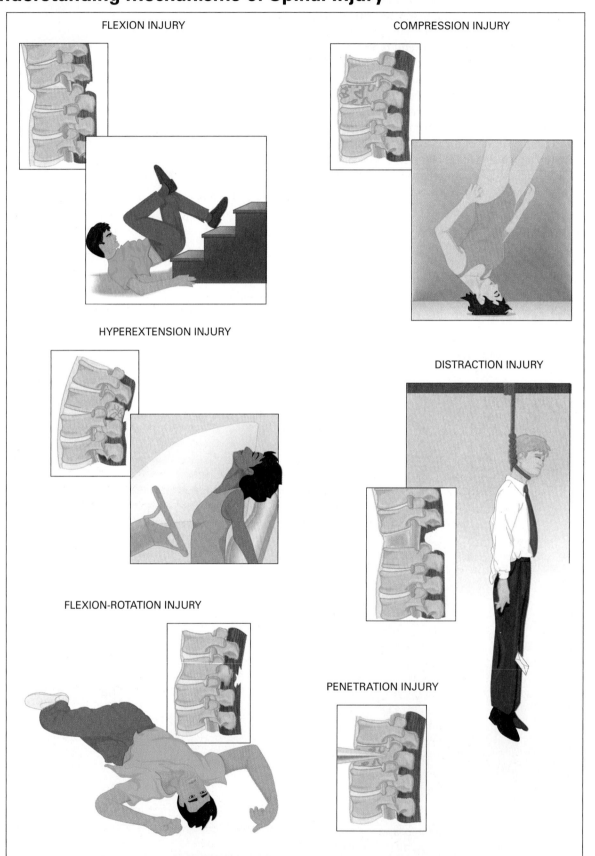

Understanding Mechanisms of Spinal Injury

FLEXION INJURY

COMPRESSION INJURY

HYPEREXTENSION INJURY

DISTRACTION INJURY

FLEXION-ROTATION INJURY

PENETRATION INJURY

If the MOI suggests that an injury to the head, neck, or spine could exist, then you must care for your patient accordingly. If the patient is unable to provide an account of what happened, then you must check with witnesses or bystanders for this information. When in doubt, provide care as if head and/or spinal injury exists. Be highly suspicious of head/spinal injury if the MOI includes any of the following:

- Falls
- Forces that caused excessive flexion (bending) or extension (stretching) of the neck or spine
- Pulling or hanging forces that caused spinal stretching
- Compression injuries from diving
- Motor vehicle crashes
- Significant blunt trauma
- Penetrating trauma such as that caused by gunshots or stabbings
- Any trauma situation in which the patient is unresponsive

Young children are very prone to head injuries. One reason is that, in children, the head is disproportionately large compared to the size of the body. This makes the head more difficult to support and protect during falls.

Injuries to the Head and Face

| LO6 | Differentiate between an open and closed head injury.

Injuries to the head and face can be some of the most challenging to manage for the Emergency Medical Responder. Having to manage the potential for neck injuries while trying to maintain an open airway is just one of the challenges you will face.

Injuries to the Head

Injuries to the head are commonly caused by blunt trauma. Blunt trauma can occur when an object strikes the head or when the head strikes a hard object such as the ground after a fall or the inside of a vehicle during a collision. Blunt trauma to the head can cause a **traumatic brain injury** (TBI).

Head injuries can be either closed or open. Closed injuries occur when the bones of the cranium remain intact (Figure 21.4). Signs and symptoms of closed head injuries can present hours and even days after the injury occurs. In a closed head injury, the skull remains intact, but the brain can be injured by the force of something striking the skull. Such a force can cause the brain to bounce off the inside of the skull. The resulting injuries to the brain may include:

- *Concussion.* A **concussion** occurs when a blow to the head causes minor and temporary damage to the brain. The injury may be so minor that it does not cause a loss of consciousness; or it may be mild, causing a headache after a brief loss of consciousness; or it may be severe, causing a prolonged loss of consciousness and abnormal vital signs. Sometimes short-term memory is lost. Any signs and symptoms of concussion are an indication of brain injury.
- *Traumatic brain injury.* Trauma that results in the alteration of normal brain function.
- *Hemorrhage (contusion).* If the mechanism of injury is severe enough, it can cause the rupture of blood vessels in the brain. Cerebral contusion occurs when the energy of the impact translates directly to the tissue of the brain (not just the capillaries) and causes the cerebral tissue to swell. The cell membranes become damaged, resulting in swelling. The swollen cerebral tissue does not work as efficiently, leading to the myriad of symptoms seen in concussion.

traumatic brain injury ▶ brain injury that occurs when a sudden, external force damages one or more areas of the brain. Abbrev: TBI.

concussion ▶ type of traumatic brain injury that causes temporary loss of normal brain function.

REMEMBER

Sometimes the terms *head injury* and *traumatic brain injury* are used interchangeably. You should be less concerned about the obvious superficial trauma to the skin covering the head and face than you are for the potential injury to the brain, which you cannot examine directly.

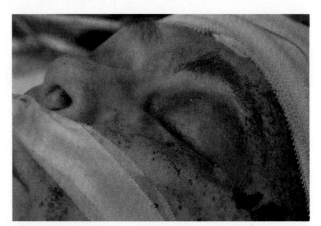

Figure 21.4 Bruising around the eyes can be a sign of a closed head injury.
(© Edward T. Dickinson, MD)

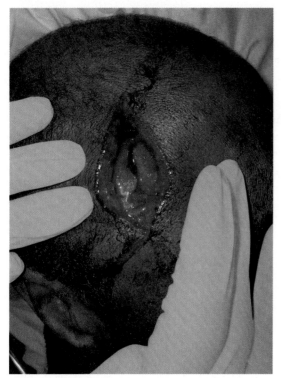

Figure 21.5 Open head injuries are characterized by a break in the skin and the underlying skull.
(© Edward T. Dickinson, MD)

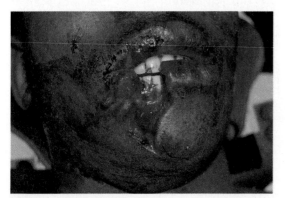

Figure 21.6 Be alert to possible airway compromise with injuries to the jaw and mouth.
(© Edward T. Dickinson, MD)

Open injuries occur when the cranium and overlying soft tissue are broken, exposing the meninges or brain (Figure 21.5). It is often difficult to determine if a head injury is open or closed because the soft tissues of the scalp can be damaged and bleeding without obvious injury to the cranium. It is always best to assume that a head injury is open and care for it accordingly.

Injuries to the Face

Facial injuries can be very serious because of the potential for airway obstruction (Figure 21.6). Blood and other fluids, blood clots, bone or bone fragments, and teeth may cause partial or complete airway obstruction. Consider the possibility of airway obstruction when you find any of the following signs:

- Blood in the airway (nose or mouth)
- Deformity or depression of any part of the face
- Swelling or discoloration around the eyes
- Swelling or discoloration of any part of the face
- Poor jaw function or inability to move the jaw
- Teeth that are loose or have been knocked out or broken dentures

Signs and Symptoms of Head (Brain) Injury

LO7 Describe the signs and symptoms of a head injury.

Injuries to the head can range from minor lacerations to the scalp and face to severe skull fractures and significant injury to the brain. While it is difficult to know the true extent of damage when the brain is injured, one of the best immediate indicators is the mental status of the injured individual. An individual who is alert and oriented following a head injury is likely to have less damage than an individual who is unresponsive or who has experienced a brief period of unconsciousness.

The following are common signs and symptoms of a head injury:

- Significant mechanism of injury
- Bleeding of the scalp
- Deformity of the cranium
- Altered mental status
- Nausea and vomiting
- Convulsions
- Abnormal vital signs
  - Abnormal breathing patterns
  - Combative behavior
  - Repetitive questions

It is common to see abnormal vital signs in a patient with significant head injury. As pressure builds up inside the skull due to bleeding and swelling, it is common to see the blood pressure increase and the pulse rate decrease. Breathing patterns can change and become erratic as well.

It is important to always consider the possibility of a spinal injury when caring for a patient who has a head injury. The force sustained by the head also could have caused injury to the vertebrae of the neck.

In extreme cases of head injury, you may see a patient with abnormal flexion or extension of the arms (Figure 21.7). This is referred to as "posturing" and is a sign of significant head injury.

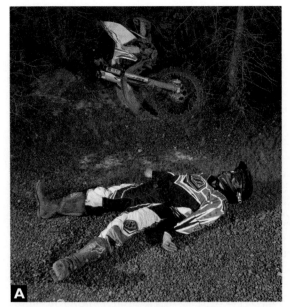
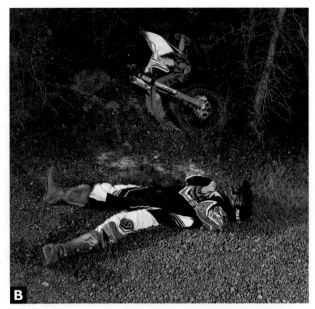

Figure 21.7 Abnormal posturing is a sign of significant head injury. (A) Abnormal extension (decerebrate posture). (B) Abnormal flexion (decorticate posture).

Caring for Head Injuries

| LO8 | Explain the appropriate assessment and care for a patient with a head injury.

When caring for someone with a head injury, it is important to suspect that they may also have sustained an injury to the cervical spine. Whenever possible, maintain manual stabilization of the head and neck when providing care. Remember that the control center for breathing is located deep within the brain. Any injury to the brain can disrupt normal breathing and cause the patient to exhibit inadequate respirations. Constantly monitor the adequacy of breathing for all patients with head injuries.

Follow these steps when caring for a patient with a suspected head injury:

1. Perform a primary assessment and ensure an open airway and adequate breathing. If the patient is unresponsive, open the airway with the jaw-thrust maneuver first. If this is unsuccessful, use the head-tilt/chin-lift method.
2. If necessary, provide rescue breaths using an appropriate barrier device.
3. Control any obvious bleeding. Be careful to apply only enough pressure to stop the bleeding but not too much pressure. Excessive pressure can injure the brain if the skull has been fractured.
4. Keep the patient still and lying flat. Maintain manual stabilization of the head and neck.
5. Administer supplemental oxygen if available. Follow local protocols.
6. Have suction prepared in case the individual vomits. If no suction is available, roll the patient onto their side while maintaining alignment of the head and neck.
7. Monitor vital signs, including mental status.

Caring for Injuries to the Face

In all cases of injury to the face, your priority is to make certain that the patient has an open and clear airway.

Injuries to the face can damage teeth and dentures. Always look for and remove avulsed (dislodged) teeth and parts of broken dental appliances such as dentures and crowns. Be careful not to inadvertently push these down the patient's airway while attempting to retrieve them. When a tooth is avulsed, there may be bleeding from the socket. Have the responsive patient bite down on a pad of gauze placed over the socket but leave several inches of gauze outside the mouth for quick removal. For the unresponsive patient, hold the gauze over the socket. This will control the bleeding and prevent the airway from becoming obstructed with blood.

SCENE SAFETY

Always wear appropriate personal protective equipment, including eye protection, when caring for someone with a suspected head injury. Injuries to the head often cause significant vomiting, exposing you to the individual's body fluids.

REMEMBER

Your first attempt at opening the airway of an unresponsive patient with a head injury should be with the jaw-thrust maneuver. If the jaw-thrust does not open the airway, use the head-tilt/chin-lift maneuver. Maintaining an open airway and providing adequate ventilations are critical priorities.

Wrap the avulsed tooth in a clean gauze dressing. If you have a source of clean water, keep the dressing moist. (Milk can also be used.) Do not attempt to clean the tooth.

Injuries to the Spine

Most patients with spinal trauma will have sustained their neurologic injury before you arrive at their side. They will have either cut or bruised the spinal cord and/or the nerves leaving the spinal column. If they are awake, they will have signs and symptoms that help you determine the presence of injury. However, if they have an altered mental status, you must assume based on the mechanism of injury that they have a spinal injury and take appropriate precautions.

Spinal injuries are caused by forces to the head, neck, back, chest, pelvis, or legs. Head injuries result in cervical spine injuries by causing severe flexion or extension of the neck. Injuries to the upper leg bones or to the pelvic bones also may cause spine injury through indirect force. Motor vehicle crashes, falls, and mishaps during activities such as diving, cycling, and skiing are common causes of spinal injuries.

paralysis ▶ loss of ability to move and sometimes loss of sensation (ability to feel).

Injuries to the cervical spine can cause **paralysis**, impaired breathing, and even death. Injuries along the rest of the spinal column can also cause paralysis and reduce normal body movement and function.

If a patient has numbness, loss of feeling, or paralysis in the legs with no problems in the arms, the injury to the spine is probably below the neck. If numbness, loss of feeling, or paralysis involves the arms and the legs, the injury is probably in the neck. Numbness, loss of feeling, and paralysis may be limited to only one side of the body as a result of penetrating trauma to the spine, but usually both sides are involved if the injury is due to nonpenetrating (blunt) trauma.

Injuries to the spine can include fractured or displaced vertebrae or swelling that presses on nerves. These injuries can produce the same signs and symptoms. In some cases, the loss of function associated with spinal injuries may be temporary if it is caused by pressure or swelling that may eventually resolve.

Signs and Symptoms of Spinal Injury

LO9 Describe the signs and symptoms of a spinal injury.

Conduct a thorough patient history during your assessment of a responsive patient. Follow these guidelines when assessing a patient with suspected spinal injury:

- Do their hands or feet feel numb or tingly? Can the patient feel you touch their hands and feet? Can the patient squeeze your hand or push your hand with their foot?
- Look and feel gently for injuries and deformities.
- Ask the patient if they can move their arms and legs.

For the unresponsive patient, ask bystanders for any information related to what they saw happen. This may help you determine the mechanism of injury. Also look and feel for injuries and deformities. See if the patient responds to pressure on or pinching of the feet and hands.

The following are the most common signs and symptoms of a spinal injury:

- Pain on palpation of the spine (point tenderness)
- Deformity of the spine
- Numbness, weakness, or tingling in the extremities
- Loss of sensation
- Paralysis
- Incontinence (loss of bladder or bowel control)
- Priapism (erection of the penis)

REMEMBER

In some cases, there may be a loss of sensation but not movement or loss of movement but not sensation. For this reason, you should check both sensation and motor function of all extremities.

Carefully check all extremities for circulation, sensation, and motor function (CSM). Any problems with sensation or motor function can be an indication of a possible spinal cord injury (Key Skill 21.2). Not all spinal injuries are immediate or permanent. The spinal cord can be damaged by direct injury or by swelling that occurs hours after the injury. Be especially careful when assessing and moving an injured individual who has a suspected spinal injury.

Assessing the Patient with a Suspected Spinal Injury

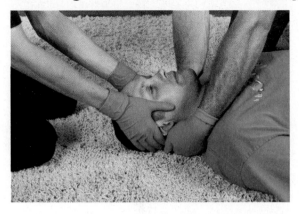

1. Palpate the neck anterior and posterior for pain and deformity.

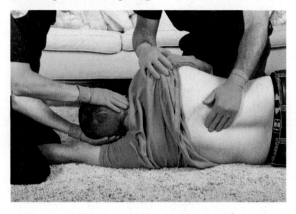

2. Palpate the spine for pain and deformity.

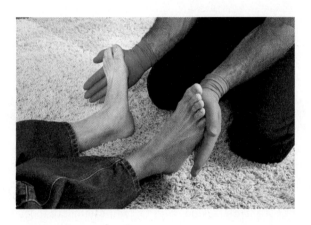

3. Assess motor function of both feet simultaneously.

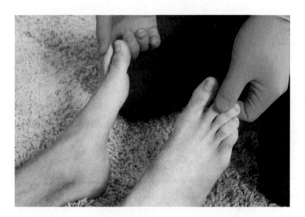

4. Assess sensation of both feet by checking for numbness and tingling in at least two toes—ideally big toe and little toe.

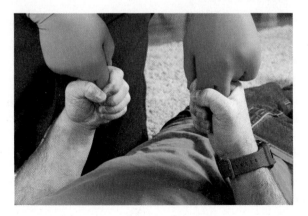

5. Assess motor function of both hands simultaneously.

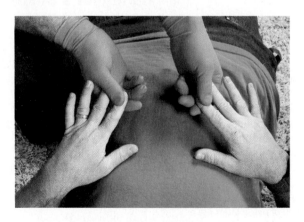

6. Assess sensation of both hands by checking for numbness and tingling in at least two fingers—ideally thumb and little finger.

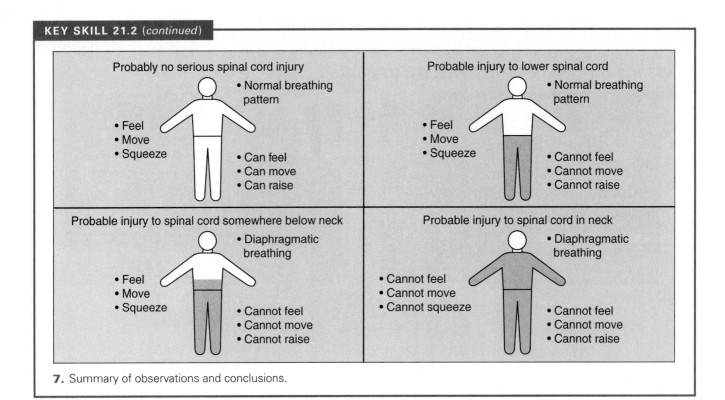

Probably no serious spinal cord injury
- Normal breathing pattern
- Feel
- Move
- Squeeze
- Can feel
- Can move
- Can raise

Probable injury to lower spinal cord
- Normal breathing pattern
- Feel
- Move
- Squeeze
- Cannot feel
- Cannot move
- Cannot raise

Probable injury to spinal cord somewhere below neck
- Diaphragmatic breathing
- Feel
- Move
- Squeeze
- Cannot feel
- Cannot move
- Cannot raise

Probable injury to spinal cord in neck
- Diaphragmatic breathing
- Cannot feel
- Cannot move
- Cannot squeeze
- Cannot feel
- Cannot move
- Cannot raise

7. Summary of observations and conclusions.

FIRST ON SCENE (continued)

"Marc, Marc, just please try and stay calm," Shelby says, securing a bandage to the side of his head. "I need to control the bleeding. We'll figure out what's going on with your legs next. I promise. Just please try not to move."

"Can you feel my hands?" Shelby asks as she grabs hold of Marc's quivering fingers. He nods, and she grips onto both of his index fingers, which he readily identifies as being held. He also squeezes tightly with both hands.

Now the legs, Shelby thinks, as she carefully palpates both of Marc's legs down to his feet, careful not to jostle him. "I'm going to check your lower extremities. Let me know what you feel."

Caring for a Suspected Spinal Injury

REMEMBER

For any patient found to be unresponsive and for whom you are unable to determine an exact mechanism of injury or nature of illness, provide care as though they have a spinal injury.

spinal motion restriction ▶ practice of using alternative methods for spinal immobilization based on mechanism of injury and patient presentation. Abbrev: SMR.

LO10 Explain the appropriate assessment and care for a patient with a suspected spinal injury.

LO11 Explain the special considerations of airway management for a patient with suspected cervical spine injury.

Injuries to the spine can result in a wide range of severity. Do not be fooled by the absence of obvious signs and symptoms during your assessment. These injuries often worsen as time passes, so be very diligent with your assessment.

When caring for a patient with a suspected spinal injury, perform a primary assessment and ensure the ABCs are intact. If you must manage the airway, attempt the jaw-thrust maneuver first, before the head-tilt/chin-lift maneuver. Then manually stabilize the head so the head, neck, and spine do not move and are kept in line (Key Skill 21.3).

The term now being used to describe the care for patients with a mechanism of injury that could be suggestive of a spinal injury is **spinal motion restriction** (SMR). SMR is a new approach to the management of patients with suspected spinal injuries that

Manual Stabilization of Head and Neck

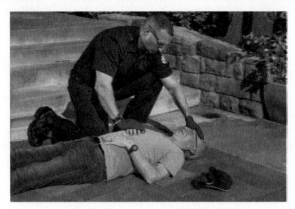

1. Using one hand to provide manual stabilization of the head when you are at the side of the injured patient.

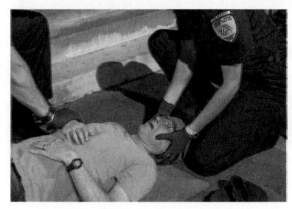

2. Using two hands to provide manual stabilization of the patient's head and neck.

better addresses the appropriate restriction required as well as the patient's comfort.[1] Those patients with a high index of suspicion for spinal injury will be managed with conventional means such as a spine board. Those patients at less risk for spinal injury may be managed with more comfortable methods, such as soft collars and manual stabilization provided by transport cots or gurneys. Professional organizations have released position statements and allocated resources advocating for discretionary use of long backboards.[2,3,4]

If the decision is made to utilize a long backboard, it should be padded with a blanket or purpose-made pad prior to placing the patient. This will minimize discomfort and help prevent development of pressure sores. Use of the long backboard may still be appropriate for patients with the following:

- Blunt trauma and altered level of consciousness
- Spinal pain or tenderness
- Neurologic complaint or deficit (such as numbness or motor weakness)
- Deformity of the spine
- High-energy mechanism of injury and any of the following:
  - Drug or alcohol intoxication
  - Inability to communicate
  - Distracting injury
  - Any patient found to be unresponsive and for whom you are unable to determine an exact mechanism of injury or nature of illness

A **distracting injury** is any injury to the body that may be preventing the patient from realizing pain in the neck or spine. For instance, a significant injury to the forearm or chest may overshadow (distract from) pain that would otherwise be felt by the patient. Even an insignificant injury can be distracting if the patient is unable to focus their attention on the questions you are asking during your exam. This results in an unreliable exam, and therefore you should assume a spinal injury is present and provide appropriate care.

distracting injury ▶ any injury to the body that may be preventing the patient from realizing pain in the neck or spine.

Research has shown that patients who are alert and oriented and who do not show signs of neurologic deficit will benefit from a soft cervical collar and placement in a position of comfort.[5]

Perform a secondary assessment, including all extremities. Obtain and monitor vital signs. Provide supplemental oxygen if available, following local protocols.

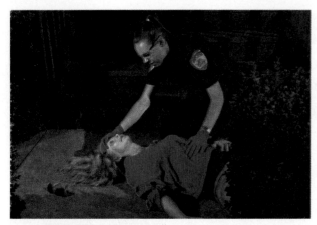

Figure 21.8 If you are alone, you may establish manual stabilization of the head by placing one hand on the patient's forehead.

You should be aware that not all injured people will present with obvious signs and symptoms of a spinal injury. Those with altered mental status and those who appear intoxicated are not able to reliably report pain. Sometimes signs and symptoms do not appear for hours. Any injured individual who appears to be intoxicated, has an altered mental status, or is found to be unresponsive should be cared for as though they have a spinal injury.

Manual Stabilization

Manual stabilization of the head and neck is an important step in caring for a patient with a suspected spinal injury. There are two basic approaches to an injured patient in the supine position (flat on the back, face up). The first is to approach the patient from the side and place your hand on their forehead to minimize movement as you begin your assessment (Figure 21.8). The second is to kneel at the top of the patient's head and use both hands to grasp the patient's head from the sides.

To perform manual stabilization of the head and neck of a supine patient, follow these steps:

1. Kneel at the top or side of the injured patient's head.
2. Introduce yourself and explain what you are going to do.
3. Grasp the patient's head by placing your hands on each side of the head and hold firmly. Do not push, pull, or rotate the patient's neck.
4. Instruct the patient to remain still and reassure them.
5. Monitor the ABCs by talking to the patient and listening to how they respond.

Follow these steps to perform manual stabilization of the head and neck of a seated patient:

1. Stand or sit directly behind the injured patient.
2. Introduce yourself and explain what you are going to do.
3. Grasp the patient's head by placing your hands on each side of the head and hold firmly. Do not push, pull, or rotate the patient's neck.
4. Instruct the patient to remain still and reassure them.
5. Monitor the ABCs by talking to the patient and listening to how they respond.

In some instances, you might arrive at the scene to find one or more injured individuals walking around. You must consider the walking wounded as patients and care for them accordingly. If you find a patient who is standing, and you have reason to suspect that they might have a neck or back injury, you must provide proper spinal immobilization. You can begin by standing behind the patient and holding manual stabilization of their head. Carefully explain to the patient why you are concerned and request their cooperation. Do not allow them to turn their head as you position yourself behind them. With the assistance of other rescuers, you will want to help the patient to a sitting then a lying position while you wait for the transport unit to arrive.

Rules for Care of Spinal Injury

Always follow these rules for the care of patients with possible spinal injuries:

- Make certain the airway is open. Assist ventilations or perform CPR as needed.
- Attempt to control serious bleeding. Avoid moving the injured part and any of the limbs when applying dressings.
- Always assume that an unresponsive patient who has experienced trauma has spinal injuries.
- Do not attempt to splint long bone injuries if there are indications of spinal injuries until you have appropriate help.

REMEMBER

Children have a very large posterior skull. This can cause the head to tilt forward when they are placed in a supine position. Carefully slipping a folded towel under the shoulders will help keep the head and neck in a more neutral or anatomical position.

- Never move a patient with suspected spinal injuries unless you must do so to provide CPR, manage the airway or assist ventilations, need to reach and control life-threatening bleeding, or must protect yourself and the patient from immediate danger at the scene.
- Keep the patient still. Tell them not to move. Position yourself to stabilize the patient's head, neck, and as much of the body as possible.
- Continuously monitor patients who have possible spinal injuries.
- Always follow local protocols because management of spinal injuries has changed based on new evidence.

Cervical Collars

When you place a patient on an immobilization device, you must first stabilize the head and neck by selecting and applying a cervical collar of the appropriate size. Also called *extrication collars*, rigid or soft cervical collars are applied to help maintain stability and alignment with the body in patients who have suspected neck and spinal injuries.

Whether or not you learn to size and place cervical collars during your training, it is vital to understand one very important concept: cervical collars will only minimize movement of the neck of a cooperative patient. A patient who is combative or otherwise uncooperative can still move their neck even with a cervical collar in place. Therefore, it is important to maintain manual stabilization of the head even after placement of a cervical collar.

Many different makes and models of cervical collars are available on the market (Figure 21.9). Some brands offer many sizes, while others offer an adjustable collar. You will be expected

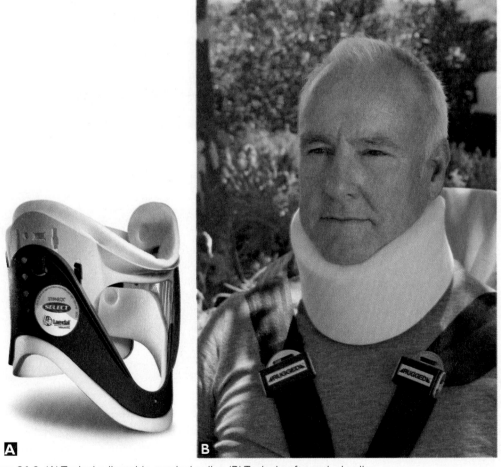

Figure 21.9 (A) Typical adjustable cervical collar. (B) Typical soft cervical collar.

to use whatever collars are currently in use in your agency or region. Whatever the case, it is best to follow the manufacturer's suggested method for sizing and application.

Regardless of the brand or type of collar, the following guidelines will ensure a proper fit for your patient (Key Skills 21.4, 21.5, and 21.6):

- Once in place, check to see that the sides of the collar do not ride too far above or below the earlobes.
- Confirm that the chin fits properly on the collar. The collar should effectively support the bony part of the chin.

KEY SKILL 21.4

Verifying the Fit of a Cervical Collar

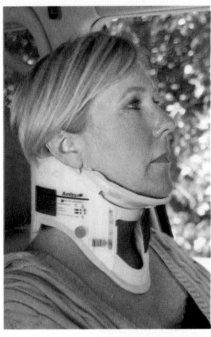

1. When properly fitted, the sides of the rigid collar should come very close to, or slightly overlap, the earlobe.

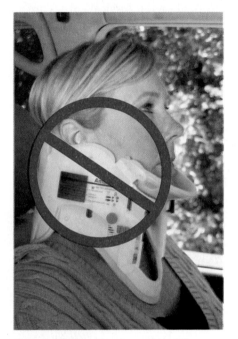

2. A rigid collar that is too big will extend way above the earlobes. Consider readjusting or selecting a smaller size collar.

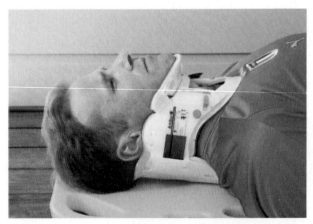

3. When properly fitted, the patient's chin will fit completely and snugly within the saddle of the rigid collar.

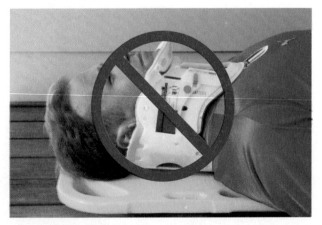

4. A collar that is too big will extend well beyond the chin, allowing for excessive movement. Consider readjusting or selecting a smaller size collar.

- The collar should be snug on all sides and not too tight or too loose. You should be able to easily slide a finger between the neck and the collar.
- Use a different size or adjust the collar if it does not fit properly.

Applying a Cervical Collar to a Seated Patient

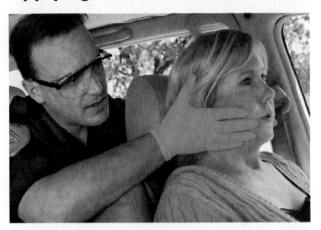

1. Establish manual stabilization of the head while your partner selects a collar.

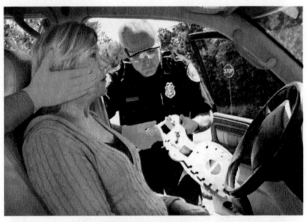

2. Select an appropriately sized collar, or adjust the collar based on the patient's size. Follow the manufacturer's guidelines for size and adjustment selection.

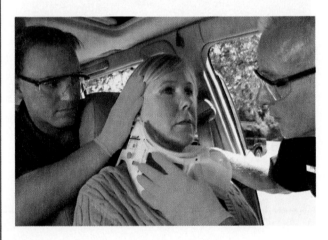

3. Place the collar beneath the patient's chin and firmly against the lower jaw. The chin should fit well within the chin saddle of the collar.

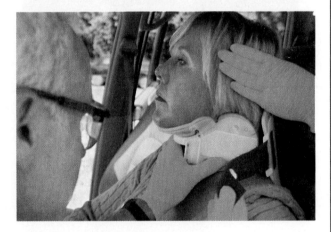

4. Secure the collar in place by overlapping the Velcro® closure at the side of the patient's neck. Confirm fit by looking at ears and chin.

CREW RESOURCE MANAGEMENT

When caring for a seated patient with a suspected spinal injury, the rescuer facing the patient should establish a relationship with them and explain exactly what is going to happen each step of the way.

Applying a Cervical Collar to a Supine Patient

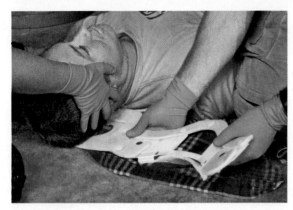

1. Slide the back portion of the collar behind the patient's neck.

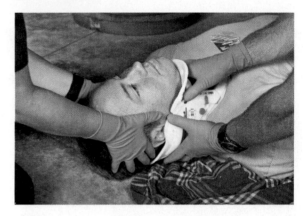

2. Secure the collar so the chin fits properly.

Alternative Method

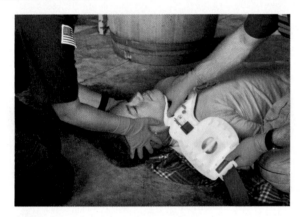

3. An alternative method of applying the collar to a supine patient is to start by positioning the chin piece and then sliding the back portion of the collar behind the patient's neck.

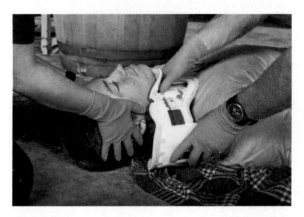

4. Hold the collar in place from the front while sliding the rest of the collar behind the patient's neck.

Helmet Removal

Helmets are designed to absorb energy forces and minimize injury to the head. However, well-fitting helmets—even the most modern ones—cannot prevent the brain from striking the interior of the skull in extreme or high-speed crash forces.

The helmet should be removed immediately if there are any issues with the ABCs, such as airway obstruction or inadequate breathing. Otherwise, consider leaving the helmet in place until you have enough help to remove it properly. For an unresponsive patient wearing a helmet, always suspect a spinal injury. Monitor the patient's ABCs and properly immobilize the spine.

For football players wearing shoulder pads, the helmet and pads left in place keep the cervical spine in alignment with the rest of the spine. Removing the helmet but keeping the shoulder pads in place causes the head to fall back in an overextended position, which pulls the spinal column out of alignment. If you choose to remove the helmet, it is best to remove the shoulder pads at the same time.

There are many types and styles of helmets. Full-face helmets cover the mouth and sometimes part of the nose and usually have a face shield. Football helmets have face guards. Bicycle helmets have no face shield or face guard. Motorcycle helmets are available in many different styles, with full-face helmets having a clear face shield or visor that moves up and down and is easy to remove. Motorcyclists who wear half-size helmets will usually wear glasses or goggles to protect their eyes. If the helmet has a face guard or face shield, remove it to gain access to the patient's airway. If any patient who is not breathing is wearing a helmet with a face guard or face shield that cannot be removed, remove the helmet to gain access to the airway. If a helmet is removed, it must be done cautiously and by two people.

Before removing a helmet, perform the following steps:

1. Remove the face piece or face shield while your partner stabilizes the head. Do not cut the chin strap. Remove the patient's glasses or goggles.
2. Check to see if the patient is breathing.
3. If the patient is breathing, check the helmet for fit. A well-fitting helmet can stay in place as long as the patient is breathing.
4. If you must clear the airway or assist the patient with breathing, remove the helmet. If the patient is wearing shoulder pads (such as football pads), remove them along with the helmet.

Provide care to any unresponsive patient as if there is a spinal injury. When you find a patient wearing a helmet lying face down or on one side, log-roll them onto their back (supine). Leave the helmet in place if you find the following:

- The helmet fits well and the patient's head does not move (or moves very little) inside of it. A well-fitting helmet keeps the head from moving, and it should be left on if there are no airway or breathing problems and the helmet does not interfere with assessment and management of the airway and breathing.
- The patient is breathing adequately and has no airway problems (e.g., fluids, obstructions).
- The patient can be placed in a neutral, in-line position for immobilization on a spine board.
- The helmet does not interfere with your ability to reassess and maintain the patient's airway or assist breathing.
- The patient is wearing shoulder pads. If the helmet is removed, remove the shoulder pads, too.

Remove the helmet if you find the following:

- The helmet interferes with your ability to assess or manage the patient's airway and breathing.
- The helmet does not fit snugly, and the patient's head moves inside the helmet.
- The helmet interferes with placing the patient on a spine board in a neutral, in-line position. When the helmet rests on the spine board, its size may force the patient's head forward (hyperflexion) and close the airway. Padding can be placed under the patient's shoulders to prevent hyperflexion and maintain an in-line position.
- The patient is in cardiac or respiratory arrest. Quickly remove the helmet while a partner stabilizes the head. Proceed with CPR steps, using the jaw-thrust maneuver.

If you must remove the helmet, remove it according to local protocols. The following steps provide general directions for removal of full-size helmets (Key Skill 21.7):

1. Rescuer 1 kneels at the head of the patient and stabilizes the patient's head by placing their hands on each side of the helmet.
2. Rescuer 2 kneels on one side of the patient at the patient's shoulders, unfastens the chin strap, removes the face guard or face shield (if not yet done), and removes the patient's glasses or goggles (if present).

3. Rescuer 2 places one hand on either side of the neck at the base of the skull and stabilizes the patient's head while Rescuer 1 removes the helmet.
4. Rescuer 1 pulls the sides of the helmet apart using the straps and slowly and carefully slips the helmet off the patient's head.
5. Rescuer 2 slowly slides their hands along the sides of the patient's head and neck to support it as the helmet is removed.
6. Rescuer 1 finishes removing the helmet, places padding under the patient's head as needed (if the patient is wearing shoulder pads), and places their hands on either side of the patient's head to take over in-line stabilization.
7. Rescuer 2 checks and clears the airway, provides ventilations with supplemental oxygen, and applies a collar.

Remember that you do not have to remove a helmet if the patient has an open airway and is breathing, the helmet is snug, and the patient can be secured to a spine board with the helmet on and the head in a neutral, in-line position with the spine.

KEY SKILL 21.7

Helmet Removal

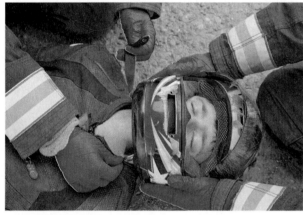

1. While holding manual stabilization, expose the neck and remove the straps that secure the helmet in place.

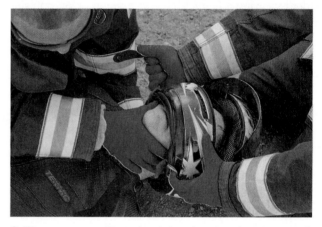

2. The rescuer at the patient's head grasps the straps and begins to pull the helmet off while the other rescuer stabilizes the head.

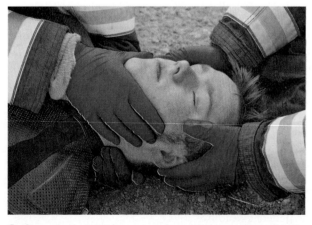

3. Once the helmet is removed, gently lower the patient's head to the ground.

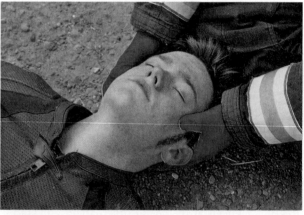

4. Maintain manual stabilization of the head while a collar is placed on the patient.

"The pinky toes," Marc says, and Shelby sighs out loud with some relief. She has checked CSM and, so far, Marc has been able to identify which toes are being touched, he can pull up on and push down with both feet, and he has a distal pulse beating faintly.

"The medics are here!" announces the loud, booming voice of the stage manager.

"Hear that, Marc?" Shelby says as she rechecks his ABCs. "We're going to hold your head still while the medics get over here, and they're going to get you to the hospital immediately."

"Thank you," says the stage manager. "I'll ride with him to the hospital."

"No," Shelby says sternly, "you will be helping me set up the safety ropes I required you to have around the stage, and we'll fill out an incident report. I'm calling a safety meeting tonight." She winks at Marc, and he smiles, wiggling his toes in relief.

Summary

- Open head injuries involve a break in the bone and overlying soft tissue. A closed head injury involves no opening of the skull. However, there may be soft-tissue damage of the scalp.
- Head injuries can range from a mild concussion to significant open fractures of the skull. A patient with a head injury will often have signs and symptoms ranging from a mild headache to bleeding of the scalp, altered mental status, deformity of the cranium, unresponsiveness, convulsions, and vomiting. A person with a head injury may also display aggressive behavior and ask repetitive questions.
- Your first concern when caring for a patient with a suspected head injury is to manage and monitor the ABCs. Consider the possibility of a neck injury and provide care accordingly. Control bleeding as appropriate.
- Management of the airway in an unresponsive patient with a suspected neck injury can be challenging, but it is important to remember that the airway is always the top priority. If you must open the airway of an unresponsive patient with a suspected neck injury, begin with the jaw-thrust maneuver. If unsuccessful, use the head-tilt/chin-lift maneuver.
- When caring for a patient with a suspected spinal injury, you must first try to identify the mechanism of injury. Always assume there is a spinal injury if the mechanism suggests it, even if the patient has no obvious signs or symptoms.
- A patient with a spinal injury may have pain and/or deformity over the injury site. They may also present with numbness, tingling, and weakness of the extremities; loss of sensation; paralysis; and incontinence.
- Once you have confirmed the ABCs are intact, your primary concern becomes stabilization of the head, neck, and spine. Provide manual stabilization of the head and neck until EMS arrives and is able to place the patient onto a long spine board.
- The practice of spinal motion restriction (SMR) allows more flexibility for the Emergency Medical Responder when choosing how to immobilize a patient with suspected spinal injury.

Take Action

Beam Me Up, Scotty

Our jobs would be much easier if every patient we came across was found lying supine and in perfect alignment. Of course, this is not the case. There will be times when it is necessary to carefully move a patient into a position that will allow you to assess the ABCs or control bleeding. It also becomes necessary to move a patient when they need to be immobilized onto a long backboard. This activity will allow you to practice this valuable skill and develop the confidence necessary to facilitate a lift onto a long backboard when necessary.

Begin by gathering at least two, and preferably four or five, of your friends or fellow classmates. Have one of them play patient and lie on the floor as if they were injured. Start by having the patient lie in a supine position. The rest of you will take your positions next to the patient in preparation for lifting them off the ground in a coordinated manner. This is known as BEAM (body elevation and movement), or BEAMing the patient. The point of this activity is to allow you to experiment with lifting a patient who may need to be placed onto a long backboard. Lifting the patient results in less movement of the spine than the traditional log-roll method. Change positions each time to get a feel for what must be done by each individual in different positions. Your goal is to keep the spine in alignment as much as possible throughout each lift.

Remember to always make the move on the count of the individual at the head. The more you practice these moves, the more confident and efficient you will become.

First on Scene Patient Handoff

Marc is a 34-year-old male who experienced a mechanical fall from approximately 12 feet onto concrete. Witnesses state that he appeared to be unconscious for 15 to 20 seconds. Upon our arrival, Marc was A&O × 3. A quick assessment revealed no obvious deformities, but he does have pain and tenderness to the back of his head. He has weakness and tingling in both lower extremities. His respirations are 20, good tidal volume and unlabored, BP of 144/78, pulse of 96, strong and regular, pupils are PERRL.

First on Scene Run Review

Recall the events of the First on Scene scenario in this chapter, and answer the following questions related to the call. Rationales are offered in the Answer Key at the back of the book.

1. What information should Shelby obtain?
2. Why did Shelby ask permission to help?
3. Why is it important to hold manual stabilization of the head?

Quick Quiz

To check your understanding of the chapter, answer the following questions. Then compare your answers to those in the Answer Key at the back of the book.

1. You are caring for a patient who you suspect has a spinal injury. Which of the following should you do first?

   a. Assess for circulation, sensation, and movement.
   b. Apply a rigid cervical collar.
   c. Transport the patient to the nearest trauma center.
   d. Manually stabilize the patient's head and neck.

2. Which of the following mechanisms of injury would cause you to suspect a spinal injury?

   a. Circular-saw amputation of fingers
   b. Fall from an anchored speedboat
   c. Bicycle crash
   d. Self-inflicted gunshot wound to the hip

3. Your patient is unresponsive, lying prone on the floor after falling off a high ladder. Appropriate care for this patient includes:

   a. completing your assessment with the patient in the prone position.
   b. using the log-roll maneuver to roll the patient into the supine position.
   c. placing the patient in the recovery position to protect the airway.
   d. immobilizing the patient in the prone position.

4. Your patient is unresponsive following a motorcycle crash. Several attempts to open the airway with the jaw-thrust maneuver are not successful. You should:

   a. maintain manual stabilization and wait for EMS to arrive.
   b. attempt the head-tilt/chin-lift maneuver.
   c. attempt to ventilate the patient anyway.
   d. begin chest compressions.

5. Combative behavior, abnormal breathing patterns, and repetitive questions are all signs of a(n):

   a. cervical spine injury.
   b. unresponsive individual.
   c. peripheral nervous system trauma.
   d. head injury.

6. You witness a low-speed ATV collision that knocks both riders from their vehicles. Neither of the men is wearing a helmet, but both quickly get back on their feet. You notice one of them is walking oddly as he retrieves his vehicle. You ask if he is okay, and he tells you his legs "are tingling." You should suspect:

   a. head injury.
   b. internal bleeding.
   c. spinal injury.
   d. hip dislocation.

7. The central nervous system consists of the:

   a. peripheral and central nerves.
   b. discs and vertebrae.
   c. brain and spinal cord.
   d. spine and nerves.

8. You are caring for a motorcycle rider who was ejected from his bike. Your physical exam reveals no crepitus or instability; however, the patient complains of a headache. He asks repeatedly "What happened?" You suspect:

   a. an open head injury.
   b. spinal trauma.
   c. a closed head injury.
   d. an ischemic stroke.

9. Your main priority when caring for a patient with a suspected head injury is to:

   a. completely immobilize the head and neck.
   b. obtain a detailed medical history.
   c. monitor vital signs.
   d. assess and manage airway, breathing, and circulation.

10. You are caring for a patient with a suspected open head injury. When attempting to control the bleeding, you should:

    a. apply firm fingertip pressure on the open wound.
    b. use only enough pressure to slow or stop the bleeding.
    c. tightly wrap a pressure bandage around the skull.
    d. keep the patient in a head-down position while holding pressure.

Endnotes

1. James F. Morrissey, Elsie R. Kusel, & Karl A. Sporer (2014) "Spinal Motion Restriction: An Educational and Implementation Program to Redefine Prehospital Spinal Assessment and Care," *Prehospital Emergency Care*, Vol. 18, No. 3 (2014): 429–432, doi: 10.3109/10903127.2013.869643

2. Fischer, P.E., Perina, D.G., Delbridge, T.R., Fallat, M.E., Salomone, J.P., Dodd, J., Bulger, E.M., & Gestring, M.L. "Spinal Motion Restriction in the Trauma Patient— A Joint Position Statement," *Prehospital Emergency Care*, Vol. 22, No. 6 (November-December, 2018): 659–661. doi: 10.1080/10903127.2018.1481476. Epub 2018 Aug 9. PMID: 30091939.

3. Joshua B. Brown, Paul E. Bankey, Ayodele T. Sangosanya, et al. "Prehospital Spinal Immobilization Does Not Appear to Be Beneficial and May Complicate Care Following Gunshot Injury to the Torso," *The Journal of Trauma*, Vol. 67, No. 4 (October 4, 2009): 774–778.

4. White, C.C., Domeier, R.M., & Millin, M.G. "EMS Spinal Precautions and the Use of the Long Backboard-Resource Document to the Position Statement of the National Association of EMS Physicians and the American College of Surgeons Committee on Trauma," *Prehospital Emergency Care*, Vol 18, No. 2 (2014): 306–331.

5. Mark Dixon, Joseph O'Halloran, and Niamh M. Cummins, "Biomechanical Analysis of Spinal Immobilisation During Prehospital Extrication: A Proof of Concept Study," *Prehospital Emergency Care*, Vol. 17, No. 1 (June 28, 2013): 106.

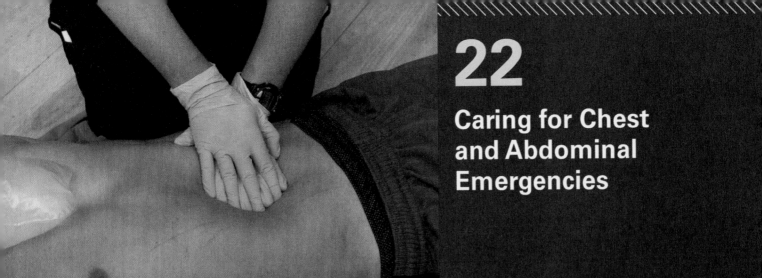

22

Caring for Chest and Abdominal Emergencies

LEARNING OBJECTIVES

Upon successful completion of this chapter, the student should be able to:

Cognitive

1 Define the chapter key terms.

2 Review the anatomy of the chest and abdomen from Chapter 4.

3 Describe the major structures of the thoracic cavity.

4 Differentiate between an open and closed chest injury.

5 Explain the relationship between a chest injury and perfusion.

6 Describe the signs and symptoms of a closed chest injury.

7 Explain the appropriate assessment of a patient with a chest injury.

8 Explain the appropriate care of a patient with a closed chest injury.

9 Explain the appropriate care of a patient with an open chest injury.

10 Describe the major structures of the abdominal and pelvic cavities.

11 Describe the signs and symptoms of internal bleeding.

12 Explain the appropriate assessment and care of a patient with abdominal pain.

13 Explain the appropriate assessment and care of a patient with an open abdominal injury.

Psychomotor

14 Demonstrate the appropriate assessment and care of a patient with a chest injury.

15 Demonstrate the appropriate assessment and care of a patient with abdominal pain.

16 Demonstrate the appropriate assessment and care of an open abdominal injury.

Affective

17 Value the importance of proper body substance isolation (BSI) precautions when assisting with chest and abdominal injuries.

Education Standards

Trauma—Chest Trauma, Abdominal, and Genitourinary Trauma

Medicine—Abdominal and Gastrointestinal Disorders

Competencies

Recognizes and manages life threats based on assessment findings for an injured or ill patient while awaiting additional emergency response

KEY TERMS

aortic dissection (*p. 472*)
closed chest injury (*p. 466*)
diaphragm (*p. 470*)
distention (*p. 471*)
evisceration (*p. 474*)
flail chest (*p. 466*)
hemothorax (*p. 466*)
kidney stone (*p. 472*)
mediastinum (*p. 465*)

occlusive dressing (*p. 468*)
open chest injury (*p. 468*)
paradoxical movement (*p. 467*)
pleura (*p. 465*)
pleural space (*p. 465*)
pneumothorax (*p. 466*)
quadrant (*p. 470*)
retroperitoneal cavity (*p. 471*)
sucking chest wound (*p. 468*)

njuries to the chest and abdomen are very common simply due to the large part of the body that the two areas make up. Chest and abdominal injuries also pose great risk to the patient because most of the body's vital organs are contained within these two cavities. This chapter discusses some of the more common injuries associated with the chest and abdomen, as well as how to properly assess and care for patients with these injuries.

FIRST ON SCENE

"Follow me! He's up here," shouts a college student who meets the campus security officers as they pull up. Liz and Jess park the vehicle, grab their response bags, and make their way up the dormitory stairs. As they enter the cramped dorm room, they see a young man lying on his bed in the fetal position.

"Hi," Liz says as she sets down her bag and kneels beside the bed. "My name is Liz. I'm trained as an Emergency

Medical Responder. I'm here to help you. Okay? Can you tell me your name?"

"It's Nico," he says, wincing. "My stomach is killing me! You've got to make it stop!" He winces again and draws his legs closer to his body.

"Jess," Liz says as she begins looking for any immediate life threats or bleeding, "go ahead and administer some oxygen while I get some vitals."

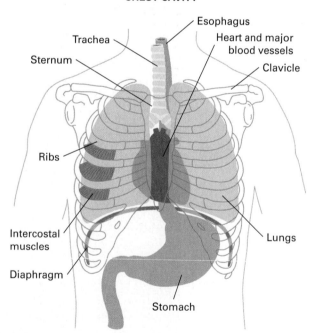

CHEST CAVITY

Esophagus
Trachea
Heart and major blood vessels
Sternum
Clavicle
Ribs
Intercostal muscles
Diaphragm
Lungs
Stomach
Parietal pleura

Figure 22.1 The chest contains the heart and lungs. The diaphragm separates the chest cavity from the abdominal cavity.

Anatomy of the Chest

LO3 Describe the major structures of the thoracic cavity.

The chest cavity, also known as the *thoracic cavity*, makes up approximately half of the torso. The torso is composed of the chest, abdomen, and pelvis. The boundaries of the chest cavity are the clavicles at the top, the diaphragm at the bottom, the sternum on the anterior side, and the spinal column at the posterior side (Figure 22.1).

The major organs contained within the chest are the heart and lungs. Major vessels such as the aorta and the vena cava either originate or terminate in the chest. The heart and lungs are well protected by the 12 pairs of ribs that make up part of the chest wall, along with skin, fat, and muscle tissue.

Within the center of the chest is a space called the **mediastinum**, which houses the trachea, esophagus, heart, vena cava, and aorta. The lungs occupy the left and right sides of the chest. The **pleura** is a thin membrane that surrounds each lung (Figure 22.2). The pleura consists of two layers: the *visceral pleura*, which is in direct contact with each lung, and the *parietal pleura*, which lines the inner wall of the chest.

The space between the visceral and parietal pleura is the **pleural space.** When the lungs are functioning normally, the two pleural layers remain in close contact with one another. They are lubricated by a fluid that allows for smooth movement between the two layers each time we breathe in and out. When injury or inflammation occurs to the visceral or parietal pleura, fluid, blood, or air can accumulate between the two layers, causing the pleural space to enlarge.

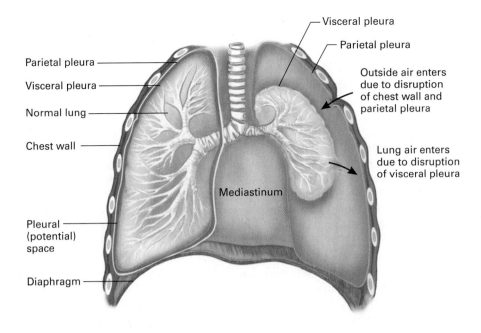

Visceral pleura

Parietal pleura

Parietal pleura

Visceral pleura

Normal lung

Chest wall

Outside air enters due to disruption of chest wall and parietal pleura

Lung air enters due to disruption of visceral pleura

Mediastinum

Pleural (potential) space

Diaphragm

mediastinum ▶ structure that divides the two halves of the chest cavity and contains the heart, trachea, esophagus, vena cava, and aorta.

pleura ▶ thin, saclike structure that surrounds each lung.

pleural space ▶ potential space that exists between the visceral and parietal pleura in the chest.

Figure 22.2 Each lung is surrounded by a thin layer of tissue called *pleura*.

Chest Injuries

LO4 | Differentiate between an open and closed chest injury.

LO5 | Explain the relationship between a chest injury and perfusion.

Like soft-tissue and head injuries, chest injuries can be classified as open or closed (Figure 22.3). Most closed chest injuries are the result of blunt trauma. Falls, contact sports, vehicle collisions, and explosions are common causes of closed chest injuries. Open chest injuries are often the result of a penetrating injury, such as from a bullet, knife or other sharp object, or some type of projectile.

The chest can be injured in several ways, including blunt trauma, penetrating objects, and compression:

- *Blunt trauma.* A blow to the chest can fracture the ribs and the sternum and damage soft tissue. Whole sections of the chest can collapse. When severe enough, blunt trauma can also damage the lungs, airways, heart, and major vessels.
- *Penetrating objects.* Bullets, knives, pieces of metal or glass, and other objects can penetrate the chest wall, damaging internal organs and impairing normal breathing.
- *Compression.* This results from major blunt trauma or from a crush injury in which the chest is severely compressed. The heart can be squeezed, the lungs can be ruptured, and the sternum and ribs can be fractured.

Closed Chest Injuries

LO6 | Describe the signs and symptoms of a closed chest injury.

LO7 | Explain the appropriate assessment of a patient with a chest injury.

LO8 | Explain the appropriate care of a patient with a closed chest injury.

Closed chest injuries are most often caused by blunt trauma to the chest or back. Closed chest injuries can cause a variety of complications, from minor to life threatening. One of the

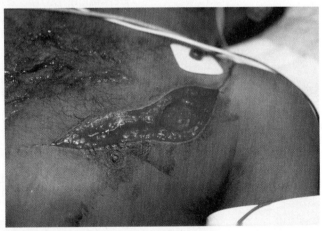

Figure 22.3 An open chest injury.
(© Edward T. Dickinson, MD)

most common types of closed chest injuries is damage to the ribs. While not usually life threatening, broken ribs can cause enough pain to keep the patient from breathing adequately. Because the chest wall moves in and out with each breath, even shallow breaths can cause pain. The patient will try to minimize the pain by taking breaths that are much more shallow than usual. Over time, this can lead to hypoxia (insufficient oxygen to tissues).

In many cases, the care for injured ribs is simply to splint the injured area with bulky dressings (Figure 22.4). If the injury is on the anterior or lateral chest, the patient will often self-splint by holding an arm tightly against the chest wall. It is appropriate to allow these patients to assume a position of comfort and provide high-flow oxygen if local protocols allow.

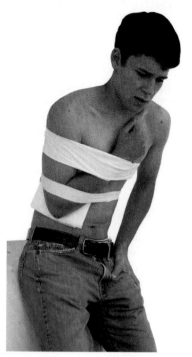

Figure 22.4 Injured ribs can be splinted by securing bulky dressings tightly over the injured area.

closed chest injury ▶ injury to the chest that is not associated with an open wound.

pneumothorax ▶ escape of air into the pleural space, often associated with trauma.

hemothorax ▶ blood in the pleural space.

flail chest ▶ traumatic chest injury in which three or more adjacent ribs are broken in two or more places.

Pneumothorax A **pneumothorax** is a common type of closed chest injury. It results when air is allowed to escape from a lung into the pleural space. This can be due to blunt trauma that causes one or more lobes to rupture or tear. A pneumothorax can also occur spontaneously, meaning that it can happen without any outside force. This is often the case when a thin spot on a lung ruptures, allowing air to enter the space between the visceral and parietal pleura.[1] A *spontaneous pneumothorax* is rarely life threatening and often presents with a sudden onset of sharp chest pain and shortness of breath. Depending on the cause, a pneumothorax may repair itself or require more intensive treatment including surgery. People between the ages of 20 and 40 who are tall and underweight are at greater risk for a spontaneous pneumothorax.

A pneumothorax caused by trauma can result in additional complications. Trauma to the chest often damages ribs, muscle tissue, and internal organs. Blood from damaged soft tissues and vessels can enter the chest cavity, a condition called a **hemothorax.**

The most obvious signs of a chest injury in the responsive patient are pain and difficulty breathing. Due to the decrease in available lung capacity, the patient will attempt to compensate by breathing faster. Injuries to the lungs may also result in sharp pain during inhalation and/or exhalation.

Flail Chest Another type of closed chest injury is a **flail chest**. It is most often the result of significant blunt-force trauma. A flail chest results when three or more adjacent ribs are broken in two or more places (Figure 22.5), causing instability of the chest wall.[2] This instability significantly decreases the patient's ability to breathe adequately.

Depending on the size of the patient, a flail chest may be difficult to discover in the field. If you suspect chest trauma, you must expose the patient's chest and palpate carefully for patches that feel soft and spongy. There may be a grating sound known as crepitus caused by bones rubbing together. The patient will experience significant pain on palpation, and you may see the flail segment move in the opposite direction as the rest of the chest wall as the patient breathes. When the patient inhales, the chest wall moves

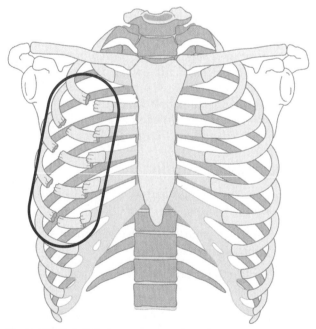

Figure 22.5 A flail chest occurs when three or more adjacent ribs are fractured in two or more places.

outward while the flail segment moves inward. When the patient exhales, the chest wall moves inward while the flail segment moves outward. This opposite movement of the flail segment is known as **paradoxical movement** and may be very difficult to see in the field.

A flail chest can be life threatening because it can greatly decrease the amount of air the patient moves with each breath (tidal volume). There is also a high likelihood for additional internal injuries, given the forces required to cause a flail chest. If the patient has sustained a blunt impact to the chest or torso and presents with any of the following signs or symptoms, suspect closed chest injuries:

- Chest wall pain
- Pain on breathing
- Increased difficulty breathing
- Accessory muscle use
- Uneven chest wall movement during breathing
- Signs and symptoms of shock

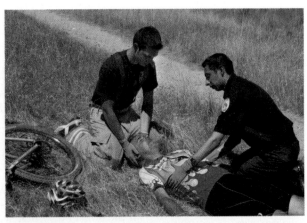

Figure 22.6 Use both hands to carefully and thoroughly palpate the chest for pain and deformity.

paradoxical movement ▶ abnormal movement of the chest wall associated with a flail chest.

Assessing the Patient with a Chest Injury Your assessment of a chest injury will begin with exposing the chest. You must remove or cut away clothing over any area where there is a complaint of pain. If the patient is unresponsive, you will want to expose the entire chest.

You must observe and palpate for any signs of deformity (Figure 22.6). Use your hands to press firmly across all areas of the chest wall. Be sure to palpate the anterior, lateral, and posterior sides of the chest wall. Note any signs of bruising or discoloration. Pay particular attention to any areas that feel soft or spongy. These could be signs of a flail chest.

The care for closed chest injuries is as follows:

1. Perform a primary assessment and ensure an open airway.
2. Consider manual ventilations if breathing rate is inadequate (less than 10 breaths per minute).
3. Administer oxygen if allowed to do so. (Follow local protocols.)
4. Place the patient in a position of comfort if there is no suspected spinal injury.
5. Provide care for shock.
6. Ensure that advanced medical care is summoned to transport the patient.

Do not attempt to stabilize the flail segment because you could further decrease tidal volume.[3] Instead, if you determine that ventilations are inadequate, attempt to ventilate the patient using a bag-mask device. This will help support good tidal volume.

> **REMEMBER**
>
> When assessing a patient who has sustained blunt trauma to the chest, you must expose the chest and palpate carefully for signs of a flail segment.

FIRST ON SCENE (continued)

Liz removes her stethoscope and says to Jess, "Nico's blood pressure is 130 over 78, and his pulse is 120, strong and regular."

Liz turns to the patient. "Okay, Nico, your pulse is a little fast, but your breathing rate and blood pressure are in the normal range. Tell me again about the pain you said started about 45 minutes ago."

Nico remains still on his right side, guarding his abdomen with his hands. "I thought I was having stomach cramps. I called my mom and she suggested mint tea, but the pain just keeps getting worse. I feel like I need to throw up, but I haven't."

Jess is in the hallway, on the phone with Nico's very worried mother. Liz says to Nico, "I'm going to check your abdomen now, all right?"

Nico clenches his arms even tighter over his abdomen. Liz reassures him, "But I'm going to be very careful, and it will take just a minute, okay?"

Nico considers this for a moment and then moves his hands to his sides.

Open Chest Injuries

LO7 Explain the appropriate assessment of a patient with a chest injury.

LO9 Explain the appropriate care of a patient with an open chest injury.

open chest injury ▶ injury to the chest associated with an open wound.

An injury that penetrates the chest wall is an **open chest injury**, which can result in specific problems that must be identified and properly cared for.

Open Pneumothorax When the mechanism of injury causes the chest wall to be penetrated, there is great risk for lung collapse and for air and blood to enter the pleural space (Figure 22.7). Common causes include gunshot wounds, blast injuries, and stabbings. It is common for the lung beneath the injury to be punctured, allowing air to enter the pleural space. Blood from the damaged tissues will begin to fill this space. If the hole in the chest wall is large enough, it may allow air to pass through into the chest cavity with each inspiration. This is referred to as a **sucking chest wound** because air can often be heard as it is being sucked through the wound when the patient breathes in. If air from a sucking chest wound becomes trapped, pressure can build inside the chest and result in the development of a *tension pneumothorax*. If left untreated, this pressure will cause respiratory and circulatory compromise as well as collapse of the remaining lobes of the lungs.[4] An early sign that pressure may be building up inside the chest is an increased work of breathing, increased respiratory and heart rates, and pain with breathing. A late sign of this pressure is a shift in the trachea to the opposite side, called *tracheal deviation*. Be sure to assess the trachea by palpating it with your fingers for normal alignment. This should be done for all patients with a chest injury. Other signs of a tension pneumothorax include bulging of the neck veins, known as *jugular vein distension*, and hypotension (abnormally low blood pressure).

sucking chest wound ▶ open chest wound characterized by a sucking sound each time the patient inhales.

REMEMBER

When air escapes into the chest cavity, it can sometimes escape outward into the tissues of the chest and neck. This is referred to as *subcutaneous air* (air under the skin). Its presence is noted by a snapping or crackling sound when the skin is palpated. This can be found during chest wall examination and is associated with both blunt and penetrating chest trauma.

Caring for an Open Chest Injury You must always inspect the torso on all sides for wounds, depending on the mechanism of injury. In the case of gunshot wounds, there may be an exit wound on the opposite side of the body from the entrance wound. However, the location of the exit wound, if present, depends on the direction the projectile took through the body. If present, both wounds must be cared for equally. The exit could be on the chest or abdomen or even an extremity. For this reason, it is important to examine all areas of the body.

Open chest wounds should be managed initially with direct pressure with a gloved hand. As soon as is practical, you must apply an **occlusive dressing** (Figure 22.8).[5]

occlusive dressing ▶ type of dressing that will not allow air to pass through; also called a *nonpermeable dressing*.

Commercially available chest seals are specifically designed to manage open chest wounds. They are available with and without a built-in one-way valve (Figure 22.9).

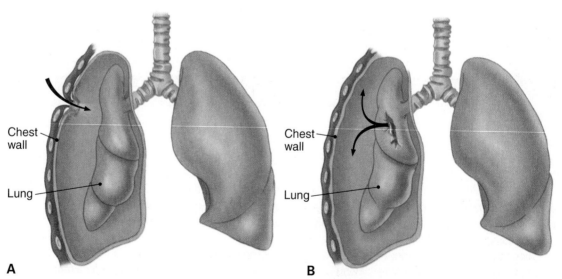

Chest wall

Lung

A

Chest wall

Lung

B

Figure 22.7 (A) Penetrating chest injuries can allow air and blood to enter the chest cavity. (B) A collapsed lung (spontaneous pneumothorax) can occur without outside trauma.

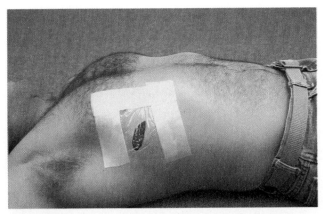

Figure 22.8 An improvised occlusive dressing may be the standard of care in some EMS systems. Follow local protocols.

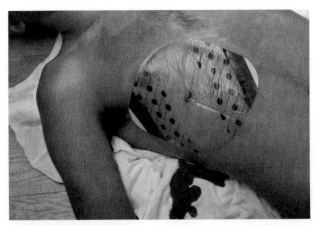

Figure 22.9 The SAM® Chest Seal is an example of a commercial chest seal.

If blood or perspiration prevents the tape from sticking to the patient's skin, you may have to hold the dressing in place with your hands. You must monitor the patient's breathing status very closely. It is possible that pressure may build up if the dressing becomes saturated with blood. If the work of breathing continues to worsen, release the dressing momentarily to see if air will escape through the wound.

The following steps should be followed when caring for an open chest wound:

1. Take appropriate BSI precautions.
2. Ensure an open airway, and cover open wounds with a gloved hand. Be sure to inspect the patient, front and back, for additional open wounds.
3. Assist ventilations if necessary.
4. Provide high-flow oxygen (if allowed by local protocols).
5. Provide care for shock.
6. When practical, apply an occlusive dressing.
7. Initiate transport as soon as possible.

FIRST ON SCENE (*continued*)

"Ow! Stop!" Nico cries out, knocking Liz's hands away. "I'm sorry," Nico says through clenched teeth. "That's where it hurts most. It's so sharp, like a jabbing knife."

Liz notes that the pain is restricted mostly to the lower right quadrant of the abdomen, but the area is free of any signs of trauma or swelling.

The responding ALS team enters the room, and Jess relays Nico's vitals to the lead medic. "Were there any other findings besides the abdominal pain?" he asks.

"No," Jess responds. "There were no remarkable findings from his secondary assessment or medical history. The onset and progression of pain were pretty rapid."

The medic positions himself beside the bed and addresses Nico: "I'm thinking you may be experiencing appendicitis, which as you know by now is pretty painful. We need to get you to a hospital quickly!"

Impaled Chest Wounds Injuries to the chest may result in an object becoming impaled in the chest. Impaled objects must be stabilized as soon as possible to minimize further injury to internal structures.

An impaled object must be left in place unless it interferes with performing CPR. Even though it created the wound, the impaled object is also sealing the wound. If it is removed, the patient may bleed profusely. The object must be stabilized with bulky dressings or pads (Figure 22.10). Begin by placing bulky dressings around the object. You may also cut a

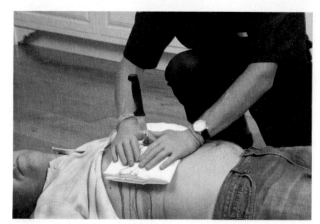

Figure 22.10 Stabilize impaled objects using bulky dressings.

hole in a large trauma dressing and slip it over the object. Place several layers to build up support around the object. You may use tape or cravats to hold the dressings and pads in place, or it may be more effective to have someone hold the dressings/pads in place.

Follow these steps when caring for a patient with an impaled object in the chest:

1. Take appropriate BSI precautions.
2. Perform a primary assessment and ensure an open airway.
3. Assist ventilations as necessary.
4. Immediately stabilize the object.
5. Provide high-flow oxygen (if allowed by local protocols).
6. Provide care for shock.
7. Initiate immediate transport.

diaphragm ▶ primary muscle of respiration that separates the chest cavity from the abdominal cavity.

quadrant ▶ one of four areas of the abdomen; used to identify the location of pain during palpation.

Abdominal Emergencies

Much like injuries to the chest, the abdominal and pelvic areas are susceptible to the same types of forces and injuries. In addition to injury, abdominal emergencies include a variety of nontraumatic problems as well. Abdominal pain, regardless of the speed and severity of its onset or association with trauma, should be considered a serious emergency. This is due to the variety of organs and structures contained within the abdomen and the fact that serious bleeding can go undetected, leading to shock and death.

Anatomy of the Abdomen and Pelvis

LO10 Describe the major structures of the abdominal and pelvic cavities.

The abdominal cavity is separated from the chest cavity by the diaphragm, which extends downward into the pelvis. Since there is no anatomic division between the abdomen and pelvis, they are often considered to be one cavity. The abdomen and pelvis contain many organs, which can be categorized as solid or hollow. Solid organs include the liver, spleen, pancreas, kidneys, and ovaries (in females). Hollow organs include the stomach, gallbladder, urinary bladder, small and large intestines, and the uterus (in females). Solid organs generally contain a richer blood supply and may result in significant blood loss when damaged. Hollow organs often contain fluids that, when allowed to spill out into the abdomen, will cause pain.

The aorta and inferior vena cava pass through the abdomen, dividing into the left and right iliac vessels in the pelvis, then becoming the femoral artery and vein in each lower extremity. These vessels supply blood to all the organs of the abdomen and pelvis.

For assessment purposes, the abdomen is commonly divided into four **quadrants**, with the navel at the center (Figure 22.11). Organs may be contained in one or more quadrants, depending on their size.

The abdomen is also divided into three regions known as the suprapubic (above the pubic bone) regions. These three regions are: the epigastric (above the navel to below the sternum), the periumbilical (around the navel), and the superpubic (below the navel to the pubic area).

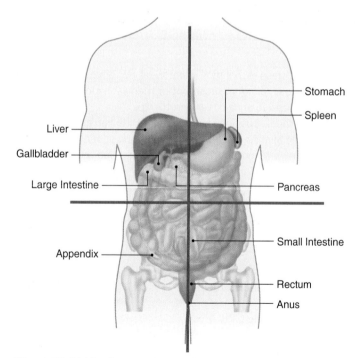

Figure 22.11 The four quadrants of the abdomen.

Liver
Gallbladder
Large Intestine
Appendix
Stomach
Spleen
Pancreas
Small Intestine
Rectum
Anus

Similar to the lungs, a thin layer of tissue called the *visceral peritoneum* lines the internal organs of the abdomen Another thin layer of tissue called the *parietal peritoneum* lines the inner surface of the abdominal/pelvic cavity. It is important to point out that the kidneys are not contained inside the same space as the other abdominal organs. They lie in a space called the **retroperitoneal cavity**, which is posterior to (behind) the abdominal cavity. Pain associated with the kidneys may present to the side and rear, near what are commonly called the flank areas.

Generalized Abdominal Pain

A sudden or gradual onset of abdominal pain can occur for many reasons and must be cared for as a true emergency. Because there are so many potential causes, it is not important or possible for the Emergency Medical Responder to determine the exact cause. Common causes of acute (sudden) abdominal pain include:

- Bleeding
- Infection
- Ulcers
- Indigestion
- Constipation
- Food poisoning
- Menstrual cramps
- Diabetic emergencies
- Kidney stones
- Pancreatitis
- Gallstones
- Appendicitis
- Ectopic pregnancy

Any woman of childbearing age who experiences acute abdominal pain should be considered pregnant until proven otherwise. It is possible for a woman to not be aware that she is pregnant (or not want to believe that she is), and a pregnancy may ultimately be confirmed.

Signs and Symptoms of Acute Abdominal Pain

LO11 Describe the signs and symptoms of internal bleeding.

Abdominal pain can present suddenly (acute) or slowly over many hours or days. The pain can be described as sharp or dull, depending on the underlying cause. In most cases, the pain can be localized to a specific area within the abdomen. It is best to start out by asking the patient if they can point with one finger to where it hurts the most. Often a patient who has abdominal pain will attempt to protect their abdomen by curling up on one side in the fetal position, lying on their back with knees drawn up, or holding their hands over the painful area (Figure 22.12). These behaviors are called *guarding* and are important signs when assessing a patient with abdominal pain.

Common signs and symptoms of acute abdominal pain include:

- Pain that is sharp or dull
- Tenderness on palpation
- Rigid or tight abdomen
- Abdominal **distention**
- Nausea/vomiting
- Cramping
- Pain that radiates to other areas
- Guarding (protecting the abdomen)

retroperitoneal cavity ► area behind the abdominal cavity that contains the kidneys and ureters.

REMEMBER

Many potentially life-threatening conditions are manifested by a sudden or gradual onset of abdominal pain. Such patients should be considered unstable and receive immediate care from advanced providers.

REMEMBER

The visceral pleura contain nerves that are stimulated when stretched, while the parietal pleura contain nerves that are stimulated by the presence of air, blood, and infection. Pain from the visceral pleura is referred to as *visceral pain*, and pain associated with irritation of the parietal pleura is referred to as *somatic pain*. Visceral pain is usually vague and poorly localized, while parietal pain is usually sharp and well localized.

---

distention ► enlargement or swelling due to internal pressure.

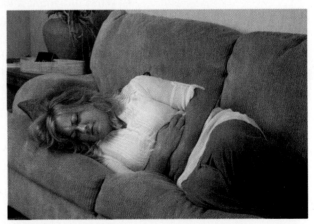

Figure 22.12 A patient experiencing acute abdominal pain will often lie on their side and guard the abdomen.

Bleeding within the gastrointestinal system can occur for many reasons, with or without injury or pain. Ulcers and colitis are examples of conditions that can cause GI bleeding. A patient who vomits bright red blood or has bright red blood in their stool likely has an active internal bleed and should be considered unstable. Blood that is old and digested will appear like dark coffee grounds when vomited. Blood that has passed through the intestines and makes its way out in the feces will appear very dark, like tar. It is always appropriate to ask a patient about recent bowel movements and if they appeared normal.

Pain caused by organs and structures located in the retroperitoneal space, such as the abdominal aorta and the kidneys, may present as back pain or flank pain (pain on one side of the body between the abdomen and the back). **Kidney stones** are small, pebble-like formations created from an excess of minerals in the urine; they occur more frequently in males than in females. Pain from kidney stones can be severe and can radiate from the flank region to the inner thigh.

An **aortic dissection** is a tear in the inner wall of the aorta most often caused by a genetic weakness in the vessel. Depending on where the tear occurs, it can present as chest pain or, more commonly, as upper or lower back pain. It is often described as a very sharp stabbing pain.

Assessing the Patient with Acute Abdominal Pain

LO12 Explain the appropriate assessment and care of a patient with abdominal pain.

Your assessment of the patient with acute abdominal pain must begin by ruling out any history of trauma. Ask the patient if they sustained any blunt-force trauma to the upper body within the past few hours or days. Many times, the patient forgets about a recent fall or injury and will not associate it with the current complaint. Injuries to the abdomen can cause bleeding that is very slow. Signs and symptoms can be delayed for hours or sometimes days.

Your assessment will focus on a thorough medical history. Using the OPQRST assessment tool, you should ask the following questions during your secondary assessment:

- When did the pain begin?
- Did the pain start suddenly or gradually?
- How bad is the pain (using a 1 to 10 scale with 10 being the most pain)?
- Is the pain sharp or dull?
- Can you point with one finger to where the pain is the worst?
- Does the pain radiate anywhere?
- Have you had a fever?
- Did you experience any injury or trauma?
- When did you last eat or drink? What did you eat or drink?
- Are you experiencing nausea or vomiting?
- Does anything make the pain better or worse?
- Is there any possibility that you could be pregnant?
- When was your last menstrual period?
- Has there been any blood in your vomit or stool?

Signs and symptoms of internal abdominal bleeding include:

- Sharp or dull pain in the abdomen
- Blood in the stool
- Blood in the vomit
- Rigid abdomen
- Signs of shock
- Abdominal distention

Abdominal Injuries

LO11 Describe the signs and symptoms of internal bleeding.

LO12 Explain the appropriate assessment and care of a patient with abdominal pain.

Injury to the abdomen can produce life-threatening emergencies that must be cared for immediately. Damage to internal organs can cause them to stop functioning normally. In addition to organ failure, bleeding from damage to organs and soft tissues can result in hemorrhagic shock and death if not identified and cared for promptly.

The following signs and symptoms may indicate injury to organs of the abdomen and pelvis:

- Pain and/or tenderness
- Bruising over the area
- Guarding (protecting the abdomen)
- Lying with legs drawn up against the abdomen (fetal position)
- Rigid and/or distended abdomen

Injuries to the abdomen and pelvis can be either open or closed. Closed injuries are most often caused by blunt trauma and may have little or no obvious signs of injury. In those cases, you will have to rely on the mechanism of injury and maintain a high index of suspicion for internal injuries. The most common symptom of a closed injury will be pain over one or more abdominal quadrants.

Caring for a Closed Abdominal Injury

Caring for a patient with a closed abdominal injury is relatively simple. You must perform a thorough assessment of the abdomen and palpate all quadrants to determine precisely where the pain is and where it is not (Figure 22.13). Always expose the abdomen to observe for any signs of injury, such as abrasions (as with a seat-belt injury) or bruising. If there is no reason to suspect a spinal injury, allow the patient to maintain a position of comfort. This will likely be lying down either on the back with knees raised or on the side with knees bent.

Open Abdominal Injuries

LO13 Explain the appropriate assessment and care of a patient with an open abdominal injury.

Open injuries to the abdomen are most often caused by sharp objects such as knives and sharp metal. The abdomen is also susceptible to penetrating injury, as in a gunshot wound. Regardless of the mechanism, the likelihood of damage to internal organs and severe bleeding is high, so you must always consider these patients unstable and in need of immediate transport.

Generally speaking, the organ directly under the penetrating wound is the one most likely to be injured. However, depending on the path of the wound, multiple organs could be involved.

Treat penetrating trauma to the abdomen and pelvis the same as you would for penetrating trauma to the chest. Cover open wounds with a sterile dressing and, in the case of gunshots, examine all areas of the patient's body to identify and manage all open wounds. Remember that exit wounds may be in the back, chest, or extremities, depending on the direction of the projectile.

Impaled objects in the abdomen are treated the same as in the chest, with proper stabilization of the object. Do not remove impaled objects!

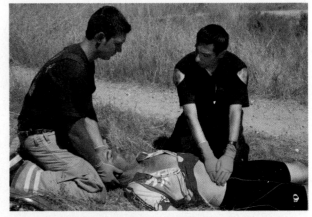

Figure 22.13 Use both hands to palpate the abdomen one quadrant at a time.

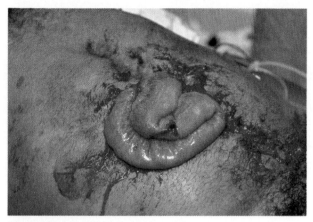

Figure 22.14 Abdominal evisceration.
(© Edward T. Dickinson, MD)

evisceration ▶ open wound of the abdomen characterized by protrusion of the abdominal contents through the abdominal wall.

Abdominal Evisceration

A common type of open abdominal injury is an **evisceration**. This type of injury occurs when the abdominal wall is penetrated by a sharp object and the contents of the abdomen are allowed to spill out (Figure 22.14). Never attempt to place spilled abdominal contents back into an open wound. This could cause many complications and introduce infection into the wound.

Care for an individual with an abdominal evisceration should include the following steps (Key Skill 22.1):

1. Take appropriate BSI precautions and ensure the scene is safe.
2. Expose the wound and any organs that may have spilled out by removing or cutting away clothing.
3. Position the patient on their back. If no spinal injury is suspected, have the patient bend their knees. This will put less tension on the abdominal muscles.
4. Place a large sterile dressing soaked with sterile water or saline over the exposed abdominal contents.

KEY SKILL 22.1

Dressing an Abdominal Evisceration

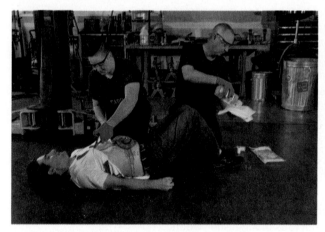

1. Cut away clothing to expose the entire injury.

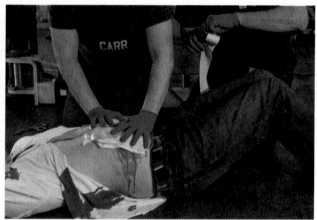

2. Place a large sterile dressing moistened with sterile water or saline over the exposed abdominal contents.

3. Place plastic wrap or a plastic sheet over the dressing and secure it in place.

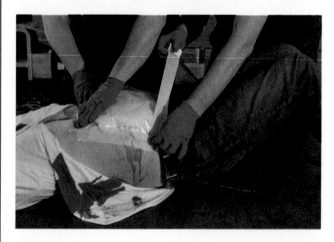

5. Cover the moist dressing with plastic wrap or a plastic sheet and secure in place. This will help contain the moisture and keep the exposed tissue from drying out.
6. Provide high-flow oxygen if allowed by local protocols.
7. Provide care for shock.
8. Initiate transport as soon as possible.

REMEMBER

Minimize any direct contact with exposed abdominal contents, and cover the wound as soon as practical with a sterile dressing. This will help minimize the likelihood of infection.

CREW RESOURCE MANAGEMENT

Managing a patient with an abdominal evisceration requires good coordination from the entire team. The abdominal dressing is best applied with a rescuer on each side of the patient.

FIRST ON SCENE WRAP-UP

"I thought for sure he was going to pass out," Jess says as the doors to the ambulance close.

"I know," Liz says as she places the oxygen tank into its case. "He cried out with every lift, bump, or shift of the gurney. It's a shame his room wasn't on the ground floor."

"Well, we did a pretty good job, I guess," Jess says, reviewing her notes. "The medic was able to get Nico in the rig pretty quickly by confirming our impression and assessment."

"I have to admit, though," Liz says, "I think I better review the abdominal cavity again so I know for sure where the organs are for future calls."

Summary

- Injuries to the chest can affect the ability of the patient to breathe adequately as well as cause damage to internal organs such as the heart and lungs.
- Injuries to the chest can be classified as open or closed.
- Common types of closed chest injuries are broken ribs with collapse of a lung (pneumothorax) and blood in the chest cavity (hemothorax).
- Signs and symptoms of closed chest injuries include pain on breathing, difficulty breathing, discoloration, deformity, and paradoxical movement of the chest wall.
- A flail chest is caused when three or more adjacent ribs are broken in two or more places. This compromises the integrity of the chest wall and makes it very difficult for the patient to breathe adequately.
- When assessing a patient with a chest injury, be sure to expose all areas and palpate thoroughly with both hands. Consider high-flow oxygen when local protocols indicate.

- Open chest injuries can result in a sucking chest wound and must be covered immediately with an occlusive dressing.
- Stabilize all impaled objects and do your best to secure the object in place. Do not attempt to remove an impaled object.
- The abdomen and pelvis contain both solid and hollow organs. Injuries to those organs can cause organ failure and severe internal bleeding.
- Signs and symptoms of an abdominal emergency include pain, rigidity, distention, and blood in the vomit or feces.
- Abdominal injuries can be classified as closed or open. Closed injuries can result in organ damage and/or severe bleeding.
- An abdominal evisceration is an open wound that has allowed the abdominal contents to spill out. These should be covered with a sterile, moist dressing and covered with plastic wrap to minimize the chances that the exposed organs will dry out.

Take Action

Hide and Seek

The cornerstone of a good assessment of the patient with chest or abdominal pain is the physical exam. You must be as thorough as possible and palpate all areas. This activity will help you become better at performing a physical assessment of the chest and abdomen.

To begin, you will need a fellow student or willing family member to serve as patient. Next, take several objects such as large paperclips, large coins, erasers, or similar objects. The individual who will play patient must go into another room and carefully tape several items to different areas around their torso or abdomen.

When the patient has secured the objects, they return and lie down on the floor. Begin by having them lie supine. Now perform your usual assessment of the chest and abdomen, attempting to locate all the items.

To make this a bit more challenging, you can tape different-sized coins to the patient's body. Of course, the smaller the coin, the more difficult it will be to palpate beneath the clothing.

First on Scene Patient Handoff

Nico is a 19-year-old male with a complaint of a sharp abdominal pain, which began approximately 1 hour ago. He denies any recent trauma or history of abdominal pain. The pain is a 9 out of 10 and has been steadily getting worse for the past hour. The pain is located in the right lower quadrant. His mother states that Nico has never had any abdominal surgery. His vitals are respirations 24, good tidal volume and unlabored, BP of 130/78, pulse of 120 strong and regular. His abdominal assessment appears normal other than the pain, and we have him on oxygen by nonrebreather mask at 10 LPM.

First on Scene Run Review

Recall the events of the First on Scene scenario in this chapter, and answer the following questions related to the call. Rationales are offered in the Answer Key at the back of the book.

1. What medical history would you want to get from Nico?
2. As an Emergency Medical Responder, how would you treat this individual?
3. What information would you like to get from his mother? What information would you give to his mother?

Quick Quiz

To check your understanding of the chapter, answer the following questions. Then compare your answers to those in the Answer Key at the back of the book.

1. You are caring for a patient who was struck in the lateral chest by a blunt object. You palpate a flail segment on the right lateral chest. This type of injury is most likely to affect the patient's:
   a. ability to breathe normally.
   b. heart and lungs.
   c. pulse rate.
   d. ability to cough.

2. Your patient has an open wound to her chest. The wound is bubbling and making "sucking" noises as she breathes. You should:
   a. cover it loosely with a cloth bandage.
   b. cover the wound with an occlusive dressing.
   c. instruct the patient to breathe deeply.
   d. pack the opening of the wound with clean gauze.

3. A 29-year-old man is complaining of difficulty breathing after being tackled while playing football. Appropriate assessment of this patient includes doing all of the following EXCEPT:
   a. palpating the chest wall.
   b. palpating the abdomen.
   c. listening to lung sounds.
   d. encouraging the patient to cough forcefully.

4. Your patient has been shot in the chest. You have sealed the wound with an occlusive dressing. Which of the following signs would cause concern that the patient is developing a tension pneumothorax?
   a. Equal chest rise
   b. Midline trachea
   c. Increasing respiratory rate
   d. Pulse rate of 90

5. The purpose of placing an occlusive dressing over an open chest wound is to:
   a. control the bleeding.
   b. keep chest contents from spilling out.
   c. keep air from entering the chest cavity.
   d. make it easier for the patient to breathe.

6. You are caring for a patient with an open chest wound and have covered the wound with an occlusive dressing. The patient becomes increasingly short of breath. You should:
   a. add another dressing to the wound.
   b. partially remove the dressing to allow air to escape.
   c. apply more pressure to the wound.
   d. remove the dressing altogether.

7. You are caring for a patient who appears to have injured a rib. There is no flail segment, and the patient is alert and oriented. What is the most likely potential complication from a simple rib injury?
   a. Hypoxia from shallow respirations
   b. Puncture of the heart or lung
   c. Internal bleeding
   d. Pneumothorax

8. Which of the following is the most appropriate care for an open abdominal injury?
   a. Pack the inside of the wound with clean dressings.
   b. Pour sterile saline over the wound.
   c. Cover the wound with a dry, clean dressing.
   d. Cover the wound with a moist, sterile dressing.

9. You are caring for a patient who has had abdominal pain for the past 2 days. She states that she had a bowel movement this morning that was very dark and tarry. Those signs and symptoms are consistent with:
   a. internal bleeding from the GI tract.
   b. ingestion of a toxic substance.
   c. appendicitis.
   d. evisceration.

10. A patient has been shot in the right upper quadrant of the abdomen. You should assume which of the following organs may have been injured?
   a. Stomach
   b. Liver
   c. Spleen
   d. Pancreas

Endnotes

1. Shi-ping Luh. "Diagnosis and Treatment of Primary Spontaneous Pneumothorax," *Journal of Zhejiang University—Science B,* Vol. 11, No. 10 (2010): 735–744.

2. Dogrul B.N., Kiliccalan I., Asci E.S., Peker S.C. "Blunt Trauma Related Chest Wall and Pulmonary Injuries: An Overview," *Chinese Journal of Traumatology*, Vol. 23, No. 3 (June 2020): 125–138. doi: 10.1016/j.cjtee.2020.04.003. Epub 2020 Apr 20. PMID: 32417043; PMCID: PMC7296362.

3. NAEMT and American College of Surgeons Committee on Trauma. *Prehospital Trauma Life Support*, 8th Edition (Burlington, MA: Jones & Bartlett Learning, 2014): 278.

4. Ibid., p. 281.

5. Butler F.K., et al. Management of Open Pneumothorax in Tactical Combat Casualty Care: TCCC Guidelines Change 13-02. *Journal of Special Operations Medicine*, Vol. 13, Edition 3/Fall 2013.

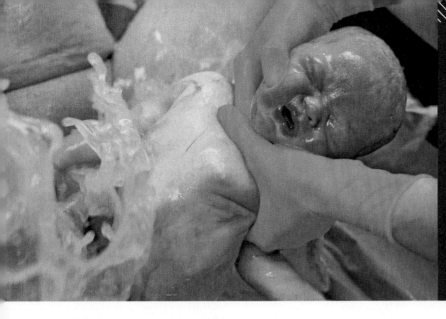

23

Care During Pregnancy and Childbirth

LEARNING OBJECTIVES

Upon successful completion of this chapter, the student should be able to:

Cognitive

1. Define the chapter key terms.

2. Describe the function of the following anatomy related to childbirth: amniotic sac, birth canal, cervix, placenta, umbilical cord, and uterus.

3. Describe the signs of an imminent delivery.

4. Describe the three stages of labor and when each begins and ends.

5. Explain the purpose of each of the items in a typical field obstetric (OB) kit.

6. Explain the steps for preparing for a field delivery.

7. Explain the steps for assisting with a field delivery.

8. Explain the priorities of care for the newborn following a field delivery.

9. Explain the priorities of care for the mother following a field delivery.

10. Explain the common causes of vaginal bleeding during the first trimester.

11. Explain the common causes of vaginal bleeding during the third trimester.

12. Explain the appropriate care for a pregnant patient with vaginal bleeding.

13. Explain the common complications related to a field delivery and how to properly care for each.

14. Describe the signs and symptoms of supine hypotensive syndrome.

15. Explain the appropriate care for a patient with signs and symptoms of supine hypotensive syndrome.

16. Describe the signs and symptoms of preeclampsia.

17. Explain the appropriate care for a patient with signs and symptoms of preeclampsia.

18. Describe the management of a pregnant woman showing the signs of preeclampsia.

19. Describe the management of a pregnant woman who has sustained a traumatic injury.

20. Describe the management of a pregnant woman with an abnormally low blood pressure.

Psychomotor

21. Demonstrate the ability to identify the signs of an imminent delivery.

22. Demonstrate the steps for preparing for and assisting with a field delivery.

23. Demonstrate the proper care of the infant following a field delivery.

24. Demonstrate the proper care of the mother following a field delivery.

25. Demonstrate the ability to identify a complicated delivery.

26. Demonstrate the proper assessment and care for a complicated field delivery.

Affective

27. Value the importance of proper body substance isolation (BSI) precautions when assisting with a field delivery.

Education Standards

Special Patient Populations— Gynecology

Competencies

Recognizes and manages life threats based on simple assessment findings for a patient with special needs while awaiting additional emergency response.

KEY TERMS

amniotic fluid (*p. 481*)

amniotic sac (*p. 481*)

birth canal (*p. 481*)

bloody show (*p. 481*)

breech birth (*p. 497*)

cervix (*p. 481*)

crowning (*p. 481*)

eclampsia (*p. 500*)

ectopic pregnancy (*p. 496*)

fallopian tube (*p. 496*)

fontanel (*p. 489*)

full term (*p. 481*)

gestation (*p. 481*)

imminent delivery (*p. 481*)

labor (*p. 481*)

meconium (*p. 497*)

miscarriage (*p. 495*)

newborn (*p. 481*)

nuchal cord (*p. 490*)

ovary (*p. 496*)

ovum (*p. 481*)

placenta (*p. 481*)

placenta abruptio (*p. 501*)

placenta previa (*p. 501*)

preeclampsia (*p. 500*)

prenatal care (*p. 485*)

prolapsed cord (*p. 498*)

spotting (*p. 495*)

supine hypotensive syndrome (*p. 500*)

trimester (*p. 481*)

umbilical cord (*p. 481*)

uterus (*p. 481*)

vagina (*p. 481*)

Childbirth is one of the most amazing events anyone can experience. Women have been delivering babies for thousands of years without sterile hospitals and sophisticated equipment. Today, it is common for pregnant women to take classes and spend many months planning for the birth of their child. Despite all this planning, situations still arise that result in an unplanned delivery or unexpected complications. Many times, EMS is called to assist.

This chapter introduces the terminology and processes involved with a normal pregnancy and childbirth. It also introduces some common complications and how to care for the mother and baby during and after delivery. There is debate within the medical field around the use of gender-neutral terms such as "birthing person" to describe an individual who is capable of giving birth. In this chapter, for simplicity we will refer to the birthing person as a female or mother. However, in the field it is always best to ask your patient their preferred pronouns.

FIRST ON SCENE

The first thing that Lucas sees, other than the blinding white of the snow swirling across the hood of his truck, is the red and blue flashing lights of a state trooper's car. The officer has blocked both lanes with his patrol car and is waving traffic toward the snow-packed off-ramp. Lucas rolls down his window and shouts above the howling wind, "What's going on?"

"Interstate is closed!" the trooper shouts back. "Pull off here and find a place to park."

Lucas sits for a moment, trying to calculate another route to Denver, then sighs, rolls up the window, and follows the officer's order.

The end of the off-ramp opens up into the parking lot of a small, crowded travel stop. As he looks for a space where his pickup will fit in the field of car-shaped mounds of snow, he begins to regret not flying to the Medical Emergency Response Team conference.

He is backing into a narrow opening when he hears a man yelling for help. The man is not dressed for the extreme weather and is running up and down between vehicles, shouting for help and knocking on windows.

"My wife!" the man shouts, his breath exploding out in white clouds. "I think she's having our baby! Somebody, please help!"

Understanding Childbirth

| LO2 | Describe the function of the following anatomy related to childbirth: amniotic sac, birth canal, cervix, placenta, umbilical cord, and uterus.

| LO3 | Describe the signs of an imminent delivery.

You may have noticed that this chapter's title refers to "childbirth" and not "emergency childbirth." In Western societies, many people consider a birth that occurs away from a hospital delivery room to be an emergency. This is just not true. In many parts of the world, babies are born at home and outside of medical facilities every day. However, complications of childbirth do occur in many settings outside of the hospital; an Emergency Medical Responder can be the key factor in the survival of a **newborn** if something does go wrong. The mother may need your help during the birth process to ensure a safe delivery, and the care provided immediately after delivery is just as important. Your assistance can make a difference for both mother and child.

Anatomy of Pregnancy

An unborn baby is called a *fetus* as it develops and grows inside of the mother. The fetus begins as an unfertilized egg, called an **ovum**. Once fertilized and implanted within the uterus, the ovum becomes an *embryo* and is referred to as such through the 7th week of pregnancy. The fetus develops inside the **uterus**, a muscular organ also called the womb (Figure 23.1). The average period of **gestation** is 38 to 40 weeks (approximately 9 months). The gestational period is divided into 3-month segments called **trimesters**. A baby who reaches the 38th week of gestation prior to delivery is referred to as **full term**.

Labor is the process the body goes through to deliver a fetus. During labor, the muscles of the uterus contract and push the baby down through the opening of the uterus, called the **cervix**. As the cervix expands to allow the head of the fetus through, the mother may notice a slight staining of blood or blood-tinged mucus. This is called **bloody show** and is normal. The fetus passes through the cervix and enters the **birth canal**, or **vagina**, before it emerges through the vaginal opening.

During your assessment of the mother, you must examine her for **crowning**, which is the showing of the baby's head at the opening of the vagina. While crowning is the most common presentation, any part of the baby may present first, including the buttocks or feet. Once the baby passes into the birth canal, more of the head (or other presenting part) will show, or appear to grow larger, with each contraction. This is a sign that delivery is imminent. An **imminent delivery** is a delivery that is likely to occur within a few minutes.

The fetus grows inside the **amniotic sac**. This sac is filled with **amniotic fluid**, which surrounds and protects the baby. Although the sac may have ruptured earlier, it usually breaks during labor, and the amniotic fluid flows out of the vagina. This is called the *rupture of membranes* and is an important milestone in the birthing process. When you are assessing the mother, you will ask her if her "water has broken." She will usually know and be able to tell you if it has or not. Sometimes the sac will break very early in the labor process. Sometimes it will break much later. The fluids help lubricate the birth canal for the passage of the baby.

During pregnancy, a special organ called the **placenta** develops in the womb. Oxygen and nutrients from the mother's blood pass through the placenta and enter fetal circulation through the **umbilical cord**. Fetal wastes pass back through the umbilical cord and the placenta to the mother's circulation to be eliminated.

Stages of Labor

| LO4 | Describe the three stages of labor and when each begins and ends.

On average, the process of labor lasts about 16 hours for the first-time mother. In some cases, labor may take longer, or it can be much shorter. The time can vary with each patient and with each delivery. It is common for the labor process to be shorter with each successive birth.

newborn ▸ infant less than 28 days old; also called *neonate*.

ovum ▸ unfertilized egg produced by the mother.

uterus ▸ muscular structure in which the fetus develops during pregnancy.

gestation ▸ development of the embryo and fetus in the uterus; the period from conception to birth.

trimester ▸ 3-month segment of a pregnancy.

full term ▸ pregnancy that has achieved a gestation of at least 38 weeks.

labor ▸ process the body goes through to deliver a baby.

cervix ▸ opening of the uterus.

bloody show ▸ normal discharge of blood-tinged fluid prior to delivery; caused by rupture of capillaries as the baby's head expands the cervix and birth canal.

birth canal ▸ passage through which a fetus passes during birth; interior aspect of the vagina.

vagina ▸ birth canal.

crowning ▸ head of the fetus showing at the opening of the vagina; sign of impending birth.

imminent delivery ▸ delivery that is likely to occur within the next few minutes.

amniotic sac ▸ fluid-filled sac that surrounds the developing fetus.

amniotic fluid ▸ fluid surrounding the baby contained within the amniotic sac.

placenta ▸ organ of pregnancy that serves as the filter between the mother and developing fetus.

umbilical cord ▸ structure that connects the baby to the placenta.

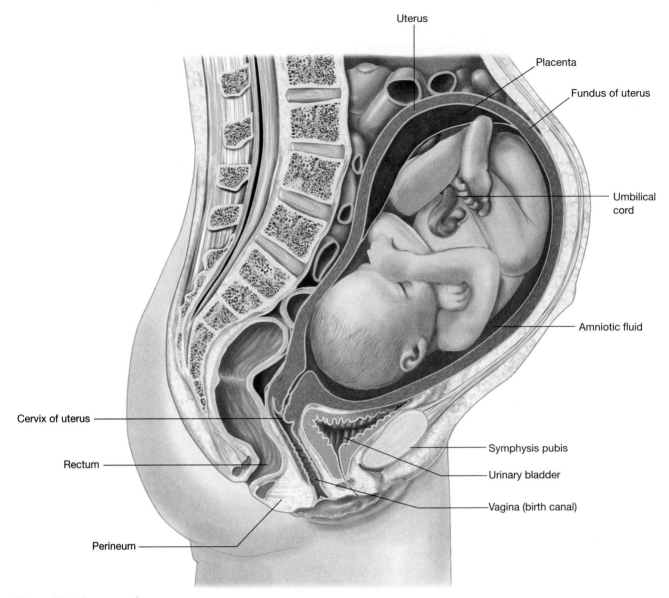

Uterus

Placenta

Fundus of uterus

Umbilical cord

Amniotic fluid

Cervix of uterus

Rectum

Symphysis pubis

Urinary bladder

Vagina (birth canal)

Perineum

Figure 23.1 Anatomy of pregnancy.

There are three stages of labor (Figure 23.2):

- Stage 1 begins with the onset of regular contractions and ends when the cervix is fully dilated (approximately 10 centimeters), allowing the baby to enter the birth canal.
- Stage 2 begins when the baby enters the birth canal and ends when the baby exits the mother's body (birth).
- Stage 3 begins when the baby is born and ends when the placenta (also called *afterbirth*), is delivered.

It is normal to have vaginal discharge throughout labor. During the first stage of labor, the first type of discharge to appear should be a watery, bloody mucus. Later, the discharge will appear as a watery, bloody fluid. This is normal and not the same as bleeding. If bleeding from the vagina occurs prior to delivery, rather than the normal blood-tinged fluids, then something may be wrong. This could be a serious problem that requires assistance from a higher level of EMS provider. Arrange transport for the mother as soon as possible.

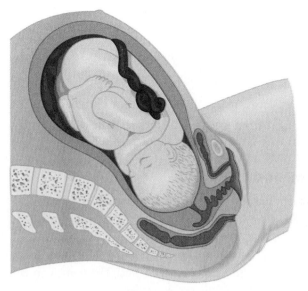

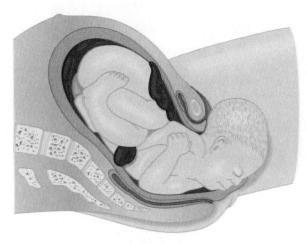

FIRST STAGE:
First uterine contraction to dilation of cervix

SECOND STAGE:
Birth of baby or expulsion

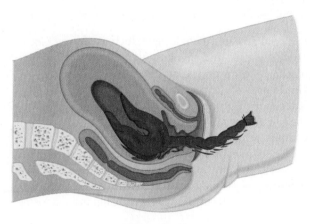

THIRD STAGE:
Delivery of placenta

Figure 23.2 Stages of labor.

Contractions of the uterus cause labor pains, and they occur in cycles of contraction and relaxation. At first, contractions are mild and spaced as much as 30 to 45 minutes apart. As the fetus is pushed into the birth canal and birth gets closer, the time between contractions becomes shorter (3 minutes or less). Pain during labor is normal and usually starts as an ache in the lower back. As labor progresses, the pain is felt in the lower abdomen. As the muscles of the uterus contract, the pain begins. When the muscles relax, the pain is usually relieved. Labor pains normally come at regular intervals and last from 30 seconds to 1 minute. It is common for the pains to start, stop for a period of time, and then start again.

Labor pains can be timed in two ways:

- *Contraction time.* The span of time from the beginning of a contraction until it relaxes is called the contraction time.
- *Interval time.* This is the span of time from the start of one contraction to the beginning of the next contraction (Figure 23.3). As labor progresses, the interval time will become shorter. This is the time that is referred to when discussing the frequency of contractions.

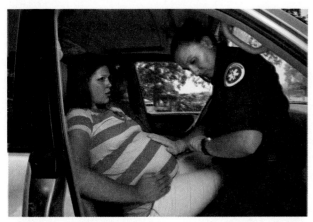

Figure 23.3 Measure the contraction intervals by counting from the beginning of one contraction to the beginning of the next contraction.

Throughout pregnancy the mother might experience light, painless, irregular contractions, which may increase gradually in intensity and frequency during the third trimester. This is known as false labor, also called Braxton Hicks contractions. False labor pains are not as regular and rhythmic as true labor contractions.

It may be difficult for you and the mother to distinguish false labor pains from true labor. Any pregnant woman who is having contractions should be evaluated by her doctor.

Supplies and Materials

LO5 Explain the purpose of each of the items in a typical field obstetric (OB) kit.

Your primary role is to help the mother deliver the baby when birth is imminent. You will need to make sure that you have the necessary supplies and materials to do this. The items you will need for preparing the mother for delivery and initial care are provided in a commercial obstetric (OB) kit (Figure 23.4). If your response unit does not carry a commercial OB kit, assemble and store the required items in a special kit and keep it on your unit. Some of these items may be available at the patient's home, but during delivery is not the time to find supplies. The items you will need include:

- Personal protective equipment such as gloves, face masks, eye shields, and gowns
- Towels, sheets, and blankets for draping the mother, for placement under the mother, and for drying and wrapping the baby
- Gauze pads for wiping mucus from the baby's mouth and nose
- Rubber bulb syringe for suctioning the baby's airway (only if the baby is not breathing normally after birth)
- Clamps and ties for use on the umbilical cord before cutting
- Sterile scissors or a single-edged razor for cutting the cord
- Sanitary pads or bulky dressings for vaginal bleeding
- A basin and plastic bags for collecting and transporting the placenta
- Red plastic biohazard bags for storing and disposing of soiled linens and dressings

Your primary and secondary assessments will help you determine if the mother is ready to deliver. If birth appears likely before a transport unit can get her to the hospital,

Figure 23.4 Contents of a commercial obstetric (OB) kit. All items are disposable.

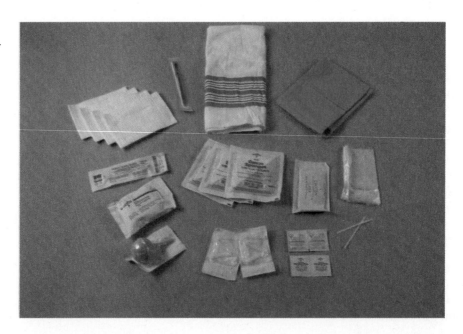

place supplies so they are within your reach during the delivery process. Don your personal protective equipment. Then prepare the mother for delivery. It may be helpful to ask the mother if she has been receiving **prenatal care** (regular care and monitoring of the fetus by a health care provider throughout the pregnancy). A woman who has been receiving regular prenatal care will be more informed if there are any expected complications with the delivery.

Delivery

The delivery of a baby is one of the most exciting calls for any EMS provider. Knowing what to expect and being properly prepared will go a long way toward making this a successful event.

Preparing for Delivery

| LO6 | Explain the steps for preparing for a field delivery.

Due to the nature of childbirth, it is important for you to wear appropriate face and eye protection and a gown, in addition to protective gloves, to minimize your exposure to the mother's body fluids during delivery. Make sure that an EMS transport unit has been activated. Let the mother know that you have called for additional assistance and that you will stay with her to help if she starts to deliver the baby. Provide emotional support throughout the entire process. Reassure the mother to help her remain calm.

If the expectant mother is in active labor (contractions that are 2 minutes apart or less) and complains that she feels as if she needs to go to the bathroom or have a bowel movement, tell her that this is normal and that it is caused by pressure on her bladder and rectum. Encourage her to remain lying down. Explain that her body is reacting normally to all the changes that are taking place. In preparation for delivery of the baby, place clean sheets or towels under her buttocks. If she does have a bowel movement or urinates, tell her that this is normal. Remove soiled linens and replace them with fresh ones.

Begin to evaluate the mother by asking for the following information:

- What is the expected due date?
- Has she been seeing a doctor during her pregnancy?
- Does she have other children?
- If so, how was her last labor? (Note that if this is her first delivery, labor will typically last about 16 hours. Labor time is usually shorter for subsequent deliveries.)
- Were previous children delivered normally or did they require a Cesarean section (C-section)?
- Is she aware of any known complications, particularly a multiple birth (twins or triplets)?
- Has there been any discharge of fluid or bloody mucus?
- How long has she been having labor pains?
- How frequent are the contractions?
- Has her water broken? If so, when, and what color? (Clear is normal. Cloudy or green indicates a stressed fetus and requires immediate transport.)
- Does she feel the need to move her bowels? If so, can she feel the baby beginning to move into the birth canal?
- Does she have any significant medical history such as seizures, diabetes, or vaginal bleeding during the pregnancy?

If the mother says she feels the urge to bear down (push), birth may be imminent. If the contractions are 2 minutes apart or less, delivery is imminent. Should she also be straining, crying out, and complaining about having to go to the bathroom, prepare to deliver very shortly. The mother will be your best source of information as to what is going on. When she says she feels the baby coming, believe her.

prenatal care ▶ routine medical care provided during pregnancy.

SCENE SAFETY

The delivery of an infant in the field setting presents a significant risk of exposure to blood and other potentially infectious materials. This is one of the rare occasions when you would employ full BSI precautions, including gloves, face mask, eye protection, and gown.

REMEMBER

A Cesarean section (also called C-section) is a surgical procedure performed to deliver a baby. An incision is made through the abdomen into the uterus, and the baby is delivered directly from the uterus instead of through the vaginal canal. This procedure is done for many reasons, including abnormality of the fetus, placenta, or uterus, or when the mother has some type of medical condition that would prevent or interfere with a vaginal delivery.

SCENE SAFETY

The baby entering the birth canal causes downward pressure on the mother's rectum. This pressure will make her feel as if she needs to have a bowel movement. She may insist on using the bathroom during the delivery process. Be prepared for this, and never allow a mother in active labor (contractions that are 2 minutes apart or less) to use the restroom because there is risk of the baby being delivered into the toilet.

Following are a few simple coaching steps:

- As each contraction begins, have the mother take a deep breath, hold it, and encourage her to gently bear down, or push.
- Encourage her to rest between each contraction and to breathe normally.
- If available, have the father or someone appropriate at the mother's head to help coach her through each contraction.

After evaluating and examining the mother and finding that birth is imminent, immediately prepare the scene and the mother for delivery:

1. Take BSI precautions.
2. Control the scene so the mother will have privacy. Ask unnecessary bystanders to leave. You may have to move her a short distance to a more private location. If labor is not too severe, it may be appropriate to allow the mother to walk. If she appears to be in early labor and this is her first child, her labor pains will typically have long contraction and interval times.
3. Position the mother on her back with her knees bent, feet flat, and legs spread wide apart. If this position causes her to feel dizzy and faint, it may be because the weight of the baby is pressing on the inferior vena cava, the vessel that returns blood from the lower part of the body to the heart, and is restricting blood flow back to the heart. Allow the mother to sit up slightly and support her back with pillows and/or blankets.
4. Palpate the mother's abdomen to feel for contractions when she says she is having a contraction. Explain what you are going to do, and place the palm of your hand on her abdomen above the navel. It is not necessary to remove any of the patient's clothing to feel for contractions. If the mother says she can feel the baby coming, skip this step. Feel for, and time, several contractions to help determine if birth is near. As birth nears, the interval time will decrease, and you will feel the uterus and the abdomen become more rigid. If the interval time between contractions is 3 minutes or less, consider that birth may be imminent.
5. Prepare the mother for examination. Tell her that you need to see if her baby has entered the birth canal. Help her to remove clothing or underclothing that obstructs your exam of her vaginal opening. Use clean sheets or towels to cover the mother. If you have a commercial obstetric (OB) kit, use the materials provided. Make sure you have enough light to see what you are doing.
6. Check for crowning. See if any part of the baby is visible at the vaginal opening. When the baby is in the normal position for birth, you will see the top of the baby's head (crowning), although any part of the baby may present first. The area of the head that you see on your first inspection may be only a couple of inches. The mother is now in the second stage of labor because the baby is in the birth canal. Do not try to transport the mother at this point.
7. Do not attempt any type of internal or vaginal exam. Touch the vaginal area only as necessary during the delivery process.

FIRST ON SCENE (continued)

"Hey, buddy!" Lucas calls as he opens his door. "Where is your wife?"

The man, hearing a response to his cries for help, runs toward Lucas. "She's in my car." The man breathes heavily. Thin strands of ice hang from his beard. "Please help her. I don't know what to do."

"Well, for starters, we've got to get her inside," Lucas says as he pulls on his heavy jacket and wool gloves. "Take me to your car." The man quickly shakes Lucas's hand, turns, and jogs back through the cars, looking back over his shoulder to make sure Lucas is following.

Like many of the other vehicles in the lot, the man's car looks like a snow sculpture. The rising exhaust smoke and the dull red glow of the buried taillights are the only clues that there is actually a vehicle there. The man knocks a clump of white powder from the door handle and opens the passenger-side door, exposing the warm interior of the car and his very pregnant, very terrified wife.

Normal Delivery

LO7 Explain the steps for assisting with a field delivery.

Constantly reassure the mother and remind her that you are there to help. Encourage her to relax between contractions. If her water breaks, remind her that this is normal.

Perform the following steps when assisting the mother in a normal delivery (Figure 23.5 and Key Skill 23.1):

1. Wash your hands with soap and water, or use a commercial hand sanitizer. Don personal protective equipment (gloves, mask with eye shield, and gown) if you have not already done so.
2. Drape the mother and place her on clean sheets or towels. Place a folded blanket, towels, or sheets under her buttocks to lift her pelvis about 2 inches. You may place a pillow under her head and shoulders for comfort.

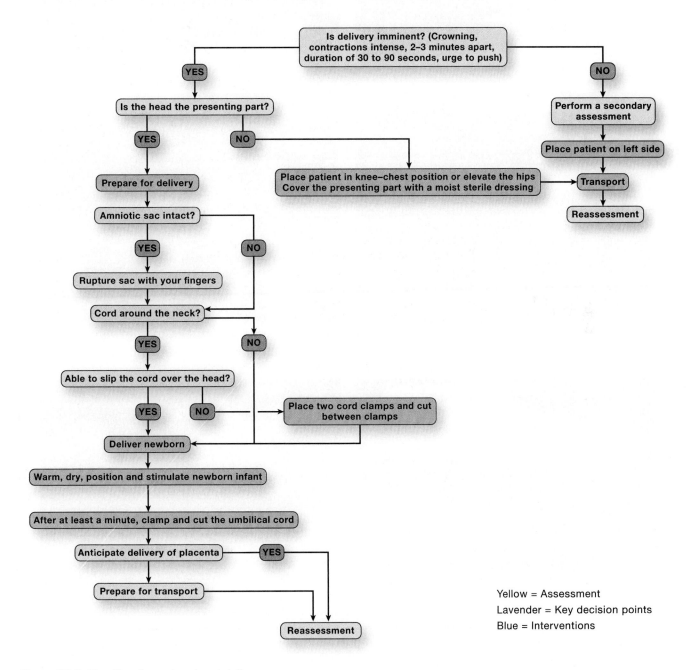

Figure 23.5 Algorithm for an imminent delivery.

Assisting with a Normal Delivery

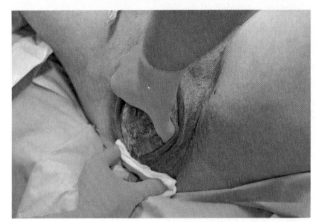

1. Crowning is evident as the head emerges from the vagina.
(Kevin Link/Pearson Education, Inc.)

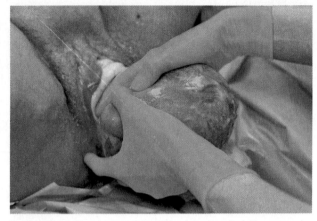

2. Use both hands to support the head as it delivers, and check the neck for presence of the umbilical cord.
(Kevin Link/Pearson Education, Inc.)

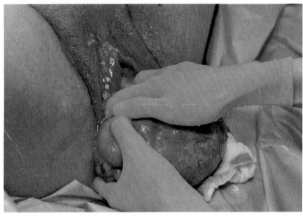

3. Guide the baby's head downward to facilitate delivery of the top shoulder.
(Kevin Link/Pearson Education, Inc.)

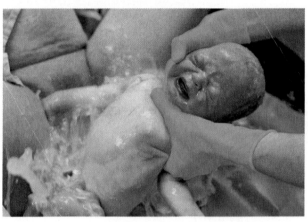

4. Use both hands to support the baby following delivery.
(Kevin Link/Pearson Education, Inc.)

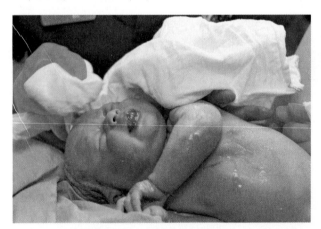

5. Carefully dry the baby and cover them to conserve heat.
(Kevin Link/Pearson Education, Inc.)

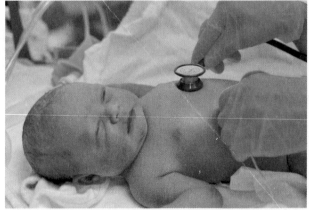

6. Assess breathing and heart rate of the newborn.
(Kevin Link/Pearson Education, Inc.)

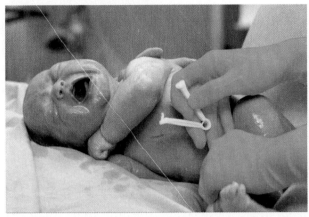

7. Once the cord has stopped pulsating, clamp it in
preparation for cutting.
(Kevin Link/Pearson Education, Inc.)

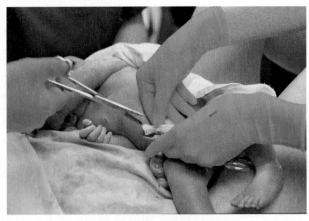

8. Cut the cord between the clamps.
(Kevin Link/Pearson Education, Inc.)

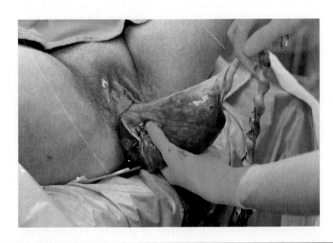

9. Expect delivery of the placenta within 20 to 30 minutes
following the delivery of the baby.
(Kevin Link/Pearson Education, Inc.)

3. Position someone near the mother's head or use the mother's coach to reassure
and offer her encouragement and to turn her head in case she vomits. If no one is
on hand to help, talk with the mother during the delivery process and be alert for
vomiting.

4. Place one hand below the baby's head as the baby emerges. Spread your fingers
evenly around the head for support but avoid pressing the soft areas known as
fontanels at the top of the skull. These are areas where the skull bones have not
completely fused together. Apply a slight pressure on the baby's head as they emerge
to control the speed of delivery. Sometimes the head can "pop out" too quickly from
the birth canal, which can tear the skin at the vaginal opening or perineum. (Some
stretching and tearing is normal.) Use your other hand to help cradle the baby's
head. Do not pull on the baby.

5. If the amniotic sac has not yet ruptured, use a cord clamp or your gloved fingers to
tear the membrane and pull it away from the baby's mouth and nose.

6. Most babies are born face down as the head emerges. Then they rotate to the right
or left. Once the head is delivered, instruct the mother to stop pushing. You need a
few seconds to check if the umbilical cord is wrapped around the baby's neck. This
is called a **nuchal cord**. If you find the cord is wrapped around the baby's neck, use

fontanel ▶ soft area on an
infant's skull where the bones
have not yet fused together.

nuchal cord ▶ condition in
which the umbilical cord is
wrapped around the baby's neck
during delivery.

two fingers and attempt to slip it over the baby's head or shoulders. (We will discuss later what to do if you are unable to easily slip the cord over the baby's head.)

7. The upper shoulder usually delivers next, followed quickly by the lower shoulder. On the next contraction, gently guide the baby's head downward, which will assist the mother in delivering the baby's upper shoulder. Then gently guide the baby's head upward to facilitate the delivery of the bottom shoulder. Newborn babies are very slippery. Make certain you have a good but gentle grip on the baby, and provide proper support throughout the delivery process. Key Skill 23.1 shows hand placement during delivery.

8. Once the baby's feet deliver (the end of the second stage of labor), lay the baby on their side with the head slightly lower than the body. This position will enable blood, other fluids, and mucus to drain from the mouth and nose. Wipe the baby's mouth and nose with gauze pads.

9. Once the baby is completely delivered, note the exact time of birth.

10. Keep the baby at the level of the vagina until the cord is cut.

11. Wait at least 1 minute following delivery, and clamp or tie the umbilical cord. The first clamp should be placed approximately 6 inches from the baby's abdomen. The second clamp should be placed approximately 2 inches away from the first clamp (farther from the baby). Then cut the cord between the clamps. If you do not have sterile equipment, do not cut the cord. Simply clamp it. Follow local protocols.

12. Monitor and record the baby's and mother's vital signs. Support the ABCs as necessary.

13. Watch for more contractions, which may signal the delivery of the placenta. It is important to save the placenta for examination. If any part of it remains attached inside the uterus, it can cause bleeding and an infection. Place the placenta in a plastic biohazard bag and label the bag with the mother's name. You will give it to EMS personnel to transport to the hospital.

14. Place a sanitary pad over the mother's vaginal opening. Lower her legs and place them together.

Caring for the Baby

LO8 Explain the priorities of care for the newborn following a field delivery.

Follow these steps to provide care for the baby immediately after birth (Figure 23.6):

1. Clear the baby's airway. Position the baby on their side with head slightly lower than the body to allow for drainage. Keep the baby's body at the level of the vagina until the cord is clamped. Use a sterile gauze pad or a clean cloth to clear mucus and blood from around the baby's nose and mouth (Figure 23.7). Throughout the rest of your care steps, be sure the baby's nose remains clear. Babies are nose breathers, and clogged nostrils may prevent adequate breathing.

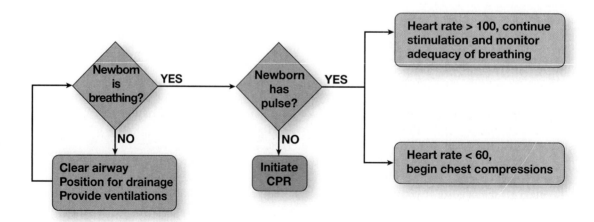

Figure 23.6 Algorithm for assessment of the newborn.

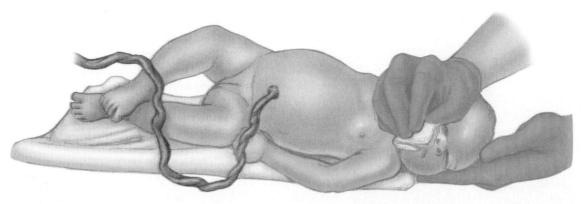

Figure 23.7 Use a sterile pad or clean cloth to wipe blood and mucus from around the baby's mouth and nose.

Following delivery, if the baby is not breathing adequately or appears to be experiencing respiratory distress, it may be helpful to suction the airway. Suctioning should be avoided if the baby is breathing normally. Suction can cause trauma to the airway and can slow the heart rate by stimulating the airway. The correct steps for using a bulb syringe to suction the airway are:

- Squeeze the bulb first.
- Insert the tip about one-half inch into the nose or 1 inch into the mouth.
- Gently release the pressure to allow the syringe to take up fluids.
- Remove the tip of the filled syringe, and squeeze out any fluids onto a towel or gauze pad.
- Repeat this process 2 or 3 times for the mouth and for each nostril.

2. Make certain that the baby is breathing. Usually the baby will be breathing on their own by the time you clear the airway, which will take about 30 seconds. If the baby is not breathing, then you must encourage them to do so. Begin by vigorously but gently rubbing the baby's back. If this fails to stimulate breathing, snap one of your index fingers against the soles of the baby's feet (Figure 23.8).

3. Once you are sure the baby is breathing, perform a quick assessment. Note skin color (blue, normal, or pale), any deformities, the strength of their cry (strong or weak), and whether they move on their own or just lie still. After a few minutes, note if there are any changes in those conditions. It is important to give this information to the transport personnel for relay to the hospital staff, who will base the baby's subsequent exam on the original assessment.

4. Clamp or tie off the umbilical cord if protocols allow.

5. Keep the baby warm. Dry the baby and discard the wet material in a biohazard bag. Wrap the baby in a clean, dry towel, sheet, or blanket, and place the baby on the mother's abdomen. Keep the baby's head covered to help reduce heat loss.

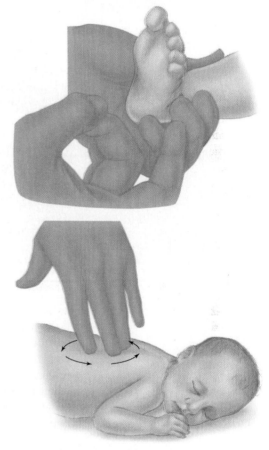

Figure 23.8 It may be necessary to stimulate the newborn baby to breathe.

The mother may want to nurse the baby. You may encourage the mother to do so because it helps contract the uterus and control bleeding.

CREW RESOURCE MANAGEMENT

One person from your team should be dedicated to ensuring that the newborn is kept warm and is breathing well, with a strong, rapid pulse following delivery. This will ensure that both mother and baby get any needed care during and after delivery.

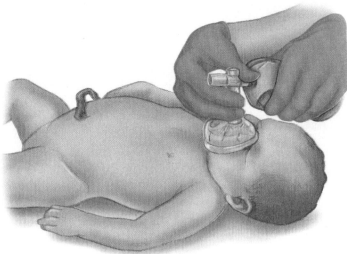

Figure 23.9 Resuscitate the newborn baby with a bag-mask device of an appropriate size.

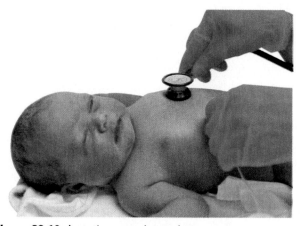

Figure 23.10 A stethoscope is used to assess a newborn's heartbeat.
(Kevin Link/Pearson Education, Inc.)

SCENE SAFETY

Do not be fooled into thinking that an infant with a pulse is doing okay. Infants have a much higher baseline heart rate than children or adults. Take time to assess the heart rate accurately and, if it is below 60 beats per minute, begin chest compressions.

Caring for the Nonbreathing Newborn If the baby is not breathing, you must provide rescue breaths. Begin with two gentle but adequate breaths using the mouth-to-barrier or bag-mask technique (Figure 23.9). Then assess breathing and heartbeat. To check the heartbeat of a newborn, listen at the chest with your stethoscope (Figure 23.10).

Do not use a bag-mask device or airway adjuncts designed for older children or adults to resuscitate a newborn. Be careful not to hyperextend the head and neck of the baby, which would close off the airway.

Provide ventilations if breaths are shallow, slow, or absent. Ventilate at 40 to 60 breaths per minute (about one breath every second). Watch for the chest to rise, which is the best indication of adequate ventilation. Reassess breathing after 30 seconds of assisted ventilations. The next step depends on the heart rate (Table 23.1):

- If the heart rate is 100 beats per minute or greater and the newborn is breathing adequately, stop ventilations but continue to provide gentle stimulation (rub the back) to help maintain and improve the baby's breathing.
- If you are allowed to provide oxygen to the baby, direct a stream of oxygen toward the baby's face, either through a face mask or by passing an oxygen tube through the bottom of a paper cup. Hold the mask or cup several inches from the baby's face, and allow the oxygen to blow by the face as the baby breathes (Figure 23.11). This is referred to as "blow-by" oxygen and is a good technique when a traditional mask or cannula is not appropriate.
- If the newborn's heart rate is below 100 beats per minute and respirations are inadequate, continue to assist ventilations with a bag-mask device.
- If the heart rate is less than 60 beats per minute, continue to assist ventilations and begin chest compressions. Perform CPR with your fingertips if you are alone or with your thumbs with your hands encircling the chest if there are two rescuers. Continue resuscitation until the baby is able to maintain adequate breathing and a pulse, or when a higher level of EMS provider relieves you. For the newborn, perform CPR using a compression-to-ventilation ratio of 30 to 2 for a lone rescuer or 15 to 2 for two rescuers. Continue to provide blow-by oxygen.

Umbilical Cord Your instructor will tell you if local protocols allow Emergency Medical Responders to clamp and cut the umbilical cord (Figure 23.12). If you are allowed to do so, remember that the baby can get an infection through the cord, so cut it only if you

TABLE 23.1	**Care for the Nonbreathing Newborn**
IF THERE IS A PULSE, BUT YOU SEE THIS:	**THEN DO THIS:**
Breathing rate is inadequate.	Ventilate at 40 to 60 breaths per minute for 30 seconds and reassess breathing.
Heart rate is at least 100 beats per minute and spontaneous breathing is present.	Stop ventilations but continue to gently stimulate the baby by rubbing the back or legs.
Heart rate is less than 60 beats per minute.	Continue to assist ventilations. Start chest compressions.

have sterile conditions. If you must cut the cord, you will need a sterile pair of scissors, single-edged razor blade, or sharp knife.

Cutting the umbilical cord is usually a low priority, and Emergency Medical Responders may provide other care until transport personnel arrive. In most cases, the transport unit should arrive before the cord needs to be clamped or tied.

Usually, it is not necessary to tie and cut the cord until the afterbirth is delivered and the cord is empty of blood and stops pulsating. If you see or feel the cord pulsating, it is still delivering oxygen to the baby from the mother. The baby will benefit from this oxygen.

However, if during the delivery you see that the umbilical cord is around the baby's neck, you must insert one or two fingers under the cord and try to slip it back over the infant's head, or you must cut the cord. If the cord cannot be slipped over the head, then quickly place clamps or ties and cut it. If this is not done and the infant delivers, the cord may strangle them.

If you are allowed, take the following steps in a normal delivery when the cord has stopped pulsating:

1. Use sterile clamps or umbilical ties found in the OB kit.
2. Apply one tie or clamp to the cord about 6 inches from the baby's abdomen.
3. Place a second tie or clamp about 2 inches farther from the baby.
4. Cut between the two ties or clamps. Never untie or unclamp the cord once it has been cut. Examine the cut ends of the cord. After trapped blood drains, bleeding should stop if the clamps or ties are secure. If bleeding continues, apply another tie or clamp as close to the original as possible.

If the afterbirth delivers while you are still providing care to the baby and protocols do not allow you to cut the cord, then place the afterbirth at the same level as the baby or slightly higher. The placenta is still the baby's blood source, and blood can continue to flow to them if the placenta is positioned as described. If the placenta is placed lower than the baby, blood can flow away from them, back into the placenta.

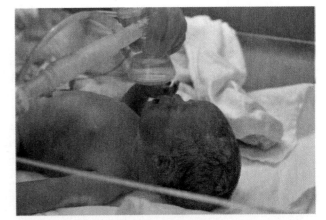

Figure 23.11 Use an oxygen face mask or a paper cup attached to an oxygen source, and hold it near the baby's face to supply blow-by oxygen.
(Kevin Link/Pearson Education, Inc.)

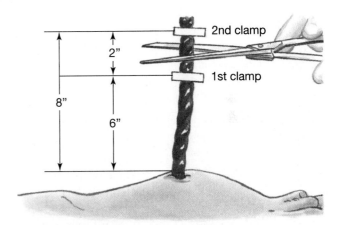

Figure 23.12 Cutting the umbilical cord.

FIRST ON SCENE (continued)

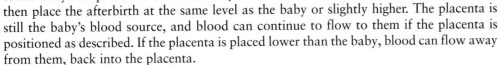

The loud conversation in the small restaurant grows silent, and the crowd parts as Lucas and the woman's husband crash through the doors, carrying her inside.

"She's having a baby," Lucas says as he grabs a tablecloth from an empty table and hands it to a man wearing a puffy down vest. "Lay that out flat on the floor, please. Quickly!"

The man complies and within moments the woman is resting on the floor. They support her head with a hastily gathered pile of coats.

"Could you get me some towels and a couple more tablecloths?" Lucas asks a waitress. She nods and disappears into the wall of people surrounding them. "And could you all please turn away and give the lady some privacy?"

"Just stay calm," Lucas says to the husband before turning his attention to the panting woman.

He then asks her, "What's your name?"

"Pamela," the woman gasps. As her face contorts in pain, she grabs her belly.

"Okay, Pamela," Lucas says, taking a stack of towels and tablecloths from the waitress. "I'm going to cover you up, and then I need to look down there to see how close the baby is. Okay?"

Her face shining with sweat, Pamela glances at the group of people—all with their backs to her—and nods quickly. She clenches her teeth as another strong contraction occurs.

Caring for the Mother

LO9 Explain the priorities of care for the mother following a field delivery.

Care for the mother includes helping her deliver the afterbirth (the placenta and other birth tissues), controlling vaginal bleeding, making her as comfortable as possible, and providing reassurance.

Delivering the Placenta The delivery of the placenta (afterbirth) is the third stage of labor. It delivers anywhere from a few minutes to 20 minutes or longer after the baby is born. Some women prefer to sit upright following delivery. You may have to remind them that they will have to remain at rest until they deliver the afterbirth. Make the mother as comfortable as possible and wait. However, if the baby requires immediate transport or the ambulance arrives, do not delay transport by waiting for the placenta to deliver. When she begins to have more contractions, it will be evident that delivery of the afterbirth is imminent. The contractions will be milder with less discomfort.

Save the placenta, all attached membranes, and all soiled sheets and towels. A physician must examine those items to ensure that the entire organ and its membranes were expelled from the uterus. Try to position a basin or container at the vaginal opening so the afterbirth will deliver into it (Figure 23.13). Place the container in a biohazard bag. If no container is available, allow the afterbirth to deliver directly into a biohazard bag, and place the bag into another biohazard bag. Label the bag with the mother's name.

REMEMBER

Once you have made sure that the infant is breathing adequately, place the baby on or against the mother's chest, skin-to-skin. If appropriate, allow the infant to begin nursing if that is the mother's desire. This causes release of a hormone that contracts the uterus and reduces bleeding. Do not be surprised if the mother chooses not to allow the baby to nurse or if the baby does not begin nursing naturally. This can initially be a difficult process for both the baby and mother and may take time and practice.

Controlling Vaginal Bleeding After Delivery Bleeding from the vagina is normal after delivery of the placenta. Perform the following steps to care for vaginal bleeding after delivery:

1. Place a sanitary pad or clean towel over the vaginal opening. Do not place anything in the vagina.
2. Have the mother lower her legs and keep them together.
3. Gently palpate the mother's abdomen until you find a grapefruit-sized object. This is the uterus. Gently but firmly massage from the pubis bone at the front of the pelvis upward only and toward the navel. This will help stimulate the uterus to contract and stop bleeding.
4. If bleeding continues, provide oxygen and maintain normal body temperature. Arrange transport as soon as possible. Continue massaging the uterus. If the mother wants to nurse, allow her to do so. Nursing stimulates contraction of the uterus and helps control bleeding.

Providing Comfort to the Mother Reassure the mother throughout the entire birth process, explaining what you are doing and what is happening. She will especially want to know about the baby's condition. Once you have completed your duties with the afterbirth, replace any soiled towels or sheets with clean, dry ones. Make sure both mother and baby remain warm and comfortable.

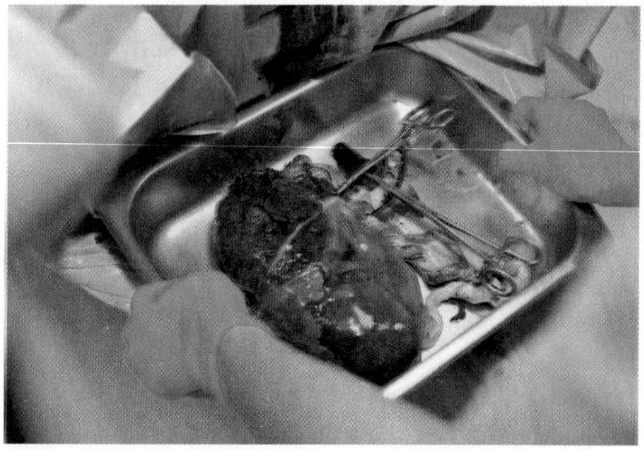

Figure 23.13 Collect the placenta following delivery and transport it to the hospital for inspection.
(Kevin Link/Pearson Education, Inc.)

Complications and Emergencies

There are a variety of complications related to pregnancy and childbirth of which you should be aware. While most of these problems are relatively uncommon, it is still possible to encounter them in the field. Complications include abnormal bleeding, miscarriage, breech delivery, premature delivery, multiple births, and stillbirths. Keep in mind that most pregnancies and births are normal. Emergency Medical Responders can often care for some of the difficulties that may arise. However, severe complications must be handled by more advanced personnel and require immediate transport to a medical facility.

The risk of complications before, during, and after delivery increases when the patient has one or more of the following factors:

- Younger than 18 or older than 35 years of age
- First pregnancy or more than five pregnancies
- Swollen face, feet, or abdomen from water retention
- High or low blood pressure
- Diabetes
- History of seizures
- Predelivery bleeding
- Infections
- Injuries from trauma
- Premature rupture of membranes (water broke more than a few hours before delivery)
- Alcohol dependency
- Illicit drug use during pregnancy

You will find out this information when you gather the patient's history during the secondary assessment. As you assess the patient, ask her the appropriate questions to determine if she is in a high-risk group.

Infections of the reproductive organs, especially sexually transmitted infections, can be transmitted to the baby during birth. Remember to take BSI precautions and wear all personal protective equipment, which will protect you as well as the mother and infant. Report to the hospital any information you receive from the mother about a history of infection.

Predelivery Emergencies

LO10 Explain the common causes of vaginal bleeding during the first trimester.

LO11 Explain the common causes of vaginal bleeding during the third trimester.

LO12 Explain the appropriate care for a pregnant patient with vaginal bleeding.

A variety of emergencies can occur during pregnancy and prior to the delivery. While most are relatively rare, you should be familiar with what they are and how they present.

Prebirth Bleeding Vaginal bleeding early in pregnancy may indicate a **miscarriage** (spontaneous abortion). Light, irregular discharges of blood, called **spotting**, are normal in early pregnancy but may concern the patient. If bleeding occurs late in pregnancy or while the patient is in labor, the problem may be with the placenta. Regardless of the cause of bleeding or stage of pregnancy, you must:

miscarriage ▶ spontaneous loss of the embryo or fetus before the 20th week of pregnancy.

spotting ▶ normal discharge of blood during pregnancy.

1. Make certain an ambulance is on the way.
2. Take BSI precautions if you have not done so already.
3. Place the patient on her back or left side, but do not hold her legs together (Figure 23.14).
4. Provide care for shock, monitor the patient's airway, and administer oxygen per local protocols.
5. Place a sanitary pad or bulky dressings over the vaginal opening.
6. Replace pads or dressings as they become soaked. Do not place anything in the vagina.
7. Save all blood-soaked pads and dressings, as well as any tissues the mother passes. Place them in a biohazard bag for transport to the hospital and examination by a physician.
8. Monitor and reassure the patient while you wait for transport personnel.

Miscarriage If the fetus delivers before it can survive on its own (before the 20th week), it is considered a miscarriage. The medical term for a miscarriage is a *spontaneous abortion*. However, because the word *abortion* may have a negative connotation, it is not a good idea to use this term with a woman who may be having a miscarriage or premature signs of labor.

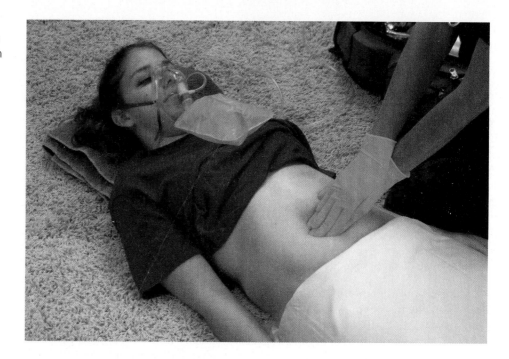

Figure 23.14 Position the patient on their back or side to control excessive prebirth bleeding.

Women having miscarriages typically have abdominal cramps and pains. Vaginal bleeding is to be expected and can be mild to severe. In many cases, there will be vaginal discharge consisting of bloody mucus and tissue particles.

When caring for a woman having a suspected miscarriage or vaginal bleeding, first perform a primary assessment, and then focus on the physical exam and patient history. Take the following steps to provide care:

1. Place the patient on her side, provide care for shock, and administer oxygen per local protocols.
2. Take a baseline set of vital signs. Then continue to take vital signs every few minutes thereafter.
3. Place a sanitary pad or bulky dressing over the vaginal opening. Do not place anything in the vagina.
4. Save all blood-soaked pads and any tissues that are passed. Place them in a biohazard bag.
5. Provide emotional support.
6. Arrange for transport immediately.

Ectopic Pregnancy A leading cause of pregnancy-related death is **ectopic pregnancy**.[1] This occurs when the fertilized egg implants somewhere other than the uterus. Ectopic pregnancies most often occur within a **fallopian tube**. Normally, just prior to conception, the unfertilized egg leaves the **ovary** and begins a journey through a fallopian tube on its way to the uterus. During conception, the sperm joins up with the egg while it is still in a fallopian tube. Eventually, the fertilized egg implants along the wall of the uterus. This is normal. However, when the fertilized egg implants along the wall of the fallopian tube, it will not take long before the developing fetus outgrows the narrow space, causing the tube to rupture. This will always result in loss of the fetus and is a life-threatening emergency for the mother.

The most common signs and symptoms of an ectopic pregnancy include:

- Abdominal pain
- Absence of normal menstrual cycle
- Vaginal bleeding

The care is the same for any woman with a general complaint of abdominal pain, including a thorough history and physical, oxygen if available, and transport to a hospital.

REMEMBER

Because ectopic pregnancies can progress for more than 4 to 6 weeks, they cause significant injury to the reproductive tract. The signs and symptoms of an ectopic pregnancy or miscarriage can be similar to several other abdominal emergencies. For that reason, it is wise to consider a woman of childbearing age with the complaint of abdominal pain to be potentially pregnant until proven otherwise.

ectopic pregnancy ▸ pregnancy in which the fertilized egg implants outside the uterus.

fallopian tube ▸ tube-like structure that connects the ovary to the uterus.

ovary ▸ one of a pair of glands in females in which eggs (ova) are produced.

Complicfcations During Delivery

LO13 Explain the common complications related to a field delivery and how to properly care for each.

A number of complications of childbirth can occur. You will want to be on the alert for potential problems and know how to address them.

Meconium Staining   A stressful or difficult delivery affects both the mother and baby. When the baby is stressed during delivery, they may defecate (empty the bowel). The fecal material is called **meconium**. When this material mixes with amniotic fluid, the normally clear fluid is stained green or brownish yellow and is called *meconium staining*. If the baby inhales this fluid on their first attempt to breathe, they can develop aspiration pneumonia, a lung infection caused by aspirating (breathing in) the meconium.[2]

meconium ▶ product of the baby's first bowel movement.

Sometimes the amniotic sac will rupture many hours before delivery. You will have to rely on information from the mother to determine if the fluids were clear or stained. Ask the mother if she noticed the color of the fluid when her water broke. If you witness the rupture, look for meconium staining. Be prepared to wipe the baby's mouth and nose. Suction the meconium only if it is significantly interfering with the baby's breathing.

Breech Birth   In a **breech birth**, the buttocks or feet present first. It is possible for the baby to be delivered; however, it usually requires the skills of an experienced physician. If, upon examination, you see anything other than the top of the baby's head presenting, initiate transport immediately. A breech birth can be a complication if the baby's head will not deliver.

breech birth ▶ birth in which the buttocks or feet deliver first.

While waiting for a transport unit to arrive, do the following:

1. Place the mother on a high concentration of oxygen.
2. Create an airway for the baby because the umbilical cord will be compressed between the infant and vaginal wall, shutting off blood flow. Tell the mother what you must do and why. Insert your gloved hand into the vagina, with your palm toward the baby's face. Form a V by placing one finger on each side of the baby's nose (Figure 23.15). Push the wall of the birth canal away from the baby's face.

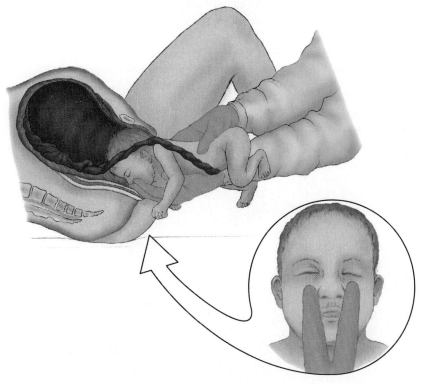

Figure 23.15 Create and maintain an airway for the baby during a breech birth.

If you cannot complete this process, then try to place one fingertip into the infant's mouth and push away the birth canal wall with your other fingers. Place the mother in the knee-chest position to reduce pressure on the birth canal.

3. Maintain the airway. Once you have created an airway for the baby, keep the airway open. Do not pull on the baby. Allow delivery to take place while you continue to support the baby's body and head. Instruct the mother not to hold her breath and to pant with each contraction.

4. Initiate immediate transport to a medical facility. Maintain the airway throughout all stages of care until higher-level EMS personnel relieve you. Expedite transport to the nearest medical facility.

Limb Presentation   The presentation of an arm or a single leg is called a *limb presentation* and is an emergency requiring immediate transport. Do not pull on the limb or try to place your gloved hand into the birth canal. Do not try to place the limb back into the vagina. Place the mother in the knee-chest position (Figure 23.16) to help reduce pressure on the fetus and the umbilical cord. Medical direction and protocols may instruct you to keep the mother in the typical delivery position. Follow your local protocols.

Prolapsed Cord   When you examine the mother for crowning, you may find the umbilical cord protruding from the vaginal opening. When the umbilical cord delivers first, this is called a **prolapsed cord** and is common in a breech birth.

A prolapsed cord endangers the life of the baby. As the baby emerges through the vaginal opening, their head presses the umbilical cord against the vaginal wall, reducing or completely cutting off blood flow and oxygen. When oxygen flow through the cord is obstructed, the baby will try to breathe. But because the baby's face is pressed against the wall of the birth canal, the mouth and nose cannot take in air. To help the baby breathe, provide an airway, using the same methods described for breech birth. Place your fingers into the vaginal opening in front of the infant's face and make a *V*. Do not try to push the cord back into the birth canal.

In addition, take the following steps (check with medical direction or your protocols to find out what Emergency Medical Responders are allowed to do):

- Place the mother in a knee-chest position to reduce pressure on the cord.
- Try to monitor a pulse in the cord by palpating the cord.
- Place wet dressings (use sterile water or saline if available) over the cord to keep it moist.
- Wrap the cord in a towel or dressings to keep it warm.
- Provide the mother with a high concentration of oxygen as soon as possible.
- Monitor vital signs and arrange for transport immediately.

Multiple Births   Multiple births are not necessarily abnormal, but they do frequently involve premature delivery. Premature infants may not be fully developed and often have respiratory complications. If the mother is giving birth to more than one infant,

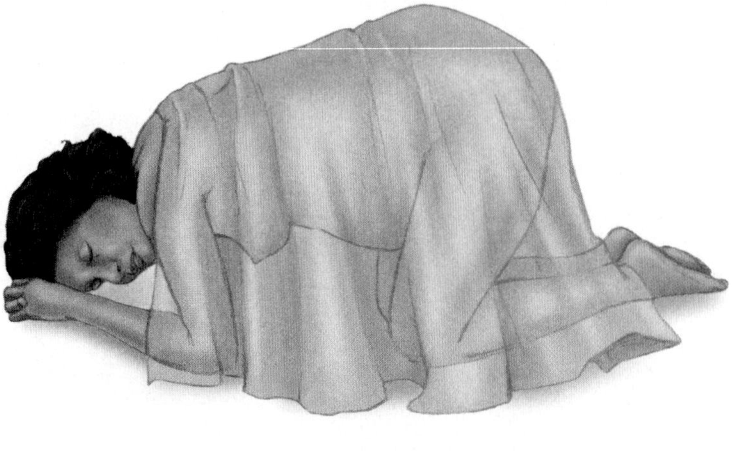

prolapsed cord ▶ delivery of the umbilical cord first; medical emergency that endangers the baby.

REMEMBER

The baby's chances for survival improve if you can keep the head from pressing on the umbilical cord and keep the cord pulsating. Check with your instructor to see if protocols allow you to insert several fingers into the mother's vagina and gently push up on the baby's head to keep pressure off the cord.

Figure 23.16 Place the mother in the knee-chest position, which will help keep pressure off the umbilical cord in a limb-presentation birth.

contractions will begin again shortly after the birth of the first baby. The contractions may lead to delivery of the afterbirth of the first baby or delivery of another baby.

The procedures for assisting the mother remain the same. If the umbilical cord has stopped pulsating, you will tie or clamp the cord of the first baby before the second baby is born. Once the babies are delivered and they are breathing, assess each one, noting skin color (blue, normal, or pale), any deformities, strength of their cries, and whether they move on their own or just lie still. When assessing the quality of skin color on dark-skinned babies, check the nail beds, lips, and palms of the hands for signs of cyanosis. After a few minutes, note if there are any changes in those conditions. If necessary, perform resuscitation. Document the time of birth for each baby. Call for assistance as soon as possible.

Preterm Births   Any baby weighing less than 5.5 pounds at birth or any baby born before the 37th week (prior to the ninth month) of pregnancy is considered a *preterm birth*. If the mother tells you the baby is early by more than 2 weeks, play it safe and consider the baby premature.

In addition to the procedures for normal births, you must take special steps to keep a premature baby warm. It is important to dry the baby. Wrap them in a blanket, sheet, or towel. A blanket covered with foil is ideal. Cover the baby's head but keep the face uncovered. Place the infant skin-to-skin with the mother for warmth. If this is not possible, transfer the baby to a warm environment (90°F to 100°F [32°C to 37°C]), but do not place a heat source too close to the baby. Ventilate a premature baby who needs resuscitation using a mouth-to-mask technique or an appropriately sized bag-mask device. Wipe or suction blood and mucus from the mouth and nose before ventilating.

Stillborn Deliveries   A fetus that is delivered dead is referred to as *stillborn*. This is a very traumatic event for the mother and father or partner, family members, and care providers. Do not feel embarrassed to show your emotions, but be prepared to continue to act professionally and provide comfort to the mother and other family members who are present.

If the infant shows no signs of life at birth or goes into respiratory or cardiac arrest, provide the resuscitation measures described earlier in this chapter. Do not stop resuscitation until the baby regains respirations and a heartbeat, other emergency care providers relieve you, or you are too exhausted to continue. If in doubt, always begin resuscitative efforts and allow the transport team to decide if further resuscitation is warranted.

There are cases in which a baby has died hours or longer before birth. Do not attempt to resuscitate a stillborn infant who has large blisters and a strong, unpleasant odor. There may be other indications that the infant died earlier in the uterus, such as a very soft head, swollen body parts, or obvious deformities.

Other Emergencies

LO14   Describe the signs and symptoms of supine hypotensive syndrome.

LO15   Explain the appropriate care for a patient with signs and symptoms of supine hypotensive syndrome.

LO16   Describe the signs and symptoms of preeclampsia.

LO17   Explain the appropriate care for a patient with signs and symptoms of preeclampsia.

LO18   Describe the management of a pregnant woman showing the signs of preeclampsia.

LO19   Describe the management of a pregnant woman who has sustained a traumatic injury.

LO20   Describe the management of a pregnant woman with an abnormally low blood pressure.

A few other complications that affect the mother and developing fetus include supine hypotensive syndrome, preeclampsia and eclampsia, trauma, vaginal bleeding, and sexual assault.

> **REMEMBER**
>
> It is not uncommon for a baby to be born prior to reaching 38 weeks' gestation yet appear at birth to be fully developed and healthy. For that reason, many refer to such births as *preterm* instead of premature. A mother with good prenatal care will know how her baby is developing. In the absence of such care, it is appropriate to consider the birth to be premature and be prepared for complications.

supine hypotensive syndrome ▶ abnormally low blood pressure that results when the mother is supine and the fetus puts pressure on the vena cava.

Supine Hypotensive Syndrome   **Supine hypotensive syndrome** is a condition that can occur during the last 2 months of pregnancy. It is caused when the mother lies on her back and the weight of the fetus and other organs press on the mother's inferior vena cava, the large vessel in the abdomen that returns blood to the heart. The pressure on the vena cava restricts blood return to the heart, causing signs of shock such as low blood pressure, increased pulse, pale skin, and in some cases, an altered mental status.[3]

Care for supine hypotensive syndrome is usually as simple as repositioning the mother to more of a seated position (semi-Fowler's) or having her lie on her left side. The weight of the fetus will shift to the left and off the vena cava, allowing better blood flow (venous return) to the heart.

preeclampsia ▶ potentially life-threatening condition that affects the mother during the third trimester and is characterized by high blood pressure and fluid retention.

Preeclampsia and Eclampsia   Another potentially dangerous condition that affects approximately 5% of all pregnant women is known as **preeclampsia**. While its exact causes are not well understood, it most often occurs after the 20th week of pregnancy and seems to affect women in their teens, women over 40, and women who are pregnant for the first time.

Signs and symptoms of preeclampsia include:

- Abnormally high blood pressure
- Fluid retention causing swelling of the arms, hands, legs, and face
- Headache
- Nausea

eclampsia ▶ life-threatening condition characterized by seizures, coma, and eventually death of both the mother and baby.

If left untreated, preeclampsia can lead to **eclampsia**, which is characterized by seizures, coma, and eventually death of both the mother and baby.[4]

The only treatment for preeclampsia is the delivery of the baby. If you should see signs of either condition in a pregnant woman, rapid transport to a hospital is essential. While waiting for transport, provide the following care:

- Support the ABCs as necessary.
- Provide high-flow oxygen, if protocols allow.
- Have suction ready and be prepared for seizures.

Trauma   Vital signs of a pregnant woman are usually different from those of a woman who is not pregnant. A pregnant woman's blood volume increases up to about 45%, a natural protection and preparation for the loss of blood during delivery. Her heart rate increases by about 15 beats per minute, and blood pressure falls 10 to 15 mm Hg. Do not mistake the high pulse rate and low blood pressure for signs of shock in the normal nontrauma pregnant woman. But in a trauma situation, the mother's larger blood volume allows her body to compensate for blood loss and, therefore, she may not show early signs of shock.

A pregnant woman can lose almost 40% of her blood volume before she shows any signs of shock. In shock, the mother's body shunts blood away from the uterus first. Less blood to the uterus affects the fetus, causing harm well before the mother shows any signs. Blood loss may be internal and not obvious to the Emergency Medical Responder. Always suspect internal bleeding in any pregnant trauma patient, even if she seems to be initially unharmed and shows normal vital signs for a pregnant woman. Even if the mother is not injured, the fetus may be injured in an advanced pregnancy.

During the scene size-up, look carefully at the environment, the patient, and the mechanism of injury. Try to determine what injuries might have been caused. Two common types of trauma that can cause significant harm to the mother and the fetus are:

- *Blunt-force injuries*, which are common in falls, vehicle crashes, abuse, and assaults.
- *Penetrating injuries*, which are usually a result of gunshot wounds, stabbings, or punctures from debris of auto wreckage.

During the early months of pregnancy, when the fetus is small, the fluids in the amniotic sac provide some protection from blunt-force trauma. As the fetus grows, blunt trauma can cause more damage to the fetus, especially in the last two months of pregnancy. As a result, Emergency Medical Responders should provide direct care for the mother and indirect care for the fetus.

The greatest danger to both the mother and baby is bleeding and shock. First, ensure an open airway and adequate breathing and look for and control external bleeding. Provide a high concentration of oxygen as soon as possible, and keep the patient warm but do not overheat her. The steps that prevent or care for shock will also assist the fetus. Arrange for immediate transport and, while waiting for transport personnel to arrive, provide appropriate care based on the mechanism of injury, such as immobilization for possible spinal injuries, splinting for possible fractures, and dressing of wounds.

Vaginal Bleeding There are many reasons for excessive vaginal bleeding during pregnancy. Emergency Medical Responders must be aware of them and look carefully for the mechanism of injury that caused them, including the following:

- Blunt-force and penetrating trauma
- Intercourse
- Sexual assault
- Reproductive organ problems
- Abnormal pregnancy
- Placental tears and uterine rupture

There are two types of placental tears. In **placenta previa**, the placenta lies low in the uterus and attaches itself over the opening to the cervix, meaning it would have to emerge prior to the fetus during birth. In this position, the placenta tears and bleeds when the cervix dilates during labor. **Placenta abruptio** can occur in a trauma situation when the force of the trauma abruptly tears the placenta partially or completely away from the wall of the uterus. The pregnant woman may have major internal blood loss because blood can be trapped between the placenta and the uterine wall. She may also lose blood vaginally.

The only indications you may have of internal blood loss and developing shock are changes in vital signs, feeling a hard uterus when examining the abdomen, and the mother's complaint that her abdomen is painful or tender. Get a set of baseline vital signs as soon as possible in your assessment, and monitor the vital signs by retaking them every few minutes. Provide high-concentration oxygen as soon as possible (if protocols allow) and maintain body temperature to help reduce the effects of shock. Arrange for immediate transport.

The care for controlling vaginal bleeding includes:

- Place sanitary pads or bulky dressings over the vaginal opening.
- Replace pads or dressings as they become soaked.
- Do not place anything in the vagina.
- Save all blood-soaked pads and dressings. Place them in a biohazard bag for transport to the hospital and examination by a physician.

Sexual Assault Sexual assault or rape is always a psychologically and physically traumatic experience. The Emergency Medical Responder's professional manner, attitude, and emotional support are important steps in the care of the expectant mother who has been assaulted.

As the woman struggles or resists the attacker, and as the attacker uses force against her, she can receive many types of injuries to the external soft tissues, the vaginal canal, and the internal organs. The fetus is also a victim in the assault. The injuries the fetus receives may be direct from blows to the abdomen or indirect as a result of injuries to the mother.

You may have multiple roles to perform when caring for a pregnant woman who is the victim of a sexual assault. If one of the responders is a woman, it may be best for her to manage the patient. You may have to provide care for injuries, including spinal immobilization, extremity splinting, and wound dressing. In sexual assault cases, you will need to provide emotional support and protect the patient's privacy by shielding her from

placenta previa ▶ placenta grows in the lowest part of the uterus, covering all or part of the opening to the cervix.

placenta abruptio ▶ premature separation of the placenta from the uterus.

onlookers. Do not clean the vaginal area. Advise the patient to not wash or go to the bathroom. You should advise her that hospital personnel may be able to collect evidence from her that will help with the investigation. Emergency Medical Responders should collect clothing and any items that were used during the assault for examination and legal needs. Transport anything that may be evidence in a paper bag or wrap it in a towel. Do not place such items in plastic, because plastic can promote the growth of bacteria.

It is important to provide care that will prevent or manage shock and arrange transport as soon as possible. Provide both emotional support and physical comfort. Listen to your patient and talk to her throughout all procedures.

 FIRST ON SCENE WRAP-UP

As snow continues to fall outside the steamed up windows of the restaurant, Pamela's cries are replaced by the small wails of a newborn.

"It's a boy," Lucas says, wiping sweat from his forehead as the child's father proudly smiles down at the small, bloody infant.

"You did a great job," the waitress says as she leans in close to see the baby. "But it looks like the ambulance can't get here for an hour or more."

"That's fine," Lucas replies. He finishes wiping down the baby and wraps him in several clean, warm towels. "There's absolutely nothing wrong with this little guy." He gently passes the bundled child to Pamela and stands to stretch his back.

As he watches husband and wife gazing in amazement at their tiny son, Lucas is suddenly very glad he didn't take that plane to Denver after all.

Summary

- The normal gestation period for a human fetus is 38 to 40 weeks or approximately 9 months. An infant is considered premature if delivered prior to the 37th week of gestation.
- Labor is the normal process the body uses to deliver a baby. The average labor is 16 hours but can be much shorter or much longer.
- Labor has three stages. The first begins with the onset of labor and ends with full dilation of the cervix. The second stage begins with dilation of the cervix and ends with delivery of the baby. The third stage begins after delivery of the baby and ends with delivery of the placenta.
- Signs of an imminent delivery include contractions that are less than 3 minutes apart, the mother's feeling of needing to bear down, and crowning at the vaginal opening. When the signs of an imminent delivery are obvious, you must prepare for delivery at the scene.
- Upon delivery of the head, you must check for the presence of the umbilical cord around the neck. If present, gently slip it over the baby's head. Suction the nose and mouth prior to delivery of the baby.
- After delivery, stimulate the baby by drying them with a clean, dry cloth. The baby should begin breathing on their own. If breathing or pulse is inadequate, provide the appropriate care immediately.
- Immediately call for ALS backup for any delivery that appears to be abnormal or complicated, such as a breech presentation or prolapsed cord. Place the mother in the knee-chest position and provide high-flow oxygen if available. Follow local protocols.
- The possibility of a spontaneous abortion (miscarriage) is quite common during the first trimester of pregnancy. The patient most often presents with abnormal vaginal bleeding and pain. It is important to remain compassionate and professional at all times.
- In cases of sexual assault, a female responder should manage the patient if possible. Be sure to not disturb anything that could be used as evidence by authorities.

Take Action

Know Your Tools!

As an Emergency Medical Responder, you will learn many skills that cover a wide variety of emergencies. Some emergencies are fairly common, and others you may see only once or twice in your career. Delivering a child in the field does not occur very often. For that reason, it is important to occasionally review the steps necessary to care for a mother in labor as well as the specialized tools you will need to assist the delivery of the baby.

For this activity, borrow a commercial OB kit from your instructor and explore its contents item by item. Invite a classmate to join you, and discuss the specific use for each item in the kit. Write the name of each item on an index card. On the back of the card write an explanation of the use of the item. Later on, the cards can be used as a tool when reviewing the steps for caring for a woman in labor.

First on Scene Patient Handoff

Pamela is a 34-year-old who was in active labor when I was called to her car by her husband. Upon arrival, contractions were approximately 1 minute apart so we brought her inside here to deliver. She states that she has been receiving prenatal care throughout her pregnancy and that she is 37 weeks along. Upon examination, I could see crowning so we set up for a field delivery. I instructed her through what turned out to be a normal delivery of a baby boy at 9:47 a.m. I have been monitoring the baby's and mother's breathing and heart rate until EMS arrived.

First on Scene Run Review

Recall the events of the First on Scene scenario in this chapter, and answer the following questions related to the call. Rationales are offered in the Answer Key at the back of the book.

1. Do you need to ask permission before treating this woman? Why or why not?
2. What are the stages of labor?
3. What information would you want from the woman about her pregnancy?
4. What information would you need to record about the baby following delivery?

Quick Quiz

To check your understanding of the chapter, answer the following questions. Then compare your answers to those in the Answer Key at the back of the book.

1. The organ that serves as a filter between the mother and the developing fetus is the:

   a. placenta.
   b. uterus.
   c. vagina.
   d. cervix.

2. You are caring for a woman who is 39 weeks pregnant. She complains of regular, intense contractions and asks to use the bathroom before leaving for the hospital. You should:

   a. allow her to use the bathroom while you prepare the gurney.
   b. move the patient to the ambulance and initiate transport.
   c. check for crowning and prepare for immediate delivery.
   d. recognize the signs of an emergency and call for ALS backup.

3. The first stage of labor begins at the onset of contractions and ends:

   a. when the baby is delivered.
   b. when the baby enters the vaginal canal.
   c. after the delivery of the placenta.
   d. when the amniotic sac ruptures.

4. A typical field obstetrics kit contains all of the following EXCEPT:

   a. umbilical cord clamps.
   b. bulb syringe for suctioning.
   c. plastic bag for biohazard disposal.
   d. infant size blood pressure cuff.

5. A woman in her third trimester of pregnancy believes she is about to deliver her baby. Your exam reveals crowning. You should:

   a. immediately move the patient to the ambulance and transport.
   b. tell the woman not to push and wait for EMS to arrive.
   c. get the OB kit, don BSI, and prepare to assist the mother.
   d. call for medical direction and obtain a set of vital signs.

6. You are assisting a woman in active labor. As the baby's head begins to deliver you should:

   a. apply gentle pressure and support the head during delivery.
   b. attempt to turn the baby face up.
   c. firmly press against the head and tell the mother not to push.
   d. prepare to administer oxygen to the baby.

7. Immediately following delivery, the newborn appears limp and cyanotic. You should:

   a. dry, warm, and stimulate the baby.
   b. immediately begin CPR.
   c. ventilate with a bag-mask device.
   d. initiate rapid transport.

8. You have just assisted in the uncomplicated delivery of a healthy newborn. You notice moderate vaginal bleeding from the mother. You should:

   a. pack the vaginal canal with sterile dressings.
   b. prepare for the mother to go into shock.
   c. place a sanitary pad at the vaginal opening.
   d. initiate rapid transport.

9. You are caring for a 38-year-old woman who states that she is 8 weeks pregnant. She is experiencing heavy vaginal bleeding and abdominal cramping. You suspect:

   a. ectopic pregnancy.
   b. placenta previa.
   c. miscarriage.
   d. preeclampsia.

10. Your patient is in her 38th week of pregnancy and is experiencing light, painless vaginal bleeding. She is very concerned for the baby. Which of the following would be an appropriate response?

   a. "I'm sure everything is fine; bleeding is completely normal at this stage."
   b. "This may be normal; however, let's call for the ambulance so a doctor can examine you."
   c. "This is a bad sign; we need to rush to the hospital right away."
   d. "You're right to be concerned; you could be having a miscarriage."

11. While examining a mother for crowning, you notice that the umbilical cord is protruding from the vaginal opening. You should:

   a. insert a gloved hand into to vaginal canal and lift the baby off the cord.
   b. tug gently on the cord to encourage delivery.
   c. push the cord back into the vaginal opening.
   d. encourage the mother to push hard with each contraction.

12. During a breech delivery, the baby appears to be stuck with the buttocks and legs presenting. You should:

   a. firmly pull on the baby.
   b. tell the mother not to push.
   c. insert a gloved hand into the birth canal to create an air passage for the baby.
   d. gently massage the mother's belly to encourage strong contractions.

13. A woman in her third trimester of pregnancy complains of dizziness and nausea when lying on her back. You suspect:

   a. eclampsia.
   b. supine hypotensive syndrome.
   c. gestational diabetes.
   d. placenta previa.

14. A woman late in pregnancy called 911 after feeling dizzy and "lightheaded." You should:

   a. position her on her back.
   b. elevate her feet and legs.
   c. position her on her left side.
   d. position her on her right side.

15. Your patient is a 35-year-old female in her third trimester of pregnancy. She complains of a headache and swollen feet, and says that her vision is "spotty." You recognize:

   a. a non-life-threatening situation requiring routine care.
   b. signs of imminent delivery.
   c. a life-threatening situation requiring immediate transport.
   d. signs of gestational diabetes.

16. You are caring for a woman who is 34 weeks pregnant and is complaining of a headache and nausea. Her pulse is 140, strong and regular, and her blood pressure is 174/96. Her condition is most likely caused by:

   a. supine hypotensive syndrome.
   b. ectopic pregnancy.
   c. preeclampsia.
   d. placenta previa.

17. You are caring for a woman who states she is 36 weeks pregnant. She slipped and fell down three stairs, and while she says she isn't in any pain, she is concerned for her baby. You should:

   a. check for crowning.
   b. apply oxygen, take vital signs, and call for transport.
   c. palpate her abdomen to check for contractions.
   d. fully immobilize her to a backboard.

18. You are caring for an 18-year-old woman with a complaint of severe abdominal pain and vaginal bleeding. You should:

   a. apply low-flow oxygen.
   b. inspect the vagina.
   c. inquire about the possibility of pregnancy.
   d. find out what she had to eat.

Endnotes

1. Mummert T., Gnugnoli D.M., *Ectopic Pregnancy*. [2022 Aug 8]. In: StatPearls [Internet]. Treasure Island (FL): StatPearls Publishing; 2022 Jan–. PMID: 30969682.
2. Sayad E., Silva-Carmona M., *Meconium Aspiration*. [2022 May 8]. In: StatPearls [Internet]. Treasure Island (FL): StatPearls Publishing; 2022 Jan–. PMID: 32491357.
3. Al-Jameil N., Aziz Khan F., Fareed Khan M., Tabassum H., "A brief overview of preeclampsia," *Journal of Clinical Medicine Research*, Vol. 6, No. 1 (February 2014): 1–7.
4. Ibid.

24

Caring for Infants and Children

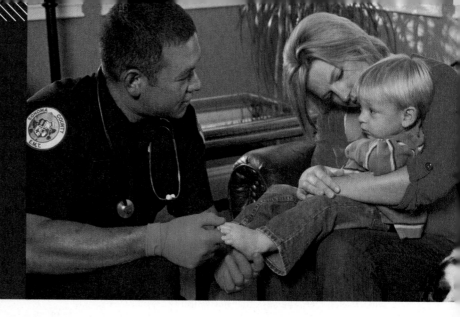

Education Standards

Special Patient Populations—Pediatrics, Neonatal Care, Patients with Special Challenges

Competencies

Recognizes and manages life threats based on simple assessment findings for a patient with special needs while awaiting additional emergency response.

LEARNING OBJECTIVES

Upon successful completion of this chapter, the student should be able to:

Cognitive

1. Define the chapter key terms.
2. Review the major stages of lifespan development for the pediatric patient (Chapter 4).
3. Explain the components of the pediatric assessment triangle.
4. Explain various techniques that can be employed to maximize successful assessment of the pediatric patient.
5. State the most common cause of cardiac arrest in the pediatric patient.
6. Explain the assessment and management of the following emergencies in pediatric patients: respiratory emergencies (including airway obstruction), difficulty breathing, and respiratory infection; seizures; altered mental status; shock; fever; hypothermia; diarrhea and vomiting; poisoning; and drowning.
7. Differentiate between sudden unexpected infant death (SUID) and sudden infant death syndrome (SIDS).
8. Explain the appropriate steps for management of a suspected SIDS death.
9. Describe the proper management of a child with burn injuries.
10. Describe the rule of nines as it applies to an infant.
11. Describe common signs and symptoms of abuse and neglect.
12. Explain the role of the Emergency Medical Responder in cases of suspected abuse and/or neglect.

Psychomotor

13. Demonstrate the ability to properly assess and care for a pediatric patient.
14. Demonstrate various techniques that can be employed to maximize successful assessment of the pediatric patient.
15. Demonstrate the application of the pediatric assessment triangle.

Affective

16. Demonstrate sensitivity for the feelings of the family while caring for an ill or injured pediatric patient.
17. Recognize the emotional impact responding to pediatric patients can have on the Emergency Medical Responder.
18. Value the role of the Emergency Medical Responder with respect to patient advocacy.

KEY TERMS

abuse (*p. 526*)
adolescent (*p. 509*)
croup (*p. 519*)
epiglottitis (*p. 519*)
neglect (*p. 526*)
pediatric assessment triangle
  (PAT) (*p. 514*)

retractions (*p. 515*)
shaken-baby syndrome (*p. 529*)
sudden infant death syndrome
  (SIDS) (*p. 524*)
sudden unexpected infant death
  (SUID) (*p. 524*)
toddler (*p. 509*)

This chapter introduces methods used in providing care for medical and trauma emergencies that involve the pediatric patient. Infants and children must be managed and cared for differently than adults because of their age, physical and mental development, personalities, and their responses to unfamiliar experiences. Children respond well to familiar, normal routines. Many have difficulty handling strange situations and unfamiliar adults, including Emergency Medical Responders. Seriously ill and injured children also provoke strong emotions in those who provide care for them. Through proper training and practice, EMRs can increase their confidence and manage pediatric emergencies calmly while providing empathetic and effective care.

FIRST ON SCENE

City police officer Bryn backs the cruiser into an empty parking space and opens her laptop, hoping to catch up on paperwork for what is turning out to be a very busy swing shift.

Just as the computer connects to the department server, the radio blares to life. "Adam 8, priority call on tach 3." The dispatcher's voice is monotone.

Bryn hits the radio's channel button several times and announces that she is ready for the call. "Adam 8."

A different voice answers. "Respond priority 1 for shots fired at the 43rd Street subway station entrance. We're trying to clear a backup unit for you but for now, you're it."

"Adam 8, copy." Bryn slides the laptop back into its case and shifts the car into drive. Her stomach is immediately tense and nauseated, and she must force herself to breathe evenly while maneuvering the patrol car in and out of the Friday night traffic.

As she navigates the final turn to the scene, she sees that the street is in chaos. People are crouching against buildings, lying flat on the pavement, and running in all directions. The front

windows of several businesses are shattered, and large shards of broken glass hang in the frames like jagged teeth. A woman huddled next to a low concrete wall bordering the subway station stairs sees Bryn's patrol car, scrambles to her feet, and runs directly toward her carrying a small bundle. As Bryn climbs from the car, gun drawn, the woman reaches her and screams about an ambulance.

"Who was shooting?" Bryn demands, looking directly into the woman's terrified eyes.

"I don't know. It was from a . . . a car!" The woman is bordering on losing complete control.

"So, the shooter drove away?" Bryn notices that blood is dripping at the feet of the crying woman.

"Yes!" she screams. "It was a green van, and they just kept shooting. Then they . . . they drove that way. Please! I need help for my baby!" The woman shifts the dark blanket she is carrying, and Bryn's stomach drops as she sees the small, pale face spattered with bright red drops of blood.

Caring for the Pediatric Patient

Responding to a call for a child's illness or injury can be stressful. Some situations will make you feel sad or angry. You must learn to keep your emotions in check, especially in front of a child or parent. When faced with the assessment and care of an infant or a child, you may feel at first that you do not know what to do or where to start. An anxious or frightened child who cannot be comforted may further add to your stress level. Remember that many of the assessment and care techniques used for adults are similar for children, with some modifications. Those modifications consider the child's age, physical development, and emotional response.

Emergency Medical Responders who are unsure of what to do in pediatric emergencies are likely to have a stronger emotional response during and after an incident than those who are prepared and confident in their actions. By training, practicing, and drilling to prepare for pediatric incidents, you will not only improve your confidence and decrease your stress, but you will improve patient outcomes as well.

Your Approach to Infants and Children

Everyone has some fear of the unknown. Because so many things are unknown to children, it is easy to see why emergencies can be so frightening for them. A severe illness or injury is a new and unknown experience for most children, and it is an experience that increases their anxiety, especially if their parents are not present. For most children, security comes from their parents or primary caregivers. The desire to be with their parents may be a child's first priority, even above having you offer help, comfort, or relief of pain.

When dealing with children, you need to gain their trust. Attempt to calm and reassure them using the following techniques:

- Approach them slowly, establish eye contact from a safe distance, and ask permission to get closer.
- Get down at eye level with the child. Standing makes you appear large and frightening.
- If a parent or caregiver isn't present, let the child know that someone will call them.
- Let them see your face and expressions. You want to appear friendly, concerned, and willing to listen. Speak directly to them. Speak clearly and slowly so they can hear and understand you. Keep your voice gentle and calm even when you need to be firm. Try not to raise your voice or talk loudly to a crying or screaming child. Some children are shy or uncomfortable with strangers and may not look at you. Try to maintain eye contact (Figure 24.1).
- Pause frequently to find out if the child understands what you have said or asked. Even if you communicate easily with your own children, never assume that other children understand you. Find out by asking questions.
- Quickly determine if there are any life-threatening problems, and care for them immediately. If there are no immediate life threats, continue with patient assessment at a relaxed pace.
  - Responsive, alert young children may become frightened if you start your exam with the head and face. If children show fear as you reach out to touch them and there are no critical injuries, begin the physical examination at the feet and slowly work your way up to the head. While you are performing the toe-to-head assessment, look for the same signs of illness and injury as you do when assessing the adult patient.
  - Always tell children what you are going to do before each step of your assessment. Do not try to explain the entire procedure at once. Explain one step, do it, and then explain the next step.
  - Never lie to a child. Tell them if it will hurt when you are examining them. If children ask if they are sick or

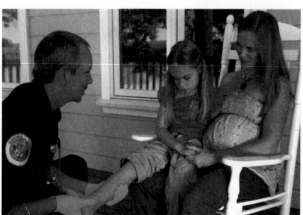

Figure 24.1 Approach at eye level and speak directly to the child.

hurt, tell the truth, but reassure them by saying that you are there to help and other people will also be helping.

- Offer comfort to children by stroking their foreheads or holding their hands. Children will let you know if they do not want to be touched. Children will show their acceptance of you by their reactions to your touch. Do not expect rapid acceptance. Use your smile and gentle words to provide comfort.
- When appropriate, talk to the child. Do not direct all your conversation to the parent or caregiver. If you are at the scene of an emergency in which the parents are also injured, let the child know that other people are caring for their parents.

While assessing and caring for children, you will have to consider and work with the reactions of the parents or primary caregivers. Usually, the responses of parents or guardians are positive and helpful even though they are concerned. Sometimes parents will react with strong emotional responses that can hinder your care. Both types of reactions are natural.

Ask the anxious caregiver to help you with tasks such as holding and reassuring the child, holding a dressing in place, holding the oxygen mask, or assisting with any other device you need to use. If this does not work to calm the parent, have a friend, neighbor, or other team member distract the parent with questions about the child's history or with getting the child's toy, favorite blanket, or clean clothes. It is usually best to keep the child and parent within eyesight of one another.

Age, Size, and Response

You will find that you instinctively treat infants and children differently from adults. You will know that an infant needs to be handled and cared for differently than a **toddler**, and that a toddler is spoken to and cared for differently than an older child or **adolescent**. Through proper training and experience, you will become familiar with the age ranges, mental and physical development, and varying needs of pediatric patients so you can assess and care for them appropriately.

When assessing and caring for pediatric patients, recall the following developmental stages described in Chapter 4 (Table 24.1):

- Neonate (birth to 28 days)
- Infant (birth to 1 year old)
- Toddler (1–3 years old)
- Early childhood (3–6 years old)
- Middle childhood (6–12 years old)
- Adolescence (12–18 years old)
- Early, middle, and late adulthood (18 to end of life)

The specific definition of an infant or child will vary depending on the context in which you are providing care. For the purpose of performing CPR, newborns are from birth to 1 month of age, infants are from 1 month to 1 year, and children are from 1 year up to the onset of puberty (about age 11 to 12 but can vary). After that, CPR is performed the same as it is performed on an adult. Some procedures will change according to the child's physical size more so than the exact age.

Each of the developmental stages requires a slightly different approach to assessment. However, in some situations, you may be unable to determine the age of an infant or child. Some are large or small for their age, and parents may not be there to provide the information. You will have to estimate age based on physical size, emotional responses, interaction with you, and language skills.

Special Considerations

You already realize that infants and children differ from adults in terms of physical size, emotional maturity, and responses. You should be aware that there are important anatomical differences, as well. These are described in the following subsections.

REMEMBER

Children are very sensitive to the feelings of those around them. If you are fearful, they will sense it and their discomfort will worsen. Be aware of your feelings. Take the opportunity to reassure yourself and your fellow rescuers as to their responsibilities, and make every effort to remain calm.

toddler ▶ child between the ages of 1 and 3 years.

adolescent ▶ child between the ages of 12 and 18 years.

JEDI

Children with special needs such as those with Down syndrome, cerebral palsy, autism, and attention-deficit/hyperactivity disorder (ADHD) often progress through developmental stages at a slower rate than children without these conditions. You will have to take that into consideration and not rely solely on chronological age when assessing them.

TABLE 24.1   Developmental Characteristics of Infants and Children

Age Group	Characteristics	Assessment and Care Strategies
Neonate (birth to 28 days)	Infants do not like to be separated from their parents.	Have the parent or caregiver hold the infant while you examine them.
Infant (birth to 1 year)	They have minimal stranger anxiety.	Be sure to keep the infant warm. Also, warm your hands and stethoscope before touching the infant.
	They are used to being undressed but like to feel warm, physically and emotionally.	It may be best to observe the infant's breathing from a distance, noting the rise and fall of the abdomen for normal breathing and the chest for respiratory distress, the level of activity, and the infant's color.
	The younger infant follows movement with their eyes.	
	The older infant is more active, developing a personality.	Examine the heart and lungs first and the head last. This is perceived as less threatening and therefore less likely to cause crying.
	They do not want to be "suffocated" by an oxygen mask.	A pediatric nonrebreather mask may be held near the face to provide blow-by oxygen.
Toddler (1 to 3 years)	Toddlers do not like to be touched or separated from their parent or caregiver.	Have a parent or caregiver hold the child while you examine them.
	They may believe that their illness is a punishment for being bad.	Assure the child that they were not bad.
	Unlike infants, they do not like having their clothing removed.	Remove an article of clothing, examine the toddler, and then replace the clothing.
	They frighten easily, overreact, and have a fear of needles and pain.	Examine in a toe-to-head approach to build confidence. (Touching the head first may be frightening.)
	They may understand more than they communicate.	Explain what you are going to do in terms they can understand. (Taking the blood pressure may be a "squeeze" or a "hug on the arm.")
	They begin to assert their independence.	Offer the comfort of a favorite toy.
	They do not want to be "suffocated" by an oxygen mask.	Consider giving the child a choice: "Do you want me to look at your belly first or your feet first?"
		A pediatric nonrebreather mask may be held near the face to provide blow-by oxygen.
Early childhood (3 to 6 years)	Children in this age group do not like to be touched or separated from their parent or caregiver.	Have a parent or caregiver hold the child while you examine them.
	They are modest and do not like their clothing removed.	Respect the child's modesty. Remove an article of clothing, examine them, then replace the clothing.
	They may believe that their illness is a punishment for being bad.	Have a calm, confident, reassuring, and respectful manner.
		Be sure to offer explanations about what you are doing.
	They have a fear of blood, pain, and permanent injury.	Allow the child the responsibility of giving the history.
		Explain as you examine.
	They are curious, communicative, and can be cooperative.	A pediatric nonrebreather mask may be held near the face to provide blow-by oxygen.
	They do not want to be "suffocated" by an oxygen mask.	Do not lie. Explain that what you do to help may hurt.
Middle childhood (6 to 12 years)	Children in this age group cooperate but like their opinions to be heard.	Allow the child the responsibility of giving the history.
		Explain as you examine.
	They fear blood, pain, disfigurement, and permanent injury.	Present a confident, calm, and respectful manner.
	They are modest and do not like their bodies exposed.	Respect the child's modesty.
		Do not lie. Explain that what you do to help may hurt.

(Continued)

TABLE 24.1 (Continued)

Age Group	Characteristics	Assessment and Care Strategies
Adolescent (12 to 18 years)	Adolescents want to be treated as adults. They generally feel they are indestructible but may have fears of permanent injury and disfigurement. They vary in their emotional and physical development and may not be comfortable with their changing bodies.	Although they want to be treated as adults, they may need as much support as younger children. Present a confident, calm, respectful manner. Be sure to explain what you are doing. Respect their modesty. You may consider assessing them away from their parent or caregiver. Have the physical exam done by an Emergency Medical Responder of the same sex as the patient if possible. Do not lie. Explain that what you do to help may hurt.

Head and Neck   A child's head is disproportionately larger and heavier in relation to the body than that of adults. The body will catch up with the size of the head at about age 6. Because of the size and weight of the head, the child can be considered top heavy and is more likely to land head first in a sudden fall or stop.

Always handle the head of the newborn with caution because of the fontanels (soft spots). The largest soft spot, on the top of the head, does not close completely until about 18 months of age. This soft spot is flat when the infant is quiet, and you may see it pulsate with each heartbeat. If the soft spot is sunken, the child may have lost a lot of fluids (dehydration) because illness has caused inadequate fluid intake or diarrhea and/ or vomiting. If the soft spot is bulging, it may indicate that there is increased pressure inside the skull. This can be due to brain swelling from trauma or from an illness such as meningitis. Because the fontanels also can also bulge when the infant is agitated and crying, they should be assessed when the infant is quiet.

When assessing a head injury, look for blood and clear fluids leaking from the nose and ears, just as you would in adults.

When infants and small children sustain head injuries and also show signs of shock, suspect and assess for internal injuries as well.

Airway and Respiratory System   The airway and respiratory system of the infant and child are not fully developed. The tongue is large relative to the size of the mouth, and the airway is narrower than that of an adult and, thus, more easily obstructed.

When a child is lying on their back, the shape of the head may cause the airway to flex forward and close. Place a folded towel under the child's shoulders to help keep the head in line with the body and the airway open (Figure 24.2). There are some unique points to remember about children's breathing. Infants prefer to breathe through the nose. Make sure the nostrils are clear of secretions, so the infant can breathe freely.

> **SCENE SAFETY**
>
> In a young infant, fontanels are soft spots at the top of the head where the bones of the skull have not yet fused together. These areas are not quite as fragile as some may believe. Although you certainly should not poke, prod, or apply firm pressure to these areas, they can be gently palpated without causing harm to the infant.

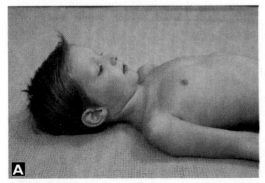
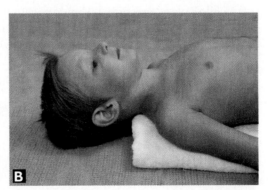

Figure 24.2 (A) When an infant or young child is supine, the head will flex forward, obstructing the airway. (B) To keep the airway in a more neutral position, place a folded towel under the shoulders.

REMEMBER

Infants are primarily nose breathers. They will not automatically open their mouths when the nose is obstructed.

Remember the child's trachea (windpipe) is also softer, more flexible, and narrower than that of an adult and will obstruct easily. Overextending a child's neck during airway management can cause the trachea to collapse and obstruct the airway.

Chest and Abdomen   Because the diaphragm is the major muscle of breathing, you will see more movement in the abdomen than in the chest. But the chest is more elastic, so when the child's breathing is labored or distressed, chest movement is obvious in the muscles between the ribs and in the muscles above the sternum around the neck and shoulders. The use of the accessory muscles for breathing is important to note and indicates that the child is in respiratory distress.

The child's less developed and more elastic chest has both advantages and disadvantages when compared to that of an adult. In a crushing mechanism of injury, the bones of the child's chest may not break, but they will flex. The disadvantage is that the more flexible chest offers less protection to the vital organs underneath. In the physical exam, the mechanism of injury is important and will help you determine the possibility of internal injury, especially if there is no obvious external injury. Some signs to look for are loss of symmetry (unequal appearance on both sides of the chest), unequal chest movement with breathing, and bruising over the chest and abdomen.

Injury to the abdomen can result in tenderness, distention, and rigidity, just as it can in adults. The abdominal muscles are not as well developed as they are in the adult and offer less protection. The abdominal organs (especially the liver and spleen) are large for the size of the cavity and are more susceptible to injury. A child who sustains a blunt abdominal injury can bleed out within minutes. Injury that causes distention or swelling can restrict movement of the diaphragm muscle and make it difficult for the child to breathe.

Body Surface Area   Infants and children have a large amount of total surface area (skin) in proportion to total body mass. The large surface area can easily lose heat and cause the pediatric patient to become chilled, or hypothermic, even in an environment in which an adult feels comfortable. It is important to keep infants and children covered and warm, especially if there is trauma and blood loss or illness and fluid loss.

Blood Volume   The smaller the patient, the less blood volume they have. The newborn may have slightly less than 12 ounces, or about a cup and a half, of blood and cannot afford to lose much. As children grow, their blood volume increases. By age 8, they will have about 2 liters (roughly one-half gallon) of blood. Moderate blood loss in an adult may not concern you if it is easily controlled, but the same amount of blood loss in an infant or small child can be life threatening.

SCENE SAFETY

Never assume that a child is stable or otherwise healthy based on just one set of vital signs. The signs and symptoms of children and infants must be continually assessed for changes. Those changes will reveal important trends in the child's condition.

Vital Signs   Pulse and respiratory rates vary with the size of the child. The smaller the child, the higher the rates. Tables 24.2 and 24.3 list the average pulse and respiratory rates for infants and children.

Blood pressure also varies in children and depends on their sex, age, and height (Table 24.4). Boys tend to have slightly higher blood pressure than that of girls the same age.

If you are trained to take blood pressure, use the appropriate size cuff when you take a child's blood pressure. It should cover about one-half of the child's upper arm. Cuffs that are too small or too large may give inaccurate readings. It is not necessary to measure a blood pressure on a child younger than age 3 in the prehospital setting.

TABLE 24.2   **Average Pulse Rate in Infants and Children**

Age Group	Beats Per Minute
> 10 years	60 to 100
2 to 10 years	60 to 140
3 months to 2 years	100 to 190
Newborn to 3 months	85 to 205

(Continued)

TABLE 24.2 (*Continued*)

Pulse Quality	Significance/Possible Causes
Rapid	Exertion, anxiety, pain, fever, dehydration, blood loss, shock
Slow	Head injury, drugs, some poisons, some heart problems, lack of oxygen
Irregular	Arrhythmia (abnormal electrical activity in the heart)

Note: In infants and children, a high pulse is not as great a concern as a low pulse. A low pulse may indicate imminent cardiac arrest.

Source: Data gathered from the American Heart Association's Pediatric Advanced Life Support (PALS) Provider Manual (Dallas, TX: American Heart Association, 2015).

TABLE 24.3 Average Respiration Rate in Infants and Children

Age Group	Breaths Per Minute
Adolescent: 12 to 18 years	12 to 16
Middle childhood: 6 to 12 years	18 to 30
Early childhood: 3 to 6 years	22 to 34
Toddler: 1 to 3 years	24 to 40
Infant: < 12 months	30 to 60

Source: Data gathered from the American Heart Association's Pediatric Advanced Life Support (PALS) Provider Manual (Dallas, TX: American Heart Association, 2015).

TABLE 24.4 Average Blood Pressure in Infants and Children

Age Group	Systolic (mm Hg)	Diastolic (mm Hg)
Adolescent: 12 to 18 years	113 to 131	64 to 83
Middle childhood: 6 to 12 years	96 to 115	57 to 76
Early childhood: 3 to 6 years	88 to 106	42 to 63

Source: Data gathered from the American Heart Association's Pediatric Advanced Life Support (PALS) Provider Manual (Dallas, TX: American Heart Association, 2015).

Assessment of Infants and Children

LO3 Explain the components of the pediatric assessment triangle.

LO4 Explain various techniques that can be employed to maximize successful assessment of the pediatric patient.

Certain aspects of the assessment of the pediatric patient need to be handled differently than when assessing an adult patient.

Scene Size-up

Size up the scene just as you would a scene involving an adult, but approach slowly so you do not frighten the child. Determine scene safety and the number of patients involved in the emergency. Determine the mechanism of injury or the nature of illness. Prepare for patient care by putting on appropriate personal protective equipment. If you think you may need additional resources, call for them immediately.

Primary Assessment

Forming a *general impression* involves looking at the child and the environment as you approach. Quickly gather critical information that will help you decide whether to hurry or take your time. From a short distance or from across a room, you can see if the child is alert, struggling to breathe, crying, quiet and listless, or unresponsive to your approach. Is the skin pale, bluish, or flushed? How is the child interacting with the environment, with those around them, and to you as you approach? What is the child's body position? From those clues, you can get a general impression of the child's status. In children, the general impression is an important indicator of the severity of illness or injury.

Pediatric Assessment Triangle   A very effective tool used for establishing a general impression of a pediatric patient is the **pediatric assessment triangle (PAT)** (Figure 24.3). The PAT uses three criteria to help make a quick determination of the seriousness of the child's condition during the general impression. When combined with other signs and symptoms, as well as the experience of the Emergency Medical Responder, it can be very effective for quickly forming an accurate first impression. The three criteria of the PAT are:

* *Appearance.* As you enter the scene and approach the patient, quickly assess the child's appearance. Are they alert and looking around? Is the child's behavior consistent for their age and the environment? A toddler will likely look frightened and may be crying at the sight of the EMS crew entering their home or the scene. This would be normal behavior for this age. On the other hand, a child who is still and listless might be quite ill and feeling so poorly that they show no interest in what is going on around them. Characteristics to consider when evaluating the appearance of an ill or injured child are muscle tone, interactivity, consolability, gaze, and speech or cry.

pediatric assessment triangle ▶ tool used to form a general impression of a pediatric patient; its elements are appearance, work of breathing, and circulation (perfusion). Abbrev: PAT.

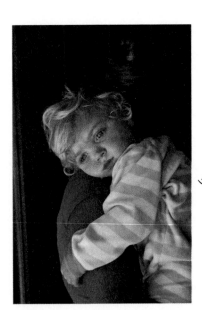
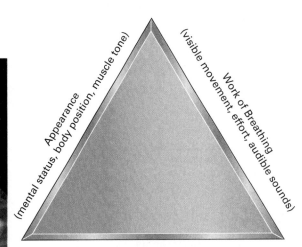
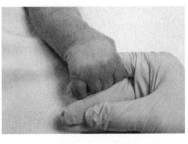
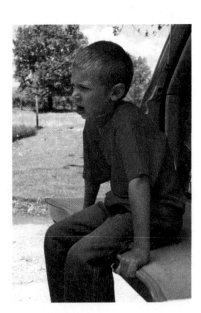

Appearance
(mental status, body position, muscle tone)

Work of Breathing
(visible movement, effort, audible sounds)

Circulation
(skin color)

Figure 24.3 Pediatric assessment triangle.
(Based on Episode 93—PALS Guidelines, https://emergencymedicinecases.com/pals-guidelines/)

- *Work of breathing.* Recall that work of breathing refers to the effort required for an individual to breathe. Normally, a child displays little to no work when breathing is normal. When a child is hypoxic or in distress, the work of breathing will increase and become more obvious. Typically, this can be seen as you approach the child. You will see obvious movement of the chest and abdomen with each breath, nasal flaring, and possibly **retractions**. Retractions are the inward movement of the soft tissue between the ribs (intercostal muscles) when a child breathes in. They are a sign of significant distress. You must bare the chest to see retractions. You may also hear sounds such as stridor (a high-pitched sound) or wheezing as the child breathes. These, too, are strong signs of an ill child.

- *Circulation.* This refers to how well the child is perfusing, as evidenced by the presence of pulses and the color of the skin. Notice the general color of the skin. Compare the arms and legs with the trunk of the body. In light-skinned patients, all areas should be an even shade of pink. For dark-skinned patients, you will look for pink tissues inside the mouth and at the nail beds. Notice if the skin is mottled (blotchy and not a uniform color), pale, or cyanotic (bluish). You must also check capillary refill time at the extremities as well as the trunk of the body. A delayed capillary refill time anywhere on the body is a possible sign of serious illness.

retractions ▶ inward movement of the soft tissues between the ribs (intercostal muscles) when a child breathes in.

Once you reach the child, you can quickly determine mental status using the AVPU scale. Is the child alert? Are they responsive to your voice or only to a painful stimulus, such as squeezing their shoulder? Or is the child unresponsive? Are they oriented to individual, place, and time? An infant or a very young child is not able to answer questions about their name, where they are, or what day it is; however, parents or caregivers can explain if the child's actions are as they would normally expect them to be.

Next, quickly assess the child's ABCs. If the child is crying, you may assume that they have an airway and adequate breathing and circulation. For the quiet or unresponsive child, check the airway. Is it open? Check breathing. Is the child breathing normally or with effort? What is the rate? Is chest expansion adequate and equal? Are there noises such as grunting or stridor associated with the child's respiratory efforts? Is the skin pale or cyanotic? Check circulation. Is the pulse strong and regular? Is there any obvious bleeding?

CREW RESOURCE MANAGEMENT

It can be helpful to assign one crew member to take a parent or caregiver aside to obtain more information about the child and the recent medical history.

For all children, you will want to determine:

- Is the skin warm and dry, indicating normal circulation? Or is it cool and moist, suggesting blood loss and shock?
- Which skin areas are most accessible for you to determine cool and moist skin?
- Is capillary refill time less than 2 seconds?
- Are there any life-threatening conditions that affect the ABCs present? If so, care for those first. Remember that the unresponsive child needs immediate care.

When you determine priority of transport, you will recognize the high-priority infant or child patient as one with:

- Poor general impression
- Altered mental status
- Airway problem
- Respiratory distress or inadequate breathing
- Pale or mottled skin.
- Evidence of bleeding that may soon result in shock

Managing the Airway   The airway is your first concern in the care of any patient. Always ensure the airway is open and clear and the patient is breathing adequately or is receiving appropriate ventilations and supplemental oxygen when necessary. Follow local protocols.

Opening the Airway   When a child lies on their back, the tongue may fall to the back of the throat much like in an adult. Remember that, with an infant or child, the tongue is larger in relation to the body and can more easily obstruct the airway. Also, when lying on their back, the larger head of the infant may cause the head to flex or bend forward and close off the airway. In small children, if you are not careful when opening the airway, you may cause hyperextension or bend the head too far back, which also can close off the airway. You must be sure to place the head in a neutral position so the airway is open.[1]

As noted previously, you can easily position the infant or small child correctly by placing a towel under the shoulders. Check for breathing before repositioning the head. Then, if necessary, perform a slight head-tilt or a jaw-thrust maneuver to assess breathing and provide ventilations.

Clearing and Maintaining the Airway   If air does not enter easily or the chest does not rise when you are providing rescue breaths, reposition the head and try again. If you still have no success in ventilating the patient, you may assume there is an airway obstruction. Perform 30 chest compressions. Then check the mouth to see if there is an obstruction. If you see one, sweep the mouth with the little finger of your gloved hand. Do not perform blind finger sweeps.

If there are fluids in the airway, clear them by sweeping the mouth with a gauze pad or by suctioning. Check with your instructor to find out if Emergency Medical Responders in your area are allowed to use suctioning equipment. If so, your instructor will provide you with training. You may also be able to use nasopharyngeal and oropharyngeal airways in the infant and child patient. Again, your instructor will let you know and give you appropriate training.

Providing Oxygen   If you are allowed to provide oxygen to patients, your instructor will have the appropriate equipment and train you in how and when to use it with pediatric patients.

Providing oxygen may be a vital part of the emergency care procedures used in caring for children. However, it may be difficult to deliver in the prehospital setting. Children may resist having a mask placed over the face, and the flow of oxygen may even cause children to hold their breath. Oxygen can still be provided to children who need it by using a blow-by technique.

To perform the blow-by technique, hold or have the parent hold the oxygen tubing or the pediatric nonrebreather mask about 2 inches from the child's face. The oxygen will enrich the area in front of the face as it blows by and the child inhales (Figure 24.4). Oxygen tubing can be pushed through the bottom of a paper cup and provide oxygen effectively. The advantage to this method is the child will likely be curious about the cup and hold it to their face to examine it or try to drink from it. As the child is receiving oxygen, they will calm down because they have something of interest to keep their attention.

If the patient is not breathing, provide rescue breaths. For infants, provide rescue breaths at a rate of 1 breath every 3 to 5 seconds using a pediatric-sized pocket face mask or a bag-mask device of the correct size. Remember the following steps when ventilating:

- Breathe less forcefully. Watch for the chest to rise. Ventilate slowly so as not to cause stomach distention.
- Provide a gentle squeeze of the bag-mask device. Watch for the chest to rise.

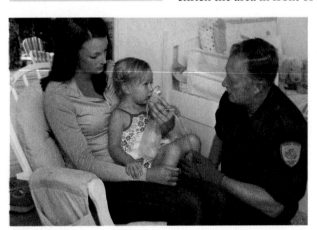

Figure 24.4 Hold the oxygen mask close to the child's face to provide blow-by oxygen.

- Use a properly sized face mask to get a good mask-to-face seal.
- If ventilations are not successful, perform the procedures for clearing an obstructed airway. Then try to ventilate again.

After requesting an ambulance and notifying dispatch of the description and direction of the suspect vehicle, Bryn quickly flips the car radio to loudspeaker mode. "Attention! This is the police! Is anyone injured?" She speaks clearly into the mic. Her voice bounces off the surrounding buildings and echoes into the distant concrete canyons of the city's west side. People are cautiously standing up all around the intersection, looking around with wide eyes.

There is no indication of other injuries, so Bryn turns her attention to the baby. She gently removes the child from the woman's arms and places the bundle onto the hood of her patrol car. The baby cries weakly as she unwraps the blanket and examines the small, pale body. There is a ragged wound to the child's lower abdomen and a small round hole in the lower back. Blood flows steadily from both wounds, and Bryn cradles the baby in one arm as she runs around to the trunk to get the Emergency Medical Responder bag.

Secondary Assessment

After completing your primary assessment, focus on getting a history and conducting a physical exam. These steps may be done at the scene with the responsive patient and while you are waiting for the ambulance to arrive. Normally, infants or very young children will not respond to your questions, but children older than 2 or 3 years will be able to answer questions requiring a yes or no response. They also can tell you or point to where it hurts. Otherwise, parents or other caregivers such as babysitters or teachers will have to give you information about the child's history and how they became sick or hurt.

While you are getting a general impression of the child, decide if they are seriously injured or sick. If so, perform a rapid assessment just as you would for an adult:

- *Patient with significant mechanism of injury (MOI).* Maintain manual in-line stabilization of the head and spine while performing a primary assessment. Inspect and palpate each body area. Get baseline vital signs and, if possible, a history.
- *Unresponsive patient.* Maintain manual in-line stabilization of the head and spine while performing a primary assessment. Inspect and palpate each body area. Get a history, if possible, from those at the scene. Get baseline vital signs.

If your general impression leads you to decide that the child is responding or acting normally, then perform a secondary assessment:

- *Trauma patient with no significant MOI.* Determine the chief complaint. Inspect and palpate the area. Get baseline vital signs. Gather a history that focuses on the injury and events that caused the injury.
- *Responsive medical patient.* Determine the chief complaint or the nature of illness. Gather a history of the events leading up to the illness and the illness itself. Focus your physical exam on the area of complaint, and inspect and palpate the part of the body involved. Get baseline vital signs.

Physical Exam

Now that you have completed a focused assessment, you may have time to perform a more detailed physical exam. This exam is similar to what you do for an adult except when caring for a frightened or crying infant or young child. In this case, the exam is performed in reverse order (toe to head). This will give the child an opportunity to get used to you and your touch if they have not done so during the short, focused assessment.

In a medical situation, examine the child in more detail from toe to head while they are in the parent's or caregiver's lap or being held. In a trauma situation with no significant MOI, let the parent or caregiver help comfort the child while you begin your exam.

Always explain to the child and parent what you are doing, and make sure both understand. Most infants are used to being dressed and undressed and examined by parents, caregivers, and health care professionals. As children get older, they are more modest and have learned that strangers should not touch them. Remove or rearrange only the clothing that must be moved for you to determine what is wrong with the child. Then replace it when you have examined that part of the body.

Children who are seriously ill or injured are usually unresponsive or too critically injured to know or care that a stranger may be assessing them. Be sure to communicate with the caregiver exactly what you are doing and why.

Reassessment

You are never finished with your patient until they have been turned over to an equal or higher level of medical care. This means that when you finish your secondary assessment, you will start again. This reassessment will continue until more advanced EMS personnel arrive. The status of a child can change rapidly and frequently, so reassess mental status, maintain airway, monitor breathing, check pulse, and reevaluate skin signs. Take and record vital signs every 5 minutes for unstable patients and every 15 minutes for stable patients. Continue to monitor the effects of interventions, provide appropriate care, and give emotional support.

Managing Specific Medical Emergencies

LO5 State the most common cause of cardiac arrest in the pediatric patient.

LO6 Explain the assessment and management of the following emergencies in pediatric patients: respiratory emergencies (including airway obstruction), difficulty breathing, and respiratory infection; seizures; altered mental status; shock; fever; hypothermia; diarrhea and vomiting; poisoning; and drowning.

Many of the specific medical emergencies listed here have been described in detail in other chapters. Much of the care you will provide to infants and children is similar to what you would provide to adults.

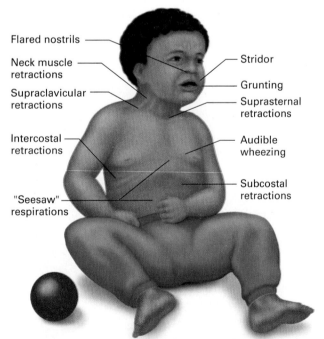

Flared nostrils

Neck muscle retractions

Supraclavicular retractions

Intercostal retractions

"Seesaw" respirations

Stridor

Grunting

Suprasternal retractions

Audible wheezing

Subcostal retractions

Figure 24.5 Signs of early respiratory distress.

Respiratory Emergencies

Emergency Medical Responders do not usually receive the in-depth training for determining different respiratory illnesses and causes of airway and breathing problems in pediatric patients. This section describes some common causes, general signs and symptoms, and the general management of respiratory emergencies in pediatric patients (Figure 24.5).

It is important to note that *the most common cause of cardiac arrest in infants and children is respiratory arrest.*[2] Identifying and caring for a respiratory problem early can minimize the chances of cardiac arrest.

Airway Obstruction You may want to review the signs and symptoms and the management of partial and complete airway obstruction for pediatric patients in Chapter 9. Continue to review and practice them during and after your training. This will enable you to act quickly to ensure an open airway and adequate breathing for all patients. Because the steps of relieving an obstructed airway in infants are different than for adults, practice the steps of back blows and chest thrusts frequently so you can perform them quickly and effectively. Remember that the unresponsive child needs immediate care.

Difficulty Breathing   Many types of airway and respiratory infections and conditions cause airway and breathing problems. A simple cold can plug the nose and make breathing difficult, but the nose can be easily cleared by blowing or suctioning. A respiratory infection can cause swelling of the respiratory tract or blocking by mucus secretions, making it difficult to breathe.

Apparent Life-Threatening Event (ALTE)   An apparent life-threatening event (ALTE) is the sudden onset of certain alarming signs such as prolonged periods of apnea (no breathing), changes in skin color or muscle tone, coughing, and gagging in children under 1 year of age. In almost all cases, apnea occurs while sleeping. For this reason, it is called *sleep apnea*. Some cases of sleep apnea are related to airway obstruction, while others are associated with failure in the central nervous system to stimulate respirations during sleep. The relationship between ALTE and sudden infant death syndrome (SIDS) is still unclear.

Respiratory Infections   Upper respiratory tract infections are very common in infants and children. One such infection is known as **croup**, and any infant or child with noisy respiration and a hoarse cough may have it. Croup is an infection caused by a virus and affects the larynx (voice box), trachea, and bronchi. It usually causes the tissues in the upper airway to become swollen, restricting airflow.

A less common problem that can affect the respiratory status of a pediatric patient is **epiglottitis**. It occurs when the epiglottis (the flap that closes over the trachea while swallowing) becomes inflamed. Epiglottitis can have a sudden onset in what seems to be an otherwise healthy child. Suspect this respiratory emergency if the child develops a rapid fever, has cold-like symptoms, has difficulty swallowing, and is drooling. Children with epiglottitis will also sit upright in a tripod position (leaning forward with arms braced on the edge of the bed or chair) with the chin thrust out and the mouth wide open. You will notice that they will use the muscles in the upper chest and those around the shoulders and neck to breathe. This effort to breathe is very tiring for the child, and you must act quickly. Although uncommon, epiglottitis is considered life threatening.

Providing Care for Respiratory Emergencies   Because it may be difficult to determine what type of respiratory emergency an infant or a child is having, consider any airway problem or breathing difficulty a life-threatening emergency. Call for transport immediately. Provide oxygen as soon as possible using a blow-by technique if you cannot get the child to accept a face mask or a nasal cannula. Do not place anything in the child's mouth (e.g., a tongue depressor) in an attempt to examine the airway. Probing the mouth can cause spasms that will further close the airway. Avoid any actions that might agitate or stimulate the child.

Signs and symptoms of respiratory distress include:

- Wheezing, stridor, or grunting
- Increased work of breathing
- Breathing that is faster or slower than normal, is inadequate, and requires assisted ventilations and oxygen
- Use of accessory muscles to breathe
- Holding a tripod position
- Drooling
- Nasal flaring
- Cyanosis (late sign)
- Capillary refill of more than 2 seconds (late sign)
- Slow heart rate (late sign)
- Altered mental status

REMEMBER

The most common cause of cardiac arrest in infants and children is respiratory arrest. The best way to minimize the chances of cardiac arrest is to support the child's breathing as best you can.

REMEMBER

Emergency Medical Responders should consider all respiratory disorders in children as serious and take action immediately. Respiratory distress and low oxygen levels in children are the primary causes of cardiac arrest not related to trauma.

croup ▸ acute respiratory condition common in infants and children characterized by a barking type of cough or stridor.

epiglottitis ▸ swelling of the epiglottis that may be caused by a bacterial infection; may cause airway obstruction.

REMEMBER

When caring for a patient with suspected croup or epiglottitis, *do not* attempt to examine the mouth by placing a tongue blade or bite stick in the mouth. Doing so could cause rapid swelling of the tissues of the throat and upper airway. This could lead to complete airway obstruction. If you see a child presenting with signs and symptoms of croup or epiglottitis, call for transport immediately and keep the child comfortable and calm.

Asthma　Asthma is a respiratory condition common to children. It can become life threatening if left untreated. Most children who have asthma use medication and/or an inhaler prescribed by their doctors. Parents or caregivers call for assistance for a child with asthma if the signs and symptoms are new and unfamiliar, do not respond to at-home care, or the child is not responding to the usual prescribed treatment. Signs and symptoms of asthma occur when the small airways in the lungs go into spasm and constrict or become too narrow for air to pass through. Many things can trigger an asthma attack. Triggers include allergies, viral infections, physical activity, cold air, and air pollutants such as cigarette smoke. Strong emotional reactions such as anger, fear, excitement, and even laughter can trigger an attack.

Signs and symptoms of asthma include:

- Increased work of breathing
- Wheezing that can be heard with a stethoscope and possibly without
- Obvious respiratory distress with easy inhalation and forced expiration
- Cough
- Faster-than-normal breathing rate
- Increased heart rate
- Sleepiness or slowed response
- Bluish (cyanotic) tint to the skin, especially around the lips

Provide emergency care to the pediatric patient who has difficulty breathing and the previously described signs and symptoms by following these steps:

1. Act calmly and with assurance, which will help calm and reassure the child and the parents or caregiver. For mild distress, the child will be agitated. For severe distress, the child will be exhausted and unable or unwilling to move. Signs of sleepiness and slow response mean low oxygen levels.
2. Place the child in a sitting position. The child will likely have taken a position of comfort that makes it easier for them to breathe—usually a tripod position.
3. Administer oxygen. (Follow local protocols.) Ask the child to breathe in normally but to blow out air forcefully, as if blowing out the candles on a birthday cake or blowing up a balloon. Show the child how and breathe with them.
4. If you are allowed to assist in giving medications, help a parent or caregiver administer the child's medication. Check local protocols and always call for medical direction before assisting a patient with medications (see Appendix 2).
5. Arrange for transport by ambulance. A severe and ongoing asthma attack that is not relieved by medication and oxygen may be *status asthmaticus*, a very serious and life-threatening condition.

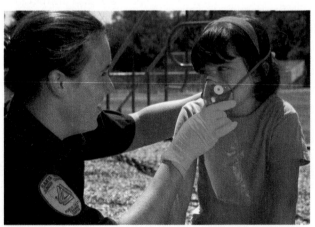

Figure 24.6 For respiratory distress, provide oxygen with a correctly sized pediatric nonrebreather mask placed on the child.

In cases of respiratory distress, provide oxygen by a pediatric-sized nonrebreather mask (Figure 24.6) or by using the blow-by technique. For severe distress and respiratory arrest, provide assisted ventilations with a pediatric-sized bag-mask device and supplemental oxygen and call for support (Figure 24.7).

Always allow the child to assume a comfortable position. The alert child will naturally find the position in which it is easiest to breathe. If you are not trained to use oxygen or do not carry it, call for transport at the first sign of respiratory distress in children.

Altered Mental Status

Any medical or trauma emergency that affects the brain can cause an altered mental status. Examples include low blood sugar (hypoglycemia), poisoning, infection, head injury, decreased oxygen levels, shock, and seizures. As you assess the child, note the mechanism of injury or nature of illness, which will give clues to causes of the child's mental status. Look for signs of poisoning (ingested, inhaled, or absorbed), and ask family members or caregivers if there is a history of diabetes or seizure disorder. While observing and examining the child, you may notice signs of sleepiness, confusion, agitation, or listlessness.

General Emergency Care As you gather information, perform the following emergency care steps:

- Provide support for the ABCs as necessary.
- Provide oxygen as soon as possible by nonrebreather mask, or assist ventilations with a bag-mask device and supplemental oxygen.
- Place the patient in the recovery position if there is no indication of a spinal injury.
- Care for shock.
- Arrange to transport as soon as possible.

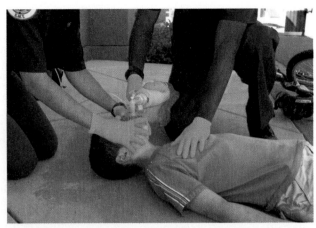

Figure 24.7 If respirations are inadequate, provide assisted ventilations with a bag-mask device.

Seizures A seizure will cause a sudden change in mental status as well as in sensation, behavior, and movement. The more severe forms of seizure cause violent muscle contractions called *convulsions*. Seizures may be the result of high fever, epilepsy, infections, poisoning, low blood sugar (hypoglycemia), or head injury. They also may occur when the brain does not receive enough oxygen because of inadequate blood circulation (shock) or inadequate oxygen in the blood (hypoxia). In some cases, there is no known cause. Many children have seizures, but they are rarely life threatening. Seizures caused by fever (febrile seizures) should be taken seriously. If a child is having prolonged or multiple seizures, consider it a life-threatening emergency and call for transport immediately.

In many cases, a patient's seizures stop before EMS arrives. After a seizure, it is normal for children to be lethargic (drowsy) and difficult to arouse. Look for signs of illness or injury, and question the child or family about symptoms. Also, get the following information:

- Has the child had prior seizures? How long did they last? What part of the body was affected?
- Has the child had a fever recently?
- Has the child had an injury or fall in which the head may have been struck?
- Is the child taking any medications, specifically medication for seizures?
- Did the child's skin (nail beds and mucous membranes) change from its normal color to pale or bluish during the seizure?

Any child who has had a seizure must have a medical evaluation. Arrange for transport as soon as possible. In the meantime, provide the following emergency care steps after the suspected seizure:

1. Maintain an open airway and insert nothing in the mouth.
2. Look for evidence of injury sustained during the seizure.
3. If you do not suspect a spinal injury, position the child on their side.
4. Be alert for vomiting.
5. Provide oxygen or assisted ventilations with supplemental oxygen if allowed to do so.
6. Monitor breathing and altered mental status.

> **REMEMBER**
>
> Frequently, rescuers are called for "child not breathing" only to be met with a crying child who is reported to have had a seizure and then stopped breathing. This is the most common presentation of a febrile seizure. The child may appear perfectly fine upon your arrival. However, it is vital that the child receives a medical evaluation to exclude any serious cause of the fever.

Shock

Common causes of shock in infants and children include losing large amounts of fluid from diarrhea and vomiting, blood loss, and abdominal injuries and other trauma. Shock from fluid loss occurs quickly in infants and is a serious emergency. Call for transport immediately.

The child's body can compensate for shock for a long time, but the body's compensating mechanisms can suddenly fail. This failure is called *decompensated shock*. It occurs when the body can no longer function or compensate for low blood volume or lack of perfusion of oxygenated blood to the brain. As a result, the child has an altered mental status and the blood pressure drops (hypotension). When a child experiences decompensated shock, signs and symptoms of shock can develop rapidly and include:

- Decreasing heart and respiratory rates
- Decreasing blood pressure
- Weak or absent pulse
- Delayed capillary refill
- Decreased urine output (information received from parents or caregiver), which indicates dehydration
- Altered mental status
- Pale, cool, moist skin
- Sunken fontanels in infants

For management of the infant or child who shows signs of shock, first provide support for the ABCs as necessary. Provide oxygen by nonrebreather mask, or assist ventilations by bag-mask device with supplemental oxygen per local protocols.

Diarrhea and Vomiting

A child can lose large amounts of needed body fluids through vomiting and diarrhea, which are normal reactions to illness (and sometimes to certain ingested poisons). This fluid loss can lead to dehydration. Infants are more susceptible to dehydration than adults because the infant has such a small circulating blood volume to start with. For example, think about losing one cup of fluid during an illness. This would be insignificant to an adult, whereas the total circulating blood volume in a newborn is only a cup and a half.

Suspect that a child is dehydrated if they have been feverish for a day or more, have been vomiting without taking in any fluids, or has had diarrhea for several days. As the child loses fluids through vomiting and diarrhea and cannot replace them, the fluid balance in the body is disturbed. A balance of fluids-in to fluids-out is needed to maintain muscle and organ function. Shock can result when large amounts of fluids are lost, even if the fluid is not blood.

If you suspect a child is dehydrated, provide support for the ABCs as necessary. Position the child on their side to help keep the airway open and clear, and administer blow-by oxygen per local protocols. Check vital signs and arrange to transport immediately.

When treating a child who wears diapers, a good thing to find out from the parents or caregiver is if the child has been going through the normal number of diapers recently. A child who is dehydrated will not soil as many diapers as usual.

Fever

The body's normal response to many childhood infections is fever (higher-than-normal body temperature). But the rise in body temperature may also be caused by heat exposure, a noninfectious disease, and even childhood immunizations. The parents or caregiver probably monitored their child's temperature and can report the temperature readings taken before you arrived. Try to find out how high the fever is and how rapidly it rose. Increased temperature is not necessarily what causes a seizure, but a rapid rise in body temperature can cause one.

A fever with a rash, long bouts of diarrhea and vomiting, little intake of fluids, or a fever that rose rapidly with or without seizure are all indications that a potentially serious medical condition may be present. Call for transport as soon as possible.

It is not necessary to take a temperature. If the skin feels very warm to the touch, report this finding along with skin color and condition. A child with a high fever will likely be flushed (reddish skin color) and dry. A mild fever may quickly elevate to a high fever and become a life-threatening problem.

If the child is hot to the touch and there is a history of recent fever reported by the parent or caregiver, take the following steps if your local protocols allow:

- Undress the child down to underwear or diaper, but do not allow them to become chilled.
- Cover the child with a towel soaked in tepid (not cold) water if the fever is the result of heat exposure. If the child starts to shiver, stop the cooling process and cover them with a light blanket.
- Place damp, cool cloths on the child's forehead.
- Call for the transport of any child who has had a seizure. If the child is seizing, monitor airway and breathing.

Be cautious about cooling a fevered child. You can cause hypothermia (reduced body temperature). Wet towels and sheets cool rapidly and become cold, which causes the child to shiver and become chilled.

Hypothermia

Children lose a lot of body heat through their heads. The surface area of the child's head is disproportionately larger than the rest of the body. The large head radiates and loses heat when it is uncovered. When the head is exposed, the body will make every effort to keep the brain warm and functioning, so it sends heat from other parts of the body to the head. Because the child cannot conserve heat well, it will not take long to use up any reserves and develop hypothermia. Keep the head covered to prevent heat loss when caring for infants and children in cool environments.

Children's bodies are unable to regulate temperature as well as adult bodies can, even in normal room temperatures (68°F, or 20°C). Many children do not have much fat stored under their skin and cannot conserve heat. They can become chilled through the environment, injury, or illness, including:

- Exposure to cool weather and water
- Damp or wet clothes or removal of clothes for medical evaluation
- Hypoglycemia (low blood sugar)
- Brain disorder or head trauma that affects the temperature regulation mechanism of the body
- Severe infection
- Shock

When you look for a mechanism of injury or try to determine the nature of illness, also think about conditions that can cause overcooling of the child. In a cold environment, warm the child by stripping off any wet clothing and by wrapping them in a blanket. Be sure the head is covered.

Poisoning

Part of a child's learning experience includes exploring and tasting things. This can sometimes lead to exposure to or ingestion of poisonous substances. Poisons can affect any or all of the body's systems and can rapidly threaten the life of a child. Much of your assessment and care will be the same as for an adult. Know your local protocols for contacting medical direction or a poison control center if there is any indication or suspicion that a child has been exposed to a poison. Be aware that some poisons may be considered hazardous materials, which will require response by specialized personnel trained to handle them.

Drowning

The child who has been submerged in water may still be alive or clinically dead (no breathing and no heartbeat) but not biologically dead (brain cells are still alive). Many patients have been revived after more than 30 minutes of submersion in cold water. Children have been

REMEMBER

In the United States, the local or regional Poison Control Center can be reached by dialing 1-800-222-1222. This national number will route your call to the nearest center. They are a valuable resource that can provide you with emergency first-aid instructions for all poisons. Copy down their instructions and give them to arriving EMS providers.

successfully revived more often than adults in these situations. When caring for a possible drowning patient:

1. Make sure the airway is clear and free of fluids.
2. Provide artificial ventilations or CPR as necessary.
3. Protect the spine in cases where you suspect spinal injury or trauma.
4. Get the patient to a warm and dry environment away from wind to prevent or care for hypothermia. Remove wet clothing.
5. Place the child in the recovery position to prevent aspiration. Administer high-concentration oxygen (per local protocols).
6. Obtain a baseline set of vital signs.
7. Arrange to transport all drowning patients, even if they have recovered and are breathing on their own. It is possible that they will deteriorate hours after they have recovered.

Sudden Unexpected Infant Death (SUID) and Sudden Infant Death Syndrome (SIDS)

| LO7 | Differentiate between sudden unexpected infant death (SUID) and sudden infant death syndrome (SIDS). |

| LO8 | Explain the appropriate steps for management of a suspected SIDS death. |

sudden unexpected infant death ▶ sudden, unexpected death of an infant less than 1 year of age without a clear cause prior to investigation. Abbrev: SUID.

sudden infant death syndrome ▶ sudden death of an infant less than 1 year of age that cannot be explained after a thorough investigation; often occurs during sleep. Abbrev: SIDS.

Each year in the United States, approximately 3,400 infants die suddenly and without any clear cause prior to investigation.[3] These deaths are referred to as **sudden unexpected infant death (SUID)**. SUID encompasses all unexpected and sudden deaths of babies less than 1 year old, including those for which the cause can be determined and those for which the cause is not immediately obvious prior to investigation. The three most common causes of SUID are **sudden infant death syndrome (SIDS)**, representing 41%, accidental suffocation and strangulation in bed (27%), and unknown cause (32%).

SIDS is defined as the sudden death of an infant less than 1 year of age that cannot be explained after a thorough investigation that includes a death scene investigation, an autopsy, and a review of the clinical history. SIDS is most likely to occur in the first 4 months of life and often occurs while an infant is sleeping. Possible causes and theories are still being researched. It is known that SIDS is not caused by external methods of suffocation or choking or by vomiting.

When Emergency Medical Responders arrive, they may see distraught parents with their infant, who is in respiratory and cardiac arrest. Because Emergency Medical Responders cannot diagnose SIDS, you must immediately start emergency care as you would for any patient in cardiac arrest. Provide resuscitation and arrange transport to the hospital. Assure the parents that everything possible is being done for the baby. Normally, you would not begin resuscitation if there is obvious stiffening of the body (rigor mortis) or if blood has pooled (lividity) along whatever side the child was lying on. Check with your instructor to learn what your protocols require for those situations. In either case, be sure to provide emotional support to the parents or caregiver.

Caring for the Pediatric Trauma Patient

Because of their size, curiosity, and lack of fear due to inexperience, infants and children are frequent victims of trauma. In the United States, unintentional injuries are the number one cause of death in people between the ages of 1 and 44 (Figure 24.8).[4]

When performing a physical exam on a stable, responsive child, you may reverse your assessment order and do a toe-to-head physical exam. For unresponsive or unstable patients, perform the head-to-toe assessment, focus on the ABCs, and determine priority for transport.

Keep in mind that children's larger head size and weight make them more prone to head and neck trauma in vehicle collisions, especially if unrestrained. This is also true of bicycle mishaps if children are not wearing helmets, those in which they are struck, and incidents involving swimming, diving, and sports. Expect abdominal and pelvic injuries in vehicle crashes in which the child is restrained and extremity injuries in falls of three times their height or greater.

General emergency care steps for the infant or child trauma patient include:

1. Ensure an open airway. Manually stabilize the head and neck. Use a jaw-thrust maneuver to open the airway and protect the spine. Place a folded towel under the shoulders and torso to maintain a neutral position for the airway and alignment of the head.
2. Make sure the airway is clear. Suction if local protocols allow. If necessary, provide ventilations.
3. Provide oxygen by nonrebreather mask, or assist ventilations with a bag-mask device with supplemental oxygen per local protocols.
4. Control bleeding by applying appropriate dressings.
5. Stabilize suspected fractures.
6. Maintain manual stabilization of the patient's head and neck until the ambulance arrives.
7. Arrange for transport as soon as possible.
8. While waiting for the EMTs to arrive or while en route, perform your secondary and ongoing assessments.

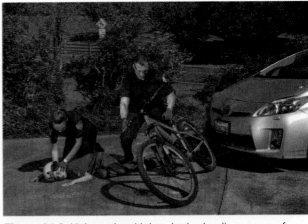

Figure 24.8 Unintentional injury is the leading cause of death for individuals ages 1 to 44.

FIRST ON SCENE *(continued)*

"Ma'am, you need to help me!" Bryn shouts at the woman, who has sunk to the pavement, crying. The woman climbs unsteadily to her feet and approaches the back of the patrol car, where her hands fly up to cover her mouth at the sight of the baby's injuries. "Ma'am," Bryn says firmly. "I need you to hold these dressings in place while I get a bandage on!" The woman takes a step toward Bryn. Her hands shake as she holds the white gauze on the baby's torso while Bryn unrolls the bandage.

"Now I need you to hold your baby close and talk to him." Bryn helps the woman hold the crying baby to her chest. "Keep talking to him, do you understand?"

The woman nods, trying to curb her own sobs as she gently rocks the child. Bryn sighs with relief as she hears the approaching sirens of both EMS and police backup.

Burns

LO9 Describe the proper management of a child with burn injuries.

LO10 Describe the rule of nines as it applies to an infant.

Burns in infants and children are assessed somewhat differently than for adults because of the child's disproportionately larger surface area of the head and significantly smaller extremities. In the rule of nines, the percentage of body surface area assigned is slightly different, and the total of 101% is close enough for estimates.

- 18% to the head and neck
- 18% to the chest and abdomen
- 18% to the entire back
- 14% to each leg
- 9% to each arm
- 1% to the genital area

If you find it is difficult to do the estimations with accuracy while you are trying to quickly care for and stabilize the patient, do not worry about precision. The safest procedure is to estimate quickly and overestimate rather than underestimate the body surface area burned.

Carefully and quickly care for the burned area with dry, sterile, or commercial nonadherent burn dressings or sheets. Dry dressings will keep air, foreign materials, and dirt off the burn and will help keep the child warm, which will help in preventing shock. Follow local protocols for burn management.

Arrange to transport the burned child as quickly as possible. Check local protocols for determining the type of cases (degree of severity, respiratory burns) that should be transported to a burn center. Burns are excruciatingly painful, and children are likely to be frantic. Rapid transport is important for obtaining pain relief for the child and care of the burns.

Suspected Abuse and Neglect

LO11 Describe common signs and symptoms of abuse and neglect.

LO12 Explain the role of the Emergency Medical Responder in cases of suspected abuse and/or neglect.

Abuse is the physical, emotional, or sexual mistreatment of another individual. A call involving the suspected **abuse** or **neglect** of a pediatric patient can be one of the most difficult situations for the Emergency Medical Responder to handle, both during and after the call. It is normal to experience strong emotions following a difficult call, but calls involving pediatric patients can be especially difficult emotionally. If given the opportunity, it is highly recommended that you participate in a formal debriefing for any difficult call. Remember to maintain patient confidentiality. You cannot name the child or family to anyone other than medical authorities, social services, or law enforcement agencies.

You must collect information, perform your assessments, and provide care without making a judgment or expressing your suspicion, distaste, or disbelief. Keep in mind that the abuser also needs help. Remember that your suspicions may be unfounded and that not every injury or sign of possible abuse to a child is the result of actual abuse. It is not your place to accuse a parent or caregiver because they may not be the abuser. You will need to check for patterns in responses and reports to confirm your suspicions. Report your concerns and impressions to ambulance personnel, medical direction, social services, the health department, or law enforcement, as required by local protocols. In all 50 states, *mandated reporters* are those designated by law to report cases of suspected abuse or neglect. In most states, EMS personnel are specifically named as mandated reporters. Be aware of your local laws and protocols regarding reporting abuse.

There are several different forms of child abuse, and they frequently occur in combination: psychological abuse, neglect, sexual abuse, and physical abuse (Figure 24.9).

abuse ▶ physical, emotional, or sexual mistreatment of another individual.

neglect ▶ failure of parents or caregivers to adequately provide for an individual's basic physical, emotional, social, and health care needs.

REMEMBER

You may be the only health care provider who suspects that a child may be abused or neglected. You may see things that no one else does. Always trust your instincts. If you suspect something, say something. Many states require you to alert law enforcement authorities or local child protective services. If you are wrong, the worst that can happen is to be guilty of caring. If you are right, it could mean the difference of a life.

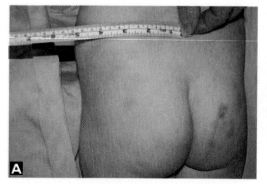 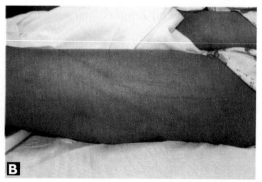

Figure 24.9 Examples of injuries caused by abuse and neglect. (A) Bruises to the buttocks, and (B) an injury from a switch on the thigh.
(© Janet M. Gorsuch, RN, MS, CRNP. Courtesy of Akron Children's Hospital)

Remind all crew members to pay close attention to the scene and the information provided by adults about what is going on with the pediatric patient. You want to be sure that the story being told is consistent with what is going on with the child. We have a duty to be the advocate for the child and to be on the alert for signs of abuse or neglect.

Psychological Abuse　It may be rare that Emergency Medical Responders are called to care for a patient who has been psychologically abused because there is no physical injury. However, there may be emotional signs and symptoms that may be difficult to assess unless you know the patient.

Psychological abuse includes emotional or verbal abuse that seriously affects the child's positive emotional development, well-being, and self-esteem. Children exposed to psychological abuse may feel rejected, degraded, or terrified. They may be forced into isolation with limited freedom or contact with others. They may be exploited or corrupted and forced to accept the beliefs of another, such as a cult or gang leader. Verbal abuse that affects emotional well-being and self-esteem and causes feelings of rejection or degradation in children includes phrases such as "You're stupid," "You are no good," "You are not like your sister," "I wish you were never born," and "I hate you." Some parents isolate their children, locking them in closets or not letting them attend school. Although psychological abuse can occur alone, victims often sustain other forms of abuse such as sexual and physical abuse.

The victims of psychological abuse, as well as other forms of abuse, are often those with the least power and resources—children and women. Possible signs of psychological abuse include:

- Depression
- Withdrawal
- Extreme anxiety
- Low self-esteem
- Feelings of shame and guilt
- Fear
- Lack of normal social skills because of isolation
- Avoidance of eye contact
- Extreme passiveness or compliance
- History or indications of self-harm
- Substance abuse
- Increased tension or anxiety when the abuser is present

Provide care and emotional support by listening to and believing what the child tells you and by expressing your understanding. Let the child know that there are people who will help and that you can get help. Arrange to have the child transported to get them away from the abuser if necessary. Be sure to report your findings to the transport personnel and to social services, the health department, or the police, as required by your protocols.

Neglect　Emergency responses are usually for the obvious trauma that occurs in physical and sexual abuse, not for neglect. However, long-term neglect can result in physical deterioration and injury or medical problems. Child neglect occurs when parents or caregivers do not provide for any or all of the basic needs of the child: food and water, appropriate shelter and clothing, medical care, and education.

On arrival, your scene size-up may reveal signs of neglect, such as a child who is dressed inappropriately for the weather; a child who is thin, lethargic, and has signs of dehydration; or an environment with unclean living conditions, particularly where the child sleeps or is confined.

Also consider the circumstances of the family. They may not be able to financially afford to provide for the basic needs of the child or even themselves, and the entire family may need help from social services. Provide appropriate care for the child's illness or injuries and arrange to transport. Follow your protocols for reporting your concerns.

Sexual Abuse   There are many forms of sexual abuse, including physical sexual contact or exposure and sexual exploitation by displaying or photographing children for sexual purposes or with sexual intent. Emergency Medical Responders usually receive a call for sexual abuse if the child is injured or showing signs of a sexually related medical condition. A child can be the victim of sexual abuse from a parent, other relative, neighbor, teacher, or trusted individual, as well as a stranger.

Do not expect the abuser to admit sexual abuse is the reason for the call. Many excuses and reasons are given for the child who has genital injuries or who has signs and symptoms of sexually transmitted diseases.

When providing care, avoid embarrassing the child or making them feel guilty. Let the child know that you and the people at the hospital will help. Signs of sexual abuse include:

- Obvious injuries to the genital area, including burns, cuts, bruises, and abrasions
- Rashes or sores around the genitals, discharges (such as seminal fluid), and bleeding from the genital openings or on underclothing
- Information from the child that they were exposed, touched, or assaulted

Be sure to report your suspicions and findings to ambulance personnel and/or to the appropriate agency, per local protocols. Use these emergency care steps:

1. Dress wounds and provide other appropriate care for injuries.
2. Save any evidence of sexual abuse, such as soiled or stained clothing. Do not let the child use the bathroom to urinate or defecate. If the child must go to the bathroom, try to collect it in a container for hospital examination. Do not let the child drink any fluids or eat anything. Do not wash the child or let the parent wash the child or change their clothes. (The parent may insist on washing the child and changing their clothing. The child may insist that they must use the bathroom. Be aware that you cannot prevent them from doing so.)
3. Minimize embarrassment by covering the child with a blanket if necessary.
4. Arrange for transport as soon as possible.
5. Provide emotional support and reassurance. Remember, you are still caring for a child. Try to engage them with toys or age-appropriate conversation or games.

Physical Abuse   Any form of violent, harmful contact with a child or any disfiguring act performed on the child is physical abuse, no matter what the intent of the adult. Indications of physical abuse include:

- Outline of marks or bruises that are the size or shape of the object used to strike the child, such as a hand, belt, strap, rope, or cord
- Areas of swelling, black eyes, loose or missing teeth, split lips
- Lacerations, incisions, abrasions
- Any unexplained bruises, broken bones, or burn marks
- Signs of injuries healing incorrectly (misshapen limbs), or a history of numerous broken bones
- Head injuries or indications of closed head injuries that could be the result of violent shaking (bulging fontanels, unresponsiveness), especially in infants and small children
- Bruises—old and new—in various stages of healing
- Abdominal injuries with signs of bruising, distention, rigidity, or tenderness that could be the result of punching or kicking
- Genital injuries with lacerations, avulsions, or bleeding
- Bite marks showing the pattern and size of an adult mouth
- Burn marks or patterns caused by cigarettes, hot irons, or stove burners; water burns or scalding marks on the legs, such as stocking burns from dipping in hot water, or a

hand mark on the buttocks where the child's skin was protected during immersion. The creases at the knees and thighs are also protected when the child flexes his or her legs while being dipped in hot water.

The child's relationship with the parents or a parent's attitude toward the child or the situation may be a clue to abuse. However, these will not always be reliable indicators of the family relationship. Look for the following:

- Story of how the injury occurred that does not match the injury found
- Child who seems afraid to say how the injury occurred
- Child who is obviously afraid of a parent or other individual at the scene
- Child who seems to expect no comfort from the parent
- Child who has no apparent reaction to pain
- Parent or caregiver who does not want to leave you alone with the child
- Parent or caregiver who tells conflicting stories or changes explanations
- Parent or caregiver who blames the child for being clumsy or incident prone
- Parent or caregiver who seems inappropriately concerned or unconcerned
- Parent or caregiver who is angry and is having trouble controlling it
- One parent or caregiver who appears depressed or withdrawn while the other parent is expressing anger or giving explanations
- Any signs of alcohol or drug abuse
- Any expression of suicidal ideations
- Parent or caregiver who is reluctant to give the child's history or to permit transport or who refuses to go to the nearest hospital

You must be the child's advocate and convince the parents that the child needs to be seen by a health care provider because of "the difficulty of determining the seriousness of injuries in the field." Do not accuse anyone of any wrongdoing.

You may respond to a call for an injured child and have no idea that the injury is related to abuse. You may observe that the child and parents or caregivers relate well and that there is a strong bond between them. There are still abuse indications that will make you suspicious over time, so be alert for:

- Repeated responses for the same child or children in the same house
- Signs of past injuries during your assessment
- Signs of poorly healing wounds
- Signs of burns that are fresh or in various stages of healing
- Many types of injuries on numerous parts of the body

Obvious abuse situations can trigger strong emotions in you. Most people feel it is their duty to protect young children. Your first reactions to an abuse situation may be anger and disgust. However, you should not display these feelings while caring for the child or dealing with the parents or other caregivers. Providing necessary care for the child's injuries, clearly documenting objective findings, and alerting the proper authorities of your suspicions are appropriate actions.

If you suspect abuse and the parent or caregiver will not allow the child to be transported, call for law enforcement assistance.

Shaken-Baby Syndrome One type of physical abuse is **shaken-baby syndrome**. It is a form of child abuse that occurs when an abuser violently shakes an infant or small child, creating a whiplash-type motion that causes acceleration-deceleration injuries. The intent, usually, is not to harm the baby. Rarely, the syndrome may be caused accidentally by tossing the baby in the air or jogging with the baby in a backpack. It is not a result of gentle bouncing.

Infants and children have large, heavy heads, weak and not fully developed neck muscles, and space between the brain and the skull to allow for growth. The skull is also soft and pliable and not yet strong enough to absorb much force. During violent shaking, the brain will rebound against the inside of the skull and bruise, swell, and bleed, which

shaken-baby syndrome ▶ form of child abuse that occurs when an abuser violently shakes an infant or small child, creating a whiplash-type motion that causes acceleration-deceleration injuries.

causes increased pressure. Shaking can also cause injury to the neck and spine and to the eyes, causing loss of vision.

If you are called to the scene of a sick or injured child, ask the parent or caregiver questions to obtain a history. Look for signs and symptoms of illness or injury in your assessment. A shaken baby may have no obvious signs of trauma, such as bruising, bleeding, or swelling. The history and some of the signs and symptoms of shaken-baby syndrome may include the following, which may also be indications of other illnesses:

- Change in behavior
- Irritability
- Lethargy or sleepiness
- Decreased alertness
- Unresponsiveness
- Pale or bluish (cyanotic) skin
- Vomiting
- Convulsions (seizures)
- Not eating normally
- Not breathing

Shaken-baby syndrome is a serious emergency. Call for transport immediately for any child with the above signs and symptoms. While waiting for them to arrive, ensure that the baby has an airway, is breathing, and has a pulse. Perform rescue breathing or CPR as needed and provide oxygen if you are trained and allowed to do so. If the child is vomiting, protect and clear the airway. Be sure to turn the infant as a unit, keeping the head in line with the body. If the infant is having seizures, protect them from further injury.

Safety Seats

Many safety seats are not installed correctly in vehicles, and children are often not secured properly by the safety straps and harnesses. Any movement of the seat or the child can throw both forward in a crash. As a result, the child receives internal injuries, which emergency care providers may not be able to initially detect. Usually, the child's body will compensate for these internal injuries and bleeding, which can lull the rescuers into thinking the child is unharmed and stable.

Any vehicle crash should lead you to suspect that the child has been injured, even if you do not see any damage to the safety seat. If the child is still secured to the car seat, leave them there and carefully assess the child in place. If there are any issues with the ABCs, maintain manual stabilization of the child's head, remove them from the seat, and provide care as appropriate.

There are many types of child safety seats, but each provides the same safety functions if used properly. You should not hesitate to act to immobilize and provide initial airway care for a child, even if you are not familiar with the safety seat found at a crash site. Use the following guidelines if you must extricate an infant or a child from a safety seat, but do not perform these steps unless you have learned and practiced them under the supervision of your instructor:

- Do a quick visual inspection of the vehicle interior. Did the crash force the safety seat from its position, even slightly? Was the safety seat in the rear or front seat? Was the safety seat a rear-facing or forward-facing seat? Is there structural damage to the seat?
- Throughout the assessment and immobilization process, be sure someone maintains manual stabilization of the infant's or child's head.
- Assess the patient for the ABCs. Assess for injuries.
- If the safety seat has a protection plate over the patient's chest, remove it (cut the straps securing it if necessary) to assess the chest. (Before performing chest compressions, move the infant onto an immobilization device.)
- As you assess the patient, check for loose straps, which would have provided little protection. Extricate the child onto an immobilization device, which can then be secured to the ambulance stretcher (Key Skill 24.1).

Rapid Extrication from a Car Safety Seat

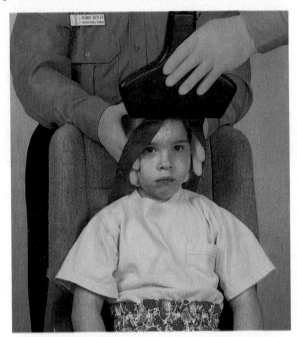

1. Rescuer 1 stabilizes the car seat in an upright position and applies manual head/neck stabilization. Rescuer 2 prepares equipment then loosens or cuts the seat straps and raises the front guard.
(Michael Gallitelli/Pearson Education, Inc.)

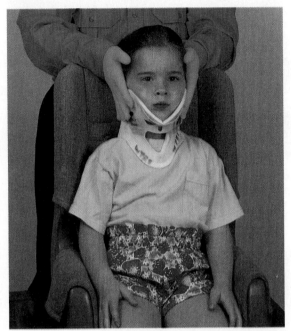

2. Cervical collar is applied to patient as Rescuer 1 maintains manual stabilization of the head and neck.
(Michael Gallitelli/Pearson Education, Inc.)

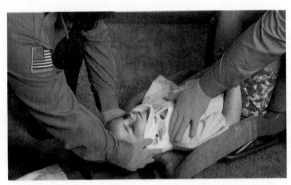

3. As Rescuer 1 maintains manual head/neck stabilization, Rescuer 2 places child safety seat on center of backboard and slowly tilts it into a supine position. Both rescuers are careful not to let the child slide out of the chair. For the child with a large head, place a towel under the area where the shoulders will eventually be placed on the board to prevent the head from tilting forward.
(Michael Gallitelli/Pearson Education, Inc.)

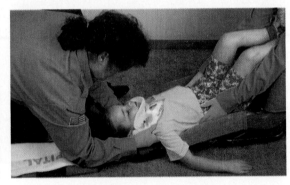

4. Rescuer 1 maintains manual head/neck stabilization and calls for a coordinated long axis move onto the backboard.
(Michael Gallitelli/Pearson Education, Inc.)

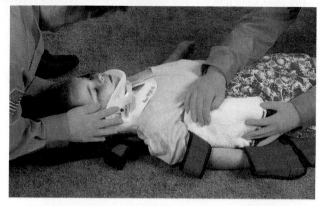

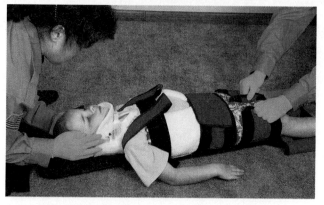

5. Rescuer 1 maintains manual head/neck stabilization. Rescuer 2 places rolled towels or blankets on both sides of the patient.
(Michael Gallitelli/Pearson Education, Inc.)

6. Rescuer 1 maintains manual head/neck stabilization. Rescuer 2 straps or tapes the patient to the board at the level of the upper chest, pelvis, and lower legs. Do not strap across the abdomen.
(Michael Gallitelli/Pearson Education, Inc.)

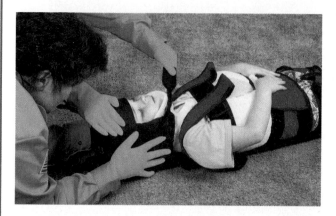

7. Rescuer 1 maintains manual head/neck stabilization as Rescuer 2 places rolled towels on both sides of the head then tapes the head securely in place across the forehead and the cervical collar.
(Michael Gallitelli/Pearson Education, Inc.)

FIRST ON SCENE WRAP-UP

The scene is suddenly awash with flashing emergency lights, and both police officers and firefighters scatter around the intersection, checking on people and securing the area. Bryn describes the child's wounds to the medical crew, who quickly give the mother an oxygen mask to hold near the baby's face and usher her to the back of the ambulance.

"It's good that he's crying," the paramedic says to the mother as he helps her into the ambulance. "But we need to get him over to the university hospital right away."

He then turns to Bryn, just before closing the back doors, and says, "You did a great job, Officer. Perfect." Bryn nods and waves weakly.

As the ambulance moves quickly across 43rd Street and down Buchanan, Bryn sits down on the bumper of her patrol car. "We caught the shooters, you know," a voice says, startling her. She looks up and sees the shift sergeant standing on the sidewalk, looking at her and the bloody gloves she is still wearing.

"How's the little one going to be?" he asks, stepping closer and putting a hand on her shoulder.

"I hope he'll be okay," she answers, standing up. "I mean, I think I did everything I was supposed to."

"You did just fine." He smiles. "Go ahead back to the station and relax. We'll all debrief when we're done here."

Summary

- Assessment and emergency care of infants and children is basically the same as for adults. However, you must consider the special characteristics of the pediatric patient's anatomy, physiology, and emotional responses when assessing and caring for them.
- Infants breathe through the nose. If it is obstructed, they may not immediately open their mouths to breathe. Be sure to clear the nostrils of secretions.
- When managing the airway of an infant, make sure the head is in a neutral position, neither hyperflexed nor hyperextended. Place a folded towel under the infant's shoulders to maintain the spine and the airway in neutral alignment.
- Care for respiratory distress in infants and children immediately. For respiratory distress, provide oxygen with a pediatric-sized nonrebreather mask or by using the blow-by technique. Follow local protocols.
- For severe distress and respiratory arrest, provide assisted ventilations with the appropriate device, such as a pocket face mask or pediatric bag-mask device and supplemental oxygen.

- Children tolerate high fevers better than adults do, but a fever that rises rapidly can cause seizures. Arrange to transport the feverish child as soon as possible. Also arrange to transport the child who is vomiting and has diarrhea.
- Care for shock early. In an infant or child, signs and symptoms of shock mean it has progressed and is in the late stages. If you suspect shock may result from the mechanism of injury or nature of illness, provide emergency care immediately.
- Because of their size, curiosity, and a lack of fear due to inexperience, infants and children are frequent victims of trauma. When assessing and providing emergency care, keep in mind that their larger head makes pediatric patients more prone to head and neck trauma.
- Be calm, professional, and discreet about suspicions of abuse or neglect in the presence of caregivers. Be an advocate for the child and remember your obligation to report any suspicions to the proper authorities.

Take Action

Child Advocate

As much as one would like to think it doesn't happen, accounts of the abuse and neglect of innocent children are reported nearly every day. All 50 states have laws and statutes defining *mandated reporters*, individuals who are identified by vocation or profession and are legally obligated to report cases of suspected abuse or neglect. While all 50 states address the subject and define who is a mandated reporter, each has a slightly different definition. Your job with this activity is to use the internet to search for the definition and requirements related to mandated reporters in your state. You can begin your search by going to the U.S. Department of Health and Human Services, Administration for Children and Families, at www.acf.hhs.gov.

First on Scene Patient Handoff

We have a 1-year-old male with multiple gunshot wounds following a drive-by shooting. He is conscious and alert to his surroundings. We have placed pressure dressings over a wound on both the anterior and posterior torso. Bleeding seems to be controlled, and we now have him on 10 liters of oxygen by nonrebreather mask. Respirations are approximately 30 and shallow, heart rate is 124, strong and regular, skin is pale, warm, and dry. We were unable to obtain a blood pressure due to not having a cuff small enough for the patient.

First on Scene Run Review

Recall the events of the First on Scene scenario in this chapter, and answer the following questions related to the call. Rationales are offered in the Answer Key at the back of the book.

1. What information would you want from the dispatcher about the scene?
2. Did Bryn do everything she could for the baby? Describe what she did or did not do.
3. Was it a good idea to have the mother help? Explain your answer.

Quick Quiz

To check your understanding of the chapter, answer the following questions. Then compare your answers to those in the Answer Key at the back of the book.

1. The components of the pediatric assessment triangle include:

   a. appearance, approximate age, and skin signs.
   b. age, sex, and position of the patient.
   c. appearance, work of breathing, and circulation.
   d. developmental stage, pulse, and respiratory rate.

2. The most appropriate approach when assessing a 10-year-old child is to:

   a. remain at eye level, explain each step of the exam, and be truthful.
   b. remain at eye level, move to a quiet location, and perform the exam.
   c. move to a quiet location, perform the exam, and call the parents.
   d. remain at eye level and perform the exam while telling jokes.

3. The most common cause of cardiac arrest in pediatric patients is:

   a. respiratory arrest.
   b. spinal injury.
   c. drowning.
   d. heart defect.

4. An infant with an airway obstruction has become unresponsive. You should:

   a. open the mouth and perform a finger sweep.
   b. open the mouth, give two slow breaths, and perform a finger sweep.
   c. provide chest compressions as quickly as possible.
   d. provide back blows and chest thrusts.

5. An infant fell into a pool. She is now unresponsive and you are unable to palpate a brachial pulse. You should:

   a. give two rescue breaths.
   b. begin chest compressions.
   c. feel for a carotid pulse.
   d. check for breathing.

6. You are caring for a child in respiratory distress. He has noisy breathing, and his mother reports that he has been sick for several days. You should first:

   a. obtain a blood pressure.
   b. call for immediate transport.
   c. feel his skin to check for a fever.
   d. obtain a medical history.

7. You have responded to a house where an infant was found unresponsive in her crib early this morning. The infant is cold, still, and has no pulse or breathing. There is no significant medical history. You suspect:

   a. child abuse.
   b. a congenital heart defect.
   c. sudden infant death syndrome.
   d. an airway obstruction.

8. An 8-year-old male has burned his hand after falling into a campfire. His hand is red and blistered, and extremely painful. You should:

   a. cover the burned hand with dry, sterile dressings.
   b. cover the burned hand with wet gauze.
   c. wrap the burned hand in petroleum gauze.
   d. leave the burn uncovered and transport.

9. A 6-month-old child has circumferential burns to his hand. His mother states that he fell into a tub of hot water, and his father states that he accidentally spilled hot coffee on the child. You should:

   a. confront the parents regarding their differing stories and call law enforcement.
   b. document what each parent says and report your suspicions of child abuse to the hospital.
   c. ask the child's older sibling what really happened.
   d. question the parents together about what happened to clear up the confusion.

10. Children less than 1 year of age are referred to as:

    a. toddlers.
    b. babies.
    c. infants.
    d. newborns.

11. A 3-year-old has a distinct-sounding cough and signs of respiratory distress. You suspect he may have:

    a. epilepsy.
    b. sepsis.
    c. croup.
    d. febrile seizures.

12. The purpose of the pediatric assessment triangle is to:

    a. gather detailed physical assessment findings.
    b. form a general impression.
    c. assess airway, breathing, and circulation.
    d. identify the need for CPR.

13. A mother reports that her 14-month-old child was "shaking uncontrollably" for about 30 seconds. The child now presents unconscious and limp. The mother states that the child has been ill and had a high fever earlier today. You suspect:

a. febrile seizures.
b. toxic exposure.
c. head trauma.
d. child abuse.

14. All of the following are common medical emergencies for the pediatric patient EXCEPT:

a. respiratory emergencies.
b. altered mental status.
c. heart attacks.
d. seizures.

15. Your patient is a 15-year-old male complaining of anxiety and difficulty breathing. You would classify this patient's developmental stage as:

a. middle childhood.
b. adolescence.
c. neonatal.
d. early childhood.

Endnotes

1. Santillanes G., Gausche-Hill M. "Pediatric Airway Management," *Emergency Medicine Clinics of North America*, Vol. 26, No. 4 (November 2008): 961–975, ix. doi: 10.1016/j.emc.2008.08.004. PMID: 19059095.

2. Bettencourt A.P., Gorman M., Mullen J.E. "Pediatric Resuscitation," *Critical Care Nursing Clinics of North America*, Vol. 33, No. 3 (September 2021): 287–302. doi: 10.1016/j.cnc.2021.05.005. Epub 2021 Jul 7. PMID: 34340791; PMCID: PMC8445069.

3. Centers for Disease Control and Prevention. *Sudden Unexpected Infant Death and Sudden Infant Death Syndrome. Data and Statistics: Fast Facts.* https://www.cdc.gov/sids/data.htm, accessed November 2022.

4. Centers for Disease Control and Prevention. *Key Injury and Violence Data.* https://www.cdc.gov/injury/wisqars/overview/key_data.html, accessed November 2022.

25

Special Considerations for the Geriatric Patient

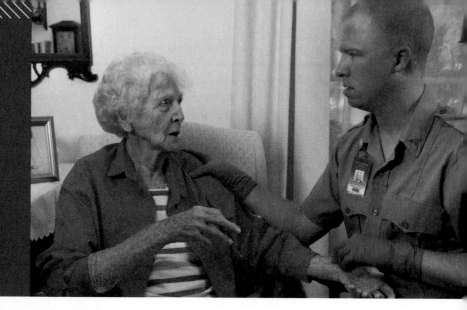

LEARNING OBJECTIVES

Upon successful completion of this chapter, the student should be able to:

Cognitive

1. Define the chapter key terms.

2. Review the major stages of lifespan development of the adult patient (Chapter 4).

3. Describe the general characteristics commonly associated with geriatric patients.

4. Describe some of the most common age-related physical changes found in geriatric patients.

5. Explain the unique challenges that can arise when assessing and caring for the geriatric patient.

6. Describe the common medical problems of geriatric patients.

7. Describe changes in the approach to care when caring for geriatric patients.

8. Describe common signs and symptoms of abuse and neglect of older adults.

9. Explain the role of the Emergency Medical Responder in cases of suspected abuse and/or neglect of older adults.

10. Describe the incidence and risk factors for suicide in older adults.

Psychomotor

11. Demonstrate the ability to properly assess and care for the geriatric patient.

12. Demonstrate various techniques that can be employed to maximize successful assessment of the geriatric patient.

Affective

13. Value the role of the Emergency Medical Responder with respect to patient advocacy.

KEY TERMS

Alzheimer's disease (*p. 544*)
elder abuse (*p. 545*)
elder neglect (*p. 545*)

geriatric (*p. 537*)
mechanical fall (*p. 545*)
self-neglect (*p. 545*)

This chapter introduces the special considerations that the Emergency Medical Responder needs to be aware of when assessing and providing care for older adult patients. In the United States, there are currently more than 35 million people over the age of 65, and that number is expected to more than double in the next two decades. Projections indicate that by the year 2060, approximately one quarter of the population will be age 65 or older.[1] Often, you will find yourself responding to calls involving older adult patients. Although some people are living healthier lifestyles, age-related changes in anatomy and physiology do make older adults more susceptible to certain illnesses and injuries.

FIRST ON SCENE

"Great match today," Tom says, smiling as he shakes his opponent's hand across the pickle ball net.

"You've really been working on that backhand, haven't you?" Mary replies, laughing, "I'll have to be prepared for that next time, but at my age I don't know how much more agile I can become."

The four players exit the pitch, making way for the next team. They make plans to play again next week.

"Does next Tuesday at 7 a.m. work for the three of you?" Tom asks.

"We can't on Tuesday," Mary replies, looking at her husband Jack. "Jack and I have our annual colonoscopy appointments that day."

The four friends smile at one another, acknowledging that at their age, 70+, these types of conversations are normal. "Can you do Wednesday instead?" Mary asks.

"Works for us!" Tom and his wife say in unison.

Suddenly a ball from the current game comes flying off the court and rolls just out of Tom's reach. He lunges for the ball and cries out in pain as his leg buckles. He hits the ground, landing on his right hip. "Owwww! My hip!" he yells. The players on the court converge on him, curious and concerned.

"I'm calling 911," Mary says, "You," she points to a player standing nearby. "Grab those towels for me."

She directs Jack, "You try to get him in a comfortable position and keep him shaded. An ambulance will be here soon."

Understanding Geriatric Patients

LO3 | Describe the general characteristics commonly associated with geriatric patients.

The term **geriatric** refers to people who are over the age of 65. This chapter uses the terms *geriatric* and *older adult* interchangeably to refer to this growing population.

There is a common misconception that most older adults are ill, hard of hearing, and altered in their mental state to the point of not being able to provide reliable information to caregivers. You should understand that this is not true. The vast majority of older adults lead healthy, active lives and can communicate clearly with those around them (Figure 25.1). Why the misconception? Most likely it is because people who are healthy and active rarely require EMS assistance. When EMS providers are summoned to help an older individual, the calls frequently come from extended-care facilities where chronically ill and/or mentally altered patients receive care. You should not let frequent calls to these types of facilities distort your view of the geriatric population as a whole.

Most older adult patients are as healthy and lucid as you are. According to surveys conducted in the United States, nearly three quarters of people aged 65 and older rate their health as good, very good, or excellent. However, there are some important differences you should keep in mind when caring for older adult patients. Those differences include unique life experiences and the accompanying concerns that come with aging and the reality of their own mortality. The differences also include anatomical and physiological changes.

geriatric ▶ of or relating to an older adult.

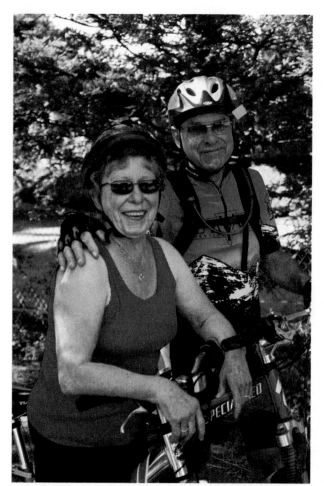

Figure 25.1 The vast majority of older adults lead healthy, active lives.

Although the bodies and illnesses of geriatric patients are unique to each individual, certain generalizations are fairly consistent across this segment of the population. Being familiar with the issues described in the following subsections will greatly assist you in understanding your geriatric patients.

Multiple Illnesses and Medications

Older adult patients are as likely to experience the same illnesses and disorders as everyone else, but their bodies are less able to defend against them and recover afterward. Older adults may have multiple medical conditions, illnesses, or diseases at one time. This number tends to increase as the individual ages. Multiple illnesses create a unique challenge for the responder who is assessing the older adult patient. The patient may be displaying signs and symptoms from a variety of illnesses, with none of them appearing to be anything specific. Do not worry; it is not your job to diagnose the patient. Your job is to perform a thorough assessment and care for the primary complaint as best you can.

Directly related to the presence of multiple illnesses, older adult patients often take numerous prescriptions and over-the-counter (OTC) medications each day (Figure 25.2). It is estimated that 90% of patients aged 65 and older use an average of one medication per week, and 40% use five or more medications per week.[2] Incorrect medication usage (sometimes caused by forgetfulness, confusion about instructions, or poor vision) can create numerous problems, from overdosing to underdosing. Overdosing will result in toxic medication levels in the patient's system. Underdosing can cause the patient's illness or disease process to worsen. Problems can also occur when multiple care providers are not coordinated when prescribing new medications, resulting in adverse reactions from one or a combination of medications (Figure 25.3).

Another common cause of medication misuse is related to the cost of some prescription medications. Older adults who live on fixed incomes may cut their medications in half or take them only every other day in an attempt to get them to last longer.

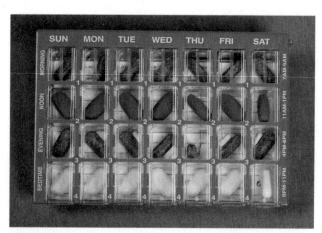

Figure 25.2 Many older adults use a pill organizer to help them remember when to take their medications.

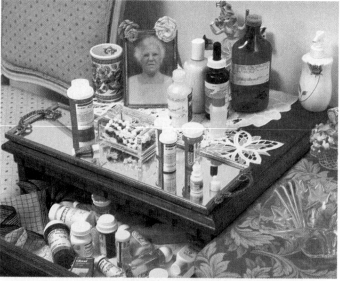

Figure 25.3 It can be challenging to keep track of multiple medications.

Some older adults take blood thinners for various conditions. This is important to know because a patient who has suffered trauma and is on blood-thinning medication is at significant risk for serious bleeding—both internal and external.

Beta blockers are another classification of drugs commonly prescribed for older adults. These medications are used to control the rhythm of the heart and control blood pressure. A common side effect of beta blockers is dizziness and lightheadedness. This side effect can make the patient more prone to injury from falls.

Mobility

Regular exercise continues to remain important as people age. It can help keep aging patients healthy and mobile. However, it is common for some older adults to live increasingly sedentary lifestyles. This can be due to illnesses such as arthritis, medications that cause excessive tiredness, or even the fear of injury as their ability to move about lessens. Having limited mobility can cause many problems for older adults, such as:

- Isolation
- Poor nutrition (Figure 25.4)
- Constipation
- Depression
- Difficulty using the bathroom
- Loss of independence
- Higher likelihood of falls or other injuries

CREW RESOURCE MANAGMENT

All crew members must keep an eye out for potential fall hazards when entering the home of a geriatric patient. One of your roles is to serve as an advocate for the patient. If a crew member identifies a hazard, there may be resources in your city or county that can assist the patient with making their home safer.

Difficulties with Communication

Age-related sensory changes are a natural part of the aging process. It is normal for older adults to experience a lower sensitivity to pain or touch, an altered sense of smell or taste, a certain amount of hearing loss, and impaired vision or blindness. Any of those can affect your ability to assess and communicate with the patient. Table 25.1 lists some strategies for effectively communicating with an older adult patient.

Incontinence

Not necessarily caused by aging, several factors predispose older adults to the inability to retain urine or feces (incontinence). Diseases such as diabetes, illnesses that cause diarrhea, and certain medications can contribute to incontinence. It is important that you *not* make a big deal out of a geriatric patient's incontinence. Maintaining the dignity of any patient is important, but for older adult patients in particular, respect and dignity are extremely vital and necessary for you to develop the level of trust necessary for a good assessment.

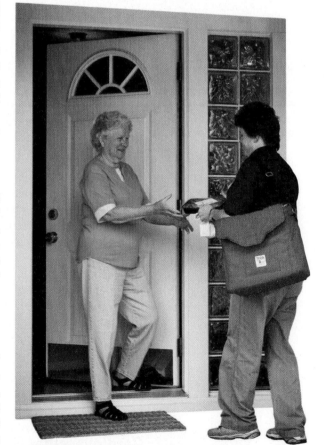

Figure 25.4 Meals on Wheels helps older adults with diminished mobility receive adequate nutrition by providing home-delivered meals.

TABLE 25.1	Age-Related Difficulties with Communication
Difficulty	**Strategy**
Poor vision	Position yourself directly in front of the patient so you can be seen.
	Put your hand on the arm of a blind patient so they know where you are.
	Locate the patient's glasses if necessary.
Decreased hearing	Speak clearly. Check hearing aids. Write notes.
	Try letting the patient wear a stethoscope and speak into the head like a microphone.
Inability to speak clearly	Consider ensuring that the patient has dentures in place if they wear them or asking a caregiver or family member to help communicate with the patient.

Confusion or Altered Mental Status

An important thing to remember when you encounter an older adult patient who seems confused or is presenting with an altered mental status is to try to determine if this is normal behavior for that individual. You want to avoid placing too much importance on a patient's confused state if this is the norm for them. Conditions such as dementia, Alzheimer's disease, and some medications may cause a patient's baseline mental status to be less than what we would consider normal. You will want to question family members or other caregivers to determine the patient's baseline mental status rather than make a wrong assumption.

Age-Related Physical Changes

LO4 Describe some of the most common age-related physical changes found in geriatric patients.

Although age-related changes can be determined by genetics and begin at the cellular level, they are greatly affected by lifestyle and environment. As anyone can see in their own community, the aging process can differ greatly from individual to individual. However, some general age-related changes will be fairly consistent throughout the older population. It is important for Emergency Medical Responders to understand these changes and how they can impact the assessment and care process (Figure 25.5).

Respiratory System

Aging creates many changes in the respiratory system. As early as age 30, without regular exercise, the lungs will begin the aging process with decreased ability to ventilate properly. For example, the mechanism that helps the body detect low levels of oxygen in the blood becomes increasingly less efficient over time. This means that a geriatric patient may become severely hypoxic before the body realizes it and attempts to compensate. Aging also leads to a decrease in the number of cilia (tiny, hair-like structures) in the airway, exposing the individual to more respiratory illnesses, such as pneumonia. Cilia line the airway and move in wave-like motions to help remove mucus and foreign material. As with any patient, it is important that you continually assess and maintain the geriatric patient's airway.

Other respiratory changes due to aging include:

- Reduced strength and endurance of respiratory muscles
- Decreased chest wall flexibility
- Loss of lung elasticity
- Collapse of smaller airway structures

Cardiovascular System

Much of what affects the cardiovascular system seems related to lifestyle. Aging does affect it to a certain degree as well. In addition, medications prescribed to older adult patients for heart conditions can prevent effective compensation for blood loss. Geriatric trauma

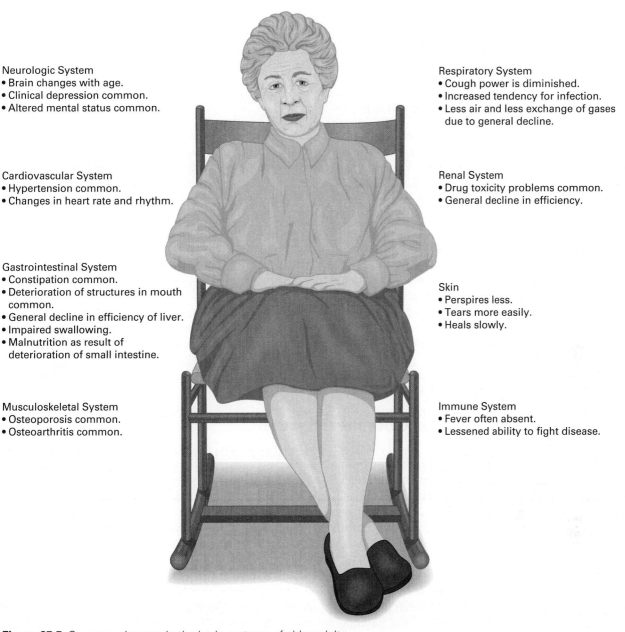

Neurologic System
- Brain changes with age.
- Clinical depression common.
- Altered mental status common.

Cardiovascular System
- Hypertension common.
- Changes in heart rate and rhythm.

Gastrointestinal System
- Constipation common.
- Deterioration of structures in mouth common.
- General decline in efficiency of liver.
- Impaired swallowing.
- Malnutrition as result of deterioration of small intestine.

Musculoskeletal System
- Osteoporosis common.
- Osteoarthritis common.

Respiratory System
- Cough power is diminished.
- Increased tendency for infection.
- Less air and less exchange of gases due to general decline.

Renal System
- Drug toxicity problems common.
- General decline in efficiency.

Skin
- Perspires less.
- Tears more easily.
- Heals slowly.

Immune System
- Fever often absent.
- Lessened ability to fight disease.

Figure 25.5 Common changes in the body systems of older adults.

patients who have lost a pint or more of blood should be treated for shock even if their signs and symptoms do not indicate it.

Age-related changes in the cardiovascular system include:

- Enlargement of the left ventricle, which can decrease the amount of blood moved by the heart
- Stiffening and elongation of the aorta, making it more susceptible to tearing
- Degeneration of the heart's electrical system, causing dysrhythmia
- Loss of elasticity in the blood vessels, which can result in high blood pressure and poor circulation

Nervous System

Aging has been shown to affect the nervous system in a few key areas. First, the brain loses about 10% of its overall weight between the ages of 20 and 90 years. Although this does *not* mean that older adult patients are less intelligent than younger ones (no relationship between brain size and intelligence has ever been found), it does mean that there is more room for destructive bleeding inside the skull following a blow to the head. Also, aging causes a substantial decrease in the overall number of nerve fibers and the speed at which the impulses travel across them. These deteriorations mean that older adult patients may experience some of the following changes over time:

- Decreased reaction times
- Difficulty with recent memory
- Psychomotor slowing

As you examine the geriatric patient, assess for sluggishness, confusion, or any mental status that appears below the level of full coherence. An altered mental status can indicate a wide range of illnesses and injuries, from infection and medication overdose to stroke and head trauma, all of which are very serious conditions. It is important that you summon advanced medical care for any older adult patient who presents with an abnormally altered mental status.

Always assume that an individual with an altered mental status is normally coherent and mentally sharp until you can determine otherwise by questioning caregivers or family members. If you operate on the assumption that a patient who seems confused, upset, or has a decreased level of consciousness always appears this way, you may fail to properly address an underlying medical problem.

Although not a normal part of aging or directly related to the effects of aging on the nervous system, depression is a common condition among older adult patients. In fact, suicides, or suicide attempts, are not unusual in the 65+ segment of the population, especially among men.[3] Be alert for signs of depression, such as poor hygiene, poor eating habits, insomnia, social withdrawal, memory problems, and disorderly living environments.

Musculoskeletal System

Age-related changes in the musculoskeletal system can lead to changes in posture, range of motion, and balance. Some older adults can even lose up to three inches of height due to deterioration of the discs between the vertebrae and the natural degeneration of muscle and connective tissues. Osteoporosis (Figure 25.6) is a disease that develops due to the loss of minerals from bones. That loss causes bones to soften and become weak, making older adults more susceptible to fractures from falls. Once they fall, the injuries can be very severe. Also keep in mind that age-related changes in the spine can result in curvatures, which can affect your ability to manage a patient's airway or effectively immobilize them following an injury.

When placing an older adult in full spinal precautions, you must take special care to use padding anywhere their body makes contact with the board. These patients often have very little skin and fat that could serve as padding. It may also be necessary to place extra padding under the patient's head, depending on the curvature of the spine.

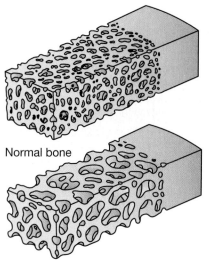

Normal bone

Osteoporotic bone

Figure 25.6 Osteoporosis causes a reduction in the quality of bone, making the skeletal tissue more brittle and less elastic.

FIRST ON SCENE *(continued)*

The man hands the towels to Mary, and she places them under Tom's head. "Do your best to remain still, Tom," Mary says as she begins to assess his pain. "Moving will only make it worse. Can you point to where you feel the most pain?"

"It's right here," Tom says, placing his hand on his right hip.

"Okay, I'm going to remove your shoes and socks so I can check the circulation in your feet." As Mary moves to Tom's feet

she notices that his right leg is somewhat shorter than his left. "Tom, can you feel me touching your feet?" she asks. "Do you feel any numbness or tingling in your feet?"

Just then, the man who brought the towels returns with a light blanket and offers it to cover Tom and keep him warm.

Integumentary System (Skin)

Age-related changes to the skin, such as thinner skin, wrinkles, or spots, are the most obvious. As people grow older, their skin loses its elasticity and thickness, causing it to be more easily torn or injured. You may notice dark areas of pigmentation on the skin, usually called "age spots" or "liver spots." The skin of a geriatric patient may be dry and flaky due to a decrease in the production of oils. The ability to perspire tends to decrease as well, making heat-related emergencies more common and the onset of shock harder to recognize. As skin grows thinner and weaker, cell reproduction slows down, so not only are skin injuries worse among older adults, but healing times can be greatly extended.

Assessment of Geriatric Patients

LO5 Explain the unique challenges that can arise when assessing and caring for the geriatric patient.

Your assessment of a geriatric patient will follow the same basic path as any other patient assessment, with a few additional considerations. As always, make sure you begin by taking appropriate BSI precautions.

Scene Size-up

In addition to ensuring that the scene is safe to enter, you also should survey the environment for evidence of the following:

- Inadequate food, shelter, or hygiene
- Lack of a functioning heating or cooling system
- Potential fall hazards
- Conditions that suggest abuse or neglect (Figure 25.7)

Primary Assessment

When you approach the patient, always focus on them instead of on caregivers or family members who may be present. This will show the patient you respect them as an individual and will give them a sense of control over the situation. If the patient is seated or in bed, position yourself at their level and make eye contact before introducing yourself (Figure 25.8).

Another way to show respect to the patient is to use their title and last name, such as Mrs. Becker or Mr. Flores. Avoid using nicknames such as "dear," "sweetie," or "honey." Also avoid using an older adult's first name (unless you are asked to use it); doing so could be considered rude or disrespectful. If appropriate, offer to shake the patient's hand during the introduction. This builds rapport while also giving you the ability to check the patient's skin signs and mobility in an unobtrusive way.

As with all patients, you will perform a complete primary assessment as the first step in the assessment process. As you approach the patient, make note of their position. Are they sitting up and alert, or are they lying in bed and unresponsive? The patient who is sitting up and aware of their surroundings clearly has a patent airway and is breathing. The patient who presents as unresponsive will require a more deliberate ABC check before you can move on to your secondary assessment.

Confirm that the patient has a clear airway and is breathing with an adequate rate and tidal volume. Confirm that they have an adequate pulse and there are no immediate threats to life before moving on to your secondary assessment.

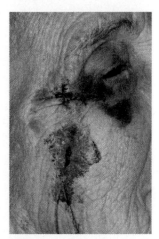

Figure 25.7 When you encounter evidence of trauma, consider the possibility of abuse until it is proven otherwise.
(Dr. P. Marazzi/Science Source)

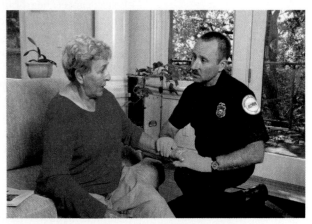

Figure 25.8 Position yourself at the patient's level, make eye contact, and speak slowly and clearly.

REMEMBER

Due to an increased risk of tuberculosis in nursing home patients, consider using a HEPA mask as part of your personal protective equipment (PPE).

REMEMBER

Geriatric patients often do not reveal problems behind the chief complaint because they either fear the loss of independence or they consider the illness "normal" for their age. The best way to determine the patient's chief complaint is to ask, "Why did you call today?" or "What is different about how you feel today?"

Obtaining a History

Unlike most younger patients, gathering a medical history for an older individual may take quite a bit of time. It is helpful to first obtain the patient's medications (prescription and over-the-counter) and then ask why each is taken. You can also get valuable information from the medication bottles such as the patient's name, health care provider's name, and directions for taking the medication. Also, be aware of the patient's surroundings. Are there medical identification tags or stickers? Oxygen supplies? Is there anything else that would indicate a medical condition? If you are unsure about a patient's answers to your questions, try to verify the information they give you with a reliable source such as a caregiver.

Physical Exam

The following considerations are important when examining a geriatric patient:

- Handle older adult patients gently.
- Histories and exams can easily tire older adult patients.
- Always explain what you are going to do before you do it.
- Anticipate numerous layers of clothing (due to problems with temperature regulation).
- Respect the modesty and privacy of older patients.

Some geriatric patients may deny or minimize symptoms during the physical exam. Often this is because they fear being hospitalized and losing their independence if the extent of their condition is "discovered."

The normal range for vital signs in the older adult is the same as that for any adult. The expectation that hypertension is a result of old age is a myth, and abnormal vital signs in the older adult should be taken as seriously as with any other patient.

Common Medical Problems of Geriatric Patients

LO6 Describe the common medical problems of geriatric patients.

LO7 Describe changes in the approach to care when caring for geriatric patients.

As we age and our bodies become less efficient, illnesses become more common. The average geriatric patient may be taking several different medications as treatment for various diseases or chronic conditions.

Illnesses

Common conditions among older adults include pneumonia; chronic obstructive pulmonary disease; cancer; heart failure; aneurysm; high blood pressure; dementia; Parkinson's disease, diabetes; bleeding in the stomach, esophagus or intestines; urinary tract infections; and reactions to medications. Due to the thinning of skin, a decreased ability to perspire, and muted physical sensations, heat- and cold-related emergencies are also common among geriatric patients.

Another illness that affects more than 5.7 million adults in the United States is **Alzheimer's disease**.[4] Alzheimer's is a progressive, degenerative disease that affects the brain and results in impaired memory, thinking, and behavior. Approximately 19% of people aged 75 to 84 have Alzheimer's, and that number is expected to reach nearly 50% by the year 2050.[5] As it progresses, the patient is less able to properly care for their own needs.

Alzheimer's disease ▶ progressive, degenerative disease that attacks the brain and results in impaired memory, thinking, and behavior.

Injuries

Trauma from falls is the leading cause of injury and death among older adults. The weakening of bones, deterioration of skin integrity, and loss of blood vessel flexibility combine to make injuries much more severe for geriatric patients. In addition, the medications taken by many older adults, including those that can prevent clotting, make controlling bleeding extremely difficult. In many cases, what might be a relatively minor injury for a young patient might actually cause serious injury or even death for an older patient.

Take extra time to investigate the details surrounding the fall. If possible, attempt to find out if the fall was "mechanical" or "medical" in nature. A **mechanical fall** is caused by a defined slip, trip, or loss of balance. Tripping on the edge of a rug or losing one's balance are examples of a mechanical fall. A person who is unable to describe a cause or does not remember falling may have experienced a medical issue such as low blood pressure, seizure, or heart dysrhythmia that ultimately led to the fall. It is important to maintain a high index of suspicion for an underlying medical problem for patients experiencing nonmechanical falls.

As an Emergency Medical Responder, you should be an advocate for injury prevention among the older adult population. As you respond to patients in their homes, you should always be looking for potential dangers, such as unsecured rugs, loose handrails, and unsafely stacked items, and make a caregiver or family member aware of the safety concerns.

Elder Abuse and Neglect

LO8 Describe common signs and symptoms of abuse and neglect of older adults.

LO9 Explain the role of the Emergency Medical Responder in cases of suspected abuse and/or neglect of older adults.

Elder and dependent adult abuse is the mistreatment or neglect of an older individual (age 65+) or an adult with a disability. A dependent adult is a person between the ages of 18 and 64 who has a physical, developmental, or emotional disability.

Elder neglect is the abandonment or deprivation of basic needs such as water, food, housing, clothing, or medical care. Another form of abuse that affects this population is **self-neglect**, characterized by the inability or unwillingness to care for oneself. Self-neglect can be a deliberate act on the part of older adults, who have purposely given up or intentionally stopped caring for themselves. It can also result from illness, dementia, or physical limitations.

Elder abuse comes in many forms, including:

- *Physical abuse*, such as hitting, pushing, causing unnecessary pain, intentional misuse of medication, causing injury, and unauthorized restraint
- *Sexual abuse*, such as inappropriate exposure, inappropriate sexual advances, inappropriate sexual contact, sexual exploitation, and rape
- *Emotional or verbal abuse*, such as humiliation, threats of harm or abandonment, isolation, noncommunication, and intimidation
- *Financial abuse*, such as undue influence to change legal documents, misuse of property, and theft or embezzlement

Signs of Abuse and Neglect   The signs of abuse and neglect are not always obvious and are sometimes difficult to identify. In many cases, the injuries or circumstances can be blamed on conditions that affect older adults such as dementia, coexisting illnesses, and more frequent falls.

Clues you might discover during your physical exam that may indicate abuse or neglect include:

- Sores, bruises, or other wounds
- Unkempt appearance
- Poor hygiene
- Malnutrition
- Dehydration
- Unrealistic or vague explanations for injuries
- An obvious delay in seeking care
- Unexplained injuries (past or present)
- Poor interaction between patient and caregiver (if applicable)

mechanical fall ▶ fall caused by a defined slip, trip or loss of balance.

REMEMBER

Many medications prescribed for older adults include those that can prevent blood clotting and, as a result, make controlling bleeding more difficult. Apply gentle pressure to bleeding wounds and elevate them above the heart. You may have to continue holding pressure on the wound longer than usual.

REMEMBER

An older adult patient who has sustained an injury has a greater likelihood of developing hypothermia, even in an environment that you would consider mild or warm. Carefully monitor body temperature and ensure that the patient is kept warm at all times.

REMEMBER

Remember that a fall often has more than one cause. When assessing an older adult who has fallen, be sure to thoroughly investigate the exact cause and interview anyone who may have witnessed the event.

elder neglect ▶ failure by caregivers to provide for the basic needs of an older adult.

self-neglect ▶ condition in which an individual fails to attend to their basic needs, such as hygiene, food, appropriate clothing, and medical care.

elder abuse ▶ physical, sexual, emotional, or financial abuse of an older adult.

A common problem for older adults who have been confined to a bed or wheelchair for extended periods of time is the development of bed sores. Bed sores, also called pressure sores or decubitus ulcers, are caused by pressure on areas of the skin that are deprived of proper blood circulation. They most often develop on skin that covers bony areas of the body, such as the heels, ankles, hips, and tailbone. Bed sores can become open sores and can easily get infected if not identified early and cared for properly. You should always be on the lookout for evidence of bed sores during your assessment. Infected bed sores can also be a sign of neglect.

REMEMBER

U.S. states have laws that require Emergency Medical Responders to report suspected cases of geriatric abuse and neglect. Make sure you are familiar with your local requirements.

Advocating for Older Adults As an Emergency Medical Responder, you have a duty to serve as an advocate for your patients, especially those who may not be able to care for or advocate for themselves. When caring for older adults, be especially diligent when obtaining a history and performing your physical exam. Be sure to evaluate for signs and symptoms that may not necessarily pertain to the chief complaint.

Much like any suspected case of abuse or neglect, you have an obligation to carefully and thoroughly document your findings objectively and report all cases of suspected abuse or neglect to the proper authorities. All 50 states have specific guidelines for reporting elder abuse and neglect, and your instructor can provide you with the details for your state.

Suicide in Older Adults

LO10 Describe the incidence and risk factors for suicide in older adults.

Suicide is a significant problem affecting older adults. Suicide rates are particularly high among older men, with men aged 85 and older having the highest rate of any group in the country.[6] Suicide attempts by older adults are much more likely to result in death than among younger persons. Reasons include:

- Older adults plan more carefully and use more deadly methods.
- Older adults are less likely to be discovered and rescued.
- The physical frailty of older adults means they are less likely to recover from a suicide attempt.

Risk factors:

- Depression and other mental health problems
- Substance use problems (including prescription medications)
- Physical illness, disability, and pain
- Social isolation

Protective factors:

- Care for mental and physical health problems
- Social connectedness
- Positive family relationships and support
- Skills in coping and adapting to change

FIRST ON SCENE WRAP-UP

"He's right over here," An observer directs the EMTs over to the court.

"Hello, Sir, my name is Jason. I'm an EMT," Jason says as he kneels beside Tom, placing his gloved hand on his radial pulse as he does so.

"My hip. I think I broke my hip," Tom says, grimacing. "Please, can I have something for the pain?"

"I'm going to do everything I can to make you as comfortable as possible and get you the help you need. Right now I'm going to walk you through how my partner and I are going to do that, okay?" Jason says.

"Okay," Tom nods, still grimacing.

"You did a great job keeping him comfortable," Jason says to Mary and the others. "Nice work on assessing his hip and leg and confirming circulation and feeling in his foot."

"We'll get you to the hospital where your hip can be scanned, and the doctors can determine the next steps," Jason tells Tom. "The fact that you're physically active is probably going to help a lot in your recovery, and we hope you'll be back out here in no time."

Summary

- The assessment and emergency care of geriatric patients can sometimes be challenging due to age-related changes in the human body.
- Many geriatric patients have multiple illnesses, take multiple prescription and over-the-counter medications, have problems with mobility, and may have issues of incontinence.
- The respiratory system can experience reduction in strength and endurance of the muscles that assist in breathing, loss of lung elasticity, and collapsing of the smaller airway structures, all of which contribute to respiratory challenges.
- The circulatory system can be affected by thickening of the walls of the heart, reduction in the effectiveness of the heart's conduction system, and loss of elasticity of the blood vessels, which can cause problems such as reduced cardiac output, dysrhythmia, and aneurysms that can burst.
- Age-related deterioration of the nervous system can cause slowing of psychomotor functioning, decreased reaction times, forgetfulness, and loss of sensation and coordination, which is often the cause of falls among older adults.
- Osteoporosis and degeneration of the musculoskeletal system can cause bone weakness and general instability, which can lead to falls and serious injuries. You also will notice degeneration-related curvature of the spine in some older adult patients, which makes immobilization and airway maintenance a challenge.
- Aging changes the skin in several important ways. The skin becomes thinner, weaker, more susceptible to tears and injuries and, due to sluggish cellular regeneration, it can be very slow to heal.
- When assessing a geriatric patient, remember to look for things in the environment such as unsafe conditions, nonworking heating and cooling systems, and signs that may indicate abuse or neglect.
- Be respectful when physically examining a geriatric patient, ensuring modesty and privacy.
- Elder abuse can come in many forms, including physical, emotional, sexual, and financial.
- As an Emergency Medical Responder, you have a legal duty to report suspected cases of elder abuse and neglect to the appropriate authorities.

Take Action

Getting to Know You

As a younger individual, it may be impossible to truly understand what it feels like to get old. However, you can strive to better understand the struggles and frustrations older adults face as a result of the aging process. For this activity, identify someone in your life who is above the age of 65 and perhaps close to 80 if possible. Make an appointment to sit down with the individual and discuss, from a medical standpoint, what the aging experience has been like. You should explain that this is part of your training as an Emergency Medical Responder. If possible, ask to be allowed to perform a patient assessment, including a history and vital signs. Your goals are to better understand the feelings, struggles, and frustrations that come with age and to better care for an older adult who may become ill or injured.

First on Scene Patient Handoff

Tom is 68 and took a mechanical fall, landing hard on his right side. He denies hitting his head and did not lose consciousness. His chief complaint is pain in the area of the right hip. I assessed both distal extremities, and circulation, sensation, and motor function all appear normal in both. We have kept him still and comfortable while waiting for EMS.

First on Scene Run Review

Recall the events of the First on Scene scenario in this chapter, and answer the following questions related to the call. Rationales are offered in the Answer Key at the back of the book.

1. How could Mary make the scene safe?
2. How should Mary assess Tom's condition?
3. What information should Mary give to the EMTs?

Quick Quiz

To check your understanding of the chapter, answer the following questions. Then compare your answers to those in the Answer Key at the back of the book.

1. Geriatric patients are often less able to defend against illness and may take much longer to recover when they do become ill. This often results in:
   a. multiple simultaneous illnesses.
   b. forgetting doctor appointments.
   c. taking the wrong medications.
   d. hearing loss.

2. Which of the following is NOT a common factor that would influence your assessment strategy for geriatric patients?
   a. Hearing loss
   b. Limited mobility
   c. Vision loss
   d. Ability to stand

3. You are caring for a 92-year-old patient who lives alone. She complains of worsening symptoms of her chronic illness. She hands you a bag of medications and states, "I have trouble reading all of these labels." This patient's presentation may be caused by:
   a. elder abuse.
   b. infectious disease.
   c. taking the wrong amount of medication.
   d. trauma.

4. The loss of mobility is a common complaint among older adults and can lead to other problems, such as:
   a. skeletal fractures.
   b. hearing loss.
   c. depression.
   d. near-sightedness.

5. The inability to retain urine or feces is called:
   a. dementia.
   b. aphasia.
   c. priapism.
   d. incontinence.

6. When performing the physical exam on a geriatric patient, remember that:
   a. older adult patients may become tired quickly.
   b. you should speak only to the patient's caregiver.
   c. older adult patents do not like to be touched.
   d. you should avoid explaining what you are doing; the patient knows what to expect.

7. All of the following are ways the respiratory system is affected by the aging process EXCEPT:
   a. increased strength of respiratory muscles.
   b. decreased flexibility of the chest.
   c. collapse of the smaller airways.
   d. loss of elasticity.

8. The aging process can cause a degeneration of the heart's electrical system, which can lead to:
   a. hearing loss.
   b. vision loss.
   c. dysrhythmias.
   d. stroke.

9. Age-related changes in the musculoskeletal system can lead to changes in posture, range of motion, and:
   a. awareness.
   b. medication usage.
   c. mental status.
   d. balance.

10. U.S. states have laws that require Emergency Medical Responders to report suspected cases of:
    a. dementia.
    b. abuse and neglect.
    c. Alzheimer's disease.
    d. overdose.

11. You have been called to the home of an older adult and discover that she is refusing care. She states that she just wants to be left alone. You observe that the patient lives alone, is wearing only undergarments, and has multiple open sores and bruises over her body. These are most likely the signs of:
    a. abuse.
    b. illegal drug use.
    c. self-neglect.
    d. Alzheimer's.

12. While caring for a geriatric patient, he tells you that his caregiver frequently leaves him alone in his bedroom for days and refuses to respond to his calls for assistance. This may be considered:
    a. physical abuse.
    b. emotional abuse.
    c. neglect.
    d. sexual abuse.

Endnotes

1. The World Bank; https://data.worldbank.org/indicator/SP.POP.65UP.TO.ZS, Accessed November 2022.

2. Sharma M., Loh K.P., Nightingale G., Mohile S.G., Holmes H.M. "Polypharmacy and Potentially Inappropriate Medication Use in Geriatric Oncology," *Journal of Geriatric Oncology*, Vol. 7, No. 5 (September 2016): 346–353. doi: 10.1016/j.jgo.2016.07.010. Epub 2016 Aug 3. PMID: 27498305; PMCID: PMC5037024.

3. Ding O.J., Kennedy G.J. "Understanding Vulnerability to Late-Life Suicide," *Current Psychiatry Report*, Vol. 23, No. 9 (July 2021): 58. doi: 10.1007/s11920-021-01268-2. PMID: 34273004; PMCID: PMC8286047.

4. Khan S., Barve K.H., Kumar M.S. "Recent Advancements in Pathogenesis, Diagnostics and Treatment of Alzheimer's Disease," *Current Neuropharmacology*, Vol. 18, No. 11 (2020): 1106–1125. doi: 10.2174/1570159X18666200528142429. PMID: 32484110; PMCID: PMC7709159.

5. Ibid.

6. Centers for Disease Control and Prevention. (2014). Fatal injury reports, national and regional, 1999–2014, https://webappa.cdc.gov/sasweb/ncipc/mortrate10_us.html, accessed November 2022.

26

Introduction to EMS Operations and Hazardous Response

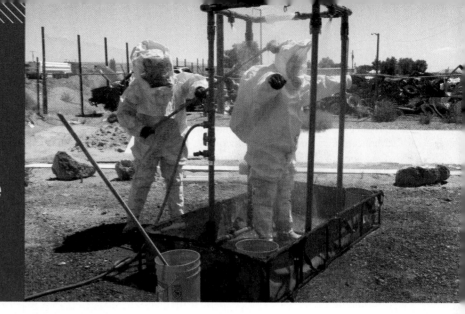

LEARNING OBJECTIVES

Upon successful completion of this chapter, the student should be able to:

Cognitive

1. Define the chapter key terms.

2. Describe the common equipment necessary to appropriately respond to an emergency.

3. Explain the importance of keeping all equipment serviceable and ready at all times.

4. Describe the phases of an emergency call.

5. Explain the appropriate use of lights and sirens when responding to or from an emergency scene.

6. Explain the concept of due regard when responding in an emergency vehicle.

7. Describe common devices used at the scene of an emergency to keep personnel and the scene safe.

8. Explain the role of the Emergency Medical Responder during extrication operations.

9. Describe common hazards during vehicle extrication operations.

10. Differentiate various methods for gaining access to an entrapped patient.

11. Differentiate simple vs. complex access as it pertains to patient extrication.

12. Discuss strategies for safely gaining entry into buildings.

13. Discuss strategies for safely managing a scene where fire is present.

14. Discuss strategies for safely managing a scene where there may be evidence of a natural gas leak.

15. Discuss strategies for safely managing a scene where high voltage electricity may be present.

16. Explain the role of the Emergency Medical Responder at a hazardous materials incident.

17. Describe the common signs of a potential hazardous materials incident.

18. Differentiate the purpose of cold, warm, and hot zones at a hazardous materials incident.

Psychomotor

19. Demonstrate the ability to identify and manage common hazards at a simulated emergency response.

20. Demonstrate the process for proper cleaning and decontamination of equipment following a simulated emergency response.

21. Demonstrate how to use the *Emergency Response Guidebook* appropriately to identify a suspected hazardous material.

Affective

22. Value the importance of always being ready and prepared for an emergency response by keeping equipment serviceable and ready for a response.

As you have undoubtedly learned by now, Emergency Medical Responders respond to a wide variety of incidents involving ill and injured patients. Each of these responses is commonly referred to as a "call," and each call is composed of several steps or phases. This chapter describes each phase of a call and the requirements for each phase. It also describes several of the more common call types and the knowledge and skills required to respond safely and efficiently. The Emergency Medical Responder's role in a hazardous materials incident is also included.

FIRST ON SCENE

"Okay, people, we're rolling!" Greg shouts into the bullhorn.

Greg is the safety supervisor for Legend Studios. He watches as the small army of technicians and pyrotechnicians don safety goggles and squint against the anticipated propane explosion. It is a cool, dark night, and once the floodlights are doused, the five-story-tall green screen is in total darkness. The only light still visible on the film set is the red light indicating the camera is on.

After a full minute of silence, somebody swears loudly and yells for the lights. The generators cough and sputter to life, and the floodlights warm and grow steadily brighter until the entire set is illuminated in harsh, white light.

"What's the problem?" Greg asks the pyrotechnician hovering above the control box.

"I don't know," the man says. "It should have gone." He is interrupted by a deafening rushing sound, like a tornado passing directly overhead. Jets of flame erupt like large, boiling clouds from the pressure valve at the far end of the pipe system.

The explosion immediately superheats the night air and sends the crew scattering in all directions as the huge green screen catches fire. The flames race up the fabric, sending burning bits fluttering downward.

"Shut it off!" Greg shouts as he tries to avoid the flames floating down from the sky like glowing snowflakes. "Everybody out!"

The lead pyrotechnician succeeds in shutting off the main propane valve, but it is too late. The green screen is fully engulfed and raining fire down onto a bank of large propane tanks on a nearby concrete pad. Greg dials 911 on his cell phone as he and the crowd of technicians run east along the main studio access road.

Safety First

Your first consideration at any emergency scene is your own safety. To ensure it, you must learn to follow standard operating procedures (SOPs), limit your actions to your specific level of training, and use the proper equipment and the required number of trained individuals for any task (Figure 26.1). SOPs are specific and different for every department,

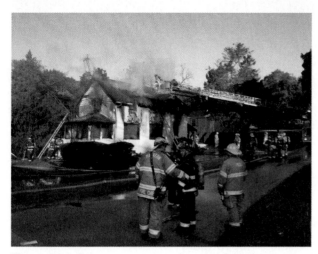

Figure 26.1 Ensure your own safety and that of your crew before entering the scene.
(© Edward T. Dickinson, MD)

service, and jurisdiction. SOPs outline how you will function operationally within your own organization.

There will always be risks associated with emergency responses, but EMS personnel must minimize those risks by learning which ones can be controlled before entering the scene. You must be able to develop a risk-vs.-benefit analysis mentality. You need to ask yourself, "Does the risk related to my actions on the scene have a measurable benefit?" There is a fine line between aggressiveness and recklessness. This is the gray area of risk management and decision making for which *all* of us in emergency services are responsible. Always remember: some risks you can avoid, some risks you can pass off to other agencies, and some risks you must face.

EMS demands effective management of risk. For example, you have no control over the chance that a drunk driver could crash into you as you provide care at the scene of a traffic collision. Through the proper use of warning devices such as reflective vests, roadside reflectors and/or flares, and positioning response vehicles properly to divert traffic, you can minimize your risk of being injured by passing cars (Figure 26.2). At any emergency scene, these rules must always be followed:

- As you approach the scene, do your best to identify any immediate and potential hazards. If you identify a hazard, make sure you can control it before you approach. If you cannot control a hazard, request assistance.
- Use the protective gear appropriate for the situation and for which you are trained and qualified to wear. Examples include firefighting turnout gear, hazmat suit, eye protection, and gloves. Federal regulations require that all emergency responders wear an approved high-visibility safety vest when working on a highway. This requirement applies to *all* emergency responders.
- Legally and ethically, you are limited by your level of training and scope of practice. If you attempt to act beyond your level of training, you may risk injury to yourself, cause harm to the patient, or add to the extent of the incident.
- If you are the first to arrive at an incident, provide dispatch with a verbal assessment of the scene and request any additional resources sooner rather than later.

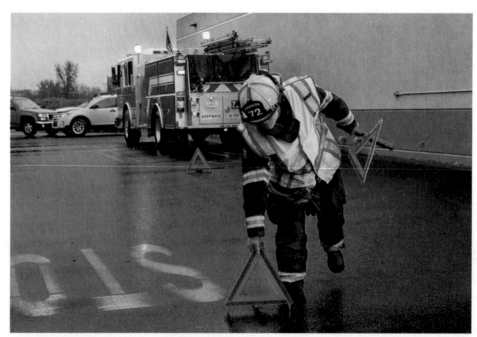

Figure 26.2 Once you arrive, there are many ways you can make the scene safer.

The Call

LO2 Describe the common equipment necessary to appropriately respond to an emergency.

LO3 Explain the importance of keeping all equipment serviceable and ready at all times.

LO4 Describe the phases of an emergency call.

You must be prepared at all times to perform your duties on any emergency call. One of your first duties at the beginning of every shift is to thoroughly check all equipment and confirm it is in working order (Figure 26.3).

All EMS responses progress through several phases. These phases may differ slightly, depending on the level of care you provide. There are six common phases to the typical emergency response:

- Preparation
- Dispatch
- En route to the scene
- At the scene
- Transfer of care
- Post-call preparation

Phase 1: Preparation

Being prepared means having the proper training, tools, equipment, and personnel ready to go at all times. In many EMS systems, there are clearly defined minimum equipment lists that specify the items that must be carried on each response vehicle.

- *Medical supplies.* Make sure that your unit is stocked with medical supplies such as airways, suctioning equipment, ventilation devices (pocket face masks, bag-mask device), and basic wound-care supplies (dressings, bandages).
- *Nonmedical supplies.* Check for other necessary items such as personal safety equipment, including gloves, masks, and eye protection. Many response vehicles also carry flares, flashlights, fire extinguishers, blankets, simple tools (e.g., screwdrivers, hammer, spring-loaded center punch), and area maps.

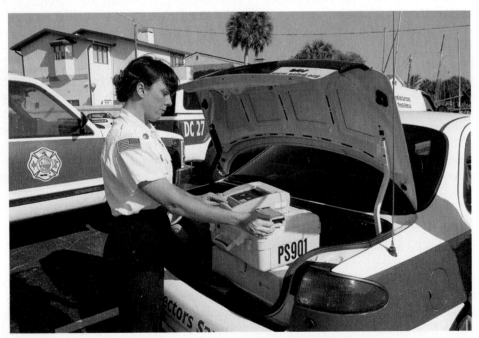

Figure 26.3 You must check all of your equipment at the start of each shift.

- *Vehicle.* Be sure to complete a thorough inspection of the vehicle and all its components at the beginning of each shift. Check the engine compartment and fluid levels of your vehicle (fuel, oil, transmission fluid, diesel exhaust fluid (DEF), coolant, windshield washer). It is also important to check the emergency equipment, including flashing lights, sirens, and radios.
- *Personnel.* Ensure that the appropriate number of qualified personnel are on duty for your shift. Each individual may be required to maintain current certifications such as CPR and driver's licenses.

Phase 2: Dispatch

Learn everything you can about your dispatch or communications system and the procedures you are to follow when dispatched. Make note of any information the dispatcher gives you about the call.

Most dispatch systems have a central dispatch or communications center with 24-hour access. Dispatch centers are staffed with personnel trained to dispatch the most appropriate units. Many dispatch centers utilize specially trained personnel who can provide prearrival instructions to the caller over the telephone while EMS personnel are en route. These dispatchers use a system called Emergency Medical Dispatch (EMD). This system allows the dispatcher to carefully screen each call with a scripted list of questions. The goal is to identify the problem so the most appropriate resources can be dispatched at the appropriate priority or code.

All dispatchers are trained to gather as much information from the caller as possible and relay that information to responding units. The nature of the call, location of the incident or patient, number of victims, and severity of illness or injury, as well as any other problems that responders might encounter at the scene, are important pieces of information and must be relayed to responding personnel.

REMEMBER

The information received from dispatch can be incomplete or incorrect. Always expect the unexpected when responding to what would otherwise appear to be a routine dispatch.

Phase 3: En Route to the Scene

LO5 Explain the appropriate use of lights and sirens when responding to or coming from an emergency scene.

LO6 Explain the concept of due regard when responding in an emergency vehicle.

Emergency Medical Responder duties while en route to an emergency scene include more than simply finding the location. State vehicle codes give special privileges to operators of emergency vehicles when responding to an emergency. However, these privileges do not relieve the operator from the responsibility of keeping everyone's safety in mind. You must always operate an emergency vehicle with **due regard** for the safety of everyone on the road. Failure to do so is risky and may result in fines and penalties from local law enforcement.

due regard ▶ appropriate care and concern for the safety of others.

Emergency lights must be on for all emergency responses. Sirens should be used when traffic is an issue and when approaching and traveling through intersections. Some jurisdictions require the use of lights and sirens for all emergency responses. Your ability to drive defensively and anticipate the actions of other drivers will help ensure a safe response.

You must communicate with dispatch and keep them informed of any delays you may encounter while en route. Be sure you have the essential information on the call, such as location, potential hazards, and number of patients. Do not hesitate to check back with the dispatcher if you need more information.

Phase 4: At the Scene

When arriving at the scene, be extra alert and approach cautiously. Look for hazards. Position your response unit where you have access to it but where it will not interfere with access to the scene by other responders. If you are the first to arrive on scene, a good rule of thumb is to position your vehicle 50 feet before the scene with emergency lights or flashers activated. Remember to always keep your eye on traffic. Do not become a victim yourself. Whenever possible, position your vehicle as if there were a hazardous materials spill—that is, upwind and uphill from the crash scene.

Notify the dispatcher of your arrival. Because dispatchers can communicate only what they are given from the reporting party, you may have to provide additional information once you arrive on scene, such as:

- Actual location of the incident if it is different from what was given on dispatch
- Type of incident and the need for additional resources (e.g., utility company, air medical helicopter, law enforcement)
- Number of victims

Size up the scene to make sure it is safe. Do your best to identify any hazards before entering. Put on your PPE (and reflective vests if working on a roadway). As you approach, look for the mechanism of injury in trauma scenes or determine if it is a medical emergency.

Always stabilize vehicles before entering them or attempting to extricate any patients. Determine if it is a multiple-casualty incident and, if so, determine the approximate number of patients. Evaluate patients quickly to determine if they are high or low priority. Do you need to move patients immediately? Can it be done safely? Will you need more assistance? Let the dispatcher know what additional resources you are going to need as soon as possible.

Phase 5: Transfer of Care

Emergency Medical Responders assess for and manage immediate life threats. They also lift, carry, and load patients on appropriate devices and assist in preparing the patients for transport. While doing so, be sure to use appropriate lifting and moving techniques. You also need to provide the transporting personnel with an accurate account of the patient's status. If practical, provide them with written documentation of your assessment findings. In some instances, you may be asked to ride along in the transport vehicle and assist the EMTs or paramedics with care en route to the hospital.

Phase 6: Post-Call Preparation

Once a call is finished, you must immediately prepare for the next call, including cleaning and disinfecting equipment, restocking supplies, and refueling the emergency vehicle. You should also complete paperwork and file reports, participate in debriefing, and finally, notify the dispatcher that you are back in service.

CREW RESOURCE MANAGEMENT

All crew members must keep an eye out for safety through every stage of every call. No one should be afraid to speak up and make others aware of a potential hazard or concern.

Motor Vehicle Collisions

LO7 Describe common devices used at the scene of an emergency to keep personnel and the scene safe.

LO8 Explain the role of the Emergency Medical Responder during extrication operations.

LO9 Describe common hazards during vehicle extrication operations.

Emergency Medical Responder responsibilities at motor vehicle collisions will vary, depending on the type of agency, jurisdiction, regulations, and SOPs. Once you ensure your own safety, your main duty at the scene of an emergency is to provide patient care. At the scene of a motor vehicle collision, you may have other duties to perform before you can reach the patients. Your responsibilities at the scene may include:

- Making the scene safe for other responders and bystanders
- Requesting additional resources as appropriate
- Gaining access to patients

- Freeing trapped patients
- Evaluating patients and providing emergency care
- Quickly moving patients who are in danger from fire, explosion, and other hazards

Many Emergency Medical Responders are injured each year as they attempt to help at vehicle collisions. They are struck by another vehicle when they do not take initial steps to make the scene safe. Your first step is to secure an area around the scene so you can work safely.

Law enforcement officers and firefighters must follow their department's SOPs when working around vehicle collisions. However, if you are an Emergency Medical Responder without a special course in collision-scene procedures, use the items listed here as guidelines. Because each collision scene is unique, you will need to proceed with caution, carefully observe the scene, and decide which actions to take to control it. Follow these steps:

1. If you are first on the scene, position your vehicle approximately 50 feet before the scene. Turn on your vehicle's emergency flashers. You may want to use your headlights to light up the scene. If so, be sure to angle your vehicle so it does not blind oncoming drivers.
2. Make certain you have parked in a safe location. Look for fuel spills and fire. If you are downhill from the scene, fuel may run in your direction. Check the wind direction. Will the wind carry smoke or fire to where you have parked?
3. If your jurisdiction or agency has SOPs for positioning your unit and using warning lights, follow those guidelines. If you turn off the unit, you cannot leave your warning lights on because the battery will be drained of all power and you will be unable to start your vehicle.
4. Set out emergency warning devices, such as cones, flashing lights, or flares, to warn others. On high-speed roads, place one of those devices at least 250 feet from the scene. On low-speed roads, set one of the devices at least 100 feet from the scene. Add at least 25 feet to those distances if the scene is on a curved road.
5. As you approach, check the scene again for safety. Is there fire or leaking fuel? Are there unstable vehicles or downed electrical wires? If any of those conditions are present, make certain to request the appropriate resources to mitigate the hazards. If a power line is down, get the nearest pole number so you may request that the power be turned off. You may need fire services and a rescue squad at the scene. Some jurisdictions automatically dispatch these units for motor vehicle collisions.
6. As you approach, observe the scene for clues. How many patients can you see? Could someone have been thrown from a vehicle? Could someone have walked away from the scene? Do you see signs indicating that children were in the vehicle (e.g., car seat, toys, backpack)? Are there signs that a pedestrian or bike rider was involved? Have someone alert the dispatcher and report the number of possible patients.
7. If the scene is safe, stabilize the vehicle by chocking the wheels (placing wedges made of sturdy material against the wheels to prevent movement), gain access to the patients, perform your assessments, and begin care on those who appear to be most critical.

Do not approach or attempt to gain access to victims if the scene is not safe. If you cannot control traffic, electrical lines are down, there is fire at the scene, or there are fuel or hazardous material spills, you are in danger. Call the dispatcher for additional resources for any of those conditions. An Emergency Medical Responder's first priority is personal safety. Your primary duty is to provide patient care once it is reasonably safe to do so. Do only what you have been trained to do.

Upright Vehicle

In most traffic collisions, the vehicles involved remain upright and are generally safer to approach than overturned vehicles. Even though the vehicles appear to be stable, with little chance of rolling or sliding away from the at-rest position, it is still necessary to take the precaution of stabilizing the vehicle.

SCENE SAFETY

As you approach the scene of a vehicle collision, perform a "windshield survey." From inside your vehicle, get a 360-degree general impression of the scene through all windows. Look carefully for signs of fluid spilling from any of the vehicles. Avoid driving through or parking over the spills or in the path of a fluid as it spreads. Consider all fluids as potentially flammable. Be very aware of changing conditions.

SCENE SAFETY

Thousands of people are injured and even killed while attempting to assist at the scene of a vehicle collision. Make certain to ensure your safety before attempting to care for patients.

Always evaluate vehicle stability when you assess the scene. As you look for traffic hazards, electrical hazards, spilled fuel, and fire, also determine if there is any chance the vehicle may roll away or flip over. If you have immediate access, make sure that vehicles are in park, the ignition is turned off, and the emergency brake is set. You may find the following situations:

- *Hills or slight inclines.* The vehicle may have come to rest on a surface that slants enough to allow forward or backward roll. To keep the vehicle from rolling, place wheel chocks, spare tires, logs, rocks, or similar objects under one or more wheels.
- *Slippery surfaces.* Ice, snow, water, or oil can produce a slippery road surface. If available, sprinkle dirt, sand, ashes, or kitty litter, or place newspapers around the wheels and chock the wheels to reduce the chances of slipping.
- *Tilted vehicle.* Even upright vehicles may be tilted to one side by their position or by the terrain. Do not work beneath a tilted vehicle or on the downhill side of one. Chocking the wheels may prevent the vehicle from tipping over but tying the vehicle in place is safer. If strong rope is available, tie lines to the frame of the car (not the bumper) in front and back or to both sides. Then secure the lines to large trees or poles, guardrails, or heavier stable vehicles while waiting for fire services to arrive.
- *Stacked vehicles.* Part of one vehicle may be resting on top of another vehicle. There are several ways to stabilize them: chock the wheels of both vehicles; insert tires, lumber, blocks, or similar sturdy items between the road surface and the vehicles; or use line or rope to tie and secure both vehicles.

Overturned Vehicle

Do not try to right an overturned vehicle. Even if you have enough help to turn the vehicle upright, moving it can cause further injury to the occupants. Stabilize the overturned vehicle while waiting for fire service units and before you try to reach the occupants. Always look for fuel spills, battery acid, and other chemical hazards around an overturned vehicle.

Vehicle on Its Side

LO10 Differentiate various methods for gaining access to an entrapped patient.

LO11 Differentiate simple vs. complex access as it pertains to patient extrication.

If you find a vehicle on its side and have some simple equipment, take the following precautions to stabilize it. You should:

1. Stabilize the vehicle with items such as tires, blocks, lumber, wheel chocks, rocks, or similar available materials. Place the items between the road surface and the roofline. Also, place stabilizing items between the road surface and the lower wheels, if the wheels are not resting on the road surface.
2. If the vehicle is still unstable, use a strong rope or line to tie the vehicle to secure objects.
3. Attempt to gain access to occupants of the vehicle. Entry through a door is dangerous because the door may be 7 feet or more off the ground, and your weight will move the vehicle as you climb on it. It will also be difficult to open the door with the vehicle on its side. Your first and more sensible entry point will be through a window. The rear window is the best approach. Never attempt access to a damaged interior through broken glass without adequate protective clothing and equipment.
4. If you open a door, tie it securely open. Do not use a prop. Props can slip or be knocked away, causing the door to slam on you or the occupants.

Vehicle Access Never try to enter or work around a vehicle until you are certain it is stable. Once you stabilize a vehicle, there are two access methods for reaching a patient: **simple access** and **complex access**. Simple access does not require equipment. Complex access requires tools and special equipment, which also calls for additional training. In most cases, you will approach an upright, stable vehicle and reach the patient by simple access.

simple access ▶ form of access to entrapped patients that does not require tools or specialized equipment.

complex access ▶ form of access to patients that requires tools and specialized equipment.

If the doors and windows are closed, there are four ways to gain access:

- *Open the doors.* Many people drive without locking the doors. However, many models automatically lock once they reach a speed of 5 to 15 miles per hour. Some lock when the driver puts the transmission in drive. Check all the doors, including side and rear doors on vans and hatchbacks, before trying another entry method. If all doors are locked, one of the occupants may be able to unlock a door. "Try before you pry."
- *Enter through a window.* If access via a door isn't possible, the patient may be able to roll down a window. If not, you will have to break a window. When you begin using tools for access, the process becomes more complex. Remember, you must wear the proper PPE for vehicle **extrication** as you will be placing yourself in danger with sharp objects. Helmet, eye protection, gloves, and turnout coat and pants are recommended.
- *Pry open the doors.* This method is very time-consuming and not very practical given the technology available today. Access through windows is usually more practical.
- *Cut through the metal.* The only other access when entry through doors and windows is not possible is cutting through vehicle roofs, trunks, and/or doors. This entry method requires special tools that Emergency Medical Responders do not usually carry unless they are members of fire services. If you cannot gain access through a door or window, it may be possible to cut around the lock of a door using a sharp tool (chisel or strong screwdriver) and a hammer.

extrication ▶ coordinated removal of entrapped patients from vehicles and structures.

Your instructor will teach you how to use these entry methods if they are Emergency Medical Responder skills in your jurisdiction.

Keep in mind that speed is sometimes crucial when you need to reach patients in a vehicle. Precious time is lost if you must return to your vehicle to retrieve tools. Take all tools with you as you approach a vehicle. Many simple tools will help you gain access to a vehicle, including a screwdriver, chisel, hammer, and pry bar. Some Emergency Medical Responder tool kits include commercial Slim Jims for unlocking doors and spring-loaded center punches for breaking glass. Access with tools and special equipment takes time, planning, and sometimes special training. It also requires taking additional safety precautions to protect yourself and the patient.

Unlocking Vehicle Doors   Tools for unlocking doors may be part of your Emergency Medical Responder kit. You might be able to unlock doors of older vehicles by slipping a Slim Jim between the window and the door. You also might be able to pry open the window with a wood wedge or pry bar and slip a wire coat hanger inside the window (Key Skill 26.1). Opening newer locks using these methods might be impossible, depending on the manufacturer. Some cars have a dead-bolt system that cannot be unlocked with special tools. Those types of locks are designed to unlock on impact and allow rescuers to gain access.

Before you attempt to unlock a door, confirm that all doors are indeed locked and windows are up, preventing access any other way. Also, be sure occupants cannot unlock it.

Check the doors for damage. A severely damaged door may not open easily even if you do unlock it. If all doors are damaged, be prepared to break glass and gain access through the window. Look in the windows to see if the car has buttons in the armrest. It will not be easy to unlock doors with this type of locking device. Vehicles with electric locks and windows cannot be unlocked if the battery is disabled.

Gaining Access Through Vehicle Windows   To gain rapid access to patients who are unresponsive or unstable when the doors are locked, use a spring-loaded center punch on the rear or side windows. A heavy hammer may work, but it requires that you aim carefully and strike forcefully (possibly several times), which may shatter and spray glass. Always wear PPE, especially goggles and gloves, when breaking glass.

REMEMBER

Don't forget to try the obvious when attempting to access an entrapped patient. Try all doors and windows before deciding to break glass or cut into a vehicle.

Unlocking Vehicle Doors

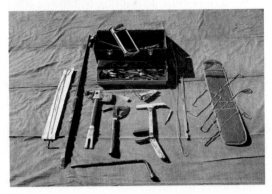

1. Various tools can be used to help unlock vehicle doors in older vehicles (check model years):

- Wire hook
- Straight wire
- Slim Jim (or similar device)
- Screwdriver
- Flat pry bar

An oil dipstick or a keyhole saw may be used to help force up a locking button.

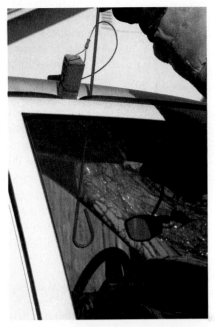

3. For flat-top locks, use a hooked wire. Snag the locking button and pull upward.

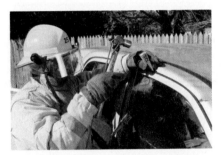

2. For framed windows, pry the frame away from the vehicle body with a wood wedge and insert a wire hook.

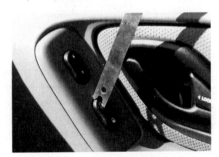

4. For rocker or push-button locks on the door panel or armrest, use a straight wire to press the lock open.

At the scene of a collision, most people consider breaking the windshield of a vehicle first if they cannot gain access through the doors. However, this is the wrong approach. Windshields are made of laminated safety glass, which has great strength. Even when shattered, the glass will still cling to an inner plastic layer. All modern cars have laminated safety glass windshields. If it is necessary to remove windshields, Emergency Medical Responders should leave that task to personnel trained in this rescue technique.

Rear and side windows are usually made of tempered glass. When this glass is broken, there is no plastic layer to hold the pieces. Tempered glass will not shatter into sharp pieces or shards. If you break it in a corner with a spring-loaded center punch, this glass will shatter into small, rounded pieces and will often drop straight down into the vehicle. The small glass pieces can cut a person, but the cuts are usually minor.

If you must use a hammer, do not bash the center of the glass with it, or you will send pieces throughout the entire passenger compartment. You must aim your tool at one of the lower corners of the window.

When gaining access through a vehicle window, you should (Figure 26.4 and Key Skill 26.2):

1. Make certain the vehicle is stable. If possible, have the driver turn off the ignition.
2. Try to open all doors and windows before attempting to break a window.
3. Protect yourself by wearing gloves and eye protection.
4. If possible, select a window that is away from the patient. Place one gloved hand flat against the window, resting the heel of your hand on the corner of the door. Place the spring-loaded center punch between two fingers in one of the lower corners of the window, as close to the door as possible. Press the center punch with your other hand. When the window breaks, the hand pressing the center punch will not go through the window.
5. After breaking the window, reach in and try to open the door. You may only have to unlock the door to open it. Often, jammed doors that will not open from the outside will open from the inside.
6. Turn off the vehicle ignition, place the transmission in park, and set the parking brake.
7. After breaking the glass, the door still may remain jammed, and you must gain access to your patient. Again, you must use proper PPE. If you do not have this equipment, wait for fire or rescue personnel.

CREW RESOURCE MANAGEMENT

Constant communication among all crew members is essential during complex operations such as stabilizing vehicles and extrications. Speak loudly and directly when issuing or confirming commands.

Patients Pinned Beneath Vehicles

When a patient is pinned beneath a vehicle, call for a rescue squad immediately. Never place yourself in danger by reaching or crawling into the area where the patient is pinned. If the scene appears too dangerous, Emergency Medical Responders can perform certain procedures to move the vehicle and free the patient, but this is often risky. Follow your department or agency SOPs in these situations.

Figure 26.4 If you can, cover the patient with a blanket prior to breaking any glass. This will prevent the patient from being hit with broken glass.

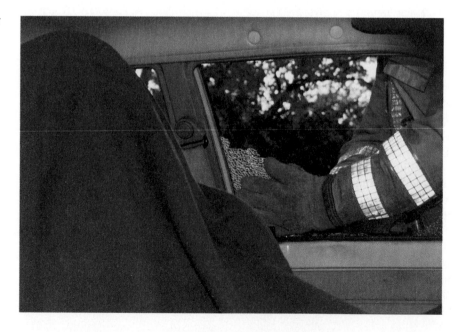

Gaining Access Through a Vehicle Window

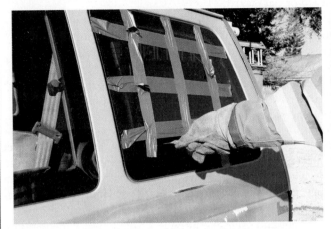

1. To break a window, first place duct tape across the window to help keep the glass intact after it is broken.

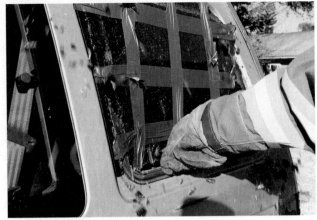

2. Use a spring-loaded center punch in one of the lower corners to break the glass.

3. Once the glass is broken, remove it from the frame.

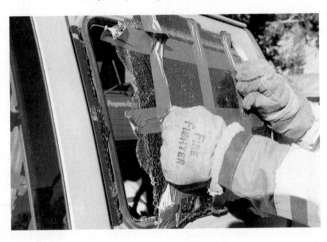

A jack or pry bar and blocks can be used to raise a vehicle, which will enable rescuers to move the patient from underneath. When lifting one side of the vehicle off the patient, be sure you are not causing the other side of the vehicle to press on another part of the patient. With enough help, you may be able to lift the vehicle off the patient. In any attempt to raise a vehicle off a pinned patient, others must shore up the vehicle as you raise it so it will not slip or fall back onto the rescuers or the patient. Use blocks, tires, lumber, or similar sturdy items at the scene. Do not attempt to enter the space to remove the victim until the entire vehicle is stable.

Patients Trapped in Wreckage

You may find patients with their arms, legs, or heads protruding through a window. Before trying to free them, you should use blankets to shield any patients who are still in the vehicle, while other rescuers continue to open the vehicle to provide better access and extrication. Use pliers, hammer claws, or a knife to carefully break or fold away glass around the patient's extremity.

When patients are trapped inside crushed vehicles, you must wait for special power tools and skilled rescue personnel. Trained personnel can quickly and easily free or disentangle patients from the wreck.

SCENE SAFETY

Most cars and trucks have airbags on both sides of the dashboard, and some may have additional airbags in other locations within the passenger compartment. It is possible for airbags to deploy after a collision. Many EMS and fire personnel have been injured when an airbag deployed while they were attempting to care for a patient. Consider this risk before deciding to enter a vehicle involved in a collision.

Emergency Medical Responders working on vehicles with occupants pinned inside will often be able to free some patients using these steps:

- Remove wreckage from on top of and around the patient.
- Carefully move a seat forward or backward.
- Carefully lift out the back seat.
- Remove a patient's shoe to free a foot, or cut away clothing caught on wreckage.
- Cut seat belts but be sure to properly support the patient during the cutting and after the tension has been released.
- Follow manufacturer and agency guidelines for working around vehicles with deployed and undeployed airbags. Check the steering wheel beneath the deployed airbag for damage indicating the patient might have struck it.

In any attempt to free patients from vehicles, you must consider the immediate need for quick access. If immediate access and patient movement is necessary to save a life, make every attempt to reach the patient. If the patient's life is not at risk but immediate movement will cause further injury, then leave the patient in place until more highly trained personnel respond to the scene.

During the wait, talk to the patient and offer reassurance. Explain why you are taking precautions. While you are talking to the patient, begin your primary assessment and provide oxygen while another Emergency Medical Responder stabilizes the head. If you must move the patient before more advanced care personnel arrive, make every attempt to maintain stabilization of the patient's spine during the move. Once EMTs and other EMS personnel arrive, report your assessment findings and provide them with any assistance they need, such as taking vital signs, controlling bleeding, gathering special equipment, or lifting and loading the patient.

Electric/Hybrid Vehicles

Ongoing incentive programs and initiatives by the U.S. government are promoting the manufacturing and sale of electric vehicles. An important consideration related to this new technology is the potential hazards that may result, and how the emergency response community will address and mitigate these hazards.

As an EMR, you will need to identify the presence of an electric vehicle. Electric vehicles will often display wording on the vehicle such as "zero emission" if the vehicle is all-electric or "hybrid" if it utilizes fuel and electric power. However, it is important to know that not all electric-powered vehicles have these markings. Also note that many electric models are built on the same chassis/platform as the conventional models, making it difficult to differentiate the two.

Safety is at the forefront of the design of these vehicles, and the likelihood of being exposed to high-voltage electricity when working around them is quite low. Regardless, use extra caution when working around electric and hybrid vehicles. The high-voltage cables are clearly identifiable by their thickness and bright coloring.

Several online resources from the National Fire Protection Administration (NFPA) provide safety information for first responders about how to identify, immobilize, and disable electric and hybrid vehicles.

Building Access

LO12 Discuss strategies for safely gaining entry into buildings.

Gaining access to a patient in a locked building may require special skills and tools outside the range of Emergency Medical Responder duties. There are many types of gates, doors, windows, and locks that restrict access to buildings. Security devices will also present barriers. In addition to access problems, older buildings may have hidden dangers such as unstable flooring or stairs.

Emergency Medical Responders are not expected to know how to open or destroy locks or have all the tools needed for the variety of windows, doors, and gates found in buildings. Unless you are trained in fire and rescue operations, you are not expected to know how to enter and make your way safely around an empty or abandoned building.

Follow your SOPs regarding notification of law enforcement prior to and following any forcible entry. Use the following guidelines for gaining access to patients inside any type of building (homes or commercial buildings such as offices, stores, and schools):

- Request additional resources if necessary.
- First, try opening and entering through unlocked doors or windows.
- Look for spare keys hidden under mats or other exterior locations.
- Ask bystanders and neighbors if they have keys.
- Break glass to unlock doors or windows.

If you know or see that someone inside needs immediate care, do not try to gain access before calling for help. Your efforts to gain entry may fail, and you will need help as soon as possible. Call the dispatcher and request additional resources immediately.

While waiting for help, try different entry points (doors and windows). If the door is locked, try opening a few low windows on your way to finding a second door. If the second door is locked, break the glass in a window or a door and enter as quickly, but as safely, as possible. Do not attempt to break through doors or windows made of large sheets of tempered glass. When attempting to break a window, you should:

1. Make certain the patient is not lying near the other side of the glass.
2. Use a hammer or similar blunt object to strike the glass near one of its edges. A nightstick or an aluminum flashlight will break most window glass. If you do not have tools, use a rock or a similar object to strike the glass.
3. Carefully clear all glass from the frame and reach in to unlock the door or window.
4. Make certain you are stepping onto a safe floor. Be sure you do not have an unusual drop when entering. Take a moment to visually inspect the floor for damage or test the floor for signs of weakness.

Hazards

A wide range of hazards can make gaining access to patients and caring for them challenging. The following sections discuss how to deal with situations involving fire, natural gas, electrical wires and transformers, various types of hazardous materials, and radiation.

Fire

LO13 Discuss strategies for safely managing a scene where fire is present.

Television and movies have led people to believe that they should enter burning buildings or run up to burning vehicles to save victims. This is a dangerous tactic. Those in the fire service are highly trained at their jobs. They are given special equipment and use proven strategies to fight fires, minimizing the risks to their safety. Firefighting requires specialized training, protective clothing, the right equipment, and usually more than one firefighter.

If you are a member of the fire service, follow SOPs for rescuing victims from vehicle and structure fires. If you are in law enforcement and have special training in rescuing victims from vehicle and structure fires, do only what you have been trained to do using proper PPE. If you are an Emergency Medical Responder without firefighting training, do not risk your life to approach a fire to provide care.

Motor vehicle collisions do not usually produce fire, and most emergency calls to buildings do not involve fire. However, these events do occur, and you must be prepared to protect yourself. Your own safety is the first priority. Emergency Medical Responders with no training or little experience at fighting fires must adhere to the following rules to ensure their safety:

- Never approach a vehicle that is in flames. Using blankets, sand, or a fire extinguisher is appropriate if you know how to evaluate the fire and the danger of explosion, you have protective clothing, and know how to attack a fire. If you do not have the proper training to perform these tasks and do not have the necessary protection, stay clear. Make sure the dispatcher knows there is a fire.
- Never attempt to enter a building that is on fire or where smoke can be seen. Even a small fire can spread toxic fumes throughout the structure. If you enter, look and smell for signs of fire. Remember that fire could be hidden within the walls, floors, and ceilings.
- Never enter a smoky room or building or go through an area of dense smoke.
- Never attempt to enter a closed building or room giving off grayish-yellow smoke. Opening a door to this building or room will cause a back draft, which immediately increases the intensity of the fire and can cause an explosion due to the sudden increase in oxygen supply.
- Do not work by yourself or enter a building unless others know that you are doing so. If you are injured or trapped, you are an unknown victim who may not be found until it is too late.
- Always feel the top of a door before opening it. If it is hot, do not open it. (Doorknobs and handles may also be hot.) If the door is cool, open it slowly and cautiously, and avoid standing in its path as you open it.
- Never use an elevator if there is a possibility of a fire in a building. The elevator shaft can act as a flue and pull flames, hot toxic gases, and smoke into the shaft. Also, the fire can cause an electrical failure, which could trap you in the elevator.
- If you find yourself in smoke, stay close to the floor and crawl to safety. If possible, cover your mouth and nose with a damp cloth.

 FIRST ON SCENE *(continued)*

As Greg is waiting for his call to be routed to the local dispatch center, he grabs two of the fleeing technicians. "I need you guys to go to the north entrance and make sure nobody gets onto the studio property." The men immediately jog off down the road toward the studio's only other gate.

"City fire dispatch, how can I help?" A man's voice comes onto the line.

"Yes, I'm calling from Legend Studios over here on Cornell Boulevard. There's a fire on the exterior west side of our main soundstage building, and there are five or six large propane tanks in the danger zone."

After answering several questions from the dispatcher, Greg hangs up and turns to the lead pyrotechnician, who is staring back at the burning building expectantly. "Hey," Greg addresses him, taking a notepad and pen from his pocket. "Is there anything at all in that area other than propane? Any chemicals or other flammable stuff? The fire department will need to know as soon as they get here."

Natural Gas

LO14 Discuss strategies for safely managing a scene where there may be evidence of a natural gas leak.

If you notice the odor of natural gas at any scene, move patients away from the area, keep bystanders away from the scene, alert dispatch so other services can be activated, and request that gas in the area be shut off or diverted.

The smell of natural gas in a building is a signal for immediate action. Evacuate the building and call dispatch to report the odor of gas. If the gas is coming from a bottled source, do not try to turn off this source unless you have experience with this type of gas system. You can vent the area by opening windows and doors as you leave. Do not enter an area to rescue a patient. You must wear a self-contained breathing apparatus (SCBA) and be trained to handle such emergencies. Remember, there is always a danger of fire or explosion from simple acts such as turning a light switch on or off or from an appliance turning on. Play it safe and request the help you will need.

Electrical Wires and Aboveground Transformers

LO15 Discuss strategies for safely managing a scene where high voltage electricity may be present.

If electrical wires are down at a scene and block your pathway to a patient, or if they are lying across a car, do not attempt a rescue. As you approach a scene with downed wires, position your vehicle at least one utility pole away from the downed wires. If the power is restored, the wires can whip and arc in a circle as wide as their free length, which can be to the next pole (Figure 26.5).

Never assume that power lines are dead or that a dead line will stay dead. Consider all downed lines to be live. Do not be fooled by the fact that lights are out in the surrounding area. Even if lights are off all around you, the wire blocking your path may be live or could be reenergized as you pass by. Call or have someone alert dispatch to call the power company and request that the power be turned off. Even if you believe the power has been turned off, it is still best to wait for trained rescue personnel to arrive.

Many communities have underground electrical wires with access through an aboveground splice box or transformer. These aboveground transformer boxes are usually green, mounted on concrete pads, and often hidden by shrubbery. It may not be safe to approach a vehicle that has collided with a transformer box. Alert dispatch immediately and ask for special rescue assistance.

If victims are in a car that is touching or near a downed wire or has crashed into a transformer box, tell them to stay in the vehicle and avoid touching any metal parts. If the victims must leave the vehicle because of fire or other danger, you must tell them to jump clear of the car without touching it and the ground at the same time. If they touch both simultaneously, they will complete a circuit and may be electrocuted.

> **SCENE SAFETY**
>
> When working in or around emergency scenes that involve utility poles and lines, be sure to evaluate the integrity of the power lines for several hundred yards in all directions. Damage to a single pole can affect the lines several poles away and create a hazard not immediately seen.

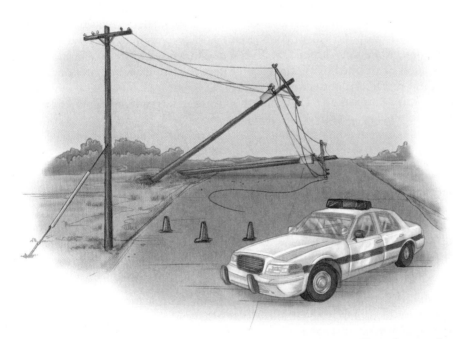

Figure 26.5 When arriving on scene, position your vehicle at least one utility pole away from the damaged pole.

Hazardous Materials

LO16 Explain the role of the Emergency Medical Responder at a hazardous materials incident.

LO17 Describe the common signs of a potential hazardous materials incident.

LO18 Differentiate the purpose of cold, warm, and hot zones at a hazardous materials incident.

hazardous materials ▸ materials that are harmful to humans when exposed.

There may be hazardous chemicals and other materials at the scene of an emergency. If so, do not attempt a rescue or perform patient care. No responders should enter a **hazardous materials** area unless they are trained to do so.

The possibility of hazardous materials incidents exists at every industrial site and every farm, truck, train, ship, barge, and airplane emergency incident. When responding to an emergency at these sites, assume there are hazardous materials until their presence can be ruled out. When in doubt, stay clear and keep others clear until trained rescuers arrive.

Hazardous materials response teams, usually called hazmat teams, consist of personnel with specialized training that goes beyond the scope of this text but may be required by your agency or department. This specialized training is regulated by the Occupational Safety and Health Administration (OSHA) Code of Federal Regulations. The regulations on how hazardous materials responders are to be trained and how hazardous materials are to be managed are *OSHA 29 CFR 1910.120* Hazardous Waste Operations and Emergency Response, commonly called **HAZWOPER**.

HAZWOPER requirements include:

HAZWOPER ▸ abbreviation for Hazardous Waste Operations and Emergency Response.

- Written SOPs and a response plan
- Use of the incident command system
- Presence of a safety officer
- Use of minimum PPE such as SCBA and full turnout gear
- Presence of backup personnel and emergency medical support

Five Levels of Hazmat Training   OSHA regulations define five levels of training for hazmat personnel. These are:

- *First Responder Awareness:* Individuals who may witness or discover a chemical release and will notify proper authorities, secure the area, and establish command.
- *First Responder Operational:* Initial responders who are dispatched to releases or potential releases of chemicals and who function in a defensive fashion without attempting to stop the leak or coming into close proximity to the product.
- *Hazardous Materials Technician:* To respond in a more aggressive fashion, these responders are trained to use chemical protective equipment and are usually members of a hazardous materials team.
- *Hazardous Materials Specialist:* A responder who has more in-depth knowledge than a technician and serves as a team leader.
- *Incident Commander:* A responder who will assume command of an incident scene beyond the level of the first responder.

Emergency Medical Responder Responsibilities   Your role as an Emergency Medical Responder in a hazardous materials situation is to first protect yourself and others around the scene. All emergency response vehicles should carry a current copy of the U.S. Department of Transportation (DOT) **Hazardous Materials: Emergency Response Guidebook**. At a hazardous materials incident, refer to the guidebook for information on the chemical or substance and the perimeter of the safe area. In general, your responsibilities are recognition and identification, notification and information sharing, isolation, and protection.

Hazardous Materials: Emergency Response Guidebook ▸ official U.S. government resource for the identification of hazardous materials; available as a smart phone app.

Recognition and Identification   Recognition and identification are the first and most essential safety factors at a hazardous materials scene. The following factors must be evaluated upon arrival at these incidents:

- Occupancy/location
- Container shape

- Markings and colors
- **Placards** and labels
- Shipping papers and Safety Data Sheets (SDS)
- Human senses

Notification and Information Sharing   Contact dispatch immediately with a description of the incident so you can get the appropriate help on the way. Advise the dispatcher of your position and stay on the line until you are told to disconnect. Ask and wait for information about the danger of the materials and for directions as to what you should do until the hazmat teams arrive. Make certain you give your name and callback number.

When possible, provide the following information:

- *Nature and location of the problem,* an estimate of when the spill occurred, and if there are other possible hazardous materials near the scene.
- *Type of material* (gas, liquid, dry chemical, or a radioactive solid, liquid, or gas) and an estimate of how much material is at the scene.
- *Name or identification number of the material.* Look for labels or placards that are visible from your safe point. Use binoculars to help in reading this information.
- *Name of the shipper or manufacturer.* From a safe point or with binoculars, look for names on railroad cars, trucks, or containers. Ask bystanders, drivers, or railroad or factory personnel.
- *Type of container.* Is the material in a rail car or a truck? Is it in open storage, covered storage, or housed storage? Is the container still intact, or is liquid leaking, gas escaping, or a powder spilled? Report if the material is stable or if it is flaming, vaporizing, or blowing into the air.
- *Weather conditions.* Rain and wind are major concerns because they will carry hazardous materials to other locations.
- *Estimate of the number of possible victims* both in the area closest to the spill and nearby.
- *Other significant problems at the scene,* such as fire, crowds, and traffic.

You may not be able to obtain and report some or most of this information, but any information you can provide is important to the responding units.

A major source of information at a hazardous materials scene is the standard materials placard required by the U.S. DOT (Figure 26.6). This placard is on the vehicle, tank, or railroad car. The numbers, symbols, and colors provide information about the material in the container. Be aware that vehicles transporting hazardous materials insert placards into brackets. They may be made of metal or plastic and are hinged so they can be flipped to indicate a different cargo. During transportation or the incident, the placard may flip and show a different material. Some hazardous materials transporters use placard stickers, which can be peeled off when the load is delivered. The driver applies another sticker for a different load of hazardous materials.

When possible, check with the driver, who must have a SDS on each hazardous material carried, to determine whether the placard information is correct. The SDS will provide you with this important information:

- Chemical and common names
- Physical and chemical properties
- Physical hazards
- Health hazards
- Primary routes of exposure
- Exposure limits
- Safe handling procedures
- Emergency and first-aid measures
- Contact individual or company

Refer to the U.S. DOT *Hazardous Materials: Emergency Response Guidebook.* You may also want to become familiar with the National Fire Protection Association (NFPA) "Standard 473 Competencies for EMS Personnel Responding to Hazardous Materials Incidents."

Figure 26.6 A typical DOT hazardous materials placard.

Isolation and Protection   For isolation of the incident, you may have to assist with the setup of *safety zones*:

hot zone ▸ at a hazardous materials incident, the area immediately surrounding the spill or release.

warm zone ▸ designated area at a hazardous materials incident where decontamination of people and equipment occurs.

cold zone ▸ designated area at a hazardous materials incident that is well beyond the incident and where patients are cared for and placed into ambulances for transport.

- **Hot zone** (exclusion) to keep all people out of the contaminated area
- **Warm zone** for contamination reduction procedures
- **Cold zone** (support), on the same level as, and upwind from, the hazardous materials incident that can be used for patient assessment, treatment, and transport

Below-grade areas, such as ditches, trenches, and basements, will often have low-oxygen environments. Many gases are heavier than oxygen and will settle in low areas. The safe zone must not be downhill or downwind from the scene or on a high point that may be exposed to vapors if the wind shifts. Avoid low spots, streams, drainage fields, sewers, and sewer openings where spills may flow and fumes may collect.

Emergency Medical Responders should assist in establishing hot and warm zones only if they have the appropriate OSHA-approved training and PPE.

Access to the zones must be controlled with an entrance point that has only one way in, called the "access corridor." The exit point from the hot zone to the warm zone for decontamination is called the "decontamination corridor." This corridor leads to the cold zone (safe zone) where the Emergency Medical Responder is allowed to assess, treat, and transport patients. The cold zone is also where the command post is located. This is where the Incident Commander coordinates resources to manage the incident (Figure 26.7).

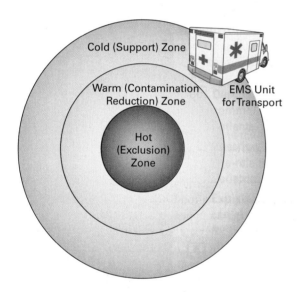

Hot (Exclusion) Zone

Contamination is actually present.
Personnel must wear appropriate protective gear.
Number of rescuers limited to those absolutely necessary.
Bystanders never allowed.

Warm (Contamination Reduction) Zone

Area surrounding the contamination zone.
Vital to preventing spread of contamination.
Personnel must wear appropriate protective gear.
Lifesaving emergency care is performed.

Cold (Support) Zone

Normal triage, stabilization, and treatment performed.
Rescuers must shed contaminated gear before entering the cold zone.

Figure 26.7 Examples of the safety zones at a hazardous materials incident.

Decontamination of Hazardous Materials   Decontamination is a chemical or physical process used to remove and prevent the spread of contaminants to prevent harm to living beings and/or the environment. The best method to accomplish decontamination is to prevent contamination.

Decontamination (decon) is performed in the warm zone by specially trained personnel. Remember, as an Emergency Medical Responder, you must remain in the cold zone and begin patient treatment and assist with transport there. It is important to note that people, equipment, and the environment all will need to be decontaminated before you come into contact with them. The Emergency Medical Responder must consider all individuals in the warm and hot zones to be contaminated. Both responders and victims are to be considered contaminated until proper decon is performed. In the cold zone, the Emergency Medical Responder must recognize that victims may be ambulatory (able to walk) or nonambulatory (not able to walk). If there are contaminated victims associated with the hazmat scene, notify receiving health care facilities of incoming patients and relay that proper decontamination has been conducted at the scene. Inform them of the chemical or substance that the patient was exposed to and of their condition, including vital signs (Figure 26.8).

Managing Patients   Remember, all contaminated victims must remain in the hot zone until the hazmat team brings them to the warm zone for decon and then to the cold zone for care by EMS personnel. If a victim of a hazardous materials incident leaves the hot zone, you must first protect yourself from exposure. Victims may have chemicals on their bodies and clothing that could be harmful to you. *Do not* attempt to care for these patients unless you have the proper protection.

Initial care includes getting the patient into fresh air and flushing with water any contaminated areas, such as the skin, clothing, and eyes, for at least 20 minutes, unless the material is dry lime. Remove contaminated clothing and jewelry as you douse the patient with water. Once dousing is complete, use blankets to protect the patient from the environment and to maintain body temperature.

Victims may be able to wash themselves, or you may wash them. Use a small-diameter hose, and make sure the individual stands in a large tub, small wading pool, or similar collection container so the contaminated rinse water does not run off into nearby sewers or streams. The hazmat team will manage the contaminated water by collecting it for transport and disposal. Perform wash operations uphill and upwind from the site if possible. Do not place yourself at risk. If it is necessary to provide artificial ventilations, use an appropriate barrier device. Use resuscitation devices with one-way valves so contaminants do not blow back into your mouth or face.

The best thing for you to do at a hazardous materials incident is to request the appropriate resources (Figure 26.9) and remain in the cold zone until the patient can be safely treated.

Radiation Incidents

Stay clear of collisions involving radioactive materials. Your first duty is to protect yourself from exposure. Your next step should be to request the appropriate resources from a safe area away from the scene.

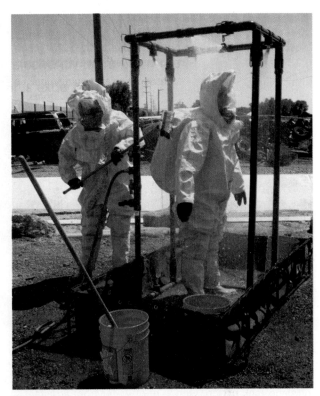

Figure 26.8 Decontamination of a fellow rescuer.

Look for radiation hazard labels (Figure 26.10). Stay upwind from any containers having these labels. Follow the same basic rules as you would when dealing with any hazardous material. The greater the distance you are from the source and the more objects that shield you from the source (concrete, thick steel, earth banks, heavy vehicles), the safer you will be.

When you are dispatched to hazardous materials and radiation incidents, position your vehicle at a safe distance. Do not approach the scene unless you are specially trained to do so and are wearing the appropriate PPE (turnout coat, pants, boots, gloves, fire-resistant hood, helmet). Your PPE will provide some protection from most types of radiation, but be aware that it does not protect you enough to work close to a high-level radiation source for any period of time.

Patients may be exposed to radiation, contaminated by it, or both. A patient who is exposed (not contaminated) was in the presence of radioactive material, but the material did not actually touch their clothing or body. Exposure to radiation may be harmful to the patient, but they are not radioactive and cannot pass on the exposure to you. However, the actual source of the radiation can be harmful to you. If the patient is still in the area of the radiation source, you must wait until the hazmat team brings them to the safe area.

Patients are contaminated when they come in contact with radiation sources, which may be gases, liquids, or particles. The radioactive materials may be on a patient's clothes, skin, or hair and will contaminate you when you touch the patient during assessment or care. The hazmat team will have to decontaminate the patient before you can provide care. Do not attempt to clean or care for patients who have been contaminated with radiation until they are in a safe area and are decontaminated.

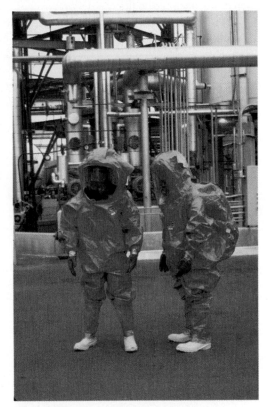

Figure 26.9 The appropriate response to a hazardous materials incident requires specialized training and equipment.

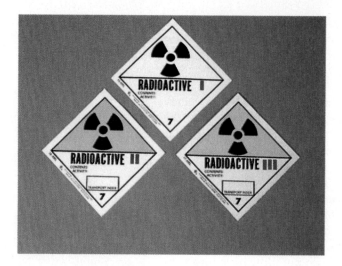

Figure 26.10 Examples of typical radiation hazard placards.

FIRST ON SCENE WRAP-UP

Within minutes, the streets leading to the studio have been closed by law enforcement, and fire services is cooling the propane tank battery with a jet of water from a distant truck. After about 15 minutes, the fabric of the green screen has burned completely from the large rectangular frame and, except for drifting gray ash and rapidly dissipating smoke, there is no sign of the once-raging fire.

"Well, Greg." The Incident Commander puts his hand on the safety officer's shoulder. "You couldn't have done anything better than you did: evacuating, blocking the two access points, and letting us know exactly what we were up against. You did a fine job managing a pretty hazardous situation."

"Thank you." Greg smiles briefly. "Next time I'm only going to make one change."

"What's that?" The IC pulls off his orange vest.

"Next time we do a shot like this," Greg says, "I'm going to have you guys already standing by."

26 REVIEW

Summary

- The phases of a typical emergency call include: preparation, dispatch, en route to the scene, at the scene, transfer of care, and post-call prep. You must know your responsibilities for each of these phases.
- As an Emergency Medical Responder, your first priority is your own safety. Before approaching a patient, make sure the scene is safe. Call for additional resources as soon as possible.
- Do not attempt to provide patient care in or around unstabilized vehicles or try to right overturned vehicles.
- Attempt to reach patients by simple access first, such as doors and windows. Wait for properly trained personnel if complex access is required.
- Remove patients from vehicles only when there is danger or if lifesaving care is required.
- If you smell natural gas, do not approach. Only trained personnel should shut off gas or electricity. If electrical wires are touching a vehicle, have passengers stay in the vehicle and instruct them to avoid touching any metal objects inside the vehicle. If they must get out, warn them to jump clear without touching the vehicle and the ground at the same time.
- The five levels of hazmat training are: awareness, operational, technician, specialist, and commander. In many areas, emergency responders must be trained to the awareness level.
- An important hazmat reference tool that should be carried on all emergency vehicles is the *Hazardous Materials: Emergency Response Guidebook*. You should become familiar with how to use this valuable resource.
- Hazmat incidents are organized into zones. The hot zone is the area immediately surrounding the incident. The warm zone is a safe distance from the incident and where decontamination operations occur. The cold zone is well beyond the incident and where patients are cared for and placed into ambulances for transport.
- Stay well clear of any scene where radioactive material may be present. Notify dispatch of the possibility based on visible placards and assist in setting up a wide barrier around the scene to keep bystanders from entering the scene.

Take Action

Hazmat Right at Home

Most people have little understanding of how many hazardous materials surround them each and every day. When things are operating properly, large quantities of hazardous materials are being transported all around them, and they have little awareness until something goes wrong. For this activity, conduct a thorough inventory of your immediate environment at home. Take a look in all the usual places, such as under the kitchen sink and in the garage, as well as not-so-obvious places, such as the home office or bathroom. Write down the name of anything that comes in a commercial container—everything from drain cleaner to dish detergent.

Next, use the internet to locate a SDS for each of those products. A simple search such as "SDS for [brand name] dishwashing liquid" will bring up a link to the appropriate SDS. Review the section titled "Hazard Identification," for the potential problems this product can cause upon exposure. Then review the "First Aid Measures" section to learn the appropriate treatment for the specific product.

Having a good understanding of the dangers associated with products in your own home and what to do should someone ingest them or handle them incorrectly will make you a better prepared Emergency Medical Responder.

First on Scene Run Review

Recall the events of the First on Scene scenario in this chapter, and answer the following questions related to the call. Rationales are offered in the Answer Key at the back of the book.

1. What precautions could Greg have taken before they began shooting the scene?
2. What information could Greg have given the dispatcher?
3. How might the *Emergency Response Guidebook* have come in handy?

Quick Quiz

To check your understanding of the chapter, answer the following questions. Then compare your answers to those in the Answer Key at the back of the book.

1. Which of the following statements is TRUE regarding equipment maintenance?

   a. Most agencies have a dedicated equipment manager who is responsible for all maintenance.
   b. At the beginning of each shift, each EMR should check all their equipment and confirm it is in working order.
   c. If there is an equipment malfunction, the EMR is never held responsible.
   d. Equipment should be checked once a month to ensure it still works.

2. The phases of an emergency call in order are:

   a. preparation, dispatch, en route to scene, at scene, transfer of care, and post-call prep.
   b. dispatch, en route to scene, at scene, transfer of care, and post-call prep.
   c. preparation, dispatch, en route to scene, at scene, transfer of care, and en route to hospital.
   d. dispatch, en route to scene, at scene, preparation, transfer of care, and post-call prep.

3. You are the first responders to arrive at the scene of a traffic accident. Where should you attempt to park your vehicle?

   a. 50 feet before the scene with lights on
   b. As close to the scene as possible with lights off
   c. 500 feet beyond the scene with lights on
   d. As far off the roadway as practical

4. An Emergency Medical Responder's first priority is:

   a. patient care.
   b. protecting property.
   c. personal safety.
   d. preventing insurance fraud.

5. Which of the following best defines both simple access and complex access?

   a. Neither simple access nor complex access requires specialized tools.
   b. Simple and complex access both require special equipment.
   c. Simple access sometimes requires special equipment; complex access often does.
   d. Simple access does not require equipment, though complex access does.

6. You are at the scene of a vehicle collision. The patient is still restrained in the driver's seat and appears to be unresponsive. To gain access to this patient, you should:

   a. call an emergency locksmith.
   b. attempt to open the car.
   c. remove the engine and enter through the dash.
   d. break the windshield.

7. The best way for the Emergency Medical Responder to manage an overturned vehicle is to:

   a. right the vehicle if enough help is available.
   b. right the vehicle before gaining access to patients.
   c. never right a vehicle because it can cause further injury to the patients inside.
   d. never right a vehicle because it can cause further damage to the vehicle.

8. When a patient is pinned beneath a vehicle,

   a. attempt to right the vehicle yourself.
   b. call for a rescue squad immediately.
   c. stabilize the vehicle then attempt to right it.
   d. use bystanders to attempt to right it.

9. You have responded to the home of an older adult woman. Her daughter called 911 after not being able to contact her. Through a window, you can see the patient, who appears to be unresponsive, on the kitchen floor. All doors and windows to the home appear to be locked. You should:

   a. enter the building and then call for help.
   b. enter the building, stabilize the patient, and then call for help.
   c. attempt to enter the building, but if you fail, call for help.
   d. request additional resources, then attempt to access the building.

10. Upon arrival at the scene of an "unknown medical problem" you see smoke billowing from a front window of the home. You should:

    a. quickly enter the home and attempt to get the patient out.
    b. open the front door but do not enter, shouting inside for people to get out.
    c. walk around the home to see if anyone has escaped.
    d. call for immediate fire department assistance.

11. While caring for a female patient who is complaining of a headache, you smell natural gas. You should:

    a. immediately leave the scene, taking the patient with you.
    b. ask the patient where the gas shut off valve is located.
    c. leave the patient and tell her you will return later.
    d. continue patient care, providing oxygen to the patient.

12. If you find yourself needing to exit a smoke-filled environment, you should:

    a. stay close to the floor and crawl to safety.
    b. run out of the building.
    c. stop, drop, and roll.
    d. not exit until you find the patient.

13. The patient treatment area and the command post are located in which zone of a hazmat incident?

a. Hot
b. Warm
c. Blue
d. Cold

14. Which of the following is NOT a sign of a possible hazardous materials incident?

a. Unusual smells
b. Vehicle crash
c. Colored smoke
d. Spilling of unknown fluid

15. At the scene of a traffic accident, patients are trapped inside their vehicle. Power lines have fallen and are draped over the car. You should:

a. shout at the people in the car to remain still and then call the power company.
b. use rubber gloves to carefully remove the downed lines from the vehicle.
c. shout at the patients to carefully exit the vehicle, being careful to not touch the power lines.
d. use leather gloves to open the car door, avoiding the downed power lines.

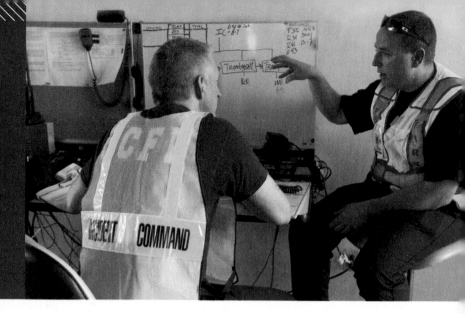

27

Introduction to Multiple-Casualty Incidents, the Incident Command System, and Triage

Education Standards

EMS Operations—
Incident Management,
Multiple-Casualty
Incidents

Competencies

Demonstrates knowledge
of operational roles and
responsibilities to ensure
patient, public, and
personnel safety.

LEARNING OBJECTIVES

Upon successful completion of this chapter, the student should be able to:

Cognitive

1. Define the chapter key terms.
2. Explain the criteria that define a multiple-casualty incident.
3. Describe common causes of multiple-casualty incidents.
4. Explain the key principles and structure of an incident command system.
5. Explain the role of the Emergency Medical Responder in the multiple-casualty situation.
6. Explain the key principles of triage at a multiple-casualty incident.
7. Differentiate patient priorities related to triage.
8. Explain the assessment criteria of the START triage system.
9. Differentiate primary and secondary triage.
10. Describe the key elements of the JumpSTART triage system for children.
11. Describe the key elements of the SALT triage system.

Psychomotor

12. Demonstrate the ability to properly categorize patients of a simulated multiple-casualty situation.

Affective

13. Recognize the importance of patient priorities during a multiple-casualty event.

KEY TERMS

incident command system (ICS) (*p. 576*)
incident commander (*p. 576*)
JumpSTART pediatric triage system (*p. 583*)
national incident management system (NIMS) (*p. 577*)

SALT triage system (*p. 585*)
START triage system (*p. 580*)
triage (*p. 577*)

This chapter discusses the role of the EMS system and that of the Emergency Medical Responder in emergencies involving multiple victims. Multiple-casualty incidents have a wide range of causes, including vehicle collisions, hurricanes and other natural disasters, acts of terrorism, and the many mass shootings we have experienced as a nation over the past few years.

FIRST ON SCENE

Lanson, a Westside Mall security guard, looks at his watch and leans on the railing that borders the mezzanine level of the huge downtown mall. He watches as the crowds down on the main level bustle from store to store, swinging shopping bags and chatting on cell phones. It is like every other Saturday afternoon at the mall.

Lanson stretches his back and walks toward the escalator that will take him down to the first floor, toward the mall's main entrance. If he doesn't check the marble entryway every few hours, it gets too crowded with loitering kids, and he'll be dealing with everything from customer complaints to fights. It is definitely better to be proactive.

Just as he steps off the escalator, it happens. A thunderous explosion from the far end of the mall sends screams and a boiling black cloud of smoke toward him. "Hey, Helen!" Lanson yells into his shoulder mic. "We just had an explosion of some kind at the north end of the mall! Call 911 right away!"

"Already on it!" comes the static-filled reply.

Lanson tries to see through the wall of rancid smoke, which is rising slowly toward the high ceiling. The mall's automated evacuation message is echoing through the enormous building. He is surprised to see the smoke fade quickly, helped by large vent fans located on the roof of the mall. Lanson stares at the scene before him.

Shattered glass, clothing, and people are scattered all over the tile floor at the end of the mall. Those who can, hurry past him to the undamaged part of the mall. As the smoke disperses, Lanson sees 15 or 20 people lying motionless on the floor—bleeding, and possibly dead.

Lanson's stomach tightens as he realizes that he is the first responder to this horrendous scene. He takes a deep breath and moves toward the closest nonmoving person.

Multiple-Casualty Incidents

LO2 Explain the criteria that define a multiple-casualty incident.

LO3 Describe common causes of multiple-casualty incidents.

Recall from Chapter 3 that a *multiple-casualty incident (MCI)* is defined as any emergency that involves more victims than can safely be cared for by the first responding units (Figure 27.1). An MCI may also be called a mass-casualty incident, and it can be the result of many different types of events. Common causes include vehicle collisions, mass shootings, earthquakes, tornadoes, floods, explosions, and building collapses.

Most fire services, rescue squads, and ambulances are prepared and capable of managing a scene with more than one patient. However, can they manage a scene with three or four? How about five or six? What if the victims are all critical and need immediate transport? It is important for the Emergency Medical Responder to remember that MCI definitions vary from one community to another. In the simplest definition, an MCI may be described as an incident that reduces the effectiveness of the standard emergency response because of the number of patients, special hazards, or a difficult rescue (Table 27.1).

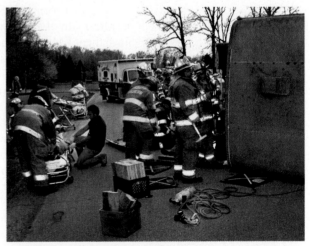

Figure 27.1 Multiple-casualty incidents require the resources of many agencies.
(© Edward T. Dickinson, MD)

TABLE 27.1	Multiple-Casualty Incidents
Type of Incident	**Incident Management**
Low-Impact Incident	Manageable by local emergency personnel
High-Impact Incident	Stresses local EMS, fire, and police resources
Disaster or Terrorism Incident	Overwhelms regional emergency response resources

In most cases, it is up to the first emergency personnel on the scene to make a judgment call and declare an MCI. If they believe they can manage the number of patients with the resources immediately available, then an MCI may not be declared. If they cannot easily manage the number of patients, then an MCI is declared and an **incident command system (ICS)** is put into action.

The role of Emergency Medical Responders at an MCI will vary depending on several factors, such as when they arrive at the scene, the type of agency for whom they are working, and their specific level of training. Emergency Medical Responders who are first on scene may be dedicated to making the scene safe and keeping bystanders from becoming injured. Thus, they may not immediately become involved in patient care. For those who arrive after the scene has been made safe, their role will likely involve the triaging of patients (discussed later in this chapter).

Other roles for the Emergency Medical Responder include treatment of patients and assisting with the transport of patients to appropriate receiving facilities. Other duties may include the setting up of landing zones if medical helicopters are used for patient evacuation.

When you are faced with multiple casualties at critical incidents, it is important to be aware of your mental and physical stress levels. Critical incident stress debriefing (CISD) sessions or other qualified psychological support should be available after a disaster or unusual emergency to address the needs of rescuers who may have been influenced by the scene and the stress generated in providing emergency care.

Incident Command System

LO4 | Explain the key principles and structure of an incident command system.

The incident command system (ICS) is a system for the command, control, and coordination of resources at the scene of a large-scale emergency involving multiple agencies. It consists of procedures for organizing personnel, facilities, equipment, and communications.

The first formal ICS was formed as a result of a mandate from Congress to analyze the aftermath of a devastating series of wildfires in Southern California in the early 1970s. Since then, EMS, fire, and police agencies across the United States continue to develop and implement such plans using ICS.

The ICS is based on well-established management principles of planning, direction, organization, coordination, communication, delegation, and evaluation. ICS is flexible enough to accommodate a single-agency or single-jurisdiction emergency, as well as multiagency or multijurisdictional events. ICS is dynamic in nature and employs a top-down modular structure that can be scaled to any size event.

The **incident commander** is the individual responsible for all aspects of the emergency response, establishing the structure and requesting resources necessary for the event. The incident commander is typically a senior fire department officer.

Some of the modules that might be included in a typical ICS are: command, operations, planning, logistics, and finance. Under each of the major modules is a complex list of responsibilities related to that functional group. For example, under operations, Emergency Medical Responders are generally assigned to the medical branch, which is a functional group under this area of responsibility.

incident command system ▶ system for the command, control, and coordination of resources at the scene of a large-scale emergency involving multiple agencies. Abbrev: ICS. Also known as *incident management system*.

incident commander ▶ individual responsible for all aspects of an emergency response.

It is easy to imagine how chaos can occur when many different agencies and departments respond to a single large-scale emergency. Designing and implementing an organized approach to such an event ensures a more positive outcome for both the rescuers and the victims.

National Incident Management System

In response to the increased terrorist threat in the United States, the Federal Emergency Management Agency (FEMA) developed its own incident management system known as the **National Incident Management System (NIMS).**[1] NIMS was developed so federal, state, local, and tribal resources could respond more efficiently to natural disasters and emergencies, including acts of terrorism. NIMS encompasses a unified approach to incident management and standard command and management structures. It puts emphasis on preparedness, mutual aid, resource management and, most important, common terminology among multiple agencies. Training in NIMS and ICS within emergency response agencies is required to receive federal funds (grants) for equipment, supplies, and personnel.

FEMA offers several free online instructional courses pertaining to both the ICS and the NIMS. You can find these courses and many others on the FEMA website.

national incident management system ▶ system that uses a unified approach to incident management and standard command and management structures, with an emphasis on preparedness, mutual aid, and resource management. Abbrev: NIMS.

Medical Branch

LO5 Explain the role of the Emergency Medical Responder in the multiple-casualty situation.

The *medical branch* of the ICS is the branch in which the Emergency Medical Responder commonly functions. This branch involves the designation and coordination of elements such as **triage**, treatment, and transport of patients. Figure 27.2 shows an example of the EMS portion of a large incident management system.

As you arrive on the scene, you will be given a specific assignment based on the needs of the incident. At a large-scale event, the Emergency Medical Responder may be assigned to one of five functional areas (groups within the medical branch). These areas are:

triage ▶ method of sorting patients for care and transport based on the severity of their injuries or illnesses.

- Triage
- Treatment
- Transport
- Staging
- Morgue

Emergency Medical Responders will be assigned to those areas and will report to group leaders who report up the chain of command to the medical group leader, who reports to the medical branch director. The medical group leader is the group's link to the medical branch director for information sharing and resource allocation.

The first responders to arrive at the scene will assume the role of triage and set up one or multiple triage divisions according to the size of the event.

REMEMBER

FEMA offers free online training for first responders. You can access this training at https://training.fema.gov/nims/.

CREW RESOURCE MANAGEMENT

The incident commander at an MCI must assign clear roles to all those working under them. This helps to ensure that all tasks are completed efficiently and contributes to saving as many lives as possible while keeping everyone safe.

Triage Group The triage group usually consists of the first responders on scene. They perform the following functions:

- Determine the location of triage areas.
- Conduct primary triage and ensure that all patients are assessed and sorted using appropriate triage protocol.

IMS EMS BRANCH

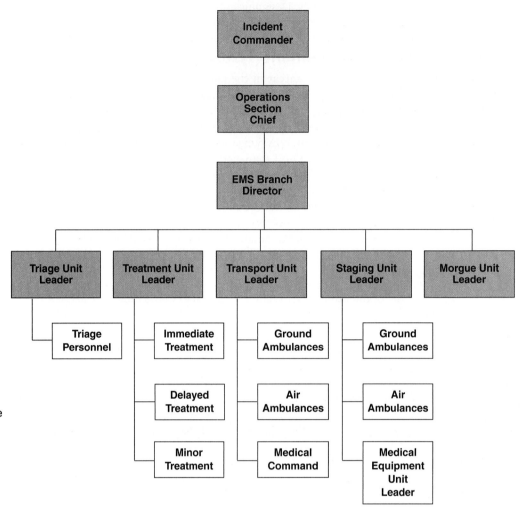

Figure 27.2 The EMS Branch of a typical ICS organizational plan.
(MISTOVICH, JOSEPH J.; KARREN, KEITH J.; HAFEN, BRENT, PREHOSPITAL EMERGENCY CARE, 10th Ed., ©2018. Reprinted and Electronically reproduced by permission of Pearson Education, Inc., New York, NY)

- Communicate resource requirements with the EMS branch director.
- Communicate with the treatment group leader to allow for movement of patients into the treatment division for care by the members of the treatment group.

Treatment Group Patients are moved from the triage group to the treatment group, where they are cared for by other EMS providers. This group is usually marked with the same color-coded indicators that match the patients' acuity levels as indicated by their triage tags. They are often marked with flags or tarps using red, yellow, green, or black. The treatment group performs the following functions:

- Determine the location for the treatment group.
- Coordinate with the triage group to move patients from the triage area to treatment areas.
- Maintain communications with the EMS branch director.
- Reassess patients—conduct secondary triage to match patients with resources.
- Direct movement to the transport division.

Transport Group The transport group coordinates transportation of patients to appropriate facilities for definitive treatment. One important function of this group is to determine the availability of receiving medical facilities. Primary responsibilities of this group include:

- Manage patient movement and accountability from the scene to the receiving hospitals.

- Work with the treatment group to establish an adequately sized, easily identifiable patient loading area.
- Designate an ambulance staging division.
- Maintain communication with the EMS branch director.

Medical Staging

The accountability of medical resources and equipment is one of the most challenging aspects of a multiple-casualty incident. With the assistance of individuals assigned to the operations group, the medical branch director can effectively meet the needs of the triage, treatment, and transport groups. Following are considerations related to staging medical resources and equipment:

- Location designated to collect available resources near the incident area
- Location that is easy for arriving resources to find
- Whether several staging divisions will be required
- Whether staging division will need to be relocated as the situation dictates

Triage

| LO6 | Explain the key principles of triage at a multiple-casualty incident.

Triage is one of the primary aspects of emergency care at a multiple-casualty incident. When there are many victims at an emergency, it is nearly impossible to provide care to all those who need it when they need it. The triage system was developed to help identify those victims who are most in need of immediate care and transport. Triage is a process for sorting injured people into groups based on their need for, or anticipated benefit from, immediate medical care. Triage is used in hospital emergency departments, on battlefields, and at emergencies when there are multiple victims and limited medical resources (Figure 27.3).

Because Emergency Medical Responders are first on the scene, they must be able to triage patients and initiate care rapidly. When additional EMS personnel arrive, Emergency Medical Responders pass on information, continue to help complete the triage process, and help provide care to the patients most in need first. You cannot begin to provide care to patients randomly. You must begin caring for those patients who have the highest priority based on their conditions. You will need to make brief notes on each patient while you are performing triage.

Triage Priorities and Process

| LO7 | Differentiate patient priorities related to triage.

Triage is a process of sorting patients into categories and prioritizing their medical care and transport based on the severity of their injuries and medical conditions. This process is commonly used at the scene of multiple-casualty incidents. When there are more victims than there are rescuers, the process of triage helps ensure that the most critical patients are cared for first. This practice allows responding personnel to do their best for the greatest number of injured patients.

For many MCIs, there may be a delay before additional help is on scene. If the emergency is large enough or in a remote area, an hour or more may pass before there are enough rescuers present to render care for all patients. Triage is also used

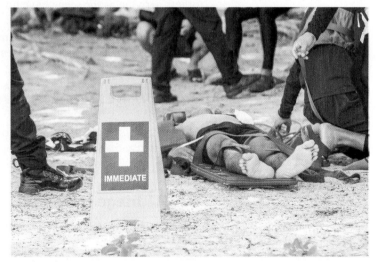

Figure 27.3 At the scene of a multiple-casualty incident, triage is the system used to identify victims who are most in need of immediate medical care.
(hooyah808/123RF)

Figure 27.4 Example of a standard triage tag, front and back.

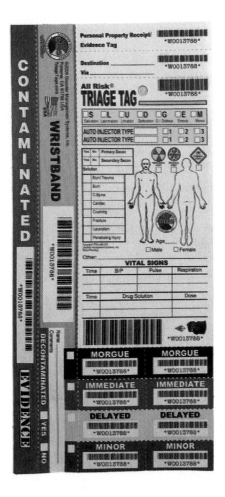
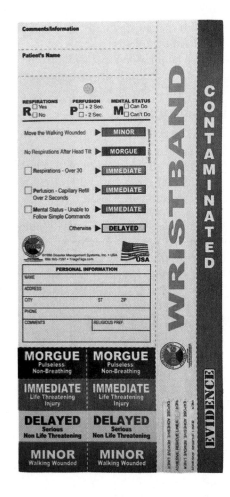

to determine the order of transport for patients. Patients who appear to have serious medical or trauma-related problems (such as heart attack, shock, or major injuries) must be transported quickly, while patients with minor injuries or illnesses can be transported later.

In some jurisdictions, Emergency Medical Responders use triage tags or colored tape to identify the different triage categories (Figure 27.4). Even if you do not carry the tags, you should be familiar with them in case you are called to help in a situation when the tags are being used. Use one triage tag per patient, and leave the tag attached to the patient so others arriving at the scene have immediate access to information. Do not delay the triage process by making elaborate notes.

There are several triage systems. Each uses slightly different criteria for classifying patients. Use the specific triage system and classifications that your jurisdiction has adopted.

CREW RESOURCE MANAGEMENT

Crew members assigned to the task of triage must stay focused on their mission and resist the urge to stop and treat every patient they encounter.

START Triage System

LO8 Explain the assessment criteria of the START triage system.

LO9 Differentiate primary and secondary triage.

One version of a triage system commonly used in the fire service and EMS is the **START triage system** developed by the Fire and Marine Department and Hoag Hospital of Newport Beach, California. START stands for Simple Triage and Rapid Treatment. START

START triage system ▶ system that uses respirations, perfusion, and mental status assessments to categorize patients into one of four treatment categories; START stands for Simple Triage and Rapid Treatment.

is based on the rapid assessment of patients using the following three criteria: respirations, perfusion, and mental status (RPM). Patients are classified into one of four categories and are tagged with the corresponding color-coded tag indicator (see Figure 27.4):

- Immediate (red)
- Delayed (yellow)
- Minor (green)
- Deceased (black)

The steps for the typical START triage process are (Figure 27.5):

1. Once the scene is safe to enter, the first rescuers on the scene begin the triage process and quickly identify and separate those patients who are probably the least injured. They are initially classified as minor. This is accomplished by directing all injured individuals who can walk to a specific location away from the immediate emergency scene. By responding to the direction to move, patients who are able will move and, therefore, self-triage into the minor category, at least initially. These patients should not be moved too far away because some of them may be able to assist with the care of more injured patients.
2. Once the ambulatory individuals have exited the immediate scene, the next step is to begin triaging the remaining patients. START triage recommends to "start where you stand." That is, begin assessing the patients closest to you and work your way out to all patients.

    Each remaining patient is assessed for the presence of respirations. It is appropriate to open the airway and check for breathing. If the patient takes a breath, they are tagged *immediate*. If they are not breathing, they are tagged *deceased*. All respiratory rates are estimates based on quick observation. It is not necessary to take actual rates during the triage process.

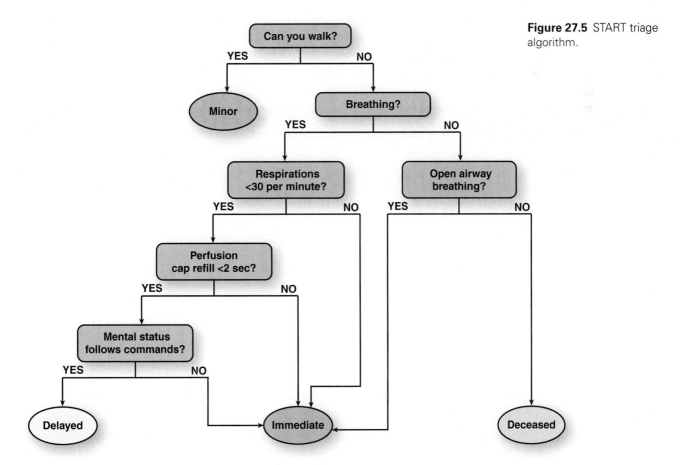

Figure 27.5 START triage algorithm.

Here is a brief overview of how a patient might be tagged based on respiratory status:

- No respirations: dead or non-salvageable (black).
- Respirations above 30 per minute: immediate (red tag). No further assessment needed.
- Respirations below 30 per minute: move on to assess perfusion.

Patients who were identified as ambulatory can assist in keeping the airway open for an unresponsive patient. If other patients cannot help, use items on the scene to position the patient's head and maintain the airway. It is important to understand that patients will constantly be reassessed as time and resources permit. *Primary triage* is when a patient is first identified and triaged. Once a patient is relocated to a treatment area, they will immediately be re-triaged by the treatment team. This is the *secondary triage*.

3. Responsive patients with respirations less than 30 per minute are assessed for perfusion status. Check the patient's radial pulse. Any patient with a radial pulse is assumed to have adequate perfusion. Therefore, assessment of mental status is the next step before categorizing the patient. Any patient without a radial pulse is assumed to have inadequate perfusion and is tagged immediate.

Some triage systems use capillary refill to assess perfusion. However, it is often unreliable because of many variables, such as age, sex, and environmental temperature. If your protocols require that you check capillary refill, the following criteria will guide you: If capillary refill is greater than 2 seconds or the radial pulse is absent, categorize the patient as immediate and move on to the next patient. If capillary refill is less than 2 seconds and the patient has a radial pulse, continue to assess mental status.

During the perfusion assessment, if you find major bleeding, do what you can to attempt to control the bleeding. Have the patient or one of the ambulatory patients hold direct pressure over the wound.

4. The final step requires assessment of the patient's mental status. This is accomplished by determining if the patient can follow simple commands, such as "open and close your eyes" or "squeeze your fingers." If the patient is able to follow simple commands, they are categorized as delayed and you will move on to the next patient. If the patient is unable to follow simple commands, they are categorized as immediate and you will move on to the next patient.

FIRST ON SCENE (continued)

Lanson checks an individual lying on the floor. The man is not breathing, and Lanson must force himself to continue. Luckily, the next five people are breathing and have signs of perfusion. Some are hurt pretty seriously, but they are definitely alive. Of the last 10—those who were obviously closest to the blast—he finds a pulse in only three. He takes the blue permanent marker from his shirt pocket and writes "Red," "Yellow," or "D" on each individual's forehead.

He is amazed at how quickly the triage training from his last Emergency Medical Responder class comes back to him.

He is just returning to the first "Red" individual to reassess him when a group of police officers emerges through the mall doors.

"I didn't have any tags, so I wrote on their foreheads," Lanson shouts as the officers stand near the mall entrance. "What are you all waiting for? These people need help!"

"Step away from the area," a police officer orders. "Go over by the escalator until we can clear the scene."

JumpSTART Pediatric Triage System

LO10 Describe the key elements of the JumpSTART triage system for children.

The START triage system works well for rapidly assessing adults, but rescuers need to use different criteria to assess pediatric patients. Using the START system, a respiratory rate of less than 30 breaths per minute in adults is a good sign, while a rate faster than 30 breaths per minute indicates a problem. Small children, especially crying infants, will normally have a respiratory rate greater than 30 breaths a minute. While a child with a respiratory rate of 8 breaths per minute would normally be categorized as delayed using the START system, they are actually in respiratory failure and should be categorized as immediate.

There are similar assessment problems when checking circulation in children. Adults usually have circulatory failure followed by respiratory arrest. Children have respiratory failure followed by circulatory failure, meaning a nonbreathing child could still have a pulse.[2] But the START system would categorize the child with no respirations as deceased. START also uses capillary refill as an assessment tool, and it can be a useful assessment for children in normal environments. However, the reliability of capillary refill as an assessment tool varies with age and the environment, and measuring it requires good lighting. The JumpSTART system does not recommend using capillary refill for assessing perfusion.

When checking mental status in children, a broad range of responses are possible, depending on the child's age. Infants will not be able to obey commands. Small children do not have the developmental ability to respond appropriately to commands. However, rescuers can check for signs of mental status using the AVPU scale (alert, responsive to voice, responsive to pain, or unresponsive).

To meet the needs of children involved in MCIs, Dr. Lou Romig, medical director for the South Florida Regional Disaster Medical Assistance Team, developed a special triage system for pediatric patients—the **JumpSTART pediatric triage system** (Figure 27.6). JumpSTART was designed to be used on children from 12 months to 8 years of age, although rescuers can use it on older children as well. The age ranges were determined by

JumpSTART pediatric triage system ▶ specialized pediatric triage system designed for patients from 1 to 8 years of age.

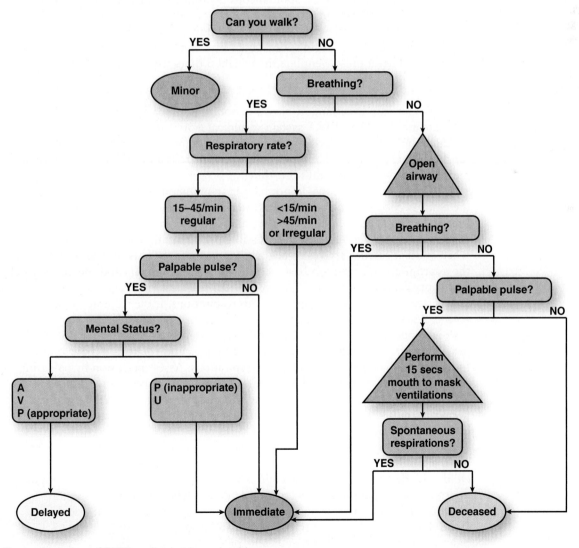

Figure 27.6 JumpSTART pediatric triage algorithm.

several criteria. Children from 12 to 18 months are beginning to walk and can be sorted as ambulatory patients. Children older than 8 years of age have airway anatomy and physiology similar to that of an adult.

Dr. Romig suggests that if the patient looks like a young adult, use START, and if the patient looks like a child, use JumpSTART. This means that JumpSTART is also used for infants and children less than 1 year old.

The assessment categories for the JumpSTART system are the same as for the START system: respirations, perfusion (peripheral pulses), and mental status (AVPU). The steps for JumpSTART are:

1. Move all children who are able to walk to an area set aside for minor injuries. There, rescuers perform a secondary triage, including respirations, pulse, and mental status. Infants are assessed during initial triage using the JumpSTART steps, or in the secondary triage area if someone carries them there. Infants and children who are ambulatory; have respirations, perfusion, and appropriate mental status; and have no significant external injury are categorized as minor.

2. Assess nonambulatory children for the presence or absence of spontaneous breathing. If there is breathing, assess the respiratory rate (see Step 3). Open the airway of any child who is not breathing or who is not breathing for more than 10 seconds. Clear a foreign body airway obstruction only if you see it. If the child begins to breathe spontaneously with an open airway, categorize the child as immediate and move on to the next patient.

   If the child does not begin spontaneous breathing when you open the airway, palpate for a peripheral pulse (radial, brachial, or pedal). If there is no peripheral pulse, categorize the patient as deceased, and move on to the next patient.

   If the child does not begin spontaneous breathing when you open the airway and the child has a pulse, ventilate the patient 5 times using an appropriate barrier device.

   Giving breaths is considered the "jump" part of the JumpSTART triage system. Children may stop breathing or have a period of not breathing (apnea) but still maintain a pulse. The START system would categorize the nonbreathing child as deceased, but the JumpSTART system modifies the process to include a pulse check for the nonbreathing child and 5 ventilations if there is a pulse. The ventilation is meant to jump-start the child's breathing.

   However, if ventilations do not trigger spontaneous respirations, categorize the child as deceased and move on to the next patient. If the child begins to breathe spontaneously, categorize the child as immediate and move on without providing further ventilations. It is possible that the child may not be breathing when another rescuer arrives to begin secondary triage. This rescuer will determine the appropriate intervention based on the number of patients and the number of rescue personnel.

3. In this step, all patients have spontaneous respirations. If the respiratory rate is 15 to 45 breaths per minute, proceed to Step 4 and assess perfusion. If the respiratory rate is slower than 15 (slower than 1 breath every 4 seconds) or faster than 45 breaths per minute or very irregular, categorize the child as immediate and move on.

4. In this step, all patients have adequate respirations. Assess perfusion by palpating peripheral pulses on uninjured limbs. Check peripheral pulses rather than capillary refill because of the many variables that affect accuracy. If the child has palpable peripheral pulses, assess mental status (see Step 5). If there are no peripheral pulses, categorize the patient as immediate and move on.

5. In this step, all patients have adequate ABCs. Check the child's mental status by using a rapid AVPU assessment. Keep in mind that the developmental age of the child will affect the results. If the child is alert, responds to your voice, or responds appropriately to pain (localizes the pain or knows where you are pressing or grasping and withdraws or pushes you away), categorize the patient as delayed. If the child does not respond to your voice and responds inappropriately to pain (makes a noise, moves sporadically, or does not localize the pain), shows

"posturing" (decorticate, with arms curled onto the chest toward the midline of the body, or decerebrate, with arms stiff at the sides and hands flexed away from the body), or is unresponsive, categorize as immediate and move on.

Alternative Triage Systems

LO11 Describe the key elements of the SALT triage system.

Other systems of triage have been developed and are in use around the country. One such system is the **SALT triage system**, which is gaining in popularity for its simplicity and ease of use. The SALT triage system has been endorsed by more than a dozen national emergency medicine and EMS organizations, as well as the Model Uniform Core Criteria for Triage, and provides a framework of clear, simple steps that field providers can use to bring order to a large incident and help improve patient outcomes.[3]

SALT stands for:

- Sort
- Assess
- Lifesaving interventions
- Treatment/Transport

SALT triage system ▶ triage system used for determining patient treatment priority during multiple-casualty incidents. SALT stands for Sort, Assess, Lifesaving interventions, and Treatment/Transport.

With the SALT method, when you assess and find a life threat you should provide a lifesaving intervention as long as it does not take longer than 1 minute and does not require you or another EMS provider to stay with the patient. For example, if you find that a patient has uncontrolled bleeding, rapidly apply a tourniquet. If a patient's airway is closed, open it. If that patient is a child or infant, consider giving them rescue breaths before moving on.

In some areas, the use of triage tags has been replaced by the use of colored plastic ribbons that can be easily tied to a patient's arm or leg to identify their triage category by color (black, red, yellow, or green).

FIRST ON SCENE WRAP-UP

Lanson sits on a bench for what seems like an eternity as the mall slowly fills—first with police officers then with people in large, clumsy bomb suits. Finally, the firefighters and EMTs are allowed in to quickly carry out the wounded. The deceased individuals Lanson had identified as "D" are left sprawled on the beige tiles where they fell after the explosion.

Lanson rubs his eyes and notices that his white uniform shirt is now covered in bloody smears and dark, pungent ash. He is taking it off when a police officer approaches him. "Let's get you out to the treatment area," the officer says.

"Oh, I'm not hurt." Lanson rolls his shirt into a ball and puts it under his arm.

"That's fine," the officer replies. "Let's just have you looked at, okay?"

Lanson can't think of any good reason to stay in the mall or to ever come back, for that matter. He walks to the door and steps out into the late-afternoon sun. He is immediately overwhelmed by the number of emergency vehicles and rescuers hustling around the entryway. He shades his eyes from the sun and sees crowds of people, including some with cameras, being held back by police barricades on the far side of the street.

"Are you the one who did the triaging in there?" A gruff voice startles Lanson, and he spins around.

"Uh, yes, sir," he answers, seeing an older firefighter wearing a white helmet.

"You did a real fine job." The man smiles, reaches out, and shakes Lanson's hand. "I bet you saved some lives in there."

Summary

- While relatively rare, multiple-casualty incidents (MCIs) can easily overwhelm the first responding units at the scene. It is up to those first units to quickly request additional resources and begin to establish command over the incident.
- An incident command system (also called incident management system) is a system used to manage overall control of large scenes involving many resources and multiple agencies.
- Triage is the sorting of patients based on the severity of their injuries or illnesses. The goal of triage is to save as many patients as possible using the available resources.
- Triage systems vary by jurisdiction, but they generally use a three- or four-category system. Typical categories include: *immediate* for the most critical but salvageable patients, *delayed* for those less critical but still in need of care, *minor* for those who are generally ambulatory at the scene, and *deceased* for those who show no signs of life.
- One version of a triage system is the START system—a Simple Triage and Rapid Treatment program that uses respirations, perfusion, and mental status assessments to categorize patients into one of four treatment categories.
- The JumpSTART system is a variation of the START triage system designed specifically to address the unique needs and presentation of pediatric patients.
- The SALT triage system provides a framework of clear, simple steps that field providers can use to bring order to a large incident and help improve patient outcomes. SALT stands for Sort, Assess, Lifesaving interventions, and Treatment/Transport.

Take Action

Volunteers Needed

Multiple-casualty incidents can be some of the most frightening and rewarding events to ever be a part of. While they are rare, if you are involved in EMS long enough, you are certain to respond to one eventually. One of the best ways to begin to get a glimpse at how these events unfold is to volunteer for a local MCI drill in your area. Fire departments, hospitals, and EMS agencies frequently conduct MCI drills as a way to prepare for the real event. There is a huge need for volunteers to play victims at those events. Contact your instructor or local EMS agency to offer your services at the next MCI drill. You will probably discover that several drills are conducted each year in your area or region.

First on Scene Run Review

Recall the events of the First on Scene scenario in this chapter, and answer the following questions related to the call. Rationales are offered in the Answer Key at the back of the book.

1. In an explosion, what is your first priority?
2. In triaging, how do you prioritize the patients?
3. What information do you want to give the arriving EMS personnel?

Quick Quiz

To check your understanding of the chapter, answer the following questions. Then compare your answers to those in the Answer Key at the back of the book.

1. A multiple-casualty incident (MCI) is best defined as a(n):
   a. situation with more than three patients.
   b. terrorist incident.
   c. incident where the number of patients overwhelms available resources.
   d. incident with more than one deceased patient.

2. An incident management system is a tool for the command, control, and _____ of resources at the scene of a large-scale emergency involving multiple agencies.
   a. constant monitoring
   b. care of victims
   c. coordination
   d. concerns of safety

3. The triage system was developed to assist in determining those victims who:

   a. will require only standard care.
   b. were the perpetrators of the incident.
   c. will likely benefit from immediate care.
   d. will be able to help with emergency response.

4. Which of the following is NOT a common component of the incident command system?

   a. Incident commander
   b. Triage
   c. Treatment
   d. Dispatch center

5. You have responded to the scene of a tour bus that has rolled over. The incident commander has assigned you to assist with triage. This means that you will:

   a. categorize patients based on injury severity.
   b. transport patients to the hospital.
   c. assist with delivering supplies.
   d. relay information to the press.

6. In the START triage system, patients are categorized based on an assessment of respirations,

   a. perfusion, and mental status.
   b. heart rate, and mental status.
   c. perfusion, and signs of shock.
   d. skin signs, and mental status.

7. While performing triage at a multiple-casualty incident, a patient walks up to you and states, "My arm hurts. I think it's broken." This patient should be tagged as:

   a. red.
   b. yellow.
   c. green.
   d. black.

8. You have just helped move a male patient who was initially tagged yellow from the scene to the treatment area. Upon arrival at the treatment area this patient should:

   a. be placed on the yellow tarp.
   b. receive a secondary triage assessment.
   c. have his blood pressure taken.
   d. be placed on the ambulance.

9. The JumpSTART triage assessment categories are:

   a. the same as those used for the START triage system.
   b. dependent on the age of the pediatric patient.
   c. very different from those used for the START triage system.
   d. dependent on the injuries of the pediatric patient.

10. You are triaging an adult patient who presents as unresponsive and breathing at a rate of 24. She should be triaged as:

   a. immediate.
   b. delayed.
   c. minor.
   d. deceased.

Endnotes

1. Federal Emergency Management Agency, "National Incident Management System," last updated March 20, 2023. Accessed May 7, 2023, at https://www.fema.gov/national-incident-management-system
2. American Heart Association, "2015 American Heart Association Guidelines for Cardiopulmonary Resuscitation and Emergency Cardiovascular Care," *Circulation*, Vol. 132 (2015): S177–S203, originally published October 14, 2015.
3. Federal Interagency Committee on EMS. National Implementation of the Model Uniform Core Criteria for Mass Casualty Incident Triage. 2014.

Patient Monitoring Devices

LEARNING OBJECTIVES

Upon successful completion of this appendix, the student should be able to:

Cognitive

1. Define the appendix key terms.
2. Explain the purpose of a cardiac monitor.
3. Describe the procedure for appropriately attaching cardiac electrode pads to a patient.
4. Explain the purpose of a pulse oximeter.
5. Explain the two values that a pulse oximeter monitors.
6. Differentiate normal and abnormal values displayed by the pulse oximeter.
7. Explain the factors that might cause a pulse oximeter to provide inaccurate readings.
8. Explain the purpose of a blood glucometer.
9. Differentiate normal and abnormal blood glucose values.
10. Explain the purpose of an end-tidal CO_2 detector.
11. Describe the procedure for using an end-tidal CO_2 detector while ventilating a patient.
12. Differentiate and discuss normal and abnormal values displayed by an end-tidal CO_2 detector.

Psychomotor

13. Demonstrate the proper method for attaching a three- and four-lead monitor to a simulated patient.
14. Demonstrate the proper method for attaching a pulse oximeter to a simulated patient.
15. Demonstrate the proper method for using an end-tidal CO_2 detector when ventilating a simulated patient.

Affective

16. Recognize the limitations of monitoring devices.
17. Value the importance of caring for the patient based on all signs and symptoms and not just those being displayed by the monitoring device.

KEY TERMS

blood glucose (*p. 592*)
cardiac monitor (*p. 589*)
end-tidal carbon dioxide (CO_2)
  detector (*p. 592*)

glucometer (*p. 591*)
pulse oximeter (*p. 590*)

A ssisting advanced-level providers such as EMTs and paramedics is
an important role of the Emergency Medical Responder. Often, the
advanced provider is busy with many duties at once, and support from an
Emergency Medical Responder can greatly enhance the efficiency and quality
of patient care. This appendix introduces you to the most commonly used
monitoring devices in the prehospital environment. It also describes the
general features of each device and explains how the Emergency Medical
Responder can best assist with their use.

Cardiac Monitor

LO2 Explain the purpose of a cardiac monitor.

LO3 Describe the procedure for appropriately attaching
cardiac electrode pads to a patient.

The **cardiac monitor** is a device used to display the electrical
activity of the heart. Cardiac monitors come in a variety
of shapes and sizes depending on the manufacturer and
features of the device. Some cardiac monitors simply
provide an image of the patient's electrocardiogram (ECG)
on a screen, while others are far more complex and allow
for the monitoring of several different signs (Figure A1.1).

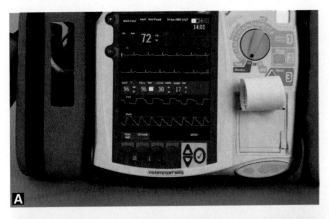

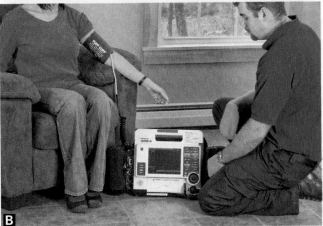

Figure A1.1 Cardiac monitors. (A) Some heart monitors
simply provide an electrical tracing of the heart. (B) More
sophisticated monitors can measure blood pressure, oxygen
saturation, and other vital signs.

These monitors are distinguished from automated external
defibrillators (AEDs) in that a trained provider is required
to interpret and act on the ECG rhythm provided by the
monitor. When using an AED, the provider does not need to
have any knowledge of cardiology or ECG interpretation;
the machine takes care of that part and instructs the
provider to either shock or continue CPR.

The typical cardiac monitor used on advanced life
support (ALS) ambulances is a multipurpose model that
can obtain both three-lead and 12-lead ECGs, provide
varying energy levels for defibrillation, and serve as an
external pacemaker for the patient's heart. Increasing
numbers of EMS systems are beginning to use models that
can monitor the patient's exhaled carbon dioxide levels
and oxygen saturation levels and automatically take blood
pressures.

The main purpose of an ECG monitor is to allow
the EMS provider to easily monitor the heart rate and,
more importantly, the heart's rhythm. Electrodes placed
on the skin pick up the electrical activity generated by the
heart. The ECG monitor can reassure the EMS provider
that the patient's heart rate is normal or alert them to an
acute condition that could require further evaluation and
treatment.

Initially, the three-lead monitor is used on the patient,
although this requires the placement of four electrodes.
The fourth electrode is the ground that allows the electrical
circuit to close. The electrical rhythm of the heart displayed
on the ECG screen does not represent the physical motion
of blood moving in and out of the heart, only the electrical
conduction. Therefore, pulse and blood pressure must
always be checked in conjunction with use of the ECG
monitor.

If the patient is having chest pain or other cardiac signs
and symptoms, EMS personnel may decide to perform a
12-lead ECG. This involves using six extra cables that are
placed on the chest wall to provide multiple images of the
electrical activity in the heart from 12 angles (Figure A1.2).
The main purpose of this is to identify if a heart attack is
occurring and where, within the heart, it is located.

The Emergency Medical Responder can assist by
connecting the cables to the ECG monitor, snapping
electrodes to the ends of each cable, and placing the
electrodes on the patient. Most monitors have labels on
the end of each cable indicating the position on the body

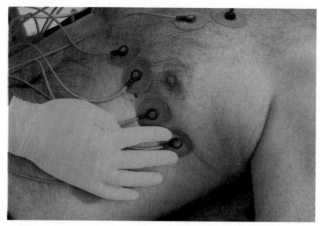

Figure A1.2 Multiple electrode pads are placed on the chest to allow the monitor to obtain a 12-lead view of the heart.

where they should be placed, such as "LL" for left leg and "RA" for right arm. Some monitors may not have this, but instead use a color-coded system. In those cases, the black lead is for the upper left extremity or chest, the red lead is for the lower left extremity or chest, and the white lead is for the right upper extremity or chest.

As a general rule, electrodes should always be placed over muscle or fat tissue, not the more bony areas.

If the patient has excess body hair, it can interfere with electrode contact. Most monitor packs will have a disposable shaving razor to use for clearing the areas where electrodes will be applied.

Another problem occasionally encountered is an extremely diaphoretic patient. Excess sweat can prevent the electrodes from sticking to the skin, leading to a poor connection. Be sure to dry the skin thoroughly before attempting to apply the electrodes.

Once the electrodes are placed on the patient and the monitor cables are plugged into the monitor, turn on the monitor and advise the paramedic that the monitor is ready. Occasionally, there may be artifact (electrical interference), which is a result of patient or vehicle movement and appears as erratic movement in the ECG baseline rhythm. If the paramedic deems the rhythm acceptable, print a 6-second strip from the monitor to capture the rhythm.

Follow these steps when applying a cardiac monitor to the patient:

1. Explain to the patient what you are doing and why.
2. Turn on the ECG monitor.
3. Take out the ECG cables and electrodes.
4. Attach the lead cable to the monitor.
5. Place an electrode on the end of each cable.
6. Expose the patient's extremities or chest as appropriate. Shave excess hair as necessary.
7. Apply the appropriate electrode to each limb, ensuring that all electrodes are firmly adhered to the skin.
8. Observe for artifact and ensure that the patient is not moving.
9. Print a 6-second ECG strip.

Even though the four leads you are placing on the patient are called "limb" leads, they are most often placed on the torso of the patient. This is typically done for convenience and is an acceptable alternative to placing the electrodes on each of the four limbs. The placement of leads on the torso will typically be near each shoulder and on the upper abdomen on the lateral side.

Pulse Oximeter

LO4 Explain the purpose of a pulse oximeter.

LO5 Explain the two values that a pulse oximeter monitors.

LO6 Differentiate normal and abnormal values displayed by the pulse oximeter.

LO7 Explain the factors that might cause a pulse oximeter to provide inaccurate readings.

A **pulse oximeter** (pulse ox for short), is a device that uses infrared technology to determine the percentage of a patient's hemoglobin that is saturated with oxygen (Figure A1.3). It does this by determining how much of the infrared and red lights that are shot through a thin area of skin are absorbed by the hemoglobin. Most commonly, the

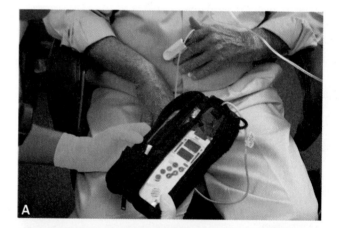

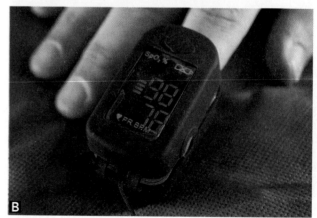

Figure A1.3 Two types of pulse oximeters. (A) This type can be attached to a finger, earlobe, or toe. (B) Style designed for fingertip use.

fingertip, earlobe, and toe are used for measurement. The pulse oximeter can be a standalone device or incorporated into cardiac monitors. The pulse oximeter displays two values: the percentage of oxygen saturation and the heart rate (Figure A1.4).

The saturation of peripheral oxygen, often abbreviated as SpO_2, is a valuable clinical tool for monitoring patients with respiratory complaints. A normal saturation is above 94%, although values as low as 90% could be normal for a patient with a chronic lung disease such as COPD. For most patients, saturations below 90% are never normal and should be corrected quickly with supplemental oxygen.

To obtain an accurate baseline saturation level, the pulse oximeter should first be applied when the patient is on room air, meaning that they are not receiving any supplemental oxygen. However, if the patient is in respiratory distress or has other indications of hypoxia, do not delay application of supplemental oxygen to obtain a pulse oximetry reading. Whenever saturation is measured for a patient on oxygen, it is important to record what type of oxygen-delivery device was being used and the rate of flow being delivered.

The pulse oximeter can give false readings in certain circumstances. The most common reason is the presence of nail polish, which will prevent the pulse oximeter probe from directing the light through the tissue. Any patient wearing nail polish should have the polish removed on the finger to be used for monitoring.

Hypothermia is a condition that will give falsely low saturation readings due to the constriction of blood vessels in the fingers or toes caused by the cold.

Falsely high readings occur in patients exposed to carbon monoxide poisoning because the carbon monoxide binds to the hemoglobin instead of oxygen. To the monitor, the hemoglobin appears saturated and will display a falsely high reading. However, the reality is that the hemoglobin is saturated with carbon monoxide and the patient may still be hypoxic. For children, a special probe is used to accommodate their smaller size.

Follow these steps when applying a pulse oximeter to a patient:

1. Explain to the patient what you are going to do. Remove the probe from the kit and connect the cable to the device (if applicable).
2. Turn on the device.
3. Identify a finger to use, and remove nail polish if necessary. Place the probe on the finger.
4. Record the percentage of saturation and heart rate. Confirm the heart rate on the device by taking a radial pulse.

Alternative sites for the application of the monitor probe are the toes and earlobe. Placement on an earlobe will require a specialized probe.

Glucometer

LO8 Explain the purpose of a blood glucometer.
LO9 Differentiate normal and abnormal blood glucose values.

The **glucometer** is a device used to measure and display the amount of glucose (sugar) in a given sample of blood. It is a portable device that allows rapid testing in the field by the EMS provider or patient (Figure A1.5). Glucometers are routinely prescribed for patients with diabetes, who learn how to check and monitor their blood sugar level at home.

To use the device, a small drop of blood must be obtained for testing. Typically, the patient's fingertip is cleaned and punctured with a small disposable needle called a *lancet*. A drop of blood is placed on a chemical test strip, which is inserted into the device either before or after the addition of blood, depending on the model (Figure A1.6).

Once the sample is collected, most glucometers will produce the result within 30 seconds. The result is given in milligrams per deciliter (mg/dL), and this is how it is traditionally reported. The chemical strip and lancet are

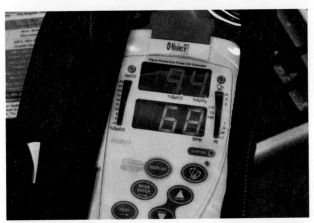

Figure A1.4 A pulse oximeter will measure and display both oxygen saturation (top display) and pulse rate (bottom display).

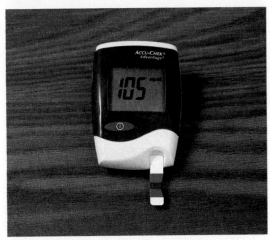

Figure A1.5 Typical blood glucometer.

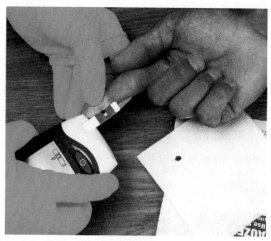

Figure A1.6 A drop of blood is placed on the test strip and is immediately analyzed by the device.

disposable, and the lancet should be placed in a sharps container after use.

Blood glucose is the level of glucose in the bloodstream at any given time. Normal blood glucose levels range from 80 to 120 mg/dL. Some patients with diabetes may run slightly higher or lower, and they will typically inform the EMS provider of this. Hypoglycemia occurs in patients with low blood glucose levels and can cause altered mental status, lethargy, and eventually unconsciousness and seizures. High blood glucose levels, or hyperglycemia, can also cause confusion but generally to a lesser extent than hypoglycemia.

In many EMS systems, Emergency Medical Responders are not allowed to use a glucometer. This must only be used by EMS providers who are trained and authorized to do so. Always follow local protocols.

End-Tidal Carbon Dioxide Detector

LO10 Explain the purpose of an end-tidal CO_2 detector.

LO11 Describe the procedure for using an end-tidal CO_2 detector while ventilating a patient.

LO12 Differentiate and discuss normal and abnormal values displayed by an end-tidal CO_2 detector.

The **end-tidal carbon dioxide (ETCO$_2$) detector** measures the amount of carbon dioxide the patient exhales with each breath. The reason it is called the end-tidal CO_2, or ETCO$_2$, is because the number it provides reflects only the amount of CO_2 at the very end of the exhalation. More advanced monitors have waveform capnography, which allows the measurement of CO_2 levels throughout the entire ventilatory cycle.

ETCO$_2$ detectors come in a variety of styles. In EMS, they are used primarily to verify proper placement of an endotracheal tube following intubation. Increasingly, the

detectors are being used on conscious and breathing patients to evaluate for the presence of certain respiratory diseases such as asthma, hyperventilation, and congestive heart failure.

Two types of ETCO$_2$ detectors are used following intubation: disposable colormetric devices (Figure A1.7) and digital sensors. The disposable colormetric devices use litmus paper that will change color in the presence of CO_2. The small plastic device has a port on either side. One side attaches to the endotracheal tube and the other to the bag-mask device. Therefore, the detector lies directly in the path of airflow. The paper is purple initially and will change to gold when it comes in contact with CO_2, indicating the tube placement is correct. If the tube is in the trachea and the lungs are being ventilated, the gas exchange will cause CO_2 to be exhaled. If the tube is misplaced, such as in the stomach, then no CO_2 will be returned and the color on the detector will not change.

Digital and waveform sensors attach similarly to the endotracheal tube and plug into the ETCO$_2$ monitor or ECG machine, depending on the model. These devices allow continuous monitoring that can be used to evaluate the efficiency of ventilation. A normal ETCO$_2$ level is 35 to 45 mm Hg. When ventilating a patient, the provider should aim to keep the level at the low end of this range. If ventilations are being given too rapidly, then the ETCO$_2$ level will drop. If ventilations are too slow, the opposite will occur and CO_2 levels will rise because the patient is not exhaling enough.

In conscious patients, the ETCO$_2$ can be monitored by a cannula-type device. The devices can measure the exhaled CO_2 from the nostril. The waveform can then be interpreted to assist in diagnosing the patient's condition, such as differentiating between an asthma attack and hyperventilation.

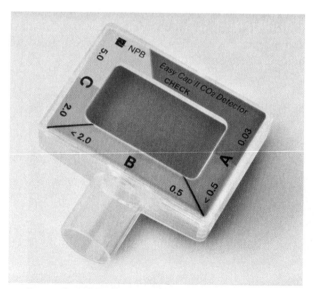

Figure A1.7 Color-changing (colormetric) end-tidal CO_2 detector.

Limitations of Monitoring Devices

The increased use of technology in medicine has greatly enhanced diagnostic and treatment abilities, but devices are no replacement for a proper and detailed physical examination. The tools are best used as supplements to traditional examination skills and can be used to support assessment findings. Various conditions can fool all the devices: carbon monoxide poisoning for the pulse oximeter, poor calibration for the glucometer, and so on. The EMS provider must always take this into account when treating the patient. Any finding on the devices should always be compared to the actual vital signs, patient complaints, and patient appearance. Remember: treat the patient, not the monitor.

Principles of Pharmacology

LEARNING OBJECTIVES

Upon successful completion of this appendix, the student should be able to:

Cognitive

1. Define the appendix key terms.
2. Describe the indications, contraindications, actions, and side effects of selected medications commonly encountered in the field environment: activated charcoal, epinephrine autoinjector, metered-dose inhalers, naloxone (Narcan), nitroglycerin, and oral glucose.
3. List the five "rights" of medication administration.
4. Explain the role of the Emergency Medical Responder when assisting a patient with administration of medication.

Psychomotor

5. Demonstrate the ability to properly assist a patient with the administration of prescribed medication.
6. Demonstrate the ability to properly assist a patient with the administration of an autoinjector.

Affective

7. Value the importance of medications being administered as prescribed.

KEY TERMS

action (*p. 595*)
autoinjector (*p. 596*)
contraindication (*p. 595*)

indication (*p. 595*)
medication (*p. 595*)
side effect (*p. 596*)

This appendix is designed to aid Emergency Medical Responders who are being trained to assist patients in taking specific prescribed medications. This training is meant to be a part of a formal training program that is under the guidance and supervision of a medical director. All EMS providers who administer or assist patients in administering their own prescribed medications must follow local protocols. Remember that you may only give or assist in giving certain medications under the supervision of medical direction.

Pharmacology is the study of medications—their origins, nature, chemistry, effects, and use. Emergency Medical Responders will assess and care for many patients whose medical history includes the medications they take and whose problems may be caused by the effects of taking or not taking these medications properly. This appendix lists and describes the few medications Emergency Medical Responders may be carrying and the few prescribed medications you may assist a patient in administering. It also discusses how to give or assist the patient in administering the medications and the effects of the medications on the patient.

Medications

LO2 Describe the indications, contraindications, actions, and side effects of selected medications commonly encountered in the field environment: activated charcoal, epinephrine autoinjector, metered-dose inhalers, naloxone (Narcan), nitroglycerin, and oral glucose.

LO4 Explain the role of the Emergency Medical Responder when assisting a patient with administration of medication.

A **medication** is a substance used for medical treatment, often a drug. Emergency Medical Responders may be trained to assist with or administer certain medications, such as oxygen, activated charcoal, and oral glucose. Many Emergency Medical Responders are allowed by their Medical Director to administer these medications under specific circumstances. Activated charcoal and oral glucose are sold over the counter in most pharmacies and are often found in many households.

The other medications described in this appendix (metered-dose inhalers, nitroglycerin, epinephrine auto-injectors, and naloxone) must be prescribed by a health care provider and are usually carried by the patient. Depending on the specific EMS system, Emergency Medical Responders may be able to assist a patient in taking one or more of these medications with the approval of medical direction and under specific circumstances.

Indications, Contraindications, Actions, and Side Effects

For each medication, the Emergency Medical Responder must know and understand the specific indications, contraindications, and actions, as well as any expected side effects the medication may have on the patient. After a medication has been administered, it will be important to monitor the patient to see how the medication is affecting them. If taken properly, a medication will usually ease the ill effects of the medical condition. But, if the medication is expired or the patient's condition is beyond the help of the medication, the medication may be ineffective.

Indications are specific signs or symptoms for which it is appropriate to use a specific medication. For example, nitroglycerin is indicated for patients experiencing suspected cardiac chest pain, and an inhaler is indicated for someone having an asthma attack.

Contraindications are specific signs, symptoms, or conditions for which it is not appropriate to use a specific medication. For example, nitroglycerin is contraindicated in patients who have a systolic blood pressure below 100. Since nitroglycerin reduces blood pressure, it is possible to cause an already low blood pressure to drop too low if it is not above 100 systolic before taking the dose. Administering oral glucose to an unresponsive patient may be contraindicated since it may cause an airway obstruction.

A medication's **action** is the specific effect it is designed to have on the patient. The action of naloxone is to block or reverse the effects of a narcotic overdose. Nitroglycerin is designed to dilate the vessels, thereby reducing the workload on the heart. The action of activated charcoal is to bind with a poison and prevent it from being absorbed by the digestive system. The action of glucose is to raise the level of sugar in the blood.

Medications sometimes have side effects. A **side effect** is any action or reaction caused by the medication other than the desired effect. Some side effects are expected and predictable. Nitroglycerin will dilate vessels, not just in the heart, but also throughout the body. This may cause a large enough drop in blood pressure to make the patient dizzy or lightheaded. Another common side effect of nitroglycerin is a headache. You must anticipate side effects and document them when they occur, especially before administering a second dose. It is good practice to advise or remind the patient about the possible side effects before administering any medication. This could minimize the chances of any surprises that could further add to the patient's anxiety. If the patient has taken any of these medications before, they will probably know what side effects to expect.

Rules for Administering Medications

LO3 List the five "rights" of medication administration.

Before you give any medication, you must check the five "rights." This is a simple checklist you must go through that will help ensure that things are done correctly. Often, you will have to rely on the patient's word. Ask the following questions:

- *Right patient?* Is this the right patient for this medication? Read aloud the name written on the medication bottle: "Is your name Bob Becker?" If the patient does not have a labeled box or bottle, simply ask if this is the patient's own medication.
- *Right medication?* Is this the right medication for this patient? For example, the patient is having chest pain but hands you a bottle of an antibiotic, or the patient has strep throat but hands you a bottle of nitroglycerin.
- *Right dose?* Is this the right dose for this patient? The dosage is usually written on the label, but the patient does not always carry the original box or bottle the medication came in.
- *Right route?* Is this the right route for taking the medication? Medications are given by different routes—swallowed by mouth, inhaled by mouth or nose, dissolved under the tongue, injected into or absorbed through the skin.
- *Right time?* Is this the right time to be giving the medication? In the case of nitroglycerin, has enough time elapsed since the last dose was given?

Routes for Administering Medications

The way a patient takes a medication influences how quickly the medication enters the bloodstream and begins to work. Medications are administered by the following routes:

- *Oral or swallowed.* Taken by mouth, these medications are in a solid form (tablet or capsule) or in a liquid form (liquid medication or a powder dissolved in or mixed with a liquid, such as the activated charcoal slurry).
- *Intramuscular.* These medications are injected into a muscle, such as the epinephrine **autoinjector**.
- *Sublingual.* These medications are dissolved under the tongue, such as nitroglycerin tablets.
- *Inhaled.* These medications are breathed into the lungs, as from an inhaler or oxygen-delivery device, such as the medication given for chronic respiratory problems, or the oxygen given for respiratory distress or other reasons.
- *Intranasal.* Medications administered via this route are sprayed directly into the nasal cavity through the nostril. Studies have shown that certain medications, such as naloxone, can be rapidly and effectively absorbed through the nasal mucous membranes and into the bloodstream.
- *Transdermal patches or transdermal infusion systems.* Patches are affixed to the skin by an adhesive backing on one side. Another chemical is mixed in with the medication, usually a form of alcohol that will carry the medication through the patient's skin into the bloodstream. These patches are slow to react and are not meant for acute attacks such as the onset of chest pain.
- *Endotracheal.* Sprayed into a tube inserted into the trachea (windpipe), this route more directly reaches the lungs and medications can be absorbed quickly. (Emergency Medical Responders will not administer medication in this form.)

Medications Carried on the Emergency Medical Responder Unit

LO2 Describe the indications, contraindications, actions, and side effects of selected medications commonly encountered in the field environment: activated charcoal, epinephrine autoinjector, metered-dose inhalers, naloxone (Narcan), nitroglycerin, and oral glucose.

LO4 Explain the role of the Emergency Medical Responder when assisting a patient with administration of medication.

Activated Charcoal

Activated charcoal (Key Skill A2.1) is not the kind of charcoal you use with a barbecue grill. It is most often found in a slurry form, which is a powder premixed with water for use in the prehospital emergency situation. Activated charcoal is administered to patients who have ingested a poison or who took an overdose of one or more oral medications. When the patient drinks the activated charcoal slurry, it binds with the poisonous substance or medication and helps prevent it from being absorbed by the body. Follow local protocols for administration. The use of activated charcoal in the prehospital setting has fallen out of favor in many EMS systems due to the difficulty of administering it and the fact that it can cause some people to vomit.

Oral Glucose

Glucose is a simple sugar found in many common foods such as candy, soda, fruit, bread, and vegetables and is the body's main source of energy. The brain, in particular, is very sensitive to abnormally low levels of glucose and functions poorly without it. A patient with abnormally low glucose levels will commonly have an altered mental status.

KEY SKILL A2.1

Administering Activated Charcoal

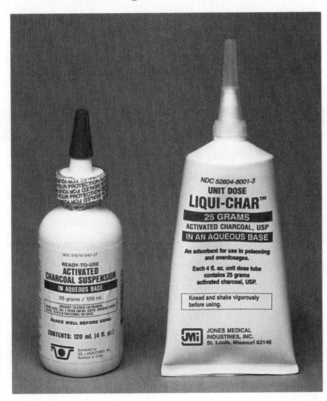

Medication Name
- Generic: activated charcoal
- Trade: SuperChar, Insta-Char, Actidose, Liqui-Char, and others

Indications

Poisoning by mouth (ingestion)

Contraindications
- Altered mental status
- Ingestion of acids or alkalis
- Unable to swallow

Medication Form
- Premixed in water, frequently available in plastic bottle containing 25 grams of activated charcoal
- Powder, which should be avoided in the field

Dosage
- Adults and children: 1 gram activated charcoal/kg of body weight
- Usual adult dose: 25–50 grams
- Usual pediatric dose: 12.5–25 grams

Steps for Administration
1. Consult medical direction.
2. Shake the container vigorously.
3. Since the medication looks like mud, the patient may need to be persuaded to drink it. Providing a covered container and a straw will prevent the patient from seeing the medication and may improve patient compliance.
4. If the patient does not drink the medication right away, the charcoal will settle. Shake or stir it again before administering.
5. Record the name, dose, route, and time of administration of the medication.
6. Perform reassessment.

Actions
- Activated charcoal binds to certain poisons and prevents them from being absorbed into the body.

Side Effects
- Causes black stools.
- Some patients, particularly those who have ingested poisons that cause nausea, may vomit. If the patient vomits, repeat the dose once.

Reassessment Strategies

Be prepared for the patient to vomit or continue to get worse. If the patient worsens, provide oxygen as you have been trained to do.

Glucose levels can be raised by giving oral glucose (Key Skill A2.2), a form of glucose that comes in a gel or chewable tablet. It is indicated for patients with an altered mental status and a history of diabetes. It is taken orally.

To assist in the administration of oral glucose, have the patient hold the tube and instruct them to squeeze small amounts into his or her mouth and swallow. You want the patient to ingest the entire tube as quickly as possible but without choking. An alternative method for administration is to apply some of the gel to a tongue depressor and spread it between the patient's cheek and gum. Continue to apply small doses until the tube is empty. The mucous membranes inside the mouth are rich in blood vessels, which quickly absorb the glucose and carry it through the bloodstream. Once the level of glucose is elevated, the patient's condition usually begins to improve.

For tablets, the typical strength is 5 grams of D-glucose (dextrose). This form of glucose passes through the mucosa (lining) of the mouth, esophagus, and stomach so no digestion is needed. It does not have to enter the small intestine to be absorbed. The manufacturer's recommended dosage is three tablets, or 15 grams. Do not try to administer glucose tablets to anyone who is unresponsive and unable to manage their own airway.

The patient should respond quickly to the tablets. Fatigue may remain for varying periods of time depending on the patient and how rapidly the blood glucose level fell during the hypoglycemic episode. Some patients have feelings of uneasiness that remain for up to half an hour. Most are able to eat additional foods that help with their symptoms. However, do not allow someone to ingest food if they have been given glucose and report nausea. The nausea should subside shortly and, if the patient requests food and remains alert, most protocols for hypoglycemic events allow it.

Oxygen

Oxygen is considered a medication (Figure A2.1). It is used to treat patients who have hypoxia (low oxygen levels in their blood). Oxygen and oxygen therapy are described in detail in Chapter 10. If your Emergency Medical Responder unit carries oxygen and oxygen-delivery devices, you must participate in a training program to learn how and when to use them properly. Be sure to follow your jurisdiction's guidelines, protocols, and medical direction.

KEY SKILL A2.2

Administering Oral Glucose

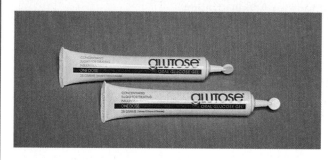

Medication Name
- Generic: glucose, oral
- Trade: Glutose, Insta-glucose, BD Glucose Tablets

Indications
- The patient has an altered mental status with a known history of diabetes.
- The patient has taken insulin but no food recently and may have been very physically active.

Contraindications
- The patient is unresponsive, unable to swallow, or otherwise unable to manage his or her own airway.
- The patient has a history of diabetes and has not taken insulin for days.

Medication Form

Gel, in toothpaste-type tubes; chewable tablets

Dosage

One tube; three 5-gram chewable tablets. This dose can be used for both adults and children. Tubes are available in 15-, 25-, and 45-gram doses.

Steps For Administration
1. Confirm signs and symptoms of altered mental status with a known history of diabetes.
2. Ensure that the patient is alert enough to swallow.
3. Administer glucose.
   a. Self-administered into mouth and swallowed.
   b. Place on tongue depressor between cheek and gum. OR
   c. Have patient chew one to three tablets.
4. Perform reassessment.

Actions

Increases blood sugar levels

Side Effects

None when given properly

Reassessment Strategies

Continue to monitor the patient's mental status and signs and symptoms. If the patient becomes less responsive, discontinue administration. Continue to provide oxygen as you have been trained to do.

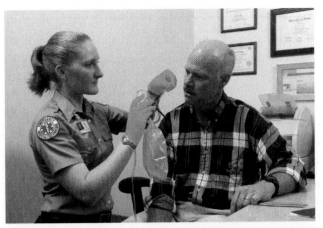

Figure A2.1 Oxygen is a useful medication for many patients.

Prescription Medications

LO2 | Describe the indications, contraindications, actions, and side effects of selected medications commonly encountered in the field environment: activated charcoal, epinephrine autoinjector, metered-dose inhalers, naloxone (Narcan), nitroglycerin, and oral glucose.

LO4 | Explain the role of the Emergency Medical Responder when assisting a patient with administration of medication.

Metered-Dose Inhalers

Many patients have chronic respiratory diseases such as asthma, emphysema, or bronchitis that cause the air passages in the lungs to narrow, or become constricted. Such patients usually carry a device called a *metered-dose inhaler* (Key Skill A2.3). It typically contains medication called a *bronchodilator*. This medication dilates the air passages so the patient can breathe easier. The inhaler device contains medication in aerosol form, which can be sprayed into the mouth and inhaled.

You must have medical direction to help a patient self-administer this medication. You must also make sure that this medication belongs to the patient and was not loaned to them by a well-meaning family member or friend with a similar problem. Also, checking for an expiration date is important since expired medication is less effective.

Naloxone (Narcan)

Narcan has been used in EMS for decades for the treatment of opioid overdose. It is now available over the counter and is being carried by many first responders and law enforcement agencies. Narcan binds to chemical receptors in the brain and acts to block or reverse the effects of any opioid. It can immediately reverse the effects of an overdose and has saved many thousands of lives over the years.

KEY SKILL A2.3

Assisting with a Metered-Dose Inhaler

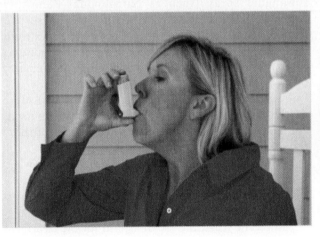

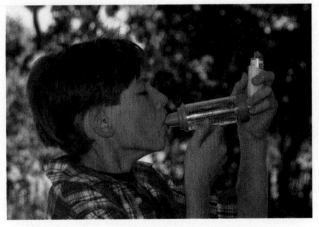

Medication Name
- Generic: albuterol, ipratropium, metaproterenol
- Trade: Proventil, Ventolin, Atrovent, Alupent, Metaprel

Indications

Meets all of the following criteria:
- The patient exhibits signs and symptoms of respiratory difficulty.
- The patient has a health care provider–prescribed inhaler.

- Medical direction gives the Emergency Medical Responder specific authorization to use it.

Contraindications
- The patient displays altered mental status (such that the patient is unable to use the device properly).
- No permission has been given by medical direction.
- The patient has already taken the maximum prescribed dose prior to the rescuer's arrival.

Medication Form

Handheld metered-dose inhaler

Dosage

The number of inhalations is based on medical directions or health care provider's order.

Steps For Administration

1. Obtain order from medical direction.
2. Confirm the patient is alert enough to use the inhaler.
3. Ensure that the inhaler is the patient's own prescription.
4. Check the expiration date of the inhaler.
5. Check if the patient has already taken any doses.
6. Shake the inhaler vigorously several times.
7. If the patient has a spacer device for use with the inhaler (attaches between inhaler and patient to allow for more effective use of medication), it should be used.
8. Have the patient exhale deeply.
9. Have the patient put their lips around the opening of the inhaler.
10. Have the patient depress the handheld inhaler when beginning to inhale deeply.

11. Instruct the patient to hold their breath for as long as is comfortable so the medication can be absorbed.
12. Allow the patient to breathe a few times and administer a second dose if so ordered by medical direction.
13. Provide oxygen as appropriate.
14. Perform reassessment.

Actions

Dilates bronchioles, reducing airway resistance

Side Effects

- Increased pulse rate
- Anxiety
- Nervousness

Reassessment Strategies

- Monitor vital signs.
- Adjust oxygen as appropriate.
- Reassess the level of respiratory distress.
- Observe for deterioration of the patient. If breathing becomes inadequate, provide artificial ventilations.

Narcan comes as a liquid that can be administered one of three ways:

- Intramuscular injection (2 mg)
- Autoinjector (2 mg)
- Nasal spray (4 mg)

The most common methods used by Emergency Medical Responders are the nasal spray and the autoinjector (Key Skill A2.4). Narcan is extremely safe and can be given to patients of any age. Indications are for use in any patient suspected of experiencing an opioid overdose and whose breathing rate is compromised. Multiple doses may be required if the first dose does not result in improved respirations.

Nitroglycerin

Nitroglycerin is a chemical that is well known as an explosive, but it also has medical uses. It decreases the workload of the heart by dilating blood vessels. It is effective in relieving certain types of pain, particularly the type caused by a heart condition called angina pectoris. Patients who have heart conditions that cause recurring chest pain or who have a history of heart attack may have a prescription for nitroglycerin (Key Skill A2.5). Nitroglycerin is available in several forms, including pill, spray, and paste.

Patients are typically instructed by their health care providers to take up to three doses—one every 5 minutes—over a 15-minute period if there has been no pain relief from the previous dose.

You will need to consult medical direction to help administer nitroglycerin or to get permission to give more after the patient has taken three doses. As with the inhalers, be sure to check that the nitroglycerin is actually the patient's medication and that it has not reached the expiration date.

The patient may have a bottle of nitroglycerin sublingual spray (such as Nitrolingual Pumpspray). Depending on local protocols, for cases of suspected cardiac chest pain, up to three metered sprays may be administered under the tongue—one every 5 minutes over a 15-minute period if there has been no pain relief from the previous dose.

The patient may have nitroglycerin transdermal patches (transdermal infusion system). These are for daily application and help prevent angina attacks, but they are not meant to relieve and correct an acute event.

Any time a patient complains of chest pain—whether it persists or not or whether the patient has a history of chest pain or not—arrange for immediate transport to a medical facility.

In recent years, the use of aspirin for the treatment of suspected heart attack has become commonplace in most hospitals and EMS systems. In fact, several pharmaceutical companies have created television and radio commercials encouraging the use of aspirin for this purpose. As an Emergency Medical Responder, you may encounter patients who have recently taken aspirin or who may want to take some while in your care. You must follow your local protocols when assisting any patient with the administration of aspirin.

Administering Naloxone (Narcan)

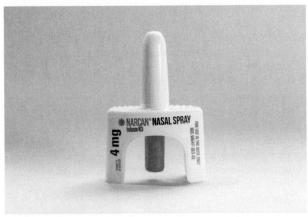

(Hanson L/Shutterstock)

Medication Name
- Generic: naloxone
- Trade: Narcan, EVZIO

Indications
Suspected opioid overdose

Contraindications
None

Medication Form
- Nasal spray (4 mg)
- Autoinjector (2 mg)

Dosage
Dependent on medication form (see below)

Steps for Administration
1. Consult medical direction.
2. Confirm respiratory status is compromised (respiratory rate 6 or less).
3. If using nasal device, firmly place in nostril and depress plunger.
4. If using the autoinjector, firmly press device against lateral side of thigh and hold in place for 10 seconds.
5. Record the name, dose, route, and time of administration of the medication.
6. Perform reassessment.
7. Monitor respiratory status and provide rescue breaths as appropriate.

Actions
Naloxone binds to the chemical receptors in the brain to block and reverse the effects of opioids.

Side Effects
May cause withdrawal symptoms such as anxiety, headache, increased heart rate and blood pressure, sweating, nausea, and vomiting.

Reassessment Strategies
Be prepared for the patient to vomit or become violent.

Administering Nitroglycerin

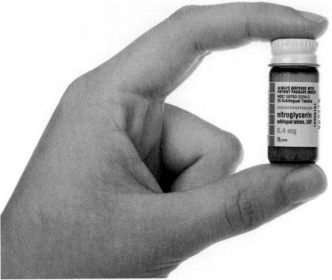

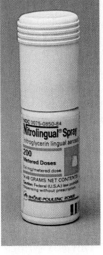

(Sheila Fitzgerald/Shutterstock)

Medication Name
- Generic: nitroglycerin
- Trade: Nitrostat, NitroTab, Nitrolingual

Indications

All of the following conditions must be met:
- The patient complains of chest pain.
- The patient has a history of cardiac problems.
- The patient's health care provider has prescribed nitroglycerin.
- The patient's systolic blood pressure is greater than 100 mm Hg. (Local protocols may vary.)
- Medical direction authorizes administration of the medication.

Contraindications
- The patient has a systolic blood pressure below 100 mm Hg. (Local protocols may vary.)
- The patient has a head injury.
- The patient has already taken the maximum prescribed dose.

Medication Form

Tablet or sublingual spray

Dosage

One dose is equal to 0.4 mg. Repeat in 3 to 5 minutes. If no relief, systolic blood pressure remains above 100 (local protocols may vary), and if authorized by medical direction, administer up to a maximum of three doses. Spray is typically prescribed for one metered spray followed by a second spray in 15 minutes.

Steps For Assisting Patient
1. Perform a focused assessment for a cardiac patient.
2. Take the patient's blood pressure. (Systolic pressure must be above 100; local protocols may vary.)

3. Contact medical direction if there are no standing orders.
4. Verify the right medication, patient, dose, and route. Check the expiration date.
5. Ensure that the patient is alert.
6. Question the patient on the last dose taken and its effects. Ensure understanding of the route of administration.
7. Ask the patient to lift their tongue. Place the tablet or spray dose on or under the tongue (while you are wearing gloves), or have the patient place the tablet or spray under their tongue.
8. Have the patient keep their mouth closed with the tablet or spray under the tongue (without swallowing) until it is dissolved and absorbed.
9. Recheck the patient's blood pressure within 2 minutes.
10. Record administration, route, and time.
11. Perform reassessment.

Actions
- Dilates blood vessels
- Decreases workload of heart

Side Effects
- Hypotension (lowers blood pressure)
- Headache
- Changes pulse rate
- Dizziness, light-headedness

Reassessment Strategies
- Monitor the patient's blood pressure.
- Ask the patient about the effect on pain relief.
- Seek medical direction before readministering.
- Record assessments.
- Provide oxygen as appropriate.

Epinephrine and Insulin Autoinjectors

Many people have allergies and will react severely to certain foods, medicines, or the poisons of insect stings or snakebites. These reactions may be life threatening when they cause the airway to become swollen and blood vessels to dilate. Epinephrine is a medication that can reverse those reactions (Key Skill A2.6). It dilates the air passages so breathing becomes easier and constricts the blood vessels.

Reactions to allergens can have a very sudden onset, and any reaction that causes breathing and circulation problems must be recognized and treated quickly. The patient must take their prescribed epinephrine immediately.

Patients who are aware of their allergies and expect severe reactions generally carry prescription medication in an autoinjector. This is a syringe with a spring-loaded needle that will release and inject epinephrine into a muscle when the patient presses it against the skin (usually in the thigh). If you need to assist the patient in taking epinephrine, first check to see if the injector is prescribed for that patient and get permission from medical direction. Remember to always check the expiration date.

Many patients with diabetes use a pen-type device to inject themselves with insulin. Be sure to check the device carefully before helping with administration.

Nerve Agent Autoinjectors

The threat of terrorism is an unfortunate reality of the times we live in. EMS systems across the country must anticipate this threat and do what they can to prepare. One of the most likely threats involves the dispersal of a deadly chemical known as a nerve agent. Nerve agents affect the nervous system and cause uncontrolled muscle activity and death.

Using an Epinephrine Autoinjector

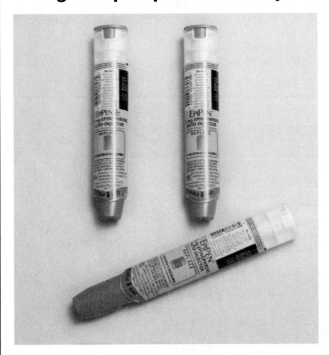

4. Place the tip of the autoinjector against the patient's lateral thigh, midway between the hip and knee.
5. Push the injector firmly against the thigh until the injector activates.
6. Hold the injector in place until the medication is injected (at least 10 seconds).
7. Record activity and time.
8. Dispose of the injector in a biohazard container.
9. Perform reassessment.

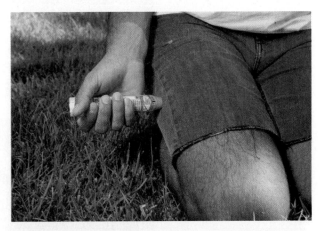

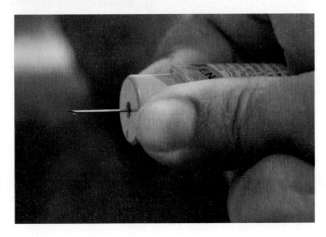

Medication Name
- Generic: epinephrine
- Trade: Adrenalin, Epi-Pen, Twinject

Indications

Must meet the following three criteria:
- The patient exhibits signs of a severe allergic reaction, including either respiratory distress or shock.
- The medication is prescribed for this patient by a health care provider.
- Medical direction authorizes use for this patient.

Contraindications

There are no contraindications when the medication is used in a life-threatening situation.

Medication Form

Liquid administered by an autoinjector (automatically injectable needle-and-syringe system)

Dosage

Adults: one adult autoinjector (0.3 mg)
Infant and child: one infant/child autoinjector (0.15 mg)

Steps for Assisting Patient

1. Obtain the patient's prescribed autoinjector. Ensure:
   a. Prescription is written for the patient who is experiencing the severe allergic reaction.
   b. Medication is not expired or discolored (if visible).
2. Obtain an order from medical direction.
3. Remove the cap from the autoinjector.

Actions
- Dilates the bronchioles
- Constricts blood vessels

Side Effects
- Increased heart rate
- Dizziness
- Chest pain
- Headache
- Nausea
- Vomiting
- Excitability, anxiety
- Pale skin

Reassessment Strategies

1. Arrange for transport.
2. Continue focused assessment of airway, breathing, and circulatory status. If the patient's condition continues to worsen (decreasing mental status, increasing breathing difficulty, decreasing blood pressure):
   a. Obtain medical direction for an additional dose of epinephrine.
   b. Provide care for shock, including administration of oxygen per local protocols.
   c. Prepare to initiate basic life support (CPR, AED).
3. If the patient's condition improves, provide supportive care:
   a. Continue oxygen.
   b. Provide care for shock.

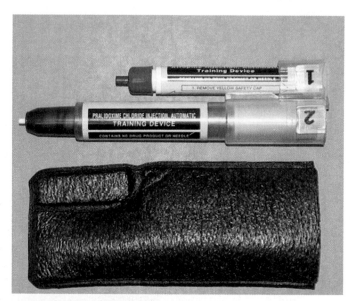

Figure A2.2 The Mark I autoinjector is used to deliver the antidote for nerve agent exposure.

Because of the potential for nerve agents to be used by terrorists, many EMS systems have assembled large supplies of an antidote. These antidotes most commonly come as an autoinjector and are designed for self-administration (Figure A2.2). As a member of the EMS team in your region or state, you will likely receive training on the indications and use of the antidote.

The autoinjectors contain two medications, atropine and pralidoxime (Protopam). They are meant to be used by EMS personnel in the event of a terrorist attack involving nerve agents. They are meant for self-administration and for administration to other EMS personnel. Administration of the antidote is like any autoinjector and should be injected into the lateral thigh muscle. In these types of incidents it is standard protocol to treat the rescuers first so that they may then move on to assist other victims.

Air Medical Transport Operations

LEARNING OBJECTIVES

Upon successful completion of this appendix, the student should be able to:

Cognitive

1 Define the appendix key terms.

2 Describe the common crew configurations within air medical transport.

3 Differentiate the benefits of fixed-wing and rotor-wing air medical transport.

4 Describe the two types of rotor-wing air medical transport missions.

5 Explain the common criteria for choosing air medical transport over ground transport.

6 Differentiate between visual and instrument flight rules.

7 Describe the characteristics of an appropriate helicopter landing zone.

8 Explain the safe principles of working around aircraft at the scene of an emergency.

Psychomotor

9 Demonstrate the ability to establish an appropriate helicopter landing zone.

Affective

10 Recognize the value of air medical transport when used properly.

KEY TERMS

fixed wing (*p. 607*)
helipad (*p. 607*)
instrument flight rules (IFR) (*p. 608*)

landing zone (LZ) (*p. 608*)
rotor wing (*p. 606*)
visual flight rules (VFR) (*p. 608*)

Education Standards

EMS Operations—Air Medical Transport

Competencies

Uses knowledge of operational roles and responsibilities to ensure patient, public, and personnel safety.

Many EMS systems across the United States use air medical resources such as helicopters (rotor wing) and airplanes (fixed wing) to transport critically ill and injured patients (Figure A3.1). Each year in the United States approximately 500,000 patients are transported by helicopter and another 150,000 are transported by airplane.

Although it is uncommon for an Emergency Medical Responder to be hired to work on an EMS aircraft, your current training can be the first step in becoming qualified to eventually gain employment with an air medical organization. However, as an Emergency Medical Responder, you may be in a position to request a helicopter or assist in the landing of a helicopter at the scene of an emergency.

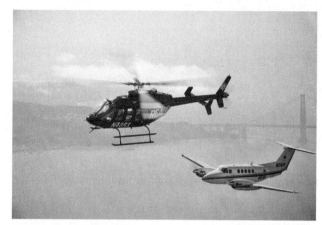

Figure A3.1 Both helicopters and airplanes are used in EMS today.
(REACH Air Medical Services)

Crew Configurations

LO2 | Describe the common crew configurations within air medical transport.

In the United States, most EMS aircraft are staffed with a nurse and a paramedic. Other common medical crew configurations are:

- Two nurses
- Two paramedics
- Doctor and nurse
- Nurse and respiratory therapist

The specific crew configuration is often determined by local regulations or the care required for the patient. These configurations are common for both helicopters and planes.

Air Medical Resources

LO3 | Differentiate the benefits of fixed-wing and rotor-wing air medical transport.

LO4 | Describe the two types of rotor-wing air medical transport missions.

Rotor-Wing Resources

The term **rotor wing** refers to the helicopter. Most EMS helicopters fly two types of missions: the *scene call* and the *interfacility transport (IFT)*. The scene call is made when a helicopter is requested to respond to the scene of an emergency, such as a vehicle collision or a near-drowning incident at a lake, river, or beach. In those cases, the helicopter is requested to respond to the scene just as

a ground ambulance might. If all goes well, the helicopter will land near the patient, allowing the medical crew to exit the aircraft, begin caring for the patient, and prepare them for transport (Figure A3.2).

The IFT occurs when a patient is already at a hospital but needs to be transported to another hospital. In most cases, the patient needs a higher level of care than the sending hospital is capable of providing. For example, a patient with significant trauma transported by ground ambulance to a hospital 5 minutes away may need to be transported to the regional trauma center 60 miles away. An IFT by aircraft would be required.

Many different types of EMS helicopters are in use today. They differ in many ways, including size, shape, number of engines, and how high or fast they can fly (Figure A3.3). Regardless of size or performance capabilities, EMS helicopters all share one very important characteristic—they are designed to carry critically ill

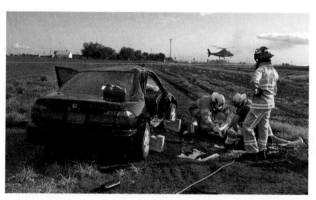

Figure A3.2 In many cases, a helicopter can land right at the emergency scene.
(REACH Air Medical Services)

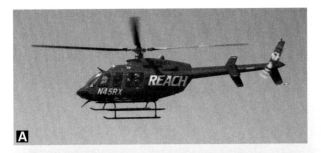

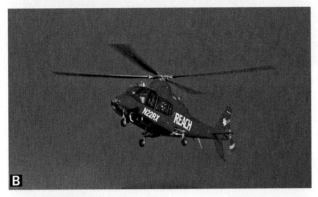

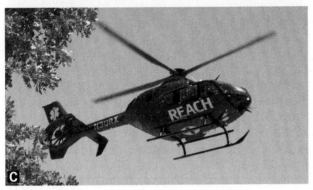

Figure A3.3 EMS helicopters come in many shapes and sizes: (A) Bell 407, (B) Agusta 109, and (C) Eurocopter EC 135.
(REACH Air Medical Services)

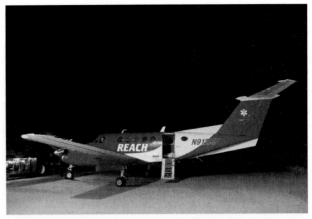

Figure A3.4 Fixed-wing aircraft (airplanes), such as this KingAir B200, are used for longer transports.
(REACH Air Medical Services)

or injured patients. The vast majority of helicopters are configured to carry just one patient lying on a stretcher. Although some can carry two patients, the ability to provide care while in flight is greatly minimized due to the limited space. Because a helicopter can fly from hospital pad to hospital pad, it is ideal for short transports (less than 200 miles).

Fixed-Wing Resources

Like helicopters, **fixed-wing** resources (airplanes) vary in size and performance capabilities; they include jets, turboprops, and piston-driven aircraft (Figure A3.4). The reason to choose an airplane over a helicopter is most often distance. Airplanes can fly much faster and farther than the typical helicopter, due largely to their ability to carry much more fuel. The airplane is ideal when there is no **helipad** (an official FAA-approved location to land a helicopter) at either the sending or receiving hospital and the two hospitals are more than 200 miles apart. Unlike the

helicopter, the airplane is capable of performing only interfacility transports. This is because it is not feasible for an airplane to land at the scene of an emergency. It can, however, land at an airport and meet a waiting ambulance.

Note that all fixed-wing transports require a ground ambulance at each end of the transport. One ambulance will be necessary to bring the patient from the sending hospital to the airport and another to take the patient from the receiving airport to the receiving hospital.

Requesting Air Medical Resources

LO5 Explain the common criteria for choosing air medical transport over ground transport.

LO6 Differentiate between visual and instrument flight rules.

In most cases, the first responding units determine the need for helicopter transport. For this reason, it is important for you as an Emergency Medical Responder to become familiar with the air medical resources in your region and understand their capabilities and limitations.

In most cases, a helicopter is appropriate whenever expedient transport is necessary or advanced providers are required but not readily available. Most helicopter medical personnel receive specialized training over and above their counterparts on an ambulance or in a hospital. This training gives them an advanced scope of practice and allows them to deliver medications and perform procedures beyond those of the typical nurse or paramedic.

Most EMS systems that have air medical resources will have specific protocols and/or guidelines for deciding when it is appropriate to activate an air resource. The protocols often define specific patient types such as severe trauma and critical medical, or they may also define areas of the region that are remote and thus may take hours for a typical ground ambulance transport. It is important that you familiarize yourself with your local protocols for the use of air medical resources.

Just because you request a helicopter does not mean that one will respond. EMS helicopters are a limited resource, and many things can prevent them from responding to your request. They could be committed to another emergency and therefore may be unable to respond to your request, or there could be weather in the area of the scene or at the receiving hospital that would prevent the pilot from completing the transport safely and legally.

Air medical transport may not be the most appropriate mode of transport for a victim of a hazardous materials incident. Despite proper decontamination, the risk of exposure for the medical crew and pilot is too great in the confined space of an aircraft.

The goal with any transport is to get the patient to definitive care as quickly as possible. Transport by air is not always faster than ground transport. The time it takes to wait for a helicopter to respond to the scene and find a suitable location to land must be considered. You must also consider whether the receiving hospital has a landing pad. If it does not and the helicopter must land at a nearby airport, the patient will have to be transferred to a ground ambulance for transport to the hospital. These transfers all add precious time to the overall transport and should be considered.

Visual Flight Rules   All pilots must operate aircraft based on specific and clearly defined rules established by the Federal Aviation Administration (FAA). The ability to fly any particular mission will depend on at least two factors: the training and capabilities of the pilot and the design and configuration of the aircraft. It is safe to say that most EMS aircraft operate under what are known as **visual flight rules (VFR)**. This means that conditions along the intended route must be clear and free of weather such as fog or clouds. A VFR mission can be flown day or night as long as there is no significant weather anywhere along the intended route of flight.

Instrument Flight Rules   Many EMS air medical programs have specially trained pilots and specially configured aircraft so they can accept a request for transport even when the weather is bad. The rules that must be followed are called **instrument flight rules (IFR)**. Being IFR capable allows the pilot to fly into and through known weather along the route of flight. There are limitations as to the type and extent of weather an IFR pilot can fly in. For instance, there must be at least some visibility on the ground for the pilot to take off and land safely. In conditions where the fog is so thick that the pilot cannot see more than a few hundred yards, they may decline the request due to extreme weather conditions.

Note that there are many more requirements that must be met for a team to safely complete a patient transport under IFR rules. The planning and preparation for an IFR flight may include extra weather checks and additional fuel, which can add to the time it takes to launch and get to the scene or hospital.

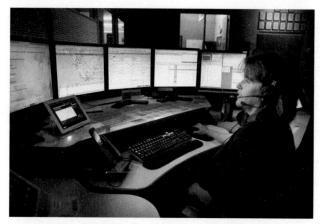

Figure A3.5 Flight Communication Specialists are responsible for dispatching and tracking EMS aircraft on each mission.
(REACH Air Medical Services)

What Happens After a Request Is Made?

EMS flight programs use specially trained dispatchers called Flight Communication Specialists (Figure A3.5). It is the Communication Specialist who receives the request for transport, provides an estimated time of arrival (ETA) to the caller, and relays the request to the flight crew in the form of a dispatch. Once the flight crew receives a dispatch, several events must take place prior to the launch of the aircraft. The pilot will perform a weather check and confirm that weather conditions along the intended route of flight are within acceptable minimums. The medical crew will gather any needed equipment and head to the aircraft. In many programs, a specific risk assessment is performed prior to each flight to ensure the highest level of safety.

If the weather is acceptable and the medical crew has everything they need, all crew members approach the aircraft and perform a series of specific preflight safety checks prior to engine start and launch. If all goes well, they will be in the air and headed to their destination within minutes.

Occasionally, there will be factors that require the team to decline a request. Some of the most common reasons a crew might decline a request are poor weather conditions, mechanical failure, or patient size and weight.

The Landing Zone

LO7   Describe the characteristics of an appropriate helicopter landing zone.

One of the characteristics that make helicopters so versatile is their ability to land nearly anywhere, but they do need a clear, flat space to set down. An appropriate space for a helicopter to land has several important characteristics and is referred to as a **landing zone (LZ)**. The following characteristics are general guidelines and may differ slightly from program to program. It is best to learn the specific requirements of the programs operating in your area. Characteristics of a good landing zone include:

- Close proximity to the incident
- 100 feet × 100 feet for daytime use or 125 feet × 125 feet for nighttime use
- Little or no slope
- Free of dry sand or dirt and loose debris
- Free of utility wires near or around the site
- Free of tall trees or poles around the site
- Free of roaming animals

Helicopter scene call operations are very risky. It is important to use an experienced individual to help choose an appropriate landing zone and assist with landing the helicopter.

One of the most important things you can do as an Emergency Medical Responder at the scene where a helicopter has been requested is to provide the dispatch center with accurate GPS coordinates (latitude and longitude). If the flight crew can readily find the scene from the air based on your coordinates, they may be able to see other areas near the scene that could serve as ideal landing zones.

Landing Zone Checklist and Procedures

Once an LZ has been selected, it is important to perform a quick checklist and report the findings to the flight crew. The acronym HOTSAW is a commonly used tool to remember this LZ checklist:

H — *Hazards.* Be sure the area is free of obvious hazards such as loose debris and traffic.

O — *Obstacles.* Confirm there are no obstacles such as tall trees, poles, or wires.

T — *Terrain.* Ensure that the area selected is firm and even.

S — *Slope.* Ensure that the area is as flat as possible.

A — *Animals.* Check to make sure there are no roaming animals in the area.

W — *Wind.* Estimate wind speed and direction and relay that information to the flight crew.

If the area chosen for the LZ is a dirt surface, try to wet the area down prior to landing. This will avoid a dust storm caused by the downwash from the rotor blades. An excessive amount of dirt or snow can cause the pilot to lose sight of the ground, which can be very dangerous.

In most instances, a single individual will be designated as the landing officer for the aircraft. This individual should maintain radio contact with the flight crew during the entire landing phase whenever possible. They should stand at one side of the LZ and wave their arms to signal to the flight crew that they are the landing officer. It is important for the landing officer and others to wear proper eye and ear protection whenever working around a helicopter. Remove any hats or loose clothing that could be blown off during the landing or departure.

If the helicopter is to land at night, *never* shine any kind of light, such as a flashlight, at the aircraft. This could temporarily blind the pilot, which could have catastrophic consequences. In most cases, the lights of your emergency vehicle will be all the pilot needs to locate the scene.

Once the aircraft is safely on the ground, maintain direct eye contact with the pilot or other flight crew members. Do not approach the aircraft until someone from the flight crew has specifically directed you to do so (Figure A3.6).

Safety Around the Aircraft

LO8 Explain the safe principles of working around aircraft at the scene of an emergency.

Depending on several factors, the pilot may decide to shut down at the scene or remain "hot" with the rotors spinning. Regardless of the circumstances, follow these important guidelines when working around an aircraft at an LZ:

- Never approach an aircraft unless specifically directed to do so by the flight crew.
- Never shine any light at the aircraft.
- Never walk behind an aircraft, regardless of whether or not it is shut down.
- If on a slight slope, never approach the aircraft from the uphill side.
- Always remove your hat before approaching the aircraft.

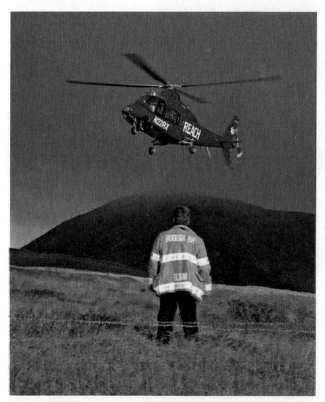

Figure A3.6 To ensure a safe landing, an Emergency Medical Responder should assist in the landing process.
(REACH Air Medical Services)

Introduction to Terrorism Response and Weapons of Mass Destruction

LEARNING OBJECTIVES

Upon successful completion of this appendix, the student should be able to:

Cognitive

1 Define the appendix key terms.

2 Describe the signs and symptoms of nuclear/radiological exposure.

3 Describe the signs and symptoms of biological agent exposure.

4 Describe the signs and symptoms for the following types of chemical agent exposures: nerve agent, vesicant agent, cyanogens agent, pulmonary agent, and riot control agent.

5 Describe the role of the Emergency Medical Responder at an incident involving weapons of mass destruction.

Psychomotor

6 Demonstrate the procedure for administering a chemical antidote autoinjector to yourself and a fellow EMS provider.

Affective

7 Recognize the importance of personal safety when working at the scene of a suspected terrorist incident.

KEY TERMS

biological agent (*p. 611*)
chemical agent (*p. 612*)
chemical antidote autoinjector (*p. 612*)
nerve agent (*p. 612*)

nuclear and radiological agents (*p. 611*)
terrorism (*p. 611*)
weapon of mass destruction (*p. 611*)

The United States Government Publishing Office defines **terrorism** as "the use of force or violence against individuals or property to intimidate or coerce a government, the civilian population, or any segment thereof to further political or social objectives." For years, the people of the United States remained somewhat insulated from the effects of terrorists and terrorism, since they viewed such events only on the news. Terrorism is no longer something that happens only in distant countries.

A **weapon of mass destruction (WMD)** is a weapon capable of causing widespread death and destruction. In recent years, the use of weapons of mass destruction and the effects of terrorism have hit home with incidents such as the World Trade Center attack in 2001 (Figure A4.1) and more recent mass shootings in Las Vegas, the Pulse nightclub in Florida, and school shootings at Marjory Stoneman Douglas High School, Virginia Tech, and Sandy Hook Elementary School.

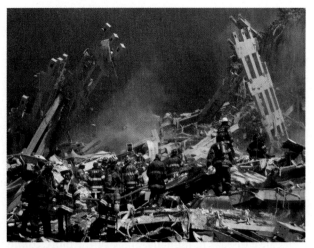

Figure A4.1 World Trade Center, September 2001.
(© Shawn Baldwin/AP Images)

Incidents Involving Nuclear/ Radiological Agents

LO2 | Describe the signs and symptoms of nuclear/ radiological exposure.

Nuclear and radiological agents are substances that contain deadly amounts of radioactive material. Until recently, the potential for a terrorist organization to obtain or develop weapons of mass destruction such as nuclear devices was thought to be minimal. With the growing supply of nuclear waste on a worldwide scale and the developing technology of third-world countries, the likelihood of a nuclear threat by a terrorist organization is ever increasing.

There are two types of potential nuclear incidents. One is the possible detonation of a nuclear device, and the other is the detonation of a conventional explosive incorporating nuclear material. A plausible scenario involves the second example. It involves the detonation of a radiological dispersal device (RDD), which would spread radioactive material throughout a wide area surrounding the blast site. Another example involves the detonation of a large explosive device (such as a truck bomb) near a nuclear power plant or radiological cargo transport.

Nuclear incidents emit three main types of radioactive particles/rays: alpha, beta, and gamma.

- *Alpha particles* are the heaviest and most highly charged of the nuclear particles. They are easily stopped by human skin but can become a serious hazard to reproductive organs if ingested or inhaled.

- *Beta particles* are smaller and travel much faster and farther than alpha particles. Beta particles can penetrate the skin but rarely reach the vital organs. While they can cause burns to the skin if exposure lasts long enough, the biggest threat occurs when they are ingested or inhaled. Beta particles can also enter the body through unprotected open wounds.

- *Gamma rays* are a type of radiation that travels through the air in the form of waves. The rays can travel great distances and penetrate most materials, including the human body. Acute radiation sickness occurs when someone is exposed to large doses of gamma radiation over a short period of time and can cause symptoms such as skin irritation, burns, nausea, vomiting, high fever, and hair loss.

Incidents Involving Biological Agents

LO3 | Describe the signs and symptoms of biological agent exposure.

Biological agents are a bacterium, virus, protozoan, parasite, or fungus that can be used purposefully as a weapon in bioterrorism or biological warfare. Biological agents pose one of the most serious threats due to their accessibility and ability to spread rapidly. The potential is also very high for widespread casualties. Biological agents are most dangerous when either inhaled (spread through the air) or ingested (through contaminated food or water supplies).

Signs and symptoms of biological agent exposure will vary by the specific agent involved, but some of the more common include:

- Fever
- Headache
- Breathing difficulty
- Nausea
- Vomiting
- Diarrhea

There are four common types of biological agents: bacteria, rickettsia, viruses, and toxins:

- *Bacteria* are single-celled organisms that can quickly cause disease in humans. Some of the more common bacteria used for terrorist activities are anthrax, cholera, the plague, and tularemia.
- *Rickettsia* is a type of very small bacteria that live inside host cells. An example is *Coxiella burnetii*, which is the organism that causes Q fever.
- *Viruses* are infectious agents that require a living host to survive. The most common viruses that have served as biological agents include smallpox, Venezuelan equine encephalitis, and Ebola.
- *Toxins* are poisonous substances that occur naturally in the environment, produced by an animal, plant, or microbe. The four common toxins with a history of use as terrorist weapons are botulism, staphylococcal enterotoxin (SEB), ricin, and mycotoxins. Ricin has been used in several well-publicized incidents in the United States and Japan. It is a toxin made from the castor bean plant, which is grown all over the world.

Incidents Involving Chemical Agents

LO4 | Describe the signs and symptoms for the following types of chemical agent exposures: nerve agent, vesicant agent, cyanogens agent, pulmonary agent, and riot control agent.

A **chemical agent** is a substance that produces chemical reactions. The primary routes of exposure for chemical agents are inhalation, ingestion, and absorption through or contact with the skin. Inhalation is the most common. The classifications of chemical agents include nerve agents, vesicant (blister) agents, cyanogen agents, pulmonary agents, and riot-control agents.

Nerve Agents

Nerve agents are substances that disrupt the nerve impulse transmissions throughout the body and are extremely toxic in very small quantities. In some cases, a single small drop can be fatal to an average human being. Nerve agents

include sarin, which has been used against Japanese and Iraqi civilians; soman, tabun, and V agent. These are liquid agents that are typically spread in the form of an aerosol spray.

These agents resemble water or clear oil in their purest form and have no odor. Sometimes small explosives are used to spread them, which can cause widespread death. Many dead animals at the scene of an incident may be a warning sign or detection clue.

Early signs of nerve agent exposure are:

- Uncontrolled salivation
- Miosis (pupil constriction)
- Urination
- Defecation
- Tearing

Later signs and symptoms include:

- Blurred vision
- Excessive sweating
- Muscle tremors
- Difficulty breathing
- Nausea, vomiting
- Abdominal pain

Many EMS systems have large supplies of antidote for nerve agent exposure. They are often self-administered by way of a **chemical antidote autoinjector**. See Appendix 2 for more information on the antidote for nerve agents.

Vesicant Agents

Vesicant agents are more commonly referred to as blister or mustard agents due to their unique smell. They can easily penetrate several layers of clothing and are quickly absorbed into the skin. Mustard and Lewisite are common vesicants. Although less toxic than nerve agents, it takes only a few drops on the skin to cause severe injury.

The signs and symptoms of vesicant exposure include:

- Reddening, swelling, and tearing of the eyes
- Tenderness and burning of the skin followed by the development of fluid-filled blisters
- Nausea, vomiting
- Severe abdominal pain
- After about 2 hours, victims will experience runny nose, burning in the throat, and shortness of breath

Cyanogens

Cyanogens are agents that interfere with the ability of the blood to carry oxygen and can cause asphyxiation in victims of exposure. Common cyanogens are hydrogen cyanide and cyanogen chloride. All cyanogens are very toxic in high concentrations and can lead to rapid death. Under pressure, these agents are in liquid form. In their pure form, they are gases. Cyanogens are common industrial chemicals used in a variety of processes, and all have an aroma similar to bitter almonds or peach blossoms. Signs and symptoms of cyanogens exposure include:

- Severe respiratory distress
- Vomiting
- Diarrhea
- Dizziness, headache
- Seizures, coma

It is essential that victims of exposure be quickly moved to fresh air and treated for respiratory distress.

Pulmonary Agents

Pulmonary agents are sometimes called choking agents. They directly affect the respiratory system, causing edema (fluid buildup) in the lungs, which in turn causes asphyxiation similar to that seen in drowning victims. Chlorine and phosgene are two of the most common of these agents and are frequently found in industrial settings. Chlorine is a familiar smell to most people due to its use in swimming pools to kill germs. Phosgene has an aroma of freshly cut hay. Both of these chemicals are in a gaseous state in their pure form and are stored in bottles or cylinders. Signs and symptoms include:

- Severe eye irritation
- Coughing
- Choking
- Severe respiratory distress

Riot-Control Agents

Riot-control agents include irritating agents, which are designed to incapacitate the victim. For the most part, they are not lethal. However, under certain circumstances, irritating agents have been known to cause asphyxiation. Common irritating agents include mace, tear gas, and pepper spray. These agents will typically cause severe pain when they come in contact with the skin, especially moist areas such as the nose, mouth, and eyes.

Signs and symptoms of exposure to irritating agents include:

- Burning and irritation in the eyes and throat
- Coughing, choking
- Respiratory distress
- Nausea
- Vomiting

Role of the Emergency Medical Responder

LO5 Describe the role of the Emergency Medical Responder at an incident involving weapons of mass destruction.

Terrorist attacks are meant to cause fear, and they are likely to occur when they are least expected. Having a high index of suspicion and recognizing the outward warning signs of a possible terrorist attack are of utmost importance for the first units on scene. Donning the appropriate personal protective equipment (PPE) early will minimize the chances of the emergency responders becoming victims themselves.

Firefighters are probably the best prepared of all Emergency Medical Responders because of the wide range of duties they are trained in and expected to perform. Ambulance personnel are probably the least equipped to respond to a terrorist attack because their personal protective equipment is primarily designed to minimize exposure to body fluids and aerosolized droplets from coughing patients.

Without the proper training and equipment, Emergency Medical Responders are likely to become victims if they enter the scene too quickly. In most cases, the best action will be to recognize the danger as soon as possible and retreat to a safe distance from the scene.

Note that many terrorists will set a secondary device that is meant to incapacitate or kill responders. The devices may be set to go off minutes to hours after the first one. By doing this, terrorists will be sure the device will go off while rescuers are caring for patients who were injured by the first one.

Decontamination

Decontamination is the process by which chemical, biological, and/or radiological agents are removed from exposed victims, equipment, and the environment (Figure A4.2). Regardless of whether the incident is a

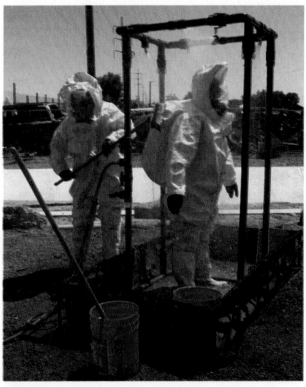

Figure A4.2 Decontamination must occur before any patients can be properly cared for.

hazardous materials release or an intentional terrorist act, prompt decontamination can be the single most important aspect of the operation to minimize exposure and limit casualties.

Depending on the size and scope of the incident, Emergency Medical Responders may be asked to assist with the decontamination process. If not a part of the decontamination process, they will certainly play an important role in the emergency care given to patients after coming out of decontamination. It will be important for Emergency Medical Responders assisting at such an event to continue to wear the appropriate PPE even after a victim has been decontaminated. This will minimize any contamination from residual agents remaining on the victim or equipment.

ANSWER KEY

CHAPTER 1

Quick Quiz

1. c   **3.** b   **5.** d   **7.** b   **9.** a
2. a   **4.** d   **6.** b   **8.** a   **10.** a

Rationale for First on Scene Run Review

1. The dispatcher is in need of pertinent information to relay to the emergency responders, who must be prepared and able to treat the patient accordingly. Examples would include, but are not limited to, what the problem is, the patient's age, signs and symptoms, location of the patient, if any first aid is being rendered, and if the caller needs any guidance to help the patient until EMS arrives.
2. They should have personal protective equipment to shield themselves against any bodily fluids. They should also have basic equipment to help the patient, including but not limited to oxygen, airway adjuncts, a bag-mask device, an AED, and bleeding-control materials.
3. It is important to do a scene size-up along with determining the patient's chief complaint so you are able to treat the patient appropriately. This way, you can be the patient's advocate and do what is best for him or her. For example, you can transfer information to the EMT, paramedic, or hospital staff. Also, consideration should be given with respect to the patient's privacy.
4. It is important to know and follow local protocols and standing orders that are established by your jurisdiction's medical director. This will ensure proper care for the patient while remaining within your scope of care for your level of training.

CHAPTER 2

Quick Quiz

1. a   **3.** d   **5.** a   **7.** b   **9.** b
2. b   **4.** d   **6.** d   **8.** c   **10.** b

Rationale for First on Scene Run Review

1. Possible reasons that Sameer doesn't wish to stop may include fear of a lawsuit, feeling unable to help, assuming someone else will stop, not wishing to make things worse, or fear for his personal safety.
2. The highest priority would be the unresponsive male in the middle of the road because he has likely suffered the most significant mechanism of injury.
3. You should never leave the scene after treatment is started because this could be considered abandonment. The only time you can leave the scene is when you realize that no one else is around to call for help. In this instance, Sameer could have gone for help if no one else were there.
4. Your report to the incoming responders should include a brief description of the number of patients and their condition, what you observed as you approached the scene, and any care you have provided.

CHAPTER 3

Quick Quiz

1. b   **4.** d   **7.** a   **10.** c   **13.** b
2. a   **5.** c   **8.** d   **11.** a
3. c   **6.** d   **9.** c   **12.** b

Rationale for First on Scene Run Review

1. It is important to always ask permission when you intend to provide care for an individual. By asking permission, you give the patient the opportunity to consent to your care. Providing care against someone's wishes can be considered battery.
2. Jake did the right thing by not immediately controlling the bleeding because he did not have proper BSI. The patient had hepatitis, which would be contagious if he had any open wounds or sores on his hands.
3. Jake could have helped her by having her control her own bleeding by giving her the materials to apply direct pressure. He could also have had someone get the first-aid kit while someone else called 911.

CHAPTER 4

Quick Quiz

1. c   **5.** a   **9.** b   **13.** d   **17.** b
2. b   **6.** c   **10.** d   **14.** b   **18.** d
3. a   **7.** b   **11.** a   **15.** c   **19.** a
4. d   **8.** c   **12.** a   **16.** a   **20.** a

Rationale for First on Scene Run Review

1. The five criteria for a proper scene size-up are ensuring scene safety, taking BSI precautions, determining the nature of illness or mechanism of injury, assessing the number of patients, and determining the need for additional resources.
2. By placing her gloved hand over the wound, Marnie helped control bleeding and prevented air from entering the chest. It is important to care for immediate life threats as you find them.
3. Gunshot wounds can cause significant damage to all organs and structures in the chest. The heart, lungs,

major vessels, muscles, and bones of the chest are all at risk for injury.

CHAPTER 5

Quick Quiz

1. a	**4.** b	**7.** a	**10.** a	**13.** c
2. d	**5.** b	**8.** a	**11.** c	
3. a	**6.** d	**9.** c	**12.** d	

Rationale for First on Scene Run Review

1. This man is in severe respiratory distress. We can tell this because he is working so hard to breathe that he is only able to speak in three- to four-word sentences.
2. This man has run out of his own supplemental oxygen and, therefore, has become hypoxic because he requires a higher concentration than just room air. Additionally, his body has released epinephrine to compensate for his hypoxic state. Epinephrine causes the vessels near the skin to constrict, giving a pale appearance.
3. By providing supplemental oxygen, you will be able to increase the oxygen concentration of the air he is breathing and thus reverse the hypoxia he is experiencing.

CHAPTER 6

Quick Quiz

1. a	**3.** b	**5.** a	**7.** c	**9.** a
2. c	**4.** b	**6.** b	**8.** a	**10.** d

Rationale for First on Scene Run Review

1. Jesse could make the scene safe by having the first passer-by pull off to the side of the road. Also, after the crash happened he could have parked his own car halfway on the road and halfway on the shoulder with his hazard lights on to alert oncoming traffic.
2. The only way Jesse could help the pickup driver would be to make sure his ABCs were intact, control any visible bleeding, and provide reassurance until the fire department arrived.
3. Jesse performed an emergent move, which is appropriate in this situation as the wrecked pickup was in an unsafe location and the driver was in danger.

CHAPTER 7

Quick Quiz

1. c	**3.** c	**5.** a	**7.** a	**9.** b
2. a	**4.** d	**6.** c	**8.** a	**10.** a

Rationale for First on Scene Run Review

1. The responders did not thoroughly assess the scene for safety. They could have done a better job looking for any signs of danger in the immediate area prior to providing care.

2. You need to be accepting and respectful of differences among cultures and belief systems. This includes allowing the patient and family to make decisions, even if you disagree with them.
3. Someone from a culture that is different than your own does not always understand your intentions. You need to be patient and communicate clearly with them to earn their trust.

CHAPTER 8

Quick Quiz

1. b	**2.** c	**3.** d	**4.** c	**5.** a

Rationale for First on Scene Run Review

1. Yes. It is possible to add additional information to a report, but you must follow proper protocols for your agency. You must ensure that your documentation gets added to all copies of the PCR.
2. If you have access to the report, you can cross out any errors with a single line and initial the changes. You may include information on additional paper and add it to the report. When amending an electronic record, you will create an addendum to the original record.

CHAPTER 9

Quick Quiz

1. b	**5.** c	**9.** a	**13.** a	**17.** d
2. a	**6.** d	**10.** b	**14.** d	**18.** a
3. a	**7.** b	**11.** c	**15.** a	
4. d	**8.** c	**12.** d	**16.** c	

Rationale for First on Scene Run Review

1. Yes. Kayla knew Camille did not have an open and clear airway and needed to be rolled onto her back. You must move someone if there are problems with the ABCs that cannot be addressed in the position in which the person is found.
2. Camille's airway is likely obstructed due to the flexed position of her neck. When the neck of a child is flexed and the chin is resting on the chest, the trachea can become occluded by the soft tissue of the airway.
3. A suspected neck injury should never take priority over an obstructed airway. You can, however, manage the airway while being mindful of a possible neck injury.

CHAPTER 10

Quick Quiz

1. b	**4.** d	**7.** d	**10.** c	**13.** c
2. d	**5.** d	**8.** d	**11.** a	**14.** b
3. b	**6.** b	**9.** d	**12.** c	**15.** a

First on Scene Run Review Rationale

1. Questions you would likely want to ask are: When did the difficulty breathing start? Do you have a history of

breathing problems? Can you estimate when you may have run out of oxygen? What were you doing prior to our arrival?

2. Possible causes of this patient's respiratory distress are chronic obstructive pulmonary diseases such as asthma, emphysema, and chronic bronchitis.

3. The handoff report should include the patient's name, age, current complaint, relevant history, and any other pertinent medical information.

CHAPTER 11

Quick Quiz

1. c	4. a	7. c	10. b	13. a
2. c	5. a	8. a	11. b	14. d
3. a	6. d	9. c	12. a	15. c

Rationale for First on Scene Run Review

1. Yes. Maria did, indeed, respond appropriately to Chris's situation. She confirmed that he was unresponsive and immediately called for an ambulance and the AED. She could tell Chris was not breathing because there was no chest rise and fall.

2. Yes. It was the right decision to place the AED immediately. Any patient who is unresponsive, not breathing normally, and without a pulse should get an AED.

3. The information you should relay is that you were talking to the patient when he collapsed and stopped breathing. You called for help and initiated CPR. You then placed the AED on the patient and shocked him one time. With that, the patient started to respond.

CHAPTER 12

Quick Quiz

1. b	5. c	9. b	13. c	17. d
2. c	6. b	10. d	14. d	18. c
3. c	7. c	11. b	15. b	19. c
4. a	8. d	12. b	16. c	20. a

Rationale for First on Scene Run Review

1. This patient had classic signs and symptoms of congestive heart failure. His respirations were rapid and "wet" sounding, and his difficulty breathing started after lying flat for a period of time. He also has high blood pressure and swollen ankles, further supporting a diagnosis of CHF.

2. First, place him in a position of comfort. Next, place him on a nonrebreather mask for his breathing difficulties and provide reassurance to calm him down and make him feel more at ease. During this time, also obtain his vital signs.

3. When a patient's lungs are filling with fluid due to heart failure, sitting them upright helps keep the fluid dependent (low) in the lungs, allowing more usable air space in the lungs.

CHAPTER 13

Quick Quiz

1. b	4. c	7. b	10. b	13. b
2. d	5. c	8. a	11. d	14. a
3. a	6. b	9. b	12. b	15. d

Rationale for First on Scene Run Review

1. It is always important to ask permission to help an individual, especially if they did not call for help. Unwanted help can be considered battery.

2. This scene poses many potentially hazardous conditions. Crowds, industrial equipment, and noisy machinery are all elements that may need to be managed during scene control.

3. The signs and symptoms this individual was exhibiting are indicative of someone having a heart attack. One of the first things you can do is to keep the patient calm and reassure him or her. Next, place the patient on oxygen and get any other past medical history that might help you in your treatment.

4. Often, patients do not want to "be a bother" or cause any trouble. At times, they may be embarrassed or in denial about the severity of their symptoms.

CHAPTER 14

Quick Quiz

1. b	3. b	5. c	7. a	9. a
2. c	4. a	6. d	8. a	10. c

Rationale for First on Scene Run Review

1. The officer could have encouraged the daughter to stay calm and reassured her that he was doing everything possible to help. He could also have told her that the paramedics were on the way.

2. This patient had substernal chest pain, poor skin signs, a rapid and irregular heart rate, and trouble breathing. All of these signs are consistent with heart problems.

3. Obtaining a full SAMPLE history, including details about when the pain started and the exact nature of the pain, would be important with this patient.

CHAPTER 15

Quick Quiz

1. b	3. c	5. b	7. b	9. a
2. a	4. a	6. a	8. c	10. a

Rationale for First on Scene Run Review

1. The OPQRST mnemonic is a good assessment tool to determine important information, such as when the problem started, what provoked it, the severity of the distress, and how long it has been going on. Because Scott did ask all of these questions, the answer would be yes.

2. The initial treatment for anxiety-induced hyperventilation would be to get her to relax and coach her on slowing her breathing. Administering oxygen may be helpful and can provide comfort to a patient who feels like they cannot breathe.
3. In most instances of respiratory distress, an ambulance should be called as soon as possible. It is just too difficult to tell if the problem will get better or worse. It is better to err on the side of caution and get the ambulance on its way sooner rather than later.

CHAPTER 16

Quick Quiz

1. d	**5.** c	**9.** d	**13.** b	**17.** d
2. b	**6.** b	**10.** d	**14.** c	
3. a	**7.** c	**11.** c	**15.** a	
4. d	**8.** b	**12.** c	**16.** c	

Rationale for First on Scene Run Review

1. The following questions would be most appropriate for any patient experiencing a seizure: Do you have a history of seizures? When did the seizure start? How long did the seizure last? Are you taking any medications? Did you experience more than one seizure? You should also look for any medical identification jewelry that may indicate pertinent medical history for the patient.
2. The treatment would be as follows: Make sure the person has a patent airway and is breathing adequately. Place her in the recovery position to help protect her airway. Provide reassurance to the patient even while the patient appears unresponsive. Be prepared should the patient experience repeated seizures. Provide supplemental oxygen if local protocols allow.
3. Any patient experiencing a seizure for the first time must seek more advanced care. A seizure could be the first sign of something more serious going on with the patient. It is not uncommon for a patient with a history of seizures to refuse to go to the hospital by ambulance.

CHAPTER 17

Quick Quiz

1. a	**4.** c	**7.** a	**10.** a	**13.** a
2. c	**5.** a	**8.** b	**11.** a	**14.** a
3. b	**6.** c	**9.** d	**12.** d	**15.** b

Rationale for First on Scene Run Review

1. Signs and symptoms of heat stroke would be altered level of consciousness and hot or warm and possibly dry skin. Sometimes the skin can be a little moist. The patient will experience weakness, nausea, vomiting, and, in extreme cases, seizures.

2. Anastasia did not need to ask permission because Juan was unresponsive. Anastasia is allowed to provide care based on implied consent.
3. Anastasia would need to tell responders that Juan has an altered level of consciousness, possibly may have had a seizure, and that they were cooling him off because he had signs of heat stroke. They will want to know of any changes in his mental status as well.

CHAPTER 18

Quick Quiz

1. b	**5.** a	**9.** b	**13.** a	**17.** d
2. c	**6.** a	**10.** b	**14.** d	**18.** b
3. a	**7.** b	**11.** a	**15.** b	**19.** c
4. d	**8.** c	**12.** c	**16.** c	**20.** b

Rationale for First on Scene Run Review

1. Given the fact that all the skin was torn away from the bone, there is a high likelihood of both venous and arterial bleeding.
2. Because the wound is not actively bleeding, the next priority is to keep the wound as clean as possible by covering it with a sterile dressing.
3. It is possible the skin can be reattached. It would depend on many factors, including how it is handled during transport to the hospital. In transport, you should make sure it is wrapped in sterile gauze and kept cool.
4. Be sure to keep Casey warm and provide care for shock, keeping him supine and providing supplemental oxygen. You would then transport to the nearest trauma center.

CHAPTER 19

Quick Quiz

1. c	**3.** b	**5.** d	**7.** b	**9.** b
2. c	**4.** d	**6.** c	**8.** d	**10.** c

Rationale for First on Scene Run Review

1. The information that you will need from dispatch is the location of the call, what happened, if any first aid is being administered, and if someone will be meeting you at the call.
2. For an individual who is feeling weak, lightheaded, and dizzy from the injury, you would want to lay them down; this prevents them from hitting their head in the event that they pass out. It is also important to keep the patient warm and provide high-flow oxygen if local protocols allow.
3. The best way to control bleeding would be to apply direct pressure and a pressure bandage. If the gauze becomes saturated, apply fresh dressings and continue with direct pressure. If necessary, apply a tourniquet.

CHAPTER 20

Quick Quiz

1. a	5. b	9. d	13. b	17. d
2. a	6. a	10. a	14. a	18. b
3. b	7. d	11. d	15. b	19. a
4. c	8. b	12. d	16. b	20. b

Rationale for First on Scene Run Review

1. If the injury has compromised blood flow or nerve function to the distal part of the extremity, you must make one attempt to realign the extremity to restore blood flow.

2. Yes. By splinting the leg, you immobilize the bone ends so there will be no further damage; splinting also helps to relieve the pain.

3. Ron will want to tell the ambulance crew how the injury occurred, if the patient lost consciousness, that the leg needed to be straightened to get a distal pulse, and that he applied the splint to help keep it from moving and to make the patient more comfortable.

CHAPTER 21

Quick Quiz

1. d	3. b	5. d	7. c	9. d
2. c	4. b	6. c	8. c	10. b

Rationale for First on Scene Run Review

1. Shelby will want to find out if anyone saw what happened, if the patient lost consciousness, any past medical history, and why an individual was holding the patient's head.

2. The person in need of care was conscious and alert. When possible, it is important to obtain consent from the patient prior to initiating any care.

3. With this type of injury, there was a possibility of neck injury. You always want to hold the head in line with the body to avoid further injury. With Shelby's assessment, it became apparent that there was a possibility of a spinal injury.

CHAPTER 22

Quick Quiz

1. a	3. d	5. c	7. a	9. a
2. b	4. c	6. b	8. d	10. b

Rationale for First on Scene Run Review

1. You should obtain OPQRST information from Nico. Ask: When did this pain start? Does anything make it worse? Does the pain radiate anywhere? Rate the pain on a scale of 1 to 10. How long have you had this pain?

2. Place the patient in a position of comfort. Talk to the patient and obtain any past medical history. If you have oxygen, administer it and do a secondary assessment. Be prepared in the event the patient vomits.

3. From the patient's mother, you would like to know if Nico had experienced this stomach pain before. If so, was he seen by a doctor, and what did the doctor say was the cause? You would give the mother information about her son's condition that will calm her down and reassure her that you are doing everything you can for her child.

CHAPTER 23

Quick Quiz

1. a	5. c	9. c	13. b	17. b
2. c	6. a	10. b	14. c	18. c
3. b	7. a	11. a	15. c	
4. d	8. c	12. c	16. c	

Rationale for First on Scene Run Review

1. It is always best to obtain consent directly from the patient whenever possible.

2. When a woman is delivering a baby, there are three stages of labor. The first stage is dilation of the cervix. The second stage is delivery of the baby. The third stage is delivery of the placenta.

3. You would want to know if this is her first pregnancy. If not, how many times was she pregnant before? How many children does she have? Has she been receiving prenatal care? Are/were there any issues/complications in this or her past pregnancies?

4. The most important detail that you would need to record would be the exact time of birth.

CHAPTER 24

Quick Quiz

1. c	4. c	7. c	10. c	13. a
2. a	5. b	8. a	11. c	14. c
3. a	6. b	9. b	12. b	15. b

Rationale for First on Scene Run Review

1. The information you would want to obtain from the dispatcher would be: Is the scene safe? What is happening at the scene? Is more backup being sent? Are there any individuals injured?

2. Bryn did everything she could for the baby by covering the wounds in an effort to control the bleeding before the ambulance arrived.

3. It is always a good idea to have the parents help if they are able. Not only does this help keep a pediatric patient as calm as possible, it allows the parents to feel more involved in the care of their child.

CHAPTER 25

Quick Quiz

1. a	**4.** c	**7.** a	**10.** b
2. d	**5.** d	**8.** c	**11.** c
3. c	**6.** a	**9.** d	**12.** c

Rationale for First on Scene Run Review

1. To make the scene safe, Mary would have to ensure that play on the court has stopped and that everyone present is aware that someone is hurt.
2. Mary should begin by making sure Tom did not hit his head or lose consciousness. Next, she could help Tom into a comfortable position to allow for a good assessment of where the pain is and the distal circulation, sensation, and motor function of the foot.
3. She should tell the EMTs Tom's chief complaint and the mechanism of injury (mechanical fall). She should also advise that there was no loss of consciousness, give her assessment findings, and describe any care she provided prior to their arrival.

CHAPTER 26

Quick Quiz

1. b	**4.** c	**7.** c	**10.** d	**13.** d
2. a	**5.** d	**8.** b	**11.** a	**14.** b
3. a	**6.** b	**9.** d	**12.** a	**15.** a

Rationale for First on Scene Run Review

1. Greg could have prepared for a potential incident by requesting a standby fire or EMS unit.
2. Greg should tell the dispatcher that the area of the fire contained propane tanks and had other structures involved. He should also relay that someone at the scene would direct the fire department where to go upon arrival.
3. The *Emergency Response Guidebook* would have come in handy because it would give the individuals at the scene a start on how to evaluate and handle emergencies dealing with propane. It would describe the criteria for evacuation from the site and from the surrounding areas. It would also describe how to handle any first-aid situations related to exposure to propane or other hazardous materials at the scene.

CHAPTER 27

Quick Quiz

1. c	**3.** c	**5.** a	**7.** c	**9.** b
2. c	**4.** d	**6.** a	**8.** b	**10.** a

Rationale for First on Scene Run Review

1. Your first priority is your personal safety. You would then call dispatch to give them all the information so they can dispatch the proper help. You could then begin evacuating the mall to ensure the safety of others. Next, you would evaluate the scene to determine if you need more help and, if possible, obtain a rough estimate of the number of patients who need help.
2. The priority of triage is red for immediate, yellow for delayed, green for ambulatory injured, and black for deceased. The way you determine the priorities is to use the START triage system. You determine respiratory rate, perfusion, and mental status.
3. You would want to inform the oncoming resources that you had completed one round of triage. You could also inform them as to whether more resources were needed, and provide an approximate number of patients.

GLOSSARY

A

abandonment to leave a sick or injured patient before equal or more highly trained personnel can assume responsibility for care.

ABCs patient's airway, breathing, and circulation as they relate to the primary assessment.

abdominal cavity anterior body cavity that extends from the diaphragm to the pelvic cavity.

abdominal quadrants four divisions of the abdomen used to pinpoint the location of pain or injury: right upper quadrant (RUQ), left upper quadrant (LUQ), right lower quadrant (RLQ), and left lower quadrant (LLQ).

abdominal thrusts manual thrusts delivered to create pressure that can help expel an airway obstruction in an adult or child; also called the *Heimlich maneuver*.

abuse physical, emotional, or sexual mistreatment of another individual.

accessory muscle use use of the muscles of the neck, chest, and abdomen to assist with breathing effort.

accessory muscles muscles of the neck, chest, and abdomen that can assist during respiratory difficulty.

action intended effect of a drug on the body.

adolescent child between the ages of 12 and 18 years.

advance directive legal document that allows a patient to define in advance what their wishes are should they become incapacitated due to a medical illness or severe injury.

Advanced Emergency Medical Technician member of the EMS system whose training includes basic-level EMT training plus responsibility for a minimal level of advanced life support. Additional skills include starting intravenous (IV) lines, inserting certain advanced airways, and administering certain medications. Abbrev: AEMT.

advanced life support prehospital emergency care that involves the use of intravenous fluids, drug infusions, cardiac monitoring, defibrillation, intubation, and other advanced procedures. Abbrev: ALS.

aerobic metabolism cellular process by which oxygen is used to metabolize glucose and energy is produced in an efficient manner with minimal waste products.

agonal breaths abnormal breathing pattern characterized by slow, shallow, gasping breaths that typically occur following cardiac arrest; also called *agonal respirations*.

agonal respirations abnormal breathing pattern characterized by slow, shallow, gasping breaths that typically occur following cardiac arrest; also called *agonal breaths*.

altered mental status state characterized by a decrease in the patient's alertness and responsiveness to their surroundings. Abbrev: AMS.

Alzheimer's disease progressive, degenerative disease that attacks the brain and results in impaired memory, thinking, and behavior.

amniotic fluid fluid surrounding the baby contained within the amniotic sac.

amniotic sac fluid-filled sac that surrounds the developing fetus.

amputation cutting or tearing off of a body part.

anaerobic metabolism cellular process by which glucose is metabolized without oxygen and energy is produced in an inefficient manner with many waste products.

anaphylactic shock form of distributive shock caused by a severe allergic reaction.

anaphylaxis severe and potentially life-threatening allergic reaction.

anatomical position standard reference position for the body in the study of anatomy; the body is standing upright (erect), facing the observer, arms are down at the sides, and the palms of the hands are facing forward.

anatomy study of body structure.

angina chest pain caused by a lack of sufficient blood and oxygen to the heart muscle.

angulated refers to an injured limb that is deformed and out of normal alignment.

anterior front of the body or body part.

aortic dissection tear in the inner wall of the aorta.

apnea absence of breaths. See also *respiratory arrest*.

arteries vessels that carry blood away from the heart (typically oxygenated blood).

asthma condition affecting the lungs, characterized by narrowing of the air passages and wheezing.

asystole no electrical activity within the heart; also called *flatline*.

auscultation listening to internal sounds of the body, typically with a stethoscope.

autoinjector device used to self-administer medication by way of a needle injection.

automated external defibrillator electrical device that, when applied to the chest, can detect certain abnormal heart rhythms and deliver a shock to the patient's heart. This shock may allow the heart to resume a normal pattern of beating. Abbrev: AED.

AVPU scale memory aid for the classifications of levels of responsiveness; the letters stand for *alert, verbal, painful*, and *unresponsive*.

avulsion tearing loose of skin or other soft tissues.

B

bag-mask device device made up of a face mask, self-refilling bag, and one-way valve that is used to provide manual ventilations; also called a *bag-valve mask* or *BVM*.

bandage material used to hold a dressing in place on the body.

base station radio high-powered two-way radio located at a dispatch center or hospital.

baseline health status preemployment medical examination to determine overall health status prior to beginning a job.

baseline vital signs first set of vital signs obtained on a patient.

battery unlawful physical contact.

behavioral emergency situation in which an individual exhibits abnormal behavior that is unacceptable or intolerable to the patient, family, or community.

biological agent microorganism or toxin that can be used in biological warfare to cause death.

biological death occurs approximately 4 to 6 minutes after onset of clinical death and results when there is an excessive amount of brain cell death.

birth canal passage through which a fetus passes during birth; interior aspect of the vagina.

blanket drag method used to move a patient by placing them on a blanket or sheet and pulling it across the floor or ground.

blood glucose level of glucose in the blood; also called *blood sugar*.

blood pressure measurement of the pressure inside the arteries, during and between contractions of the heart.

bloody show normal discharge of blood-tinged fluid prior to delivery; caused by rupture of capillaries as the baby's head expands the cervix and birth canal.

blunt trauma injury caused by impact with large objects or surfaces; nonpenetrating trauma. Also called *blunt force trauma*.

body language communication using body movements and position.

body mechanics how we hold our body when we sit, stand, and move; proper body mechanics minimize the risk of injury.

body substance isolation precautions practice of using specific personal protective equipment to minimize contact with a patient's blood and bodily fluids. Abbrev: BSI precautions.

BP-DOC memory aid used to recall what to look for in a physical exam of a trauma patient; the letters stand for *bleeding, pain, deformities, open wounds,* and *crepitus.*

brachial pulse pulse that can be felt in the medial side of the upper arm between the elbow and shoulder.

breech birth birth in which the buttocks or feet deliver first.

bronchitis lung condition characterized by inflammation of the bronchial airways and mucus formation; a form of COPD.

burnout extreme emotional state characterized by emotional exhaustion, a diminished sense of personal accomplishment, and cynicism.

C

capacity refers to patients' legal rights and ability to make decisions concerning their medical care.

capillaries smallest blood vessels in the body.

capillary refill time it takes for the capillaries to refill after being blanched. Normal capillary refill time is 2 seconds or less.

cardiac arrest absence of a heartbeat.

cardiac compromise general term used to describe signs and symptoms that indicate some type of emergency relating to the heart.

cardiac monitor device used to display electrical activity of the heart.

cardiac output amount of blood ejected from the heart in 1 minute. Abbrev: CO.

cardiogenic shock form of shock caused when the heart is unable to pump blood efficiently.

cardiopulmonary resuscitation combined chest compressions and rescue breaths that maintain circulation and breathing. Abbrev: CPR.

carotid pulse pulse that can be felt on either side of the neck.

Centers for Disease Control and Prevention U.S. government agency charged with identifying, preventing, and controlling diseases and other health problems. Abbrev: CDC.

central nervous system composed of the brain and spinal cord; responsible for voluntary and involuntary control of all bodily functions.

cervix opening of the uterus.

chain of survival adult: activation of EMS, high-quality CPR, defibrillation, advanced resuscitation, post–cardiac arrest care, and recovery.

chain of survival pediatric: prevention, activation of EMS, high-quality CPR, advanced resuscitation, post–cardiac arrest care, and recovery.

chemical agent noxious substance used in chemical warfare to cause death.

chemical antidote autoinjector device used to self-administer a chemical antidote, primarily for nerve agents.

chest compressions rapid, deep, regular compressions on the center of the chest in an attempt to circulate blood to the brain, lungs, and heart.

chest thrusts manual thrusts delivered to create pressure that can help expel an airway obstruction in an infant or in pregnant or obese patients.

chief complaint primary problem that causes a patient to seek or need medical care.

chronic obstructive pulmonary disease general term used to describe a group of lung diseases that cause respiratory distress and shortness of breath. Abbrev: COPD.

clinical death moment when breathing and heart actions stop.

clonic muscle activity violent jerking of the muscles during a generalized seizure.

closed chest injury injury to the chest that is not associated with an open wound.

closed fracture broken bone that does not have an associated break in the outer layers of the skin.

clothing drag emergent move in which the rescuer pulls the patient by their clothing, usually holding on near the shoulders.

cold zone designated area at a hazardous materials incident that is well beyond the incident and where patients are cared for and placed into ambulances for transport.

communication sharing or exchanging of information or news.

compensated shock mechanisms used by the body, such as increased pulse rate and increased breathing rate, to compensate for a lack of adequate perfusion.

competence patient's mental ability to comprehend the situation and make rational decisions regarding their medical care.

complex access form of access to patients that requires tools and specialized equipment.

concussion type of traumatic brain injury that causes temporary loss of normal brain function.

conduction pathway route of electrical impulses within the heart.

conduction loss of body heat through direct contact with an object or the ground.

confidentiality refers to the treatment of information that an individual has disclosed in a relationship of trust and with the expectation that it will not be divulged to others.

consent legal term that means to give formal permission for something to happen.

continuity of care thorough and consistent delivery of care among all providers involved in caring for an individual patient.

continuous quality improvement continuous improvement in the quality of the product or service being delivered. Abbrev: CQI.

contraindication reason that a medication should not be given to a patient because of the potential for harmful effect.

convection loss of body heat when air that is close to the skin moves away, taking body heat with it.

convulsions uncontrolled muscular contractions.

core temperature temperature of the internal organs of the body's core.

cranial cavity space inside the skull that houses the brain.

cranium the skull.

cravat triangular bandage folded to a width of 2 to 3 inches used to secure dressings and splints in place.

crepitus grating noise or the sensation felt when broken bone ends rub together.

crew resource management effective use of all available resources, allowing on-scene personnel to ensure a safe operation, increase efficiency, reduce/prevent errors, and avoid stress. Abbrev: CRM.

criminal law body of law dealing with crimes and punishment.

critical incident stress debriefing formal process in which teams of professional and peer counselors provide emotional and psychological support to those who have been involved in a critical incident. Abbrev: CISD.

critical incident stress management broad-based approach involving several strategies designed to help emergency personnel cope with critical incident stress. Abbrev: CISM.

critical incident any situation that causes a rescuer to experience unusually strong emotions that interfere with the ability to function either during the incident or after a highly stressful incident.

croup acute respiratory condition common in infants and children characterized by a barking type of cough or stridor.

crowning head of the fetus showing at the opening of the vagina; sign of impending birth.

cyanosis bluish discoloration of the skin and mucous membranes; a sign that body tissues are not receiving enough oxygen.

cyanotic describes bluish coloration of the skin caused by an inadequate supply of oxygen. Typically seen at the mucous membranes and nail beds.

D

decompensated shock life-threatening condition in which the body can no longer compensate for a lack of adequate perfusion.

defibrillation application of an electric shock to a patient's heart in an attempt to convert a lethal rhythm to a normal one.

diabetes refers to diabetes mellitus, a disease in which individuals either do not produce enough insulin or their body cannot use insulin effectively.

diaphoretic excessively sweaty. Commonly caused by exertion or a medical problem such as heart attack or shock.

diaphragm primary muscle of respiration that separates the chest cavity from the abdominal cavity.

diastolic pressure within the arteries when the heart is at rest; *diastole* is the resting phase of the cardiac cycle.

direct carry carry performed to move a patient with no suspected spinal injury from a bed or from a bed-level position to a stretcher.

direct ground lift standard lift in which three rescuers move a patient from the ground or floor to a bed or stretcher.

Disaster Medical Assistance Team specialized team that provides medical care following a disaster. Abbrev: DMAT.

dislocation pulling or pushing of a bone end partially or completely free of a joint.

distal farther away from the torso.

distention enlargement or swelling due to internal pressure.

distracting injury any injury to the body that may be preventing the patient from realizing pain in the neck or spine.

dorsalis pedis pulse pulse located on the top of the foot.

draw sheet method method for moving a patient from a bed to a stretcher.

dressing material used to cover an open wound, typically made of absorbent gauze that may be sterile or nonsterile.

drowning respiratory impairment due to submersion in water or other liquid.

due regard appropriate care and concern for the safety of others.

duty to act requirement that Emergency Medical Responders, at least while on duty, must provide care according to a set standard.

duty legal obligation to act; for EMRs, the legal obligation to provide needed medical care.

dyspnea difficult or labored breathing, shortness of breath.

E

eclampsia life-threatening condition characterized by seizures, coma, and eventually death of both the mother and baby.

ectopic pregnancy pregnancy in which the fertilized egg implants outside the uterus.

elder abuse physical, sexual, emotional, or financial abuse of an older adult.

elder neglect failure by caregivers to provide for the basic needs of an older adult.

electronic documentation refers to using technology such as laptop or tablet computers and cell phones to document patient condition and care.

emancipated minor minor whose parents or guardian(s) have surrendered the right to their care, custody, and earnings and no longer are obligated to support the minor.

emergency care assessment and basic care for an ill or injured patient in an emergency situation.

Emergency Medical Dispatcher specially trained member of the EMS system dispatch team capable of providing prearrival instructions to callers, thereby helping to initiate lifesaving care before EMS personnel arrive. Abbrev: EMD.

Emergency Medical Responder member of the EMS system who has been trained to render first-aid care for a patient and to assist higher-level providers at the emergency scene. Abbrev: EMR.

emergency medical services system chain of human resources and services linked together to provide continuous emergency care at the scene and during transport to a medical facility. Abbrev: EMS system.

Emergency Medical Technician member of the EMS system whose training emphasizes assessment, care, and transportation of the ill or injured patient. Depending on the level of training, emergency care may include starting intravenous (IV) lines, inserting certain advanced airways, and administering some medications. Abbrev: EMT.

emergent move patient move carried out quickly when the scene is hazardous, care of the patient requires immediate repositioning, or you must reach another patient who needs lifesaving care; also called *emergency move*.

emphysema progressive condition of the lungs characterized by destruction of the alveoli; a form of COPD.

end-tidal carbon dioxide (CO_2) detector device used to detect carbon dioxide (CO_2) in the exhaled breath of a patient.

epiglottis flap of cartilage and other tissues located above the larynx; helps close off the airway when a person swallows.

epiglottitis swelling of the epiglottis that may be caused by a bacterial infection; may cause airway obstruction.

epilepsy disorder of the brain that causes seizures.

ethics moral principles that define behavior as right, good, and proper.

evaporation loss of body heat when perspiration (sweat) on the skin turns from liquid to vapor.

evidence-based practice integrating clinical expertise with the best available clinical evidence from systematic research.

evisceration open wound of the abdomen characterized by protrusion of the abdominal contents through the abdominal wall.

exhalation process of breathing out.

exposure condition of being subjected to a fluid or substance capable of transmitting an infectious agent.

expressed consent competent adult's decision to accept emergency care.

extremity lift standard move performed by two rescuers, one lifting the patient's arms and one lifting the patient's legs.

extrication coordinated removal of entrapped patients from vehicles and structures.

F

fallopian tube tube-like structure that connects the ovary to the uterus.

febrile seizure seizure in a young child triggered by a fever.

fibrillation disorganized electrical activity within the heart that renders the heart incapable of pumping blood.

fixed wing airplane (describes type of aircraft).

flail chest traumatic chest injury in which three or more adjacent ribs are broken in two or more places.

focused secondary assessment examination conducted on stable patients, focusing on a specific injury or medical complaint.

fontanel soft area on an infant's skull where the bones have not yet fused together.

Fowler's position patient is placed fully upright in a seated position, creating a 90-degree angle.

fracture bone that is broken, chipped, cracked, or splintered.

frostbite localized cold injury in which the skin and underlying tissues are frozen.

full term pregnancy that has achieved a gestation of at least 38 weeks.

G

gag reflex reflex spasm at the back of the throat caused by stimulation of the back of the tongue or the soft tissue near or around the oropharynx.

gastric distention inflation of the stomach.

general impression first informal impression of the patient's overall condition.

generalized seizure seizure characterized by loss of consciousness and generalized muscle contractions.

geriatric of or relating to an older adult.

gestation development of the embryo and fetus in the uterus; the period from conception to birth.

glucometer device used to measure and display the amount of glucose in a blood sample.

Good Samaritan laws state laws designed to protect certain care providers if they deliver the standard of care in good faith, to the level of their training, and to the best of their abilities.

guarding protection of an area of pain by the patient; spasms of muscles to minimize movement that might cause pain.

H

hazardous materials incident release of a harmful substance into the environment; also called a *hazmat incident*.

hazardous materials materials that are harmful to humans when exposed.

Hazardous Materials: Emergency Response Guidebook official U.S. government resource for the identification of hazardous materials; available as a smart phone app.

HAZWOPER abbreviation for Hazardous Waste Operations and Emergency Response.

head-tilt/chin-lift maneuver technique used to open the airway of a patient with no suspected neck or spine injury.

health care literacy degree to which an individual has the ability to obtain, understand, and use health information and services to make appropriate health-related decisions.

Health Insurance Portability and Accountability Act law that dictates the extent to which protected health information can be shared. Abbrev: HIPAA.

heart failure condition that develops when the heart is unable to pump blood efficiently, causing a backup of blood and other fluids within the circulatory system; also called *congestive heart failure*.

heart rate number of heartbeats in 1 minute.

heat cramps muscle cramps, most often in the lower limbs and abdomen, associated with the loss of fluids and electrolytes while active in a hot environment.

heat exhaustion body's response to overheating, which may include heavy sweating, rapid pulse, and moist, pale skin that may feel normal or cool to the touch.

heat stroke life-threatening emergency that results from prolonged exposure to heat.

helipad designated location for landing a helicopter, typically at a hospital or airport.

hemodialysis process of mechanically filtering the blood to remove wastes and excess fluid.

hemorrhagic shock form of hypovolemic shock that occurs when the body loses a significant amount of blood.

hemostatic dressing dressing that has been treated with a specialized chemical that when placed onto a wound promotes clotting.

hemothorax blood in the pleural space.

hot zone at a hazardous materials incident, the area immediately surrounding the spill or release.

humidifier device used to increase the moisture content of supplemental oxygen.

hydrostatic test process of testing high-pressure cylinders.

hypercarbia abnormally high level of carbon dioxide in the blood.

hyperglycemia abnormally high blood-sugar level.

hypertension high blood pressure.

hyperthermia abnormally high core body temperature.

hyperventilation temporary condition characterized by uncontrolled, rapid, deep breathing that is usually self-correcting; often caused by anxiety but may have more serious causes.

hypoglycemia abnormally low blood-sugar level.

hypoperfusion decreased blood flow to an organ or tissues.

hypotension abnormally low blood pressure.

hypothermia abnormally low core body temperature.

hypovolemic shock category of shock caused by an abnormally low fluid volume (blood or plasma) in the body.

hypoxia insufficient supply of oxygen in the blood and tissues.

I

immediate life threat any condition that may pose an immediate threat to the patient's life, such as problems with the airway, breathing, circulation, or safety.

imminent delivery delivery that is likely to occur within the next few minutes.

implied consent legal form of consent that assumes that a patient who lacks the capacity or competency to provide consent would consent to receiving emergency care if they were able. This form of consent may apply in situations where the patient is a minor, is unresponsive, or lacks capacity.

incident command system for the command, control, and coordination of resources at the scene of a large-scale emergency involving multiple agencies. Abbrev: ICS. Also known as *incident management system*.

incident commander individual responsible for all aspects of an emergency response.

indication reason that a medication should be given to a patient.

infant child between 1 month and 1 year of age.

infection condition in which the body is invaded by a disease-causing agent.

inferior toward the feet.

informed consent consent granted by a patient after they have been appropriately informed of the care being suggested and associated consequences.

inhalation process of breathing in.

inspiration refers to the process of breathing in, or inhaling.

instrument flight rules Federal Aviation Administration rules regarding operation of an aircraft in inclement weather.

interpersonal communication communication between three or fewer participants who are in close proximity to one another.

interventions actions taken to correct or stabilize a patient's illness or injury.

J

jaundice medical condition that causes yellowing of the skin and whites of the eyes. Typically caused by liver failure or obstruction of the bile duct.

jaw-thrust maneuver technique used to open the airway of a trauma patient with possible neck or spine injury.

jugular vein distention abnormal bulging of the veins of the neck indicating cardiac compromise or possible injury to the chest. Abbrev: JVD.

JumpSTART pediatric triage system specialized pediatric triage system designed for patients from 1 to 8 years of age.

K

kidney stones small, pebble-like formations created from an excess of minerals in the urine.

L

labor process the body goes through to deliver a baby.

landing zone temporary location for landing a helicopter, typically at the scene of an emergency.

laryngectomy total or partial removal of the larynx.

larynx section of the airway between the throat and the trachea that contains the vocal cords.

lateral recumbent patient is lying on their side; also called *recovery position*.

lateral to the side, away from the midline of the body.

liter flow measure of the flow of oxygen being delivered through a mask or cannula.

log roll method used to move a patient from the prone position to the supine position.

M

mandated reporter any individual required by law to report (or cause a report to be made) whenever financial, physical, sexual, or other types of abuse or neglect have been observed or are suspected.

manual stabilization restricting the movement of an injured individual or body part by using one's hands.

mechanical fall fall caused by a defined slip, trip, or loss of balance.

mechanism of injury force or forces that may have caused injury. Abbrev: MOI.

meconium product of a baby's first bowel movement.

medial toward the midline of the body.

mediastinum structure that divides the two halves of the chest cavity and contains the heart, trachea, esophagus, vena cava, and aorta.

medical director physician who assumes the ultimate responsibility for medical oversight of the patient care aspects of the EMS system.

medical history previous medical conditions and events for a patient.

medical oversight supervision related to patient care provided for an EMS system or one of its components by a licensed physician.

medical patient one who has or describes symptoms of an illness.

medication substance given to treat injury/disease, alleviate symptoms, or prevent disease.

mental status general condition of a patient's level of consciousness and awareness.

message thought, concept, or idea being transmitted.

metabolism chemical reactions within each cell that provide energy for vital processes.

midline imaginary vertical line used to divide the body into right and left halves.

minimum data set minimum information required by U.S. Department of Transportation standards for data collection on each patient; typically, applies only to 911 calls.

miscarriage spontaneous loss of the embryo or fetus before the 20th week of pregnancy.

multiple-casualty incident single incident that involves multiple patients. Also called a *mass-casualty incident*. Abbrev: MCI.

multisystem trauma trauma to the body that affects multiple organ systems.

myocardial infarction when one or more areas of the heart muscle do not get enough oxygen and cells begin to die; commonly called a *heart attack*. Abbrev: MI.

N

nasal cannula device used to deliver low concentrations of supplemental oxygen to a breathing patient.

nasopharyngeal airway flexible tube inserted into a patient's nose to provide an open airway; also called *nasal airway*. Abbrev: NPA.

National EMS Education Standards education and training standards developed by the National Highway Traffic Safety Administration (NHTSA) for the four nationally recognized levels of EMS training.

National Fire Protection Association nonprofit organization that develops codes and standards for the prevention of fire, electrical, and related hazards. Abbrev: NFPA.

national incident management system system that uses a unified approach to incident management and standard command and management structures, with an emphasis on preparedness, mutual aid, and resource management. Abbrev: NIMS.

nature of illness what is medically wrong with the patient; a complaint not related to an injury. Abbrev: NOI.

neglect failure of parents or caregivers to adequately provide for an individual's basic physical, emotional, social, and health care needs.

negligence failure to provide the expected standard of care.

neonate baby less than 4 weeks (1 month) of age.

nerve agent toxic substance inhaled, ingested, or absorbed through the skin that causes harmful effects to the nervous and respiratory systems.

neurogenic shock form of distributive shock resulting from spinal-cord injury.

newborn infant less than 28 days old; also called *neonate*.

nonrebreather mask device used to deliver high concentrations of supplemental oxygen.

nuchal cord condition in which the umbilical cord is wrapped around the baby's neck during delivery.

nuclear and radiological agent substance containing radioactive material in a quantity large enough to threaten human life.

O

occlusive dressing type of dressing that will not allow air to pass through; also called a *nonpermeable dressing*.

Occupational Safety and Health Administration U.S. government agency charged with ensuring a safe work environment. Abbrev: OSHA.

off-line medical direction EMS system's written standing orders and protocols, which authorize personnel to perform particular skills in certain situations without actually speaking to the medical director or their designated agent.

on-line medical direction orders to perform a skill or administer care from the on-duty physician given to the rescuer in person by radio or by phone.

open chest injury injury to the chest associated with an open wound.

open fracture broken bone in which bone ends or fragments protrude through the skin.

OPQRST assessment tool mnemonic used as a reminder during a secondary assessment to help assess the patient's chief complaint; the letters stand for *onset, provocation, quality, region/radiate, severity*, and *time*.

O-ring gasket used to seal a regulator to the oxygen cylinder.

oropharyngeal airway curved plastic device inserted into the patient's mouth to minimize obstruction of the airway caused by the tongue; also called *oral airway*. Abbrev: OPA.

ovary one of a pair of glands in females in which eggs (ova) are produced.

overdose excessive and potentially dangerous dose of a drug or prescribed medication.

ovulation discharge of eggs from an ovary.

ovum unfertilized egg produced by the mother.

oxygen concentration percentage of oxygen being delivered to a patient.

oxygen saturation measurement of how much oxygen is in a patient's blood.

oxygen supply tubing tubing used to connect a delivery device to an oxygen source.

P

palpate to examine by feeling with one's hands.

palpation using one's hands to touch or feel the body.

paradoxical movement abnormal movement of the chest wall associated with a flail chest.

paralysis loss of ability to move and sometimes loss of sensation (ability to feel).

paramedic member of the EMS system whose training includes advanced life support care, such as inserting advanced airways and starting IV lines. Paramedics also administer medications, interpret electrocardiograms, monitor cardiac rhythms, and perform cardiac defibrillation.

partial seizure seizure characterized by a localized area of muscle contractions.

patent open and clear; free from obstruction.

patent airway open and clear airway.

pathogen disease-causing organism such as a virus or bacterium.

pathophysiology study of how disease processes affect the function of the body.

patient assessment standardized approach for performing a physical exam and obtaining a medical history on a patient.

patient care report document that provides details about a patient's condition, history, and care, along with information about the event that caused the illness or injury. Abbrev: PCR.

pediatric assessment triangle tool used to form a general impression of a pediatric patient; its elements are appearance, work of breathing, and circulation (perfusion). Abbrev: PAT.

pediatric patient refers to an infant or child. For the purposes of CPR, patients from birth to 1 year of age are considered infants. Patients from the age of 1 year to the onset of puberty are considered children.

pelvic cavity anterior body cavity surrounded by the bones of the pelvis.

penetrating trauma injury to the body caused by any object that punctures the skin.

perfusion circulation of blood through tissues.

pericardial tamponade accumulation of fluid in the sac surrounding the heart, restricting the heart's ability to expand and contract.

peripheral nervous system nerves that extend from the spinal cord throughout the body; transmits signals between the brain and the rest of the body.

personal protective equipment equipment such as gloves, masks, eyewear, gowns, turnout gear, and helmets that protect rescuers from infection and/or from exposure to hazardous materials and the dangers of rescue operations. Abbrev: PPE.

pharynx the throat.

physiology function of the body and its systems.

pin index safety system safety system used to ensure that the proper regulator is used for a specific gas, such as oxygen.

placard sign used to display information pertaining to the contents of transport containers.

placenta organ of pregnancy that serves as the filter between the mother and developing fetus.

placenta abruptio premature separation of the placenta from the uterus.

placenta previa placenta grows in the lowest part of the uterus, covering all or part of the opening to the cervix.

pleura thin, saclike structure that surrounds each lung.

pleural space potential space that exists between the visceral and parietal pleura in the chest.

pneumothorax escape of air into the pleural space, often associated with trauma.

pocket face mask device used to help provide ventilations. Most have a one-way valve and HEPA filter. Some have an inlet for supplemental oxygen.

portable radio handheld device used to transmit and receive verbal communications.

position of function refers to placement of a hand or foot; the natural position of the body at rest.

positional asphyxia potentially life-threatening lack of oxygen that results from securing an individual in the prone position, limiting their ability to breathe adequately; also called *restraint asphyxia*.

positive pressure ventilation process of using external pressure to force air into a patient's lungs, such as with mouth-to-mask or bag-mask ventilations.

posterior back of the body or body part.

postictal phase of a seizure following convulsions.

power lift technique used to lift a patient who is on a stretcher or cot.

preeclampsia potentially life-threatening condition that affects the mother during the third trimester and is characterized by high blood pressure and fluid retention.

prenatal care routine medical care provided during pregnancy.

pressure gauge device on a pressure regulator that displays the pressure inside an oxygen cylinder.

pressure regulator device used to lower the delivery pressure of oxygen from a cylinder; also called an *oxygen regulator*.

primary assessment quick assessment of the patient's airway, breathing, circulation, and bleeding to detect and correct any immediate life-threatening problems.

prolapsed cord delivery of the umbilical cord first; medical emergency that endangers the baby.

prone patient is lying face down.

protocols written guidelines that direct the care EMS personnel provide for patients.

proximal closer to the torso.

psychogenic shock form of distributive shock that results in a sudden, temporary dilation of blood vessels.

public health system local resources dedicated to promoting optimal health and quality of life for the people and communities they serve.

public safety answering point a designated 911 emergency dispatch center. Abbrev: PSAP.

pulmonary embolism blockage of an artery in the lungs.

pulse pulsation of the arteries felt with each heartbeat.

pulse oximeter device used to measure and display the percentage of oxygenated hemoglobin in the blood (oxygen saturation).

Q

quadrant one of four areas of the abdomen; used to identify the location of pain during palpation.

R

radial pulse pulse that can be felt on the anterior aspect of the wrist on the same side as the thumb.

radiation loss of body heat to the atmosphere.

rapid secondary assessment quick head-to-toe assessment of the most critical patients.

reassessment last step in patient assessment, used to detect changes in a patient's condition; includes repeating the primary assessment, reassessing and recording vital signs, and checking interventions. To be repeated as time allows until higher-trained EMS personnel assume care of the patient.

receiver individual for whom the message is intended.

recovery position position in which a patient with no suspected spinal injuries may be placed, usually on their left side; also called the *lateral recumbent position*.

repeater fixed antenna that is used to boost a radio signal.

rescue breathing act of providing manual ventilations for a patient who is not breathing or is unable to breathe adequately on their own.

research systematic investigation to establish facts.

reservoir bag device attached to an oxygen delivery device that temporarily stores oxygen.

respiration exchange of oxygen and carbon dioxide within tissues and cells; sometimes used to describe the process of breathing.

respiratory arrest absence of breathing.

respiratory compromise general term used to describe when a patient is not breathing adequately.

respiratory distress refers to breathing that becomes difficult or labored.

respiratory failure inadequate respiratory rate and volume secondary to poor oxygenation.

restraint process of securing a combative patient's body and/or extremities to prevent injury to themselves or others.

retractions inward movement of the soft tissues between the ribs (intercostal muscles) when a child breathes in.

retroperitoneal cavity area behind the abdominal cavity that contains the kidneys and ureters.

rotor wing helicopter (describes type of aircraft).

S

SALT triage system triage system used for determining patient treatment priority during multiple-casualty incidents. SALT stands for *Sort, Assess, Lifesaving interventions,* and *Treatment/Transport.*

SAMPLE history tool acronym used as a reminder in obtaining a patient history during the secondary assessment; SAMPLE stands for *signs/symptoms, allergies, medications, past pertinent medical history, last oral intake,* and *events* leading to the problem today.

scene size-up overview of the scene to identify any obvious or potential hazards; consists of taking BSI precautions, determining the scene safety, identifying the mechanism of injury or nature of illness, determining the number of patients, and identifying the need for additional resources.

Scope of Practice Model national model that defines the scope of care for the four nationally recognized levels of EMS provider.

scope of practice care that an Emergency Medical Responder, Emergency Medical Technician, or paramedic is allowed to provide according to local, state, or regional regulations or statutes; also called *scope of care*.

secondary assessment complete head-to-toe physical exam, including medical history.

self-neglect condition in which an individual fails to attend to their basic needs, such as hygiene, food, appropriate clothing, and medical care.

semi-Fowler's position patient is placed in a semi-seated position, reclining at a 45-degree angle.

sender individual introducing a new thought or concept or initiating the communication process.

sepsis potentially life-threatening condition caused by the body producing an extreme and damaging response to an infection.

septic shock form of distributive shock caused by severe sepsis, the body's extreme overreaction to an infection.

shaken-baby syndrome form of child abuse that occurs when an abuser violently shakes an infant or small child, creating a whiplash-type motion that causes acceleration-deceleration injuries.

shock position elevation of the feet of a supine patient 6 to 12 inches; recommended for shock not caused by injury.

shock life-threatening condition in which there is insufficient blood flow to tissues.

side effect undesirable action/effect of a medication.

sign something that can be observed or measured when assessing a patient.

simple access form of access to entrapped patients that does not require tools or specialized equipment.

sling large, triangular bandage or other cloth device used to immobilize the elbow and support the forearm.

sniffing position slight extension of the neck and head.

specialty hospital hospital that is capable of providing specialized services, such as trauma care, pediatric care, cardiac care, stroke care, or burn care.

spinal motion restriction practice of using alternative methods for spinal immobilization based on mechanism of injury and patient presentation. Abbrev: SMR.

splint any device used to immobilize an injured extremity.

spotting normal discharge of blood during pregnancy.

sprain partial or complete tearing of the ligaments and tendons that support a joint.

standard move preferred choice when the situation is not urgent, the patient is stable, and you have adequate time and personnel for a move.

standard of care care that should be provided by responders at each level of training based on local laws, administrative orders, and guidelines and protocols established by the local EMS system.

standard precautions steps to take to protect against exposure to bodily fluids.

standing orders component of a protocol that allows EMS personnel to provide specific interventions to a patient.

START triage system system that uses respirations, perfusion, and mental status assessments to categorize patients into one of four treatment categories; START stands for *simple triage and rapid treatment*.

status epilepticus life-threatening condition that occurs when an individual has very long seizures or seizures that occur in quick succession.

stethoscope device used to auscultate sounds within the body; commonly used to obtain blood pressure.

stoma surgically created opening from an area inside the body to the outside.

strain overstretching or tearing of a muscle.

stress emotionally disruptive or upsetting condition that occurs in response to adverse external influences.

stressor any emotional or physical demand that causes stress.

stridor abnormal, high-pitched breathing sound caused by disrupted airflow.

stroke volume volume of blood ejected from the heart in one contraction. Abbrev: SV.

stroke medical emergency that occurs when an area of the brain does not receive an adequate blood supply, leading to death of brain cells.

sucking chest wound open chest wound characterized by a sucking sound each time the patient inhales.

sudden infant death syndrome sudden death of an infant less than 1 year of age that cannot be explained after a thorough investigation; often occurs during sleep. Abbrev: SIDS.

sudden unexpected infant death sudden, unexpected death of an infant less than 1 year of age without a clear cause prior to investigation. Abbrev: SUID.

superior toward the head.

supine hypotensive syndrome abnormally low blood pressure that results when the mother is supine and the fetus puts pressure on the vena cava.

supine patient is lying face up.

supplemental oxygen supply of 100 percent oxygen for use with ill or injured patients.

swathe bandage or cloth folded into a narrow band used to secure a sling or splint to the body.

symptom something the patient complains of or describes during the secondary assessment.

systolic pressure within the arteries when the heart beats; *systole* is the contraction phase of the cardiac cycle.

T

tension pneumothorax accumulation of air in the pleural space, increasing pressure in the chest and reducing the amount of blood returned to the heart.

terrorism use of violence against persons/property to intimidate or coerce a government or population to further political or social objectives.

therapeutic communication face-to-face communication process that focuses on advancing the physical and emotional well-being of a patient.

thoracic cavity anterior body cavity that is above (superior to) the diaphragm, also called the *chest cavity*.

tidal volume amount of air being moved in and out of the lungs with each breath.

toddler child between the ages of 1 and 3 years.

tonic muscle activity stiffening of the muscles during a generalized seizure; most evident in the arms and legs.

tourniquet device used to cut off all blood supply past the point of application.

trachea tubelike structure that carries air into and out of the lungs.

tracheal deviation shifting of the trachea to either side of the midline of the neck caused by the buildup of pressure inside the chest (tension pneumothorax).

tracheostomy surgical opening on the anterior neck into the trachea to create an airway for breathing.

track marks small dots of infection, scarring, or bruising that form a track along a vein; may be an indication of IV drug abuse.

transfer of care physical and verbal handing off of care from one health care provider to another.

trauma patient one who has a physical injury caused by an external force.

traumatic brain injury brain injury that occurs when a sudden, external force damages one or more areas of the brain. Abbrev: TBI.

trending act of comparing three or more sets of signs and symptoms over time to determine if the patient's condition is worsening, improving, or remaining the same.

triage method of sorting patients for care and transport based on the severity of their injuries or illnesses.

trimester 3-month segment of a pregnancy.

tripod position body position characterized by sitting forward with hands on knees or standing, leaning forward, with hands on knees, in an attempt to ease breathing.

U

umbilical cord structure that connects the baby to the placenta.

universal precautions component of standard precautions that involves the philosophy that all patients are considered infectious until proven otherwise.

unresponsive having no reaction to verbal or painful stimuli; also referred to as *unconscious*.

uterus muscular structure in which the fetus develops during pregnancy.

V

vagina birth canal.

values personal beliefs that determine how an individual actually behaves.

veins vessels that return blood to the heart, (typically deoxygenated blood).

ventilation process of breathing in and out; also called *respiration*.

ventricular fibrillation disorganized electrical activity, causing ineffective contractions of the lower heart chambers (ventricles). Abbrev: VF.

ventricular tachycardia abnormally rapid contraction of the heart's lower chambers, resulting in very poor circulation; also called *V-tach*.

visual flight rules Federal Aviation Administration rules regarding operation of an aircraft when weather is not a factor.

vital signs six most common signs used to evaluate a patient's condition (respirations, pulse, blood pressure, skin, pupils, and mental status).

W

warm zone designated area at a hazardous materials incident where decontamination of people and equipment occurs.

weapons of mass destruction weapons with widespread effect that can kill a large number of people and cause great damage to structures and/or the environment.

wheezing coarse whistling sound often heard in the lungs when a patient with respiratory compromise exhales. May also be heard on inspiration.

work of breathing increase in the effort it takes to breathe.

INDEX

Page numbers in **bold** indicate definitions. Page numbers followed by *f* or *t* indicate figures or tables, respectively.

suction devices, 176–178, 176f, 178f
sudden infant death syndrome (SIDS), **524**
sudden unexpected infant death (SUID), **524**
suffixes (medical terminology), 61t
suicide, in older adults, 546
superficial burns, 389, 389f
superior, **61**
supine, **61**
supine hypotensive syndrome, **500**
supplemental oxygen, **183–184**. *See also* oxygen therapy equipment
supplies. *See* equipment
swallowing
    medications, 596
    tongue, 156
swathe, **419**, 425f
swine flu (H1N1), 45
sympathetic division (nervous system), 72, 100
symptoms, **226**, 250, 265
syncope, 405–406
synthetic gloves, 42
systolic, **235–236**

T

tachycardia, 99
temperature regulation, 344, 345f, 545
tension pneumothorax, **402**, 468
terminally ill patients, rescue breathing on, 161
terrorism, **611**
    biological agents, 611–612
    chemical agent, 612–613
    decontamination, 613–614
    nerve agent autoinjectors, 602, 604
    nuclear and radiological agents, 611
    role of EMR, 613
therapeutic communication, **129**
thermal (heat) burns, 385, 392, 393f
third-service EMS model, 8
thoracic cavity, **64**, 464, 464f
throat, 153
thrombolytics, 323
tidal volume, **69**, 96, **155**
toddlers, 85, 86, **509**, 510t
tongue, swallowing, 156
tonic muscle activity, **318**
tools. *See* equipment
tourniquets, **370**, 372–373
toxins, 612
trachea, **153**, 299
tracheal deviation, **276**, 468
tracheostomy, **161**
track marks, 276
transdermal infusion systems, 596
transdermal patches, 291, 596
transfer of care, **135**, 555
transgender patients, 130
translation services, 134
transport group, 578–579
trapped patients, 561–562
trauma patients, **251**
    assessing, 252, 254f, 255, 255f
    children as, 524–532
    CPR on, 214
    mechanism of injury (MOI), 257
    multisystem trauma, 376–377
    older adults as, 544–545
    pregnancy and, 500–501
    primary assessment, 259f–260f

rescue breathing on, 162
scene safety, 414
scene size-up, 256f
secondary assessment, 266–267, 266t, 269, 273, 273f–275f, 276
traumatic amputation, 379
traumatic brain injuries (TBI). *See* head injuries
treatment group, 578
Trendelenburg position, 61
trending, **231**
triage, **577**, 579–585
    JumpSTART pediatric triage system, 582–585, 583f
    priorities for care, 579–580
    SALT triage system, 585
    START triage system, 580–582, 580f, 581f
triage group, 577–578
trimester, **481**
tripod position, **301**
tuberculosis (TB), 44, 544
twisting force, 414, 415f–416f
two-rescuer bag-mask ventilation, 173–174, 174f
two-rescuer CPR, 209–210, 211f

U

umbilical cord, **481**, 492–493, 493f, 498
undeployed airbags, 557, 562
universal precautions, **40**
unlocking vehicle doors, 558, 559f
unresponsive patients, 27, 261f
unstable patients
    assessing, 252, 253f–254f, 255
    stable versus unstable, 252
upper arm injuries, 429–430
upper extremities, 412f, 413t
    elbow injuries, 430, 431f
    finger injuries, 432–433
    forearm, wrist, hand injuries, 430–432, 432f
    shoulder injuries, 428–429
    splinting, 421f–422f, 427f–428f
    upper arm injuries, 429–430
upper leg injuries, 434–435
upper respiratory tract obstructions, 96
upright vehicles, 556–557
urinary system, 78, 82f
uterus, 74, **481**

V

vaccinations, 14, 39
vagina, **481**
vaginal bleeding
    after delivery, 494
    during pregnancy, 501
values, **25**
vehicle collisions, 555–562
    breaking vehicle windows, 558–560, 561f
    electric/hybrid vehicles, 562
    overturned vehicles, 557–560
    patients pinned beneath vehicles, 560–561
    patients trapped in wreckage, 561–562
    scene safety, 555–556
    unlocking vehicle doors, 558, 559f
    upright vehicles, 556–557
    vehicle access, 557–558
veins, 72, 98, **368**

vena cava, 368
venous bleeding, 369, 369f
ventilation, **151**, 212
    process of, 151–153
    respiration, compared, 151
    See also respiration
ventilation cycle, 154
ventricular fibrillation (VF), **215**
ventricular tachycardia, **215**
Venturi mask, 189
venules, 72, 98, 368
verbal abuse, 545
verbal communication, 129
vesicant agents, 612
Vial of Life program, 34, 228
victims, 13
violence. *See* crime scenes
violence potential, assessing, 336–337
viruses, 612
visceral pain, 471
visceral peritoneum, 471
visceral pleura, 464
visual communication, 129
visual flight rules (VFR), **608**
vital signs, **230**
    blood pressure, 235–240
    capillary refill, 242
    mental status, 231–232
    of older adults, 544
    of pediatric patients, 512, 512t–513t
    pulse, 233–235
    pupils, 242–243, 243t
    respiration, 232–233, 232t
    secondary assessment, 271–272
    skin signs, 240–242, 241t
    types of, 230–231
    See also primary assessment
volatile chemicals, 331t, 332
vomiting
    during CPR, 213
    drowning and, 357
    with oropharyngeal airway, 169
    by pediatric patients, 522
    during rescue breathing, 158, 162–163

W

warm zone, **568**, 568f
water, AED usage and, 217
water-related incidents, 355–360, 358f
    emergency care, 357–359
    of pediatric patients, 523–524
    reaching victim, 356, 356f
    submersion injuries, 359–360
weapons of mass destruction (WMD), **611**
    biological agents, 611–612
    chemical agent, 612–613
    decontamination, 613–614
    nuclear and radiological agents, 611
    role of EMR, 613
West Nile virus (WNV), 45
wheeled stretchers, 114f
wheezing, **301**, 307, 520
work of breathing, **151**, 155, 232, 299, 515
wrist injuries, 430–432, 432f
written communication, 129

Z

Zika, 45
zygotes, 74